D1609240

Nutritional Care for High-Risk Newborns

Revised Third Edition

Nutritional Care for High-Risk Newborns

EDITED BY

Sharon Groh-Wargo, M.S., R.D., L.D.

Melody Thompson, M.S., R.D., L.D.

AND **Janice Hovasi Cox,** M.S., R.D.

CONSULTING EDITOR **John V. Hartline,** M.D.

PRECEPT PRESS, INC.
CHICAGO, ILLINOIS

04 03 02 01 00   5   4   3   2   1

Library of Congress Control Number: 00-106141

International Standard Book Number: 1-56625-133-8

Precept Press, Inc.
160 East Illinois Street
Chicago, Illinois 60611

Printed in the United States of America

The material contained in this volume was submitted as previously unpublished material, except in instances in which some of the illustrative material was derived.

Materials appearing in this book prepared by individuals as part of their official duties as U.S. Government employees are not covered by the above-mentioned copyright.

DISCLAIMER

The information presented in this book has been obtained from authentic and reliable sources. Although great care has been taken to ensure the accuracy of the information presented, the authors, editors, and the publisher cannot assume responsibility for the validity of all the materials or the consequences of the use of information provided in this book.

TABLE OF CONTENTS

SECTION I.
NUTRITIONAL ASSESSMENT

SECTION II.
PARENTERAL NUTRITION

SECTION III.
ENTERAL NUTRITION

SECTION IV.
MEDICAL/SURGICAL PROBLEMS

SECTION V.
DISCHARGE AND FOLLOW-UP

APPENDIXES

FOREWORD

The challenge to nourish the newly born, especially those who are sick and/or premature, has grown exponentially in recent years. One reason is the phenomenal advances in neonatal medicine that have allowed the increased survival of ever smaller and less mature infants. The other reason is that our expectations have changed. We are no longer content to provide *some* nutrition within a *few days* and to *gradually* increase nutrient intake over several *weeks*. Advances in methods used to deliver nutrients, earlier achievement of optimal nutrition, safer use of enteral feedings, and better support for breast-feeding have given us the opportunity to improve growth and nutritional status. Although ethical standards and the complex nature of studies in this population preclude definitive proof, it is not immodest and not without scientific basis to surmise that the generally improved outcomes among premature infants have something to do with improved nutritional support.

At the forefront of the struggle to provide better nutritional support for preterm babies have been the neonatal nutritionists/dietitians. Without their efforts, we would not be where we are today. Nutritional Care for High-Risk Newborns has been written by practicing neonatal nutritionists for practicing neonatal nutritionists, as well as for physicians, nurses, neonatal nurse practitioners, pharmacists, lactation consultants, occupational therapists — indeed all of us who are concerned with and about nutritional support for neonates. The authors combine a thorough and updated literature review with their wisdom gained through many years of experience to give us a resource that is comprehensive and research-based yet concise and practical. Whether establishing standard guidelines to ensure best nutrition care practices in the neonatal intensive care unit, devising strategies to address nutritional problems associated with specific diseases or conditions, or simply retrieving current recommendations for an individual nutrient, this new edition should prove even more useful than the previous edition to all those who are involved in nourishing our newly born.

Ekhard E. Ziegler, MD
Professor of Pediatrics
University of Iowa
Iowa City, Iowa

PREFACE

In its inception, *Nutritional Care for High-Risk Newborns* was written by the members of the Ohio Neonatal Nutritionists (ONN) to provide a scientific, literature-based, and practical reference for nutritionists, nurses, pharmacists, physicians, or others who were new to the field of neonatal nutrition. Particular attention was given to the explanation of terms and the specific methods of nutrition assessment and surveillance for neonates. Brief descriptions of diseases and conditions that most frequently occur during the neonatal period were also included, not as complete or extensive medical reviews, but rather to provide information that was significant from a nutritional perspective. A broad range of scientific reports and recommendations was reviewed and incorporated into one convenient reference.

In the revised edition published in 1994, as in this third edition, *Nutritional Care for High-Risk Newborns* has grown in authorship, scope, and purpose along with our growth in understanding of neonatal nutrition through experience and the constant flow of scientific reports.

In 1997, our publisher had all but run out of copies of the book and asked us to update and revise it so that a new and enhanced *Nutritional Care for High-Risk Newborns* could be printed. It has taken us a little longer than we expected and a lot of hard work—truly a labor of love—but we think you will find the newly revised edition worthwhile. A new chapter has been added to include issues such as nutrition screening, clinical pathways, and outcomes research. Each of the other chapters includes revised or additional information to reflect current research and practice. The chapter that describes the use of computer programs in the management of nutrition information for neonates has grown along with the recent growth in computer applications. The enteral nutrition and lactation issues chapters have been expanded to provide additional information about the use of human milk in neonates. Since there are several excellent references that address lactation, a comprehensive review of this topic is not included, but a conscious effort has been made to incorporate breastfeeding information more consistently throughout the text. The appendixes have been reorganized and updated with new growth charts and new product information.

With all the additions and revisions, we hope that we have continued to achieve our original purpose: to compile a convenient and concise, yet comprehensive reference of neonatal nutrition information.

Heartfelt appreciation is extended to all those who have encouraged us along the way with your positive response to the book. Neonatal nutrition and the role of the dietitian/nutritionist in the care of high-risk newborns has grown remarkably over the past 20 years.

Sharon Groh-Wargo
Melody Thompson
Janice Hovasi Cox

ACKNOWLEDGMENTS

The editors wish to thank all of the contributors for their willingness to participate in this project, in spite of deadlines imposed on their already busy schedules. We appreciate the forbearance of some authors for our frequent phone calls or misunderstandings regarding the preparation of chapters. Additionally, we would like to thank all members of the Ohio Neonatal Nutritionists (ONN) both past and present for their contributions to this and prior editions.

We thank the staff at Precept Press, especially Aaron Cohodes and Devon Freeny, for welcoming this project, for believing in us, for invaluable advice, and for patiently awaiting the final manuscript. We would additionally like to acknowledge our Precept editor, Rex Olsen, for his unfailing attention to detail and clarity.

Finally, we appreciate the patience, love, and support of our families and friends during the long hours required for the preparation of this book. We are glad to put behind us the pressure, isolation, library time, red pens, frozen dinners, and moments of insanity that this process has involved. We look forward to seeing movies, reading magazines, playing in parks, and, most of all, to hearing once again that our efforts have been worthwhile.

ABOUT THE EDITORS

Sharon Groh-Wargo, MS, RD, LD, is senior clinical nutritionist in the neonatal intensive care unit at the MetroHealth Medical Center, Cleveland, Ohio. She also instucts MetroHealth dietetic interns in neonatal nutrition and is adjunct instructor in neonatal nutrition at Case Western Reserve University, Cleveland. Ms. Groh-Wargo serves as a nutrition consultant for the Cleveland Regional Perinatal Network. She earned a bachelor of science degree in dietetics at University of Dayton (Ohio), a master's degree in medical dietetics at Ohio State University, Columbus, and completed a dietetic internship at Cook County Hospital in Chicago. A frequent speaker and writer on neonatal nutrition subjcts, she was a contributor to prior editions of this book and an editor of the previous edition.

Melody Thompson, MS, RD, LD, is a clinical nutrition specialist in the Pediatric Medical Department of Ross Products Division, Abbott Laboratories. Prior to 1998, she was the neonatal nutritionist at Columbus Children's Hospital and a clinical instructor in medical dietetics at Ohio State University, Columbus. She continues to retain active affiliations at both institutions. Ms. Thompson did her undergraduate work in nutrition and food science at the University of Kentucky, Lexington, and holds a master's degree in medical dietetics from the Ohio State University, Columbus. She completed a dietetic internship at the University of Iowa Hospitals and Clinics. She was a contributor to the first two editions of this book and has served as a faculty member for many regional and national educational programs for nutritionists and other health field professionals.

Janice Hovasi Cox, MS, RD, is neonatal/pediatric nutritionist at Bronson Methodist Hospital Kalamazoo, Michigan, a position she assumed in 1980 after having served for three years as a neonatal nutritionist at Columbus (Ohio) Children's Hospital. She also has had experience as a renal dietitian at the Ohio State University Hospitals, Columbus. Ms. Cox holds an undergraduate degree in food and nutrition from Notre Dame College, Cleveland, and a master of science degree in the same specialty from Case Western Reserve University, Cleveland. She completed her dietetic internship at Mount Sinai Hospital, Cleveland. She is a familiar speaker at regional and national forums and has been a contributor to six books on nutrition subjects, including the prior editions of this book. Ms. Cox has recently edited a book entitled *Nutrition Manual for At-Risk Infants and Toddlers*, published by Precept Press, Inc., Chicago.

The consulting editor of this book, John V. Hartline, MD, is neonatologist and co-director of the neonatology service at Bronson Methodist Hospital in Kalamazoo, Michigan. Among his academic appointments are positions as Clinical Professor in the Department of Pediatrics and Human Development at Michigan State University, and as an Adjunct Professor in the Department of Philosophy (Medical Ethics) at Western Michigan University, Kalamazoo. He is a graduate of the Northwestern University School of Medicine, Chicago; his further training included a fellowship in neonatal perinatal medicine at the University of Wisconsin, Madison. Active in many professional organizations on the local, state, and national levels, Dr. Hartline has served in various leadership capacities, including terms as president of the National Perinatal Association and the Perinatal Association of Michigan. He is a popular speaker at seminars on infant health care for physicians, nurses, and the public. He is also the author or co-author of many articles published in medical and health journals.

CONTRIBUTORS

KAREN AMORDE-SPALDING, MS, RD, CSP, Children's Hospital Oakland, Oakland, California

DIANE M. ANDERSON, PhD, RD, CSP, FADA, Baylor College of Medicine, Houston, Texas

JANINE M. BAMBERGER, MS, RD, CSP, CD, Sinai Samaritan Medical Center, Milwaukee, Wisconsin

SUSAN J. CARLSON, MMSc, RD, LD, CNSD, Children's Hospital of Iowa at the University of Iowa Hospitals and Clinics, Iowa City, Iowa

KARYN F. CATRINE, MS, RD, LD, CNSD, Miami Valley Hospital, Dayton, Ohio

JACQUELYN L. CHAMBERLIN, MA, OTR/L, Children's Medical Center, Dayton, Ohio

JANICE HOVASI COX, MS, RD, Bronson Methodist Hospital, Kalamazoo, Michigan

DENISE DOORLAG, OTR, Bronson Methodist Hospital, Kalamazoo, Michigan

MARY JO FINK, MEd, RD, LD, Rainbow Babies and Children's Hospital, Cleveland, Ohio

BONNIE FOSTER GAHN, RNC, MA, MSN, Ross Products Division of Abbott Laboratories and Children's Hospital, Columbus, Ohio

SHARON GROH-WARGO, MS, RD, LD, Case Western Reserve University and MetroHealth Medical Center, Cleveland, Ohio

JOHN V. HARTLINE, MD, Michigan State University, Western Michigan University, and Bronson Methodist Hospital, Kalamazoo, Michigan

REBECCA L. HOAGLAND, BSN, RNC, CNSN, Children's Hospital, Columbus, Ohio

SUSAN K. HOOY, RD, Children's Hospital, Medical Center of Northern California, Oakland, California

GERRI KELLER, MEd, RD, LD, Children's Hospital Medical Center of Akron, Akron, Ohio

SUSAN K. KRUG, MS, RD, LD, Children's Hospital Medical Center, Cincinnati, Ohio

JOY G. KUBIT, RN, BSN, IBCLC, Cleveland Clinic Foundation, Cleveland, Ohio

BARBARA KUZMA-O'REILLY, RD, LD, LPCC, St. Vincent Mercy Medical Center, Toledo, Ohio

KAY S. KYLLONEN, BS (Pharm), PharmD, Cleveland Clinic Foundation, Cleveland, Ohio

MARNIE I. LEVIN, PharmD, Rutgers University, St. Barnabas Hospital, New Jersey

LAURIE J. MOYER-MILEUR, PhD, RD, CD, University of Utah, Salt Lake City, Utah

NANCY L. NEVIN-FOLINO, MEd, RD, LD, CSP, FADA, Children's Medical Center, Dayton, Ohio

ELAINE POOLE-NAPP, MS, RD, LD, Toledo Hospital, Toledo, Ohio

PAMELA T. PRICE, PhD, RD, CNSD, University of Texas, Austin, Texas

JEAN M. RYAN, RD, LD, CNSD, Children's Hospital of Iowa at the University of Iowa Hospitals and Clinics, Iowa City, Iowa

AMY L. SAPSFORD, RD, CSP, LD, Children's Hospital Medical Center, Cincinnati, Ohio

NANCY S. SPINOZZI, RD, Children's Hospital, Boston, Massachusetts

LEA THERIOT, MS, LDN, RD, Children's Center, Our Lady of the Lake Regional Medical Center, Baton Rouge, Louisiana

MELODY THOMPSON, MS, RD, LD, Ross Products Division of Abbott Laboratories and Children's Hospital, Columbus, Ohio

CHRISTINA J. VALENTINE, MS, RD, LD, Baylor College of Medicine, Houston, Texas

JACQUELINE JONES WESSEL, MEd, RD, LD, CNSD, Children's Hospital Medical Center, Cincinnati, Ohio

KEY TO CREDENTIALS

CD	Certified Dietitian
CNSD	Certified Nutrition Support Dietitian (American Society of Parenteral and Enteral Nutrition)
CNSN	Certified Nutrition Support Nurse (American Society of Parenteral and Enteral Nutrition)
CSP	Certified Specialist in Pediatrics (Commission on Dietetic Registration, American Dietetic Association)
FADA	Fellow of the American Dietetic Association
IBCLC	International Board of Certified Lactation Consultants
LD	Licensed Dietitian (Also LDN)
LPCC	Licensed Professional Clinical Counselor
OTR/L	Occupational Therapist, Registered/Licensed
RD	Registered Dietitian (Commission on Dietitian Registration, American Dietetic Association)
RNC	Registered Nurse, Certified

SECTION I

NUTRITIONAL ASSESSMENT

Nutritional Care for High-Risk Newborns (Rev. 3d. Ed.)
S. Groh-Wargo, M. Thompson, J. Cox, editors
© 2000, Precept Press, Inc., Chicago

1

NUTRITIONAL IMPLICATIONS OF PREMATURE BIRTH, BIRTH WEIGHT, AND GESTATIONAL AGE CLASSIFICATION

Diane M. Anderson, PhD, RD, CSP, FADA

NEWBORNS ARE CLASSIFIED BY gestational age, birth weight, and weight for age to assess maturity and intrauterine growth. These definitions aid in the anticipation of specific clinical problems, selection of appropriate feeding modality, and determination of nutrient requirements. Definitions are listed in Table 1.1.[1-3]

Methods of Classification

Prenatally, gestational age of the infant is estimated by maternal dates, uterine fundal height, presence of quickening and fetal heart tones, and ultrasound evaluation.[4,5] These estimates may be inaccurate, however, due to an irregular menstrual period, early trimester bleeding, or inadequate prenatal care.[4,5]

With the newborn infant, the New Ballard Score is used to assess gestational age.[1,6] The examiner evaluates the infant by scoring the infant against six physical characteristics and six neurological signs.[6] The New Ballard Score is a modification of the previously developed Ballard and Dubowitz examinations.[7,8] The scoring system of the newer evaluation tool has been expanded to more accurately determine gestational age of all newborn infants, which includes infants of less than 26 weeks gestation.[6] The precision of this test is highest when performed within the first 12 hours of life for the

Table 1.1. Classification Definitions

Classification	Definition
Gestation	
Preterm	< 37 wk gestation
Term	37-42 wk gestation
Postterm	> 42 wk gestation
Birth weight	
Low birth weight	< 2,500 g
Very low birth weight	< 1,500 g
Extremely low birth weight	< 1,000 g
Size for gestational age	
Small	weight < 10%ile
Appropriate	weight ≥ 10%ile & ≤ 90%ile
Large	weight > 90%ile

infant of less than 26 weeks gestation, but for the older infant it can be used up to 96 hours of life.[6]

The Denver Growth Chart reported by Lubchenco and group is one intrauterine chart employed to assess growth by gestational age[9] (see Appendix D). This chart is based on the birth weight of infants born at various gestational ages, and statistical analyses are applied to give the different growth percentiles. Normal growth is defined as between the 10th and 90th percentiles. Growth parameters that fall below the 10th percentile identify infants who are small for gestational age (SGA). Growth parameters falling above the 90th percentile identify infants who are large for gestational age (LGA). Infants whose weight, length, and head circumference are disproportionate can also be identified. A problem with the Denver Growth Chart is that the infants on which it is based were born at a high altitude and may be smaller than infants born at a lower altitude.[10] These infants also represent a lower socioeconomic population.[3]

The Babson/Benda Intrauterine and Postnatal Growth Chart can also be used to classify infants by weight for gestational age.[11] Small or large for gestational age is defined as two standard deviations from the mean birth weight for age (see Appendix D). When two standard deviations are used to define altered growth, 6% is classified as SGA or LGA instead of 20% when using the 10th and 90th percentile criteria.

Both the Denver and the Babson/Benda Growth Charts are consistently used, perhaps reflecting their availability from pharmaceutical companies.[2] These charts may not accurately represent the

Table 1.2. Neonatal Mortality Rate

Deaths per 1,000 live births

Birth weight (g)	No. deaths	Gestational age (wk)	No. deaths
500-749	454.4	< 28	418.8
750-999	128.9	28-36	14.9
1,000-1,249	57.6	37-41	2.9
1,250-1,499	35.8	42 or >	3.4
1,500-1,999	18.8		
2,000-2,499	6.6		
2,500-2,999	2.0		
3,000-3,499	0.9		
3,500-3,999	0.7		
4,000-4,499	0.7		
4,500-4,999	0.9		

population today due to their geographic limitations, relatively small sample sizes, and their age of 30 years, which does not reflect the obstetric and maternal nutritional practices of today.[12]

Additional tables and charts are available.[13-15] However, many contain only information on weight, so that the evaluation of symmetrocal or asymmetrical growth cannot be completed; they are geographically limited; or the birth weight data are old.[13-15] The ideal chart would be specific for gender, race, gestational age, genetic potential, and geographic regions for each infant to be accurately plotted against.[2] Reference weight curves for 1989 and 1991 births in the United States have been reported for use in epidemiological research.[12,16] The 1989 curve contains information by gender, race and singleton birth, and the 1991 curve is by singleton birth.[12,16] These reference curves do not represent optimal standards to assess infant growth, since gestational age was not consistently reported.[12]

Birth weight data from Canada have also been used to classify newborns by their weight for gestational age.[17,18] The Canadian data are presented in table form.[17] These tables offer several advantages. They contain a large sample size, weight is presented by sex, and infants born in the 1980s are represented. These contemporary tables reflect the increased average birth weight of infants in the United States and Canada.[17,18]

Table 1.3. Etiologies for Factors Related to Altered Length of Gestation or Intrauterine Growth

Preterm/LBW/SGA	
Multiple gestation	Maternal alcoholism
Pregnancy-induced hypertension (PIH)	Maternal drug addition
	Maternal cigarette use
Chronic hypertension	High altitude
Intrauterine infections	Maternal diabetes with vascular complications
Congenital malformations	
Placental insufficiency	
Poor maternal nutritional status	

LGA
Hyperinsulinemia
Infant of a diabetic mother
Genetic influences

Incidence and Mortality Statistics

In the United States, the incidence of premature birth is 11%.[19] The low-birth-weight rate is 7.4% and the very low birth weight rate is 1.4%.[19] Thirty to forty percent of low-birth-weight infants are small for gestational age (SGA).[20] The mortality rate of infants with the same birth weight but different gestational ages does not differ.[21] However, at the same gestational age, the SGA infant has a higher mortality rate than the AGA (appropriate for gestational age) infant.[21] Neonatal mortality decreases with increasing birth weight and gestational age until birth weight reaches 4500 or the infant becomes postterm.[22] These trends are shown in Table 1.2.[22]

Etiologies of Variations from Normal

Altered growth or length of gestation occurs for many reasons. Prematurity, low birth weight, and/or SGA often occur together, so only one etiology list is provided for these growth classifications in Table 1.3.[3,20]

SGA infants represent a heterogeneous population.[20] Although the exact cause of growth retardation cannot always be determined,

Table 1.4. Clinical Conditions Associated with Classification

Preterm (< 37 wk gestation)

Asphyxia	Osteopenia
Hypothermia	Hyperkalemia
Respiratory distress syndrome	Hyper- and hyponatremia
Apnea	Acidosis
Patent ductus arteriosus	Alkalosis
Infection	Azotemia
Intraventricular hemorrhage	Uncoordinated suck and swallow
Necrotizing enterocolitis	Fat malabsorption
Limited renal function	Small gastric capacity
Anemia	Decreased gastric motility
Hyperbilirubinemia	Retinopathy of prematurity
Hypo- and hyperglycemia	Bronchopulmonary dysplasia
Hypocalcemia	

Postterm (> 42 wk gestation)

Asphyxia	Hypoglycemia
Meconium aspiration	Persistent pulmonary hypertension (PPHN)
Polycythemia	

SGA / LGA

SGA	LGA
Asphyxia	Asphyxia
Hypoglycemia	Beckwith-Wiedemann syndrome
Polycythemia	Hypoglycemia
Meconium aspiration	Polycythemia
Congenital anomalies	Transposition of aorta
Hypothermia	RH isoimmunization
Congenital infections	Hyperbilirubinemia
	Birth fractures (clavicle, humerus, femur)

assessment of head circumference and total body length can aid in determining the length and/or etiology of growth deprivation. Asymmetrical growth, in which the weight is stunted but the head circumference and body length are normal, indicates a shorter duration of growth retardation than symmetrical growth retardation. Symmetrical retardation refers to birth weight, length, and head circumference below the 10th percentile. Intrauterine growth charts used to plot birth weight, length, and head circumference are shown in Appendix D. Asymmetrical growth abnormalities are usually associated with placental insufficiency and symmetrical growth retardation with congenital infections or syndromes. Infants with asymmetrical growth retardation have a better prognostic prediction for growth and neurological development than infants with symmetric growth retardation.[23]

Medical and Nutritional Problems

The incidence of neonatal morbidity increases when gestational age or birth weight deviates from the physiological norm of full-term gestation or appropriate weight for gestational age.[19] Listed in Table 1.4 are conditions that often occur in infants of specific classifications.[2,3,23-28] The newborn can be provided more effectively with appropriate screening, treatment, and supportive care when problems can be anticipated.

Nutrient requirements vary by gestational age, for the premature infant has nutrient needs that are different from those of the full-term neonate (see sections II and III of this book). The choice of feeding method is influenced by gestational age. Coordinated suck and swallow is not developed until 32-34 weeks' gestation, so young infants require tube feedings to prevent formula aspiration[26] (see Chapter 18).

Weight for gestational age indicates altered nutrient needs. SGA infants have a higher basal metabolic rate than infants of the same weight but younger gestational age.[26,29] Various clinical conditions associated with prematurity or low birth weight may alter the infant's nutrient requirements and the feeding methodology (Table 1.4). SGA, LGA, preterm and postterm infants who are at risk for hypoglycemia should receive early and frequent feedings. If enteral feedings are contraindicated, I.v. dextrose should be administered. Blood glucose should be monitored. (See section IV of this book for additional information on medical problems and nutrition management.)

In summary, gestational age, weight for age, and clinical condition must be considered when assessing nutrition needs and developing a nutrition care plan. By anticipation of clinical dilemmas typical of a specific newborn classification, appropriate nutrition can be provided safely.

References

1. American Academy of Pediatrics, American College of Obstetricians and Gynecologists. Guidelines for Perinatal Care. 4th ed. Evanston, Ill.: American Academy of Pediatrics, 1997.
2. Fletcher MA. Physical Diagnosis in Neonatology. Philadelphia: Lippincott-Raven Publishers, 1998.

3.   Sparks JW, Ross JC, Cetin I. Intrauterine growth and nutrition. In: Poland RA, Fox WW, eds. Fetal and Neonatal Physiology. 2nd ed. Philadelphia: WB Saunders, 1998; 267.

4.   Pittard WP. Classification of the low-birth-weight infant. In: Klaus MH, Fanaroff AA, eds. Care of the High-Risk Neonate. 4th ed. Philadelphia: WB Saunders, 1993; 86.

5.   Alexander GR, Allen MC. Conceptualization, measurement, and the use of gestational age. I. Clinical and public health practice. J Perinatol 16:53, 1996.

6.   Ballard JL, Khoury JC, Wedig K, et al. New Ballard Score, expanded to include extremely premature infants. J Pediatr 119:417, 1991.

7.   Ballard JL, Novak KK, Driver M. A simplified score for assessment of fetal maturation of newly born infants. J Pediatr 95:769, 1979.

8.   Dubowitz LMS, Dubowitz V, Goldberg C. Clinical assessment of gestational age in the newborn infant. J Pediatr 77:1, 1970.

9.   Battaglia FC, Lubchenco LO. A practical classification of newborn infants by weight and gestational age. J Pediatr 71: 159, 1967.

10. Usher R, McLean F. Intrauterine growth of live-born Caucasian infants at sea level: Standards obtained from measurements in 7 dimensions of infants born between 25 and 44 weeks of gestation. J Pediatr 74:901, 1969.

11. Babson SG, Benda GI. Growth graphs for the clinical assessment of infants of varying gestational age. J Pediatr 89:814, 1976.

12. Alexander GR, Himes JH, Kaufman RB, et al. A United States national reference for fetal growth. Obstet Gynecol 87:163, 1996.

13. Britton JR, Britton HL, Jennett R, et al. Weight, length, head and chest circumference at birth in Phoenix, Arizona. Reprod Med 38:215, 1993.

14. Brenner WE, Edelman DA, Hendricks CH. A standard of fetal growth for the United States of America. Am J Obstet Gynecol 126:555, 1976.

15. Ott WJ. Intrauterine growth retardation and preterm delivery. Am J Obstet Gynecol 168:1710, 1993.

16. Zhang J, Bowes WA. Birth-weight-for-gestational-age patterns by race, sex, and parity in the United States population. Obstet Gynecol 86:200, 1995.

17. Arbuckle TE, Sherman GJ. An analysis of birth weight by gestational age in Canada. Can Med Assoc J 140:157, 1989.

18. Hack M, Horbar JD, Malloy MH, et al. Very low birth weight outcomes of the National Institute of Child Health and Human Development neonatal network. Pediatrics 87:587, 1991.

19. Ventura SJ, Martin JA, Curtin SC, et al. Report of final natality statistics, 1996. Monthly vital statistics report; vol. 46 no. 11, supp. Hyattsville, MD: National Center for Health Statistics, 1998.

20. Kliegman RM. Intrauterine growth retardation. In: Fanaroff AA, Martin RJ, eds. Neonatal-Perinatal Medicine Diseases of the Fetus and Infant. 6th ed. Vol. 1. St. Louis; Mosby, 1997: 203-240.

21. Piper JM, Xenakis EM-J, McFarland M, et al. Do growth-retarded premature infants have different rate of perinatal morbidity and mortality than appropriately grown premature infants? Obstet Gynecol 87:169, 1996.

22. MacDorman MF, Atkinson JO. Infant mortality statistics from the 1996 period linked birth/infant death data set. Monthly vital statistics report; 46:12 (suppl). Hyattsville, MD: National Center for Health Statistics, 1998.

23. Berstien S, Heimler R, Sasidharan P. Approaching the management of the neonatal intensive care unit graduate through history and physical assessment. Pediatr Clin No Am 45:79, 1998.
24. Fanaroff AA, Martin RJ, eds. Neonatal-Perinatal Medicine. Diseases of the Fetus and Infant. vol. 1. 6th ed. St. Louis: Mosby, 1997.
25. Fanaroff AA, Martin RJ, eds. Neonatal-Perinatal Medicine. Diseases of the Fetus and Infant. vol. 2. 6th ed. St. Louis: Mosby, 1997.
26. American Academy of Pediatrics Committee on Nutrition. Nutritional needs of preterm infants. In: Kleinman RE, ed. Pediatric Nutrition Handbook. 4th ed. Elk Grove Village, Ill.: American Academy of Pediatrics, 1998; 55.
27. Kelly JM. General care. In: Avery GB, Fletcher MA, MacDonald MG, eds. Neonatology Pathophysiology and Management of the Newborn. 4th ed. Philadelphia: Lippincott, 1994; 301-311.
28. Heird WC, Gomez MR. Parenteral nutrition in low-birth-weight infants. Annu Rev Nutr 16:471, 1996.
29. Brooke OG. Energy requirements and utilization of the low birth-weight infant. Acta Paediatr Scand (suppl) 296:67, 1982.

Nutritional Care for High-Risk Newborns (Rev. 3d. Ed.)
S. Groh-Wargo, M. Thompson, J. Cox, editors
© 2000, Precept Press, Inc., Chicago

2

ANTHROPOMETRIC ASSESSMENT

Karyn F. Katrine, MS, RD, LD, CNSD

THE USE OF WEIGHT, length, and head circumference measurements as a component of nutritional assessment is well established. Skin fold and arm circumference measurements may also be useful under specific circumstances. Growth measurements plotted on growth graphs allow comparisons with established norms. Serial measurements enable early determinations of improvements or alterations in individual growth patterns. Although growth is often the outcome measured to assess nutrition and health status, ideal growth rates and patterns for preterm infants have yet to be established. Intrauterine (fetal) growth is considered by some to be the gold standard for premature infants. Controversy exists over the feasibility of replicating intrauterine growth on an extrauterine basis.

Weight

Weight reflects the total mass of body compartments, including lean tissue, fat, and extracellular and intracellular fluid. Weight changes reflect changes in body composition as well as growth. As postnatal and gestational age increase, total body water (particularly extracellular water) decreases and protein and fat mass increase (see Figure 2.1).

Initial weight loss of ≤ 10% in the term infant and ≤ 15% in the preterm infant is expected as the body water compartments contract.[1-4] Extremely low birth weight infants (< 1000 grams) who are

The author gratefully acknowledges the contributions of Jean Crouch, MPH, RD, CNSD, author of the previous edition of this chapter.

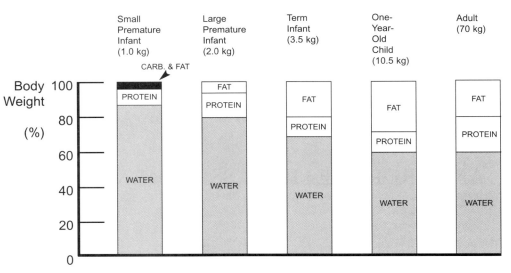

Figure 2.1.   Age-related changes in body composition.

(Reprinted by permission of Mosby Year Book. Heird WC, Driscoll JM, Schullinger JN, et al. Intravenous alimentation in pediatric patients. J Pediatr 80:351, 1972.)

(≤ 28 weeks' gestation, thus having a greater percentage of extra-cellular fluid, may lose as much as 20% of their birth weight. Small for gestational age (SGA) infants may lose a smaller percentage of weight, reflecting greater physical maturity with lower extracellu-lar fluid volumes.[5,6] Recent studies indicate that up to 50% of this ini-tial weight loss may be due to losses of endogenous glycogen and lipid stores and of lean tissues as they are used to meet metabolic demands in the absence of adequate nutrition.[7] Maximum weight loss is expected to occur by the fourth to sixth day of life.[1]

Birthweight is usually regained by two weeks of age.[1-4,7] Subsequent weight gain based on normal intrauterine growth aver-ages about 10-20 g/day for infants of < 27 weeks' gestation and 20-35 g/day for infants of 27-40 weeks' gestation (see Table 2.1).[8-11] Weight gain for preterm infants may also be expressed as a percentage of current weight as 10-20 g/kg/day.[1-3,56] Expected weight gain in term infants during the first 3 months of life averages 20-30 g/day.[12] Weight should be assessed daily. Infants are weighed nude, at the same time each day, on a regularly calibrated scale. Medical appara-tus (such as an endotracheal tube and respirator tubing) are sup-ported during measurement to improve accuracy of weight assess-ment. To further improve accuracy of weight measurements, stock medical equipment used in the individual facility may be measured and recorded. Infants' weights can then be measured without the variation caused by different techniques used in supporting medical equipment during weighing procedures.[14] Bed scales are useful in

Table 2.1. Average Daily Intrauterine Weight Gain

Age interval (wks)	Average daily weight gain[7] (g/d)	Mean weight[4] (g)	Average daily weight gain* (g/kg/d)
24-25	11.4	904-961	12.2
25-26	15.7	961-1,001	16.0
26-27	18.6	1,001-1,065	18.0
27-28	21.4	1,065-1,236	18.6
28-29	22.6	1,236-1,300	17.8
29-30	23.1	1,300-1,484	16.6
30-31	24.3	1,484-1,590	15.8
31-32	25.7	1,590-1,732	15.5
32-33	27.1	1,732-1,957	14.7
33-34	30.0	1,957-2,278	14.2
34-35	31.4	2,278-2,483	13.3
35-36	34.3	2,483-2,753	13.1
36-37	35.7	2,753-2,866	12.7
37-38	31.4	2,866-3,025	10.7
Mean	25.2		14.9

*Calculated from averaged daily gain[7] + midrange of mean weight[4]

monitoring weight for critically ill infants who cannot be moved easily to a standard scale.

Length

For preterm infants, expected incremental gain in crown-heel length based on recorded measurements of preterm infants and normal intrauterine growth, is about 0.8-1.1 cm/week.[9,10,14,56] Full-term infants gain an average of 0.69-0.75cm/week during the first three months of life.[12] Length measurements have an advantage over weight, as length more accurately reflects lean body mass and is not influenced by fluid status. Length may be more difficult to accurately measure, however, than either weight or head circumference. Length should be assessed weekly by two examiners, ideally with the infant placed in the supine, fully extended position with knees straightened and feet at right angles to the body. Recumbent length boards have been developed that add to the accuracy of measurements.*

---

*O'Leary Length Boards are available from Ellard Instrumentation Ltd., 1017 East Union St., Seattle, WA 98122; Perspective Length Boards are available from Perspective Enterprises, 7829 Sprinkle Rd., Kalamazoo, Ml 49001.

The measurement of knee-to-heel length has been proposed as a more accurate alternative to crown-to-heel length in the assessment of linear growth.[15] Knee-to-heel length can be measured with a hand-held electronic knemometer or with less expensive vernier calipers with similar measurement error.[16,17] Repeated measurement is necessary to reduce errors due to tissue compression and individual variations in technique.[16,18] Knee-to-heel length norms for 23-42 weeks' gestation have been proposed, but may have limited usefulness due to high interobserver variation, considerable differences between boys and girls, and changes in growth patterns after birth.[18] The intrauterine growth rate of the lower leg has been estimated as 0.43 mm/day with a 95% confidence interval of 0.41-0.45 mm/day using knee-to-heel measurements. Sequential measurements made by a single observer show less variation and may be used to monitor the rate of growth. For example, 10-day dexamethasone therapy appears to reduce leg growth during the time of treatment, with increased growth occurring after treatment.[19]

Head Circumference

Head growth correlates well with brain growth during fetal development, infancy, and early childhood and with later developmental achievement in preterm infants.[20] Head growth velocity changes throughout pregnancy. Peak growth velocity occurs during 12-24 weeks' gestation (1.0-1.4 cm/week) and falls linearly to lower levels near term (0.1 to 0.6 cm/week).[21,56] Preterm infants achieve similar rates of head growth. Although head circumference may decrease by about 0.5 cm during the first postnatal week as the extracellular fluid space contracts, catch-up growth occurs quickly once adequate nutrition is provided.[22,23] Average weekly gain in head circumference for term infants between birth and 3 months of age is about 0.5 cm/week.[24]

Head circumference is measured at the largest frontal occipital plane and monitored weekly along with weight, length, and nutrient intake. More frequent assessment may be indicated for infants with suspected abnormal increases in head circumference. Head growth frequently remains normal despite mild to moderate intrauterine or postnatal malnutrition which may compromise gains in weight and length.[25] Microcephaly with normal weight and length is suggestive of significant brain pathology.[25,26] Rapid increases in head circumference (> 1.25 cm/week[22]) may suggest intraventricular hemorrhage or hydrocephalus.[27]

Table 2.2. A Comparison of Selected Fetal Growth Reference Data Characteristics*

Reference	Location	Source	Characteristics	Exclusions	Measurements	Stratification	Gestational age**	No. Subjects
Gibson[48]	Birmingham, England	All births 1947	Urban, white	None	BW	Sex	Completed weeks	16,749
Thomson[49]	Aberdeen, Scotland	90% of births 1948-64	Urban, white	Illegitimate and multiple births, macerated still-births, fetal malformations	BW	Sex, parity	Completed weeks	46,703
Lubchenco[8,14]	Denver, Co., USA	1 hospital 1958-61	High altitude, low socioeconomic status; white and Hispanic	Stillbirths, malformations affecting BW,* maternal diabetes, "incompatible" BW/GA	BW, length, and head circumference	None	Nearest week	5,635
Gruenwald[50]	Baltimore, MD, USA	1 hospital late 1950s-early 1960s	Not specified	Multiple births, malformations affecting BW	BW	None	Nearest week	13,732
Usher & McLean[9]	Montreal, Canada	1 hospital 1959-63	Urban, white	Stillbirths, multiple births, major congenital anomalies, maternal diabetes, severe IUGR	BW, length, head circumference, ponderal index	None	Nearest week	300
Babson[10]	Portland, Ore., USA	2 hospitals 1959-66	Urban, white, high socioeconomic status	Stillbirths, multiple births	BW	Sex	Nearest week	39,895
Brenner[51]	Cleveland, Ohio, USA	1 hospital 1962-69	Urban, white (high socioeconomic status) and black (low socioeconomic status)	Antepartum stillbirths, multiple and breech births, congenital anomalies pre-eclampsia	BW	Corrections for sex, race, and parity	Nearest week	30,722
Williams[52]	California, USA	All births 1970-76	Mixed races and socioeconomic status	None	BW	Sex, non-His-panic white, singleton vs. multiple birth	Completed weeks	2,288,806
David[53]	North Carolina, USA	All births 1975-77	Mixed races and socioeconomic status	Stillbirths	BW	None	Completed weeks	195,867
Lawrence; Niklasson[54,55]	Sweden	Healthy; 79% of all births 1977-81	Predominantly white	Stillbirths, multiple births, pregnancy complications affecting BW, major malformations	BW, length and head circumference	Sex	Completed weeks	362,280

* Reprinted with permission. World Health Organization, from Physical status: the use and interpretation of anthropometry. Report of a WHO expert committee. Geneva, Swizerland, 1995. BW = birth weight.

** Gestational age is calculated in these reports using date of mother's last menstrual period.

Table 2.3. Body Composition Reference Values*

Sex	Age (mo)	No.	C (cm)	TSF (cm)	TUA (cm²)	UFE (cm²)	UME (cm²)	Arm fat (%)
Male	1	193	10.54 ± 0.86	0.56 ± 0.12	8.91 ± 1.47	2.98 ± 0.81	5.82 ± 1.03	33.64 ± 6.20
Male	3	179	12.46 ± 0.98	0.81 ± 0.19	12.44 ± 1.95	5.14 ± 1.52	7.46 ± 1.35	40.40 ± 8.14
Male	6	196	14.01 ± 1.06	0.96 ± 0.20	15.70 ± 2.41	6.85 ± 1.75	9.07 ± 1.81	42.90 ± 8.23
Male	9	173	14.91 ± 1.10	0.97 ± 0.22	17.78 ± 2.65	7.31 ± 1.99	10.52 ± 2.26	40.98 ± 8.70
Male	12	181	15.38 ± 1.15	0.96 ± 0.21	18.95 ± 2.84	7.48 ± 1.9	11.52 ± 2.31	39.36 ± 8.20
Female	1	200	10.36 ± 0.74	0.58 ± 0.12	8.50 ± 1.20	2.98 ± 0.81	5.50 ± 0.90	35.70 ± 6.40
Female	3	166	10.07 ± 0.91	0.80 ± 0.18	11.67 ± 1.76	3.07 ± 0.70	6.82 ± 1.37	41.57 ± 8.35
Female	6	179	13.65 ± 1.09	0.96 ± 0.22	14.93 ± 2.30	4.90 ± 1.36	8.36 ± 1.58	44.00 ± 8.68
Female	9	149	14.53 ± 1.08	0.97 ± 0.25	16.91 ± 2.50	6.67 ± 1.91	9.72 ± 1.94	42.11 ± 9.66
Female	12	164	15.00 ± 1.09	0.96 ± 0.22	18.01 ± 2.60	7.09 ± 2.20	10.78 ± 2.00	40.12 ± 8.44

* Reference values for arm circumference (C), triceps skinfold thickness (TSF), total upper arm area (TUA), upper-arm fat area estimate (UFE), upper-arm muscle area estimate (UME), and percentage of arm fat in the French reference longitudinal study. TUA = $C^2/4p$, UFE = C x (TSF/2); UME = TUA - UFE; % Arm fat = (UFE/TUA) x 100.

Adapted with permission of the American Society For Clinical Nutrition from Rolland-Cachera MF, Brambilla P, Manzoni P, et al. Body composition assessed on the basis of arm circumference and triceps skinfold thickness: a new index validated in children by magnetic resonance. Am J Clin Nutr 65:1709, 1997.

Growth Charts

Charts presently available for monitoring postnatal growth are generally divided into two categories: those developed using postnatal growth data and those using intrauterine growth data. The Dancis, Hall/Shaffer, Wright, Lair/Kennedy, and Ehrenkranz growth charts found in Appendix D are examples of charts that were developed from postnatal growth data.[1-4, 28] Although the Dancis growth chart is the best known and most frequently used,[1] technological changes in neonatal care, including nutritional care, have occurred since its publication. This chart extends to only 50 days of age and does not accommodate infants born at less than 29 weeks' gestation who may remain hospitalized until 36 weeks' gestation. Postnatal growth curves published more recently by Shaffer and Brosius were developed in similar fashion to the Dancis curves.[2,3] Although these curves add to our understanding of growth patterns in preterm infants, each has limitations. The Shaffer curves are of limited use as ideal growth norms because of the compromised nutritional status of many of their subjects and because they extend to only 40 days of age.[2] The Brosius chart was developed using a study population of well-nourished preterm neonates, but the actual format in which the curves were published limits their clinical application. The Wright growth charts extend to 105 days of age but do not give data for infants > 1,500 g birthweight. These charts include length and head circumference.[4] However, lack of control over interobserver measurement variability may limit the strength of this data set. The Lair and Kennedy weight chart combines data from Wright, Shaffer and Babson. The length and head circumference charts use data from Babson.[28] These charts provide a practical monitoring system for monitoring growth through 168 days of age. Charts and graphs describing the growth of 1,660 infants with birth weights between 501 and 1,500 g from birth to age 120 days or body weight of 2,000 g have been published by the National Institute of Child Health and Human Development Neonatal Research Network.[56] Growth data from infants with major morbidities are plotted separately and generally appear to lag about two weeks behind their healthier cohorts.

In general, the greatest benefit of using charts developed from postnatal growth data is the ability to monitor weight gain on a daily basis. The greatest drawback of using these charts is that the postnatal growth data collected to generate these charts represents a variety of nutrition practices and may not represent ideal growth.

Alternatively, intrauterine growth charts are available (see Table 2.2. and Appendix D). By compiling birth weight, length, and head circumference data on infants of varying gestational ages, these cross-sectional growth charts have been developed to reflect intrauterine growth. The Babson/Benda and Lubchenco growth charts are the most widely used and incorporate weekly monitoring.[10,14] The Lubchenco charts were developed using a population of infants born at high elevations. When using these growth data, it must be noted that altitude affects growth negatively. The Babson/Benda data set was developed from a smaller sample size, but is based on a population of infants born at sea level. Despite their shortcomings, the Lubchenco and Babson/Benda intrauterine standards are useful in establishing expected weight, length, and head circumference at various gestational ages. Although it may be argued that maintaining intrauterine growth may not be realistically attainable for most preterm infants, these charts allow weekly assessment of growth in weight, length, and head circumference. Postnatal catch-up growth is easily identified when growth is compared with normal fetal growth.

Full-term infants and preterm infants who have reached a corrected age of 40 weeks can be plotted on the National Center for Health Statistics (NCHS) growth charts.[12] Corrected age (e.g., a 30 weeks' gestation infant who is 14 weeks old has a corrected age of 4 weeks postterm) is used to adjust growth and developmental expectations for the degree of prematurity. Corrected age should be used in the growth assessment of preterm infants without significant associated diseases throughout the first year of life.[29] The use of corrected age until three and one-half years of life is reported, particularly for infants with extreme prematurity and/or ongoing medical or surgical complications.[29,30]

Lubchenco charts include the ponderal index (weight in grams x 100/length in cm³) percentiles. This chart allows assessment of weight-for-length status from birth to term age against normal fetal development at various gestational ages.[14] Growth charts plotting weight-for-length and head circumference-for-length have been developed from the Infant Health and Development Program (IHDP) data for prematurely born infants who are near term age up to 3 years of age.[31,32] The IHDP charts can be used without an accurate gestational age estimation and have separate percentile curves for girls and boys.[31]

Weight-for-length assessment is particularly useful in identifying ideal weight-for-length and symmetry of growth. SGA infants may have growth retardation in weight, length and/or head circumference. In symmetric growth retardation, all parameters are affected resulting in a greater risk of neonatal morbidity, future growth problems and developmental delay at two years.[31,33] With asymmetric or disproportionate growth retardation, only one paramater displays impaired growth. If weight is low compared to length and head circumference, catch up growth often occurs quickly.[33] If head circumference is low compared to weight and length, neurological or developmental impairment may be present.[25] Large for gestational age infants may be expected to lag down in growth postnatally, with the greatest lag in weight gain.[34,35]

Assessment of Body Composition

Standards for triceps skinfold (TSF), midarm circumference (MAC) and derived arm muscle area (AMA) [AMA = (MAC - π x TSF)^2 + 4 π, where π = 3.14], and midarm circumference/head circumference ratio have been published (see Table 2.3.).[36-39] These measurements are useful in the assessment of body composition and may add to the interpretation of growth data.[40] Like weight, length, and head circumference, these measurements can be used to compare those of an individual infant to reference norms or to assess individual changes over time. When evaluating intra- and interexaminer reliability of measurement technique, weight and head circumference have been found to be the most reliable measures, with length and mid-arm circumference the least reliable.[41]

Critical illness, medical apparatus, positioning of patients, and alterations in hydration all contribute to difficulty in obtaining accurate measurements, therefore limiting interpretation. The use of calipers in obtaining TSF may not be feasible in extremely immature infants who have friable, easily punctured skin. For these reasons, body composition is generally not routinely assessed. More commonly, these measurements are used as research tools and in the sequential assessment of selected patients.

Whole-body composition analysis may be a useful tool in nutrition assessment of infants. Picaud et al. have suggested that dual-energy x-ray absorptiometry using low-level radiation accurately reflects calcium and fat content in term human neonates, although refinements would be necessary before applying this technique to preterm infants.[42] Total body electrical conductivity has been recently used as a reliable and valid method of determining fat-free mass and total body fat in infants. Centile curves have been developed for these parameters in term infants.[43] Other methods of body composition analysis have limitations when applied to infants.[42,44]

In summary, growth may be affected by many factors related to an infant's medical condition.[31] Growth charts are available for monitoring growth of term and preterm infants and infants with specific diagnoses.[45,46] Medications, especially long-term dexamethasone therapy, may impair growth.[47] The ability to provide adequate nutritional support is essential for optimal growth. Fluid restriction, organ dysfunction, or other metabolic alterations may compromise nutrition support. Growth charts not only provide a base set of information at birth, but also a way to monitor growth as a measure of nutritional status. They can be used to establish and identify changes needed in nutrition support.

References

1. Dancis J, O'Connell JR, Holt LE. A grid for recording the weight of premature infants. J Pediatr 33:570, 1948.
2. Shaffer SG, Quimiro CL, Anderson JV, et al. Postnatal weight changes in low birth weight infants. Pediatr 79:702, 1987.
3. Brosius KK, Ritter DA, Kenny JD. Postnatal growth curve of the infant with extremely low birth weight who was fed enterally. Pediatr 74:778, 1984.
4. Wright K, Dawson JP, Fallis D, et al. New postnatal grids for very low birth weight infants. Pediatrics 91:922, 1993.
5. Bauer K, Cowett RM, Howard GM, et al. Effect of intrauterine growth retardation on postnatal weight change in preterm infants. J Pediatr 123:301, 1993.
6. Costarino AT, Baumgart S. Controversies in fluid and electrolyte therapy for the premature infant. Clin Perinatol 15:863, 1988.

7. Heird WC, Wu C. Are we discharging preterm infants in a suboptimal nutritional state? In: Posthospital nutrition in the preterm infant, report of the 106th Ross conference on pediatric research. Columbus, Ohio: Ross Products Division, Abbott Laboratories, 1966.

8. Lubchenco LO, Hansman C, Dressier M, et al. Intrauterine growth as estimated from liveborn birth weight data at 24 to 42 weeks of gestation. Pediatr 32:793, 1963.

9. Usher R, McLean F. Intrauterine growth of live-born caucasian infants at sea level: Standards obtained from measurements in 7 dimensions of infants born between 25 and 44 weeks of gestation. J Pediatr 74:901, 1969.

10. Babson SG, Benda GJ. Growth graphs for the clinical assessment of infants of varying gestational ages. J Pediatr 89:814, 1976.

11. Ziegler EE, O'Donnell AM, Nelson SE, et al. Body composition of the reference fetus. Growth 40:329, 1976.

12. Hamill PVV, Drizd TA, Johnson LL, et al. Physical growth: National Center for Health Statistics percentiles. Am J Clin Nutr 32:607, 1979.

13. Hermansen MG, Hermansen MC. The influence of equipment weights on neonatal daily weight measurements. Neonatal Network 18:33, 1999.

14. Lubchencho LO, Hansman C, and Boyd E. Intrauterine growth in length and head circumference as estimated from live births at gestational ages from 26 to 42 weeks. Pediatr 37:403, 1966.

15. Michaelsen KF, Skov L, Badsberg JH, et al. Short term measurement of linear growth in preterm infants: Validation of a hand-held knemometer. Pediatr Res 38:464, 1991.

16. Skinner AM, Cieslak Z, MacWilliam L, et al. The measurement of knee-heel length in newborn infants using a simple vernier calipers. Acta Paediatr 86:512, 1997.

17. Michaelsen KM. Short-term measurements of linear growth in early life: infant knemometry. Acta Paediatr 86:551, 1997.

18. Gibson AT, Pearse RG, Wales JKL. Knemometry and the assessment of growth in premature babies. Arch Dis Child 69:498, 1993.

19. Gibson AT, Pearse RG, Wales JKL. Growth retardation after dexamethasone administration: assessment by knemometry. Arch Dis Child 69:505, 1993.

20. Hack MB, Breslan N, Weissman B, et al. Effect of very low birth weight and subnormal head size on cognitive abilities at school age. N Engl J Med 325:231, 1991.

21. Bertino E, DiBattista E, Bossi A, et al. Fetal growth velocity: kinetic, clinical and biological aspects. Arch dis Child 74:F10, 1996.

22. Manser JI. Growth in the high-risk infant. Clin Perinatol 11:19, 1984.

23. Gross SJ, Eckerman CO. Normative early head growth in very low birth weight infants. J Pediatr 103:946, 1983.

24. Guo S, Roche Af, Moore WM. Reference data for head circumference and 1-month increments from 1 to 12 months of age. J Pediatr 113:490, 1988.

25. Georgieff MK. Assessment of large and small for gestational age newborn infants using growth curves. Pediatr Ann 24 (11):599, 1995.

26. Cordes I, Roland EH, Lupton BA, et al. Early prediction of the development of microcephaly after hypoxic-ischemic encephalopathy in the full-term newborn. Pediatr 93:703, 1994.

27. Sher PK, Brown SB. A longitudinal study of head growth in preterm infants. II: Differentiation between 'catch-up' head-growth and early infantile hydrocephalus. Dev Med Child Neurol 17:711, 1975.

28. Lair CS and Kennedy KA. Monitoring postnatal growth in the neonatal intensive care unit. Nutr Clin Prac 12:124, 1997.

29. Peterson KE, Frank DA. Feeding and growth of premature and small for age infants. In: Taeusch W, Yogman M, eds. Follow-up management of the high risk infant. Boston: Little Brown, 1987.

30. Hack M, Fanaroff AA. Growth patterns in the ICN graduate, In: Bauard CA, ed. Pediatric care of the ICN graduate. Philadelphia: Saunders, 1988.

31. Guo SS, Wholihan K, Roche AF, et al. Weight-for-length reference data for preterm low-birth-weight infants. Arch Pediatr Adolesc Med 150:964, 1996.

32. Roche AF, Guo SS, Wholihan K, et al. Reference data for head circumference-for-length in preterm low-birth-weight infants. Arch Pediatr Adolesc Med 151:50, 1997.

33. Dodd V. Gestational age assessment. Neonatal Network 15:27, 1996.

34. Albertsson-Wikland K, Wennergren M, et al. Longitudinal follow-up of growth in children born small for gestational age. Acta Paediatr 82:438, 1993.

35. Smith DW, Truog W, Rogers JE, et al. Shifting linear growth during infancy: Illustration of genetic factors in growth from fetal life through infancy. J Pediatr 89:225, 1976.

36. Voucher YE, Harrison CC, Udall JN, et al. Skinfold thickness in North American infants 24-41 weeks gestation. Hum Biol 56:713, 1984.

37. Sasanow SR, Georgieff MK, Pereira GR. Mid-arm circumference and midarm/ head circumference ratios: Standard curves for anthropometric assessment of neonatal nutritional status. J Pediatr 109:311, 1986.

38. Georgieff MK, Sasanow SR, Mammel MC, et al. Mid-arm circumference/head circumference ratios for identification of symptomatic LGA, AGA and SGA newborn infants. J Pediatr 109:316. 1986.

39. Rolland-Cachera MF, Brambilla P, Manzoni P, et al. Body composition assessed on the basis or arm circumference and triceps skinfold thickness: a new index validated in children by magnetic resonance. Am J Clin Nutr 65:1709, 1997.

40. Sheng HP, Muthappa PB, Wong WW, et al. Pitfalls of body fat assessments in premature infants by anthropometry. Biol Neonate 64:279, 1993.

41. Johnson TS, Engstrom JL, Gelhar DK. Intra- and interexaminer reliability of anthropometric measurements of term infants. J Pediatr Gastrol Nutr 24:497, 1997.

42. Picaud JC, Rigo J, Nyamugabo K, et al. Evaluation of dual energy X-ray absorptiometry for body composition assessment in piglets and term human neonates. Am J Clin Nutr 63:157, 1996.

43. deBruin NC, van Velthoven KAM, de Ridder M, et al. Standards for total body fat and fat-free mass in infants. Arch Dis Child 74:386, 1996.

44. deBruin NC, van Velthoven KAM, Stijnen T, et al. Body fat and fat-free mass in infants: new and classic anthropometric indexes and prediction equations compared with total-body electrical conductivity. Am J Clin Nutr 61:1195, 1995.

45. Krick J, Murphy-Miller P, Zeger S, et al. Pattern of growth in children with cerebral palsy. J Am Diet Assoc 96:680, 1996.

46. Cronk C, Crocker AC, Pueschel SM, et al. Growth charts for children with Down syndrome. Pediatr 81:102, 1988.

47. Gilmore CH, Sentipal-Walerius JM, Jones JG, et al. Pulse dexamethasone does not impair growth and body composition of very low birth weight infants. J Amer Coll Nutr 14:455, 1995.

48. Gibson JR, McKeown T. Observations on all births (23,970) in Birmingham 1947; VI. Birth weight, duration of gestation, and survival related to sex. Brit J Soc Med 6:152, 1952.

49. Thomson AM, Billewicz WZ, Hytten FE. The assessment of fetal growth. J Obstet Gynecol Brit Commonwealth 75:903, 1968.

50. Gruenwald P. Growth of the human fetus. I. Normal growth and its variation. Amer J Obstet Gynecol 94:1112, 1966.

51. Brenner WE, Edelman DA, Hendricks CH. A standard of fetal growth for the United States of America. Am J Obstet Gynecol 126:555, 1976.

52. Williams RL et al. Fetal growth and perinatal viability in California. Obstet Gynecol 59:624-32, 1982.

53. David RJ. Population-based intrauterine growth curves from computerized birth certificates. South Med J 76:1401, 1983.

54. Lawrence C et al. Modeling of reference values for size at birth. Acta Paediatr Scand, Suppl 350:55, 1989.

55. Niklasson A et al. An update of the Swedish reference standards for weight, length, and head circumference at birth for given gestational age (1997-1981). Acta Paediatr Scand 80:756, 1991.

56. Ehrenkranz RA, Younes N, Lemons JA, et al. Longitudinal growth of hospitalized very low birth weight infants. Pediatr 104:280, 1999.

Nutritional Care for High-Risk Newborns (Rev. 3d. Ed.)
S. Groh-Wargo, M. Thompson, J. Cox, editors
© 2000, Precept Press, Inc., Chicago

3

CLINICAL ASSESSMENT

Gerri Keller, MEd, RD, LD

CLINICAL NUTRITIONAL ASSESSMENT OF THE neonate includes observation of the infant's general condition, feeding tolerance, and signs or symptoms of nutrient deficiency or excess. These observations may have an impact on the route or amount of nutrient delivery.

General Condition

The infant's initial adaptation to extrauterine life is described using the Apgar score.[1] Heart rate, respiratory effort, muscle tone, reflex irritability, and color are observed and evaluated at one and five minutes of life. Low scores may be secondary to transplacental anesthesia or may be associated with central nervous system (CNS) depression, as in asphyxia, or with neurological abnormalities caused by longstanding CNS, neuromuscular, genetic, or metabolic problems. When it reflects duration of birth asphyxia, the five-minute score is a better indicator of survival and neurological prognosis than the one-minute score.[2]

Asphyxia, evidenced by hypoxia and ischemia, is not always accompanied by low Apgar scores. If asphyxia is significant, the infant may exhibit transitory or permanent effects on organ function. Blood flow to the small and large bowel, kidneys, and lungs may be decreased and redistributed to the myocardium and CNS. As a result, serious ischemic injury to these organs can occur. The gut is especially vulnerable to damage, increasing the risk of complications such as feeding intolerance and necrotizing enterocolitis (NEC).[2] If neurological damage has occurred, the sucking reflex or the ability to establish a functional suck and swallow pattern may be affected.

Temperature Control

Temperature control may be difficult during the newborn period, especially for the low-birth-weight and preterm infant. Smaller and less mature infants have minimal subcutaneous fat stores, a larger body surface area per unit of weight, and a higher body water content. This allows greater water loss and, subsequently, greater heat loss.

Neonates adapt to cold stress by the production of heat metabolically, sacrificing calories needed for growth. During cold stress, the breakdown of brown fat stores located primarily in the mediastinum, interscapular, paraspinal, and perirenal areas provides a metabolic source of nonshivering heat production.[3,4] The metabolism of brown adipose tissue for the production of heat occurs only in the newborn period. Brown fat stores are limited in low-birth-weight and premature infants. Heat may also be generated by crying, moving, or changing body posture to decrease exposed skin surface area. This becomes impossible if the infant is unconscious, sedated, or restrained.

Neonates who are overheated also have difficulty regulating body temperature. Sweating is rarely observed in the premature infant. Heat loss may be accomplished by peripheral vasodilatation.[4]

Unfortunately, no one environmental temperature is ideal for every baby. Heat loss and overheating can be avoided by achieving a neutral thermal environment.[5] The goal of a neutral thermal environment is the maintenance of a constant internal body temperature of 35.5°-37.5°C, with minimal metabolic expenditure.[5,6] Measuring an infant's body temperature alone is of limited value, as it does not take metabolic rate into account. An infant's skin is extremely sensitive to external temperature and is thus greatly affected by environmental changes. Even if internal body temperature is constant, metabolic rate increases if the environmental temperature drops below or rises above skin temperature. To ensure a neutral thermal environment, the environmental temperature should be consistent with skin temperature.

During initial stabilization or for other complex procedures when greater access to the infant is needed, an open bed may be used. Overhead radiant heat is used with these open beds to maintain body temperature, but they increase insensible water losses, as do phototherapy lights. Clear plastic film blankets may be placed over the infant to decrease water loss and help conserve body temperature. An incubator conserves body heat by using warm circulating air that can be adjusted to meet individual needs.

Respiratory and Heart Rates

The respiratory pattern of premature infants is often periodic and irregular, but becomes more stable with age.[7] Heart rate is also related to gestational age and is affected by the infant's state of sleep or wakefulness.[8] The effects of feeding on respiratory and heart rates may influence the type and route of nutrition support chosen.

Episodes of apnea (cessation of breathing) and bradycardia (slow heart rate) may be associated with enteral feedings. Nasogastric feeding tubes may compromise the airway or lead to bradycardia with tube placement.[9] Intermittent (bolus) nasogastric or orogastric tube feedings may be associated with aspiration, an increase in respiratory rate, a mild decrease in arterial oxygenation, and a decrease in tidal volume and functional residual capacity.[9] In these cases, continuous delivery of formula at a slow, steady rate through an indwelling orogastric, nasogastric, or transpyloric feeding tube may be better tolerated. Partial or total parenteral nutrition may be necessary if enteral feedings persistently compromise respirations and heart rate. Nipple-feeding must be approached cautiously in premature infants whose respiratory rate is > 60 breaths per minute in order to minimize the risk of aspiration.[10]

Fluid Status

During the first week of life, total body water content decreases rapidly, due mainly to a reduction of extracellular volume.[11,12] This causes a weight loss of ≤ 10-15% in premature infants.[13] This diuresis is desirable, as overhydration may be associated with several compromising conditions (see Chapter 9). Clinical signs of overhydration may include periorbital, sacral, or generalized edema.

After the first week of life, continued weight loss may be an indication of dehydration or catabolism. Clinical signs of dehydration may include decreased urine output (≤ 1 ml/kg/hr), elevated urine osmolality, dry mucous membranes, or poor skin turgor.[14] Normal urine osmolality ranges ≤ 700 mOsm/L in the term infant and ≤ 550 mOsm/L in the preterm infant.[15] Osmolality is a measure of the number of particles in solution. Specific gravity measures the refractive properties of particles in solution and is often used to estimate osmolalityusing the following equation:

$$\text{urine osmolality (mOsm/L)} = (\text{specific gravity} - 1) \times 4 \times 10^4$$

For example, if the measured urine specific gravity is 1.010, urine osmolality = (1.010 - 1) x 4 x 10^4 = 400 mOsm/L. The presence of glucose, protein, or urea may increase the specific gravity of the urine and may lead to a false overestimation of urine osmolality (see Appendix H).[15]

The osmolality of nutrient solutions is determined by the presence of osmotically active particles, including carbohydrates, proteins/amino acids, minerals, and electrolytes. Osmolality may affect gastrointestinal tolerance of enteral feedings. Enterally delivered nutrient solutions are best tolerated when osmolality is < 450 mOsm/kg water. Higher solute levels may be associated with osmotic diarrhea (see Chapter 16). The osmolality of human milk and most commercial formulas is usually in the range of 260 to 320, but commonly used medications and electrolyte supplements added to feedings may increase the osmolality significantly (see Appendix H).[16]

The osmolality of parenteral nutrient solutions may affect the integrity of vessels and surrounding tissues. Parenterally delivered nutrient solutions are best tolerated when osmolality is between 600 and 1000 mOsm/L (see Chapter 12).

Not all particles that contribute to the osmolality of the solution also contribute to the renal solute load and urine osmolality. Absorbed carbohydrate is metabolized to carbon dioxide and water, neither of which normally contributes to urine osmolality. The end products of protein metabolism, sodium, chloride, and phosphorus are excreted by the kidney and potentially contribute to urine osmolality.[17] When these nutrients are used in the building of tissues during growth phases and are retained by the body, they are not excreted by the kidneys and do not contribute to renal solute load. Excess solutes must be excreted by the kidney if solute intake is greater than that used in tissue growth, if growth does not occur, if energy or protein intake is inadequate to support growth, or if periods of catabolism or stress occur. Appendix H provides specific information needed to calculate potential renal solute load of various nutrient solutions and estimate actual renal solute load.

Indirect Calorimetry

Measurement of oxygen consumption and carbon dioxide production has been used to predict resting energy expenditure (REE) in subjects of all ages. These measurements in infants, particularly low-birth-weight infants, require specific technical and methodologic considerations that are described in detail elsewhere.[18] Difficulties commonly encountered include maintaining stable inspiratory gas concentrations, especially at high oxygen concentrations; collecting and precisely measuring expiratory gases; maintaining a resting state for adequate periods of time; and controlling margins of error, which are amplified due to the relatively small gas volumes in this patient population.

Equations that have been developed to predict REE from indirect calorimetry studies in older children and adults are not often useful in predicting energy needs in neonates. For example, the Schofield equation, which uses both length and weight to predict REE, more closely correlates with measured REE in children 4 months to 20 years of age than other equations.[19] However, this equation predicts a negative value for REE for infants < 41 cm in length.

An equation using weight, heart rate, and age has been developed to predict REE using indirect calorimetry data collected from infants of 26 to 42 weeks' gestation and one to 126 days old:

$$[- 74.436 + (34.611 \times wt) + (0.496 \times HR) + (0.178 \times age)] \times 1.44 = Cal/d$$

where "wt" is weight in kg, "HR" is heart rate in beats/min, "age" is age in days, and "Cal/d" or Calories per day is REE.[20] Because infants were not made to fast during these studies, REE includes diet-induced thermogenesis. Total energy requirements are then estimated by adding factors for activity (15 Cal/kg/d), growth (5 kcal/g weight gain/day), and for enterally fed neonates, excretory losses (10%).[20,21]

Measurements of oxygen consumption, carbon dioxide production, and urinary nitrogen used to predict total energy needs in sick neonates indicate wide variability: 113 to 163 kcal/kg/day in enterally fed neonates and 61-82 kcal/kg/day in parenterally fed neonates.[22] Clinical conditions such as temperature instability, changes in cardiac output, surgery, and skin maturity may significantly alter energy requirements. Because of wide variability, if standard equations are used to estimate energy needs rather than individual measurement, careful monitoring of growth parameters is needed to assess adequacy of energy intake and to indicate when modifications in nutrient intake are needed (see Chapters 2, 4, 10 and 15).[19]

Nutrient Deficiency

Many factors place a neonate at risk for nutrient deficiency. Some of these risk factors include low nutrient stores due to premature birth or intrauterine growth retardation, prolonged periods of suboptimal nutrition support, prolonged need for parenteral nutrition, and high nutrient needs to support growth.

Alterations in growth patterns may occur when there is a nutrient deficiency, although nutrient deficiency is often first identified biochemically before clinical presentation or growth aberration occurs (see Chapters 2 and 5). Deficiencies most commonly reported include those of calcium, phosphorus, vitamin D, vitamin E, iron, zinc, carnitine, essential fatty acid, or protein. Clinical signs of deficiency of these nutrients are shown in Table 3.1.

Table 3.1. Clinical Signs of Nutrient Deficiency

Nutrient	Signs of Deficiency
Calcium[23,24]	Neonatal seizures, decreased bone density*, rickets, osteopenia, tetany
	Since bone serves as a homeostatic mechanism, hypocalcemia may or may not be present
Phosphorus[23,24]	Seizures, decreased bone density*, rickets, bone pain, decrease cardiac function
	Since bone serves as a homeostatic mechanism, hypophosphatemia may or may not be present
Vitamin D[23]	Decreased bone density*, osteopenia, rickets
Vitamin E[25,26]	Mild hemolytic anemia, usually manifesting itself by four to six weeks of life; mild edema, thrombocytosis
Vitamin K[27]	Increased prothrombin time, bleeding (petechiae, purpura, ecchymoses, intracranial)
Folate	Megaloblastic anemia, glossitis, diarrhea, irritability
Thiamin[27]	Hyporeflexia, muscle weakness, tachycardia, edema, irritability, Wernicke's encephalopathy
Biotin[28,29]	Dermatitis, alopecia, irritability, lethargy
Selenium[27]	Poor growth, cardiomyopathy
Iron[28]	Hypochromic microcytic anemia, pallor, tachycardia
Zinc[29]	Acrodermatitis enteropathica, failure to grow, hypoproteinemia with generalized edema, impaired wound healing, increased susceptibility to infection, alopecia
Carnitine[30]	Acute encephalopathy, muscle weakness, lipid myopathy, failure to thrive, recurrent infections
Essential fatty acids[31,32]	Scaly dermatitis, thrombocytopenia, increased risk of infection, poor growth, alopecia
Protein[33-35]	Slow growth, hypoproteinemia with generalized edema, anergy, decreased total lymphocyte count, increased rate of infection, and impaired wound healing

* Methods used to assess bone density are described elsewhere.[36-38]

Table 3.2. Stool Characteristics

Protein source	Stool characteristics
Human milk	Pasty, yellow, soft
Cow's milk protein	Formed, greenish brown, very little free water
Modified cow's milk protein (whey-to-casein ratio 60:40)	Small volume, pasty yellow, some free water (similar to breast milk stool)
Soy protein isolate	Soft, yellowish green
Sodium caseinate	Formed, greenish brown, little free water
Casein hydrolysate	Green, some mucus, small volume

Adapted with permission from Enteral nutrition: Support of the pediatric patient. In: Hendricks KM, Walker WA, eds. Manual of pediatric nutrition. Philadelphia: Decker, 1990

Feeding Tolerance

Prior to the delivery of enteral feedings, the infant's airway and G.I. tract are assessed for patency or structural anomaly. Choanal atresia, tracheoesophageal fistula, esophageal blind pouch or stricture, cleft lip or palate, and micrognathia are several of the findings that may preclude or alter the method of enteral feeding (see Chapters 18, 19, and 26). Gestational and developmental maturity are assessed to determine readiness for oral feedings.

Once enteral feedings can be safely initiated, many factors may contribute to feeding intolerance. These include an immature G.I. tract, immature development of enzymes, medical complications such as NEC or sepsis, hyperosmolar feedings (Appendix K), volume of feeding, and medications (Appendix E). Feeding intolerance may be characterized by one or more symptoms: increased periods of apnea and bradycardia associated with feedings; large gastric residuals; increased abdominal girth or abdominal distention; vomiting; or stools that are positive for blood, reducing substances, or fat.[39]

Early feedings are commonly characterized by gastric residuals and abdominal distention. Peristalsis (assessed by auscultation of bowel sounds) may be weak at birth but tends to improve rapidly.[40] Prior to each feeding or at specific intervals during continuous feedings, gastric residuals should be checked and abdominal girth measured. For intermittent feedings, a large gastric residual is often defined as half of the previous feeding or greater than one hour's volume when continuously fed.[41] Increased gastric residuals and abdominal girth may be result of a large feeding volume, an increase in the caloric density of the formula,[42] poor G.I. motility, NEC, or intestinal obstruction. In the first few days of life, feeding low-volume, human milk or formula, sometimes referred to as "gut priming," has been shown to stimulate G.I. function and to improve tolerance of enteral feedings.[43,44]

Regurgitation of small amounts of formula during or after a feeding is common. The volume differentiates "spitting" from vomiting. When mild "spitting" is present with no other symptoms, simple techniques such as repositioning during and after feeding or frequent burping may resolve the problem. If symptoms such as choking, apnea, respiratory problems, increased irritability, poor weight gain, or sudden refusal of oral feedings are present, a more in-depth diagnostic evaluation is warranted. Vomiting can be serious and may be the result of illness, allergy, obstruction, gastroesophageal reflux, or a too-large feeding volume (see Chapters 26 and 27). Presence of bile or blood in the vomitus may be associated with serious pathology and always needs medical evaluation.

The first stool of a newborn infant is known as meconium. It is usually greenish black to light brown and of a tarry consistency. Most healthy full-term infants will have their first stool within 24 hours after birth. A premature infant's first stool may be delayed six or seven days as a result of immature G.I. motility and withholding of enteral feedings.[45] Subsequent stool color, consistency, and volume varies depending upon the type of enteral protein that is ingested; various characteristics are described in Table 3.2. Stools positive for blood may result from maternal blood swallowed by the infant during delivery, gastric irritation from an indwelling feeding tube, formula intolerance, rectal fissures, or NEC. Grossly evident blood is of greater concern than positive laboratory findings of occult blood. The latter is present in a significant percentage of normal appearing stools in growing preterm infants.

Clinical signs of carbohydrate intolerance may include abdominal distention, explosive stools, and watery, osmotic diarrhea.[46] Lactase activity develops late in gestation and is not fully functional until term. Premature infants may display some degree of lactose intolerance, although recent studies show minimal excretion of lactose. Colonic fermentation and absorption of acetate and other short-chain fatty acids thus formed may adequately salvage unabsorbed lactose and prevent osmotic diarrhea.[47] Reducing substances of $> 0.5\%$ and a stool pH of < 5.5 indicate carbohydrate malabsorption.[48] Oligosaccharides, such as the glucose polymers that are present in many infant formulas, react only at their reducing ends. Malabsorption of these carbohydrates may be greatly underestimated by analyzing stool for reducing substances unless acid hydrolysis is used in the analysis.[49,50] If sucrose malabsorption is suspected, sugar chromatography must be performed, since sucrose is not a reducing sugar. Although carbohydrate intolerance may be due to a primary deficiency of enzymes or absorptive sites, it is more commonly encountered after acute episodes of infectious gastroenteritis and diarrhea.[50]

Protein intolerance may cause clinical symptoms of vomiting, intestinal upset, diarrhea, bloody stools, colitis, atopic dermatitis, urticaria, rhinitis, increased irritability, and/or colic. During the first few months of life, gastrointestinal barriers to antigens are immature, something that may increase the risk of systemic sensitization with ingested proteins, particularly when the mucosal barrier is further compromised by infectious diarrhea.[50]

Full-term newborn infants absorb 80-85% of ingested human milk fat, coconut oil, soy oil, or medium-chain triglycerides.[51,52] Preterm infants may absorb fat less well-about 60-75% of that ingested.[51,52] Most infants will be able to more efficiently absorb fat, up to 95%, by 4-10 months of age.[51,52] If significant fat malabsorption is present, stools may be large, bulky, oily, and unusually foul-smelling.[46] Fecal fat can be quantified using methods described elsewhere.[51,52] Fat malabsorption may result from pancreatic insufficency and/or a small bile acid pool.[53,54] Stools may appear white, grey, or clay colored if bile acids are insufficient.

In summary, the clinical assessment of the neonate requires observation of the infant's general condition as well as specific evaluation of physical signs of nutrient deficiency or excess and feeding tolerance. It is important to remember that each infant is unique and must be assessed individually. This assessment must be integrated with anthropometric, biochemical, and intake assessments to appropriately formulate the nutrition care plan.

References

1. Harper RG, Yoon JJ. Handbook of neonatology, 2d ed. Chicago: Year Book Medical Publishers, 1987; 25.
2. Fanaroff AA, Martin RJ. Neonatal-perinatal medicine. Diseases of the fetus and infant. 4th ed. St. Louis: Mosby, 1987; 364, 374-75.
3. Aherne W, Hall D. Brown adipose tissue and heat production in the newborn infant. J Pathol Bacteriol 91:233, 1966.
4. Streeter NS. High-Risk Neonatal Care. Rockville, MD: Aspen Publishers, 1986; 99-104.
5. Fanaroff AA, Martin RJ. Neonatal-perinatal medicine. Diseases of the fetus and infant. 4th ed. St. Louis: Mosby, 1987; 401.
6. Hey, EN. Thermal neutrality. Br Med Bull 31:69, 1975.
7. Fanaroff AA, Martin RJ. Neonatal-perinatal medicine. Diseases of the fetus and infant. 4th ed. St. Louis: Mosby, 1987; 617.
8. Fanaroff AA, Martin RJ. Neonatal-perinatal medicine. Diseases of the fetus and infant. 4th ed. St. Louis: Mosby, 1987; 343.
9. Lemons JA, Brady MS, Rickard K, et al. Considerations in feeding the very-low-birth-weight infant. Perinatol Neonatol May/June: 76, 1982.

10. Topper WH. Enteral feeding methods for compromised neonates and infants. In: Lebenthal E, ed. Textbook for gastroenterology and nutrition in infancy. New York: Raven Press, 1981; 647.

11. Bauer K, Boverman G, Roithmaier A, et al. Body composition, nutrition, and fluid balance during the first two weeks of life in preterm neonates weighing less than 1500 grams. J Pediatr 118:615, 1991.

12. Shaffer SG, Bradt SK, Meade VM, et al. Extracellular fluid volume changes in very low birth weight infants during the first two postnatal months. J Pediatr 111:24, 1987.

13. Fanaroff AA and Hack M. Fluid requirements of the low-birth-weight infant. In: Sunshine P, ed. Feeding the Neonate weighing less than 1,500 grams-nutrition and beyond, report on the Seventy-Ninth Ross Conference on Pediatric Research. Columbus, Ohio: Ross Laboratories, 1980; 2-6.

14. Harper RG, Yoon JJ. Handbook of neonatology, 2d ed. Chicago: Year Book Medical Publishers, 1987; 544.

15. Shaffer SG, and Weismann DN. Fluid requirements in the preterm infant. Clin Perinatol 19:233, 1992.

16. Jew RK, Owen D, Kaufman D, et al. Osmolality of commonly used medications and formulas in the neonatal intensive care unit. Nutr Clin Prac 12:158, 1997.

17. Fomon SJ, Ziegler EE. Renal solute load and potential renal solute load in infancy. J Pediatr 134:11, 1999.

18. Thureen PJ, Phillips RE, DeMarie MP, et al. Technical and methodologic considerations for performance of indirect calorimetry in ventilated and non--ventilated preterm infants. Crit Care Med 25:171, 1997.

19. Kaplan AS, Zemel BS, Nelswender KM, et al. Resting energy expenditure in clinical pediatrics: Measured versus prediction equations. J Pediatr 127:200, 1995.

20. Pierro A, Jones MO, Hammond P, et al. A new equation to predict the resting energy expenditure of surgical infants. J Pediatr Surg 29:1103, 1994.

21. Reichman B, Chessex P, Putet G, et al. Partition of energy metabolism and energy cost of growth in the very low-birth-weight infant. Pediatr 69:446, 1982.

22. Forsyth S, Crighton A. An indirect calorimetry system for ventilator dependent very low birthweight infants. Arch Dis Child 67:315, 1992.

23. Cooke R, Hollis B, Conner C, et al. Vitamin D and mineral metabolism in the very low birth weight infant receiving 400 iu of vitamin D. J Pediatr 116:423, 1990.

24. Glass EJ, Hume R, Hendry GMA, et al. Plasma alkaline phosphatase activity in rickets of prematurity. J Arch Dis Child 57:373, 1982.

25. Oski FA, Barness, LA. Vitamin E deficiency: A previously unrecognized cause of hemolytic anemia in premature infants. J Pediatr 70:211, 1967.

26. Ritchie JH, Fish MB, McMaster V, et al. Edema and hemolytic anemia in premature infants. A vitamin E deficiency syndrome. N Engl J Med 279:1185, 1968.

27. Balint JP. Physical findings in nutritional deficiencies. Pediatr Clin North Am 45:245, 1998.

28. Moya FR. Nutritional requirements of the term newborn. In: Suskind RM, ed. Textbook of pediatric nutrition. 2nd ed. New York: Raven Press, 1993; 9.

29. Pereira GR, Zucker, AH. Nutritional deficiencies in the neonate. Clin Perinatol 13:175, 1986.
30. Winter SC, Szabo-Aczel D, Curry GJR, et al. Plasma carnitine deficiency. Am J Dis Child 141:660, 1987.
31. Hansen AE, Wiese HF, Boelsche AW, et al. Role of linoleic acid in infant nutrition. Clinical and chemical study of 428 infants fed on milk mixtures varying in kind and amount of fat. Pediatr 31:171, 1963.
32. Paulsrud JR, Pensler L, Whitten CF, et al. Essential fatty acid deficiency in infants induced by fat free intravenous feeding. Am J Clin Nutr 25:897, 1972.
33. Gross SJ. Growth and biochemical response of preterm infants fed human milk or modified infant formula. N Engl J Med 308:237, 1983.
34. Fomon SJ, Ziegler EE, and Vazquez HD. Human milk and the small premature infant. Am J Dis Child 131:463, 1977.
35. The National Academy of Sciences: Recommended dietary allowances. 10th ed. Washington, D.C.: National Academy Press, 1989; 53.
36. Lyon AJ, Hawkes DJ, Doran M, et al. Bone mineralization in preterm infants measured by dual energy radiographic densitometry. Arch Dis Child 64:919-23, 1989.
37. Braillon PM, Salle BL, Brunet J, et al. Dual energy X-ray absorptiometry measurement of bone mineral content in newborns: validation of the technique. Pediatr Res 32:77, 1992.
38. Salle BL, Braillon PM, Glorieux FH, et al. Lumbar bone mineral content measured by dual energy X-ray absorptiometry in newborns and infants. Acta Paediatr 82:1, 1993.
39. Moyer-Mileur LJ. Nutrition. In: Streeter NS, ed. High-risk neonatal care. Rockville, MD: Aspen, 1986; 282.
40. Morriss FH, Moore M, Weisbrodt NW, et al. Ontogenic development of gastrointestinal motility: IV. Duodenal contractions in preterm infants. Pediatr 78:1106, 1986.
41. Warman KY. Enteral nutrition: Support of the pediatric patient. In: Hendricks KM, Walker WA. Manual of pediatric nutrition. 2d ed. Philadelphia: Decker, 1990; 104.
42. Siegel M, Lebenthal E, Krantz B. Effect of caloric density on gastric emptying in premature infants. J Pediatr 104:118, 1984.
43. Slagle TA, Gross SJ. Effect of early low-volume enteral substrate on subsequent feeding tolerance in very low birth weight infants. J Pediatr 113:526, 1988.
44. Dunn L, Hulman S, Weiner J, et al. Beneficial effects of early hypocaloric enteral feeding on neonatal gastrointestinal function: Preliminary report of a randomized trial. J Pediatr 112:622, 1988.
45. Jhaveri MK, Kumar SP. Passage of the first stool in very low birth weight infants. Pediatr 79:1005, 1987.
46. Gryboski J, Walker WA. Gastrointestinal problems in the infant. 2d ed. Philadelphia: Saunders, 1983; 594.
47. Kien CL, Kepner J, Grotjohn KA, et al. Efficient assimilation of lactose carbon in premature infants. J Pediatr Gastroenterol Nutr 15:253, 1992.
48. Lebenthal E, Tucker NT. Carbohydrate digestion: Development in early infancy. Clin Perinatol 13:37, 1986.
49. Ameen VZ, Powell GK, Jones LA. Quantitation of fecal carbohydrate excretion in patients with short bowel syndrome. Gastroenterology 92:493, 1987.

50. Kerner JA. Formula allergy and intolerance. Gastroenterol Clin North Amer 24:1, 1995.
51. Silverman A, Roy CC. Pediatric clinical gastroenterology. St. Louis: Mosby, 1983; 901.
52. Shmerling DH, Forrer JCW, Prader A. Fecal fat and nitrogen in healthy children and in children with malabsorption or maldigestion. Pediatrics 46:690, 1970.
53. Brady MS, Rickard KA, Ernst JA, et al. Formulas and human milk for premature infants: A review and update. J Am Diet Assoc 81:547, 1982.
54. Watkins JB, Szczepanik P, Gould JB, et al. Bile salt metabolism in the human premature infant: Preliminary observations of pool size and synthesis rate following prenatal administration of dexamethasone and phenobarbital. Gastroenterology 69:706, 1975.

Nutritional Care for High-Risk Newborns (Rev. 3d. Ed.)
S. Groh-Wargo, M. Thompson, J. Cox, editors
© 2000, Precept Press, Inc., Chicago

4

INTAKE ASSESSMENT

*Nancy L. Nevin-Folino, MEd, RD, LD,
and Janice Hovasi Cox, MS, RD*

SYSTEMATICALLY COLLECTING AND EVALUATING nutrient intake data is an important aspect of nutrition assessment in the management of critically ill neonates. Intake data are derived from volume and type of parenterally administered solutions, human milk, commercial infant formulas, vitamin and mineral supplements, and caloric supplements. Intakes are most often calculated per kilogram of body weight per day or total intake per day. Nutrient intake can be expressed per 100 calories to assess calorie-to-nutrient ratios. Calculations of nutrient intake are compared to generally accepted, published recommendations.[1-7] (See Chapters 10, 11, and 15 for recommended nutrient intakes.) Estimated nutrient needs often vary, depending upon the route of administration. The proportion of parenteral nutrition (PN) and enteral nutrition (EN) to total intake are included in evaluating the adequacy of nutrient intake. Intakes that vary significantly from established recommendations are investigated, as well as discrepancies between actual and ordered intakes.

An intake assessment system is established based on the specific needs of the infants, the number of infants, and the staff available to provide intake assessment. Nutrient intake assessment may be limited to only two or three nutrients, such as fluid, calories, and protein. Calculations of these nutrients can be used as part of a "nutrition screen" to identify which infants may require a more in-depth evaluation. The neonatal registered dietitian can use inpatient screening criteria to prioritize nutrition intervention. Screening is guided by hospital protocol, as determined by the neonatologist, registered dietitian, or other qualified nutrition expert. Initial screening usually occurs within 24 to 72 hours of admission, with subsequent weekly monitoring of identified parameters. Sample nutrition screening and monitoring criteria are given in Chapter 7 and Table B.1 of Appendix B. These may be modified to fit the needs of a particular facility. No set of criteria is guaranteed to identify 100% of the infants at risk for developing nutrition problems. The goal is to have reasonable parameters that can be quickly assessed and that will identify most of the patients who require nutrition intervention.

The intake of other nutrients may be assessed if indicated by clinical, laboratory, or anthropometric indexes. The units of measure commonly used for comparison with published recommendations are given in Table 4.1 for the most frequently assessed nutrients. Computer programs are available to calculate and store intake data as well as compare intake data with laboratory and anthropometric indexes (see Chapter 6).

Specific record sheets developed for an individual hospital's needs may incorporate other pertinent clinical, laboratory, and anthropometric data. Examples are shown in Figures 4.1-4.3. An intake assessment system can be incorporated into unit nutrition standards and hospital quality assurance programs.[8] When collected longitudinally, nutrition intake data can also be used for research purposes.

Monitoring the intake of parenterally delivered nutrients varies with ordering methods, nutrient solutions used, and the compounding process. Nutrients may be ordered per kilogram of body weight, per unit of solution delivered, or as the total amount delivered per day. Nutrients may be ordered in grams, milligrams, milliequivalents, millimoles, or milliliters of a specific solution. (See conversion information for selected nutrients in Appendix C.) Computer programs have been developed to simplify, reduce errors, and improve individualization of ordering parenteral nutrients.[9] Although ordering patterns may vary, nutrient intake analysis should be reported using the units described in Table 4.1 so that they can be compared to published standards (see Chapters 10, 11, and 15).

Case Study

Although methods of ordering parenteral nutrients vary, the following case study provides a demonstration of nutrient intake calculations based on a sample parenteral and enteral nutrition order. An

Figure 4.1. Daily flow sheet for nutrient intake.

Name:

Birth date:

Gestational age:

Chart number:

Date							
Day of life							
Weight (kg)							
Fluid (ml/kg/d)							
Parenteral							
Enteral							
Total							
Energy (kcal/kg/d)							
Parenteral							
Enteral							
Total							
Protein (g/kg/d)							
Parenteral							
Enteral							
Total							

Figure 4.2. Nutrient intake worksheet.

Name:______________________________ Chart number:______________________________

	Date/day of life							
	Weight (kg)							
Intake (ml)	PN #1 D___% AA___%							
	PN #2 D___% AA___%							
	Lipid _____%							
	Human milk							
	Formula __________							
	Supplement(s)							
	Total ml							
	Total ml/kg							
Calories	I.V. kcal/kg/d							
	% of total kcal							
	EN cal/kg/d							
	% of total kcal							
	Total cal/kg/d							
Protein	I.V. Pro g/kg/d							
	NPC/g N							
	EN Pro g/kg/d							
	g/100 kcal EN							
	% of total kcal							
	Total g/kg/d							
Fat	I.V. fat g/kg/d							
	% of total kcal							
Vitamins	Vitamin A IU/d							
	Vitamin D IU/d							
	Vitamin E IU/d							
	Vitamin C mg/d							
	Folic acid μg/d							
Minerals	Ca mg/kg/d							
	P mg/kg/d							
	Mg mg/kg/d							
	Fe mg/kg/d							
	Zn μg/kg/d							
	Cu μg/kg/d							

Figure 4.3. Nutrient intake assessment.

(Chart adapted with permission of Children's Center Neonatal Dietitians, Cincinnati; Dayton Infant Care Specialists; and Children's Medical Center, Dayton, Ohio.)

Name:_____ DOB:_____ Admit Date:_____ Gestational age:_____

Problem list:_____ Apgars:___1 ___5 ___10

Birth weight:_____ Birth length:_____ Birth OFC:_____

Day BW regained:_____ Max % BW lost:_____

Parenteral nutrition: DOL full PN kcal achieved:_____

    Amino Acid (AA):_____ DOL AA started:_____ DOL AA d'cd:_____

    Lipids (L):_____ DOL L started:_____ DOL L d'cd:_____

Enteral nutrition: Formula/human milk:_____ DOL full EN kcal achieved:_____

Output Anthropometrics	Date/Day of life (DOL)						
	Weight (g)						
	Weight change ⇧ or ⇩ (g/d)						
	Length (cm)						
	Head circumference (cm)						
	Abdominal girth (cm)						
	Gastric aspirate (% of feeding)						
	Stool/ostomy output (# or ml/24°)						
	Urine output (ml/24° or ml/kg/hr)						
Parenteral intake (ml/24°)	#1: D___% AA___% L___%						
	#2: D___% AA___% L___%						
	#3: D___% AA___% L___%						
	KCAL: total PN kcal/kg/d						
	CHO: mg/kg/min (% total PN kcal)						
	PRO: g/kg/d (% total PN kcal)						
	Fat: g/kg/hr (% total PN kcal)						
	Non-protein kcal/g N ratio						
Enteral Intake (ml/24°)	#1:						
	#2:						
	Modality: PO OG NG NJ OJ GT						
	KCAL: total EN kcal/kg/d						
	PRO: g/kg/d						
Totals	Total intake kcal/kg/d						
	Total intake %PN : %EN						
	Total intake PRO g/kg/d						
Supplements	Vitamin E						
	Vitamin D						
	Folic acid						
	Multivitamin (w or w/o fluoride)						
	Iron						
	Other						

infant is born at 32 weeks' gestation weighing 1,500 g. Two weeks after birth, birth weight has been regained. Although enteral feedings are progressing well, PN continues to provide much of the infant's nutrients. PN includes 15 ml of 20% lipid emulsion (2.0 fat kcal/ml) and 135 ml/day of a dextrose/amino acid solution containing the following:

12.5%	dextrose (3.4 kcal/gx 12.5 g/dl = 42.5 CHO kcal/dl)
2.5%	amino acids (4 kcal/g x 2.5 g/dl = 10 PRO kcal/dl)
35 mEq	sodium chloride/L
10 mEq	potassium acetate/L
10 mEq	potassium phosphate/L (provides 6.8 mMol or 212 mg phosphorus/L)
2,000 mg	calcium gluconate/L (provides 10 mEq or 200 mg calcium/L)
I ml	magnesium sulfate 50%/L (provides 4.1 mEq or 49 mg magnesium/L)
20 ml	pediatric multivitamin/L (provides 2 doses/L)*
2 ml	pediatric multiple trace element/L (provides 1,000 µg zinc, 200 µg copper, 50 µg manganese, and 1.7 µg chromium/L)

* 1 "dose" of parenteral pediatric multivitamin provides 80 mg ascorbic acid, 2,300 iu retinol, 400 iu ergocalciferol, 1.2 mg thiamin, 1.4 mg riboflavin, I mg pyridoxine, 17 mg niacinamide, 5 mg dexpanthenol, 7 mg dl-a-tocopherol, 20 µg biotin, 140 µg folic acid, 1 µg cyanocobalamin, and 200 µg phytonadione.

Daily EN intake includes 75 ml of Similac Special Care 20 (Ross Laboratories, Columbus, Ohio). (See Appendix K for a complete list of nutrient content.) The calculated intake of nutrients in the schedules below must then be compared with PN and EN recommendations for intake in light of the percentage of nutrient delivery by each route.

Although the nutrient intake of an individual infant is compared with the recommended nutrient intake for age, physical maturity, and route of nutrient delivery, one must also consider the anthropometric, clinical, and laboratory components of nutrition assessment in providing optimal nutrition for the individual infant.

FLUID (ML) INTAKE

PN: 135 ml dextrose/amino acid solution ÷ 1.5 kg = 90 ml/kg/d
15 ml lipid emulsion ÷ 1.5 kg = 10 ml/kg/d

EN: 75 ml Similac Special Care ÷ 1.5 kg = 50 ml/kg/d

Total fluid intake = 150 ml/kg/d

CALORIE (KCAL) INTAKE

PN: CHO: 42.5 CHO kcal/dl x 1.35 dl/d = 57 CHO kcal/d
PRO: 10.0 PRO kcal/dl x 1.35 dl/d = 14 PRO kcal/d

Fat: 2.0 fat kcal/ml x 15 ml/d   = 30 fat kcal/d

Total PN kcal/d: 101 kcal/d
Total PN kcal/kg/d: 67 kcal/kg/d
Total nonprotein PN kcal/d: 87 kcal/d

EN: 75 ml Similac Special Care 20/d x 0.67 kcal/ml   = 50 kcal/d
                          50 kcal/d ÷ 1.5 kg   = 33 kcal/kg/d

Total: 67 PN kcal/kg/d + 33 EN kcal/kg/d = 100 kcal/kg/d

Total calorie intake: 67% PN and 33% EN.

PROTEIN (PRO) INTAKE

PN: 90 ml/kg/d x 2.5 g PRO/dl   = 2.3 g PRO/kg/d
EN: 50 ml/kg/d x 1.8 g PRO/dl   = 0.9 g PRO/kg/d

Total: = 3.2 g PRO/kg/d

3.2 g PRO/kg/d x 4 kcal/g   = 12.8 PRO kcal/kg/d

12.8 PRO kcal/kg/d ÷ 100 total kcal/kg/d = 12.8% of total kcal as PRO

NONPROTEIN CALORIE-TO-NITROGEN (N) RATIO

The nonprotein calorie-to-nitrogen ratio is usually calculated only for parenterally administered nutrients, as enteral formulas are standard and appropriately balanced.

Nonprotein PN calorie intake (see above): 87 kcal/d

PN nitrogen intake:

1.35 dl/d dextrose/amino acid solution x 2.5 g PRO/di = 3.4 g PRO/d
3.4 g PRO/d ÷ 6.25 g PRO/g N = 0.5 g N/d

Nonprotein PN calorie to N ratio:

87 nonprotein kcal/d ÷ 0.5 g N/d = 174 nonprotein kcal-to-N ratio

ENTERAL PROTEIN INTAKE PER 100 KCAL

Enteral products are balanced for carbohydrate, protein, and fat content. This calculation should be done when additional nonprotein calories are added to increase the caloric density of a commercial product. For example, for a patient retaining carbon dioxide, a higher fat intake may be desired than is available in a standard formula.

If 1 ml of Microlipid is added per 100 ml of Similac Special Care 20 in the case example, the calculations would be as follows:

100 ml Similac Special Care 20 = 67 kcal and 1.8 g PRO
               1 ml Microlipid = 4.5 kcal

100 ml Similac Special Care 20 + 1 ml Microlipid = 71.5 kcal

1.8 g PRO/71.5 kcal = 2.5 g PRO/100 kcal

CARBOHYDRATE (CHO) INTAKE

The dextrose used in parenteral preparations contains water molecules so that 1 g hydrated dextrose provides only 3.4 kcal or 0.85 g anhydrous glucose. This discrepancy is not always considered when calculating glucose infusion rates (GIR), but is usually considered when calculating calorie intake.

PN: 12.5 g hydrated cHo/dl x 0.85 = 10.6 g anhydrous glucose/dl
      10.6 g glucose/dl x 0.9 dl/kg = 9.5 g glucose/kg/d

GIR: 9.5 g glucose/kg/d ÷ 1,440 min/d x 1,000 mg/g = 6.6 mg glucose/kg/min

12.5 g hydrated CHO/dl x 3.4 kcal/g = 42.5 CHO kcal/dl
      42.5 CHO kcal/dl x 90 ml/kg/d = 38 CHO kcal/kg/d

Technically, the glycerol in the PN lipid solution is metabolized as carbohydrate, and in this case provides 3 kcal/d or adds 0.5 g CHO/kg/day. This is usually insignificant and is included in the calculation of fat intake.

EN: 7.2 g CHO/dl x 0.5 dl/kg/day = 3.6 g CHO/kg/day
      3.6 mg CHO/kg/d x 4 kcal/g = 14 CHO kcal/kg/d

TOTAL:
38 PN CHO kcal/kg/d + 14 EN CHO kcal/kg/d = 52 total CHO kcal/kg/d

52 CHO kcal/kg/d ÷ 100 total kcal/kg/d = 52% of total kcal as CHO

FAT INTAKE

PN: The 20% PN lipid emulsions contain 20 g fat/dl or 0.2 g fat/mi. They provide
     2 kcal/ml, instead of the expected 1.8 kcal/ml calculated from the usual
     9 kcal/g of fat, as glycerol provides an additional 0.2 kcal/ml.

     15 ml/d x 0.2 g fat/ml = 3 g fat/d
       3 g fat/d ÷ 1.5 kg = 2 g fat/kg/d
      2 g fat/kg/d ÷ 24 hr = 0.08 g fat/kg/hr

15 ml/d x 2.0 kcal/ml = 30 kcal/d
30 kcal/d ÷ 1.5 kg = 20 PN fat kcal/kg/d

EN: 3.7 g/dl x 0.5 dl/kg/d = 1.9 g EN fat/kg/d
1.9 g EN fat/kg/d x 9 kcal/g fat = 17 EN fat kcal/kg/d

TOTAL:
20 PN fat kcal/kg/d + 17 EN fat kcal/kg/d = 37 total fat kcal/kg/d

37 fat kcal/kg/d ÷ 100 total kcal/kg/d = 37% of total kcal as fat

CALCIUM (Ca) INTAKE

One milliequivalent of calcium equals 20 mg of calcium. If calcium gluconate is used, calcium gluconate 10% contains 100 mg calcium gluconate or 10 mg (0.5 mEq) of calcium per ml. Requirements for calcium are often expressed in mEq/kg for parenteral intake and mg/kg for enteral intake.

PN: 90 ml/kg/d x 10 mEq Ca/L = 0.9 mEq Ca/kg/d (18 mg/kg/d)

EN: 50 ml/kg/d x 1,220 mg Ca/L = 61 mg Ca/kg/d (3 mEq/kg/d)

PHOSPHORUS (P) INTAKE

PN: One millimole of phosphorus equals 31 mg of phosphorus. Potassium phosphate (KPhos) contains 93 mg (3 mM) P and 4.4 mEq potassium (K) per ml; sodium phosphate contains 93 mg (3 mM) P and 4 mEq sodium per ml. Requirements for phosphorus are often expressed as mM/kg for parenteral intake and mg/kg for enteral intake.

10 mEq KPhos/L x 3 mM P ÷ 4.4 mEq K = 6.8 mM P/L (212 mg/L)
6.8 mM P/L X 90 ml/kg/d = 0.6 mM P/kg/day (19 mg/kg/d)

EN: 610 mg P/L x 50 ml/kg/d = 30.5 mg P/kg/d (1 mM/kg/d)

MAGNESIUM (Mg) INTAKE

PN: One milliequivalent of magnesium equals 12 mg of magnesium. Magnesium sulfate (MgSulf) 50% contains 500 mg magnesium sulfate heptahydrate or 4.1 mEq (49 mg) magnesium per ml.

1 ml MgSulf/L x 4.1 mEq Mg/ml = 4.1mEq Mg/L
4.1 mEq Mg/L x 90 ml/kg/d = 0.4 mEq Mg/kg/d (4.8 mg/kg/d)

EN: 81 mg Mg/L x 50 ml/kg = 4 mg Mg/kg/d (0.34 mEq/kg/d)

Table 4.1.   Calculation of Nutrient Intake for Comparison with Published Recommendations

Nutrient	Calculation of intake for comparison with published recommendations
Fluid	ml/kg/d
Calories (kcal)	Parenteral kcal/kg/d and % of total Enteral kcal/kg/d and % of total Total kcal/kgld Nonprotein kcal/g nitrogen (parenteral)
Protein	g/kg/d g/100 kcal (enteral) Nonprotein kcallg nitrogen (parenteral) % contribution total kcal intake
Carbohydrate	g/kg/d mg/kg/min (parenteral) % contribution to total kcal intake
Fat	g/kg/d g/kg/hr (parenteral glucose infusion rate) % contribution to total kcal intake
Vitamin A	IU/d
Vitamin D	IU/d
Vitamin E	IU/d IU/wk during first 1-2 wk
Vitamin C	mg/d mg/100 kcal
Folic acid	µg/kg/d µg/d
Sodium	mEq/kg/d
Potassium	mEq/kg/d
Calcium	mg/kg/d (enteral) mg calcium gluconate/kg/day (parenteral) mEq calcium/kg/d (parenteral)
Phosphorus	mg/kg/d (enteral) mMlkg/d (parenteral)
Magnesium	mg/kg/d (enteral) mEq/kg/d (parenteral)
Iron	mg/kg/d
Zinc	µg/kg/d
Copper	µg/kg/d

VITAMIN INTAKE

PN: In this example, 67% of the caloric intake is parenteral. Two doses are present in 1 L of solution. The infant receives 135 ml or 13.5% of the liter of solution, or 27% of one dose of the parenteral multivitamin preparation. The recommended intake is 40% of one dose. The parenteral multivitamin intake is:

27% of one dose ÷ recommended 40% of one dose = 68% of PN recommendation

EN: In this example, 33% of the caloric intake is enteral. Vitamin intake from Similac Special Care (Ross Laboratories) meets recommendations for all except vitamins A and D at a caloric intake of 120 kcal/kg/d. The intake in this example is:

33 kcal/kg/d ÷ 120 kcal/kg/d (full dose) = 28% of EN recommendation

TOTAL:
The total intake in this case provides 96% of recommended intake.

'THREE-IN-ONE' SOLUTIONS

If a 3-in-1 solution is used, such as:

12.5% dextrose (3.4 kcal/g x 12.5 g/dl = 42.5 CHO kcal/dl)
2.5% amino acids (4.0 kcal/g x 2.5 g/dl = 10 PRO kcal/dl)
2.0% lipid (11.0 kcal/g x 2.0 g/dl = 22 fat kcal/dl)

100 ml/kg/d will provide: 72.5 kcal/kg/d, 2.5 g PRO/kg/d, 2.0 g fat/kg/d, and 12.5 g hydrated glucose/kg/d (GIR: 8.7 mg hydrated glucose/kg/min) or 10.6 g anhydrous glucose/kg/d (GIR: 7.4 mg anhydrous glucose/kg/min).

References

1. Food and Nutrition Board Subcommittee on the 10th Edition of the RDAs. Recommended dietary allowances. 10th ed. Washington D.C.: National Academy Press, 1989.
2. Tsang RC, Uauy R, Lucas A, et al, eds. Nutritional needs of the preterm infant: Scientific basis and practical guidelines. Baltimore: Williams and Wilkins, 1993.
3. Clark D. Nutritional requirements of the premature and small for gestational age infant. In: Suskind RM, ed. Textbook of pediatric nutrition. 2nd ed. New York: Raven Press, 1993; 23.
4. American Academy of Pediatrics Committee on Nutrition. Nutritional needs of low-birth-weight infants. Pediatrics 75:976, 1985.
5. Kerner JA. Parenteral nutrition. In: Walker WA, et al, eds. Pediatric gastrointestinal disease, vol. 2. Philadelphia: Decker, 1996.
6. Groh-Wargo S. Prematurity and low birth weight. In: Lang CE, ed. Nutritional support in critical care. Rockville, MD: Aspen, 1987; 295.

7. Cox JH. High risk neonates and infants. In: Lang CE, ed. Nutritional support in critical care. Rockville, MD: Aspen, 1987; 12.
8. Wooldridge NH, ed., Spinozzi N, suppl ed. Quality assurance criteria for pediatric nutrition conditions: A model. Chicago: Am Diet Assoc, 1998.
9. Puangco MA, Nguyen HL, and Sheridan MJ. Computerized pn ordering optimizes timely nutrition therapy in a neonatal intensive care unit. J Amer Dietet Assoc 97:258, 1997.

Bibliography

Food and Nutrition Board Committee on Nutritional Status During Pregnancy and Lactation. Nutrition services in perinatal care. Washington, DC: National Academy Press, 1992.

Cowell C, Simko MD, Gilbride JA. The nutrition profile as a tool for identifying who needs nutritional care: Nutrition assessment. Rockville, MD: Aspen Systems, 1998.

Nevin-Folino N. Nutrition assessment of premature infants. Williams CP (ed). Pediatric manual of clinical dietetics. Chicago: American Dietetic Association, 1998; 3-17.

Nutritional Care for High-Risk Newborns (Rev. 3d. Ed.)
S. Groh-Wargo, M. Thompson, J. Cox, editors
© 2000, Precept Press, Inc., Chicago

5

LABORATORY ASSESSMENT

Laurie J. Moyer-Mileur, PhD, RD, CD

LABORATORY DATA ARE USEFUL as one component of nutrition assessment. Laboratory tests can be specific and may help detect nutritional deficiency or toxicity before the appearance of clinical symptoms.

Technical factors such as handling of the specimen, laboratory method, and technician accuracy may affect the validity of laboratory tests. Disease state and/or medical treatment may also affect the results. Transfusions may alter hematologic status and mask hemolytic anemia. Laboratory tests should be interpreted with caution and should be used to complement other nutritional assessment data. The cost and relative usefulness of a complex laboratory test should be taken into consideration before the test is performed.

Low-birth-weight infants cannot afford to lose much blood volume for lab tests. Total blood volume is about 90 ml/kg of body weight. An infant who weighs 1,500 g, for example, would have only 135 ml of total blood volume. The laboratory performing the tests must be capable of using techniques that require only microliters of blood.

Periodic assessment of laboratory data is necessary for the infant receiving parenteral nutrition (PN). Early detection of metabolic complications of PN is facilitated by laboratory data such as arterial blood gases, levels of sodium, potassium, chloride, calcium, magnesium, phosphorus, urea nitrogen, glucose, and triglycerides. Response to treatment may also be assessed by specific laboratory tests (see chapter 8, Table 8.2).

Laboratory assessment of the infant receiving enteral nutrition is not well delineated. In the very low birth weight and/or chronically ill infant, it may be desirable to follow serial parameters of hematologic, protein, mineral, electrolyte, and acid/base status. A proposed

Table 5.1.   Suggested Laboratory Monitoring Schedule
              for Enterally Fed Infants

Metabolic variables	Suggested frequency (days)
Acid/base balance*	7-10
Sodium, potassium, chloride*	7-10
Albumin	7-10
Prealbumin†	10-14
Calcium, phosphorus	10-14
Alkaline phosphatase	10-14
Hematocrit/hemoglobin	10-14

* Very low birth weight and/or chronically ill infants will require monitoring of
  electrolytes and acid/base status.

† If available

laboratory monitoring protocol for enterally fed infants with chronic illness or poor growth is shown in Table 5.1.[1]

The ability to use energy is influenced by the infant's acid/base balance. Acid/base balance, which refers to the control of hydrogen ion concentration, is expressed as pH. A normal pH falls between 7.35 and 7.45. Acidosis (pH < 7.35) indicates an increase in hydrogen ions, and alkalosis (pH > 7.45) reflects a decrease in hydrogen ions. Acid/base imbalances may be respiratory or metabolic in origin. Blood gases are used to determine pH and the type of acidosis or alkalosis. Normal arterial blood gas and pH values are shown in Table 5.2. Interpretation of blood gas results to determine a respiratory or metabolic imbalance is shown in Table 5.3.[2]

Serum concentrations of transport proteins are frequently used as indicators of nutritional status. Although their use as indexes of protein status has been criticized, serum concentration of transport proteins may identify patients at high risk for morbidity and mortality.[3] Albumin, transferrin, prealbumin (transthyretin), and retinol-binding protein (RBP) have been used to assess nutritional status in infants.[3-8] Both albumin and transferrin have a longer half-life than prealbumin or RBP (Table 5.4). Prealbumin and RBP concentrations appear to correlate better with nitrogen balance during nutrition therapy and have been shown to be a more sensitive measure of protein and calorie intake in small premature infants.[3-8] Serum transferrin and RBP levels may be influenced by iron or vitamin A, respectively, altering results.[3]

Liver function tests are helpful as indicators of hepatic complications of PN. Levels of direct bilirubin, serum glutamic oxaloacetic transaminase (SGOT) or aspartate amino transferase (AST), serum glutamic pyruvate transaminase (SGPT) or alanine amino trans-

Table 5.2. Normal Arterial Blood Gas and pH Values[2]

Indicator	Mean	Range
pH	7.4	7.35-7.45
pC02 (mm Hg)	40	35-45
HC03- (mEq/L)	24	22-26
p02 (mm Hg)	90	70-100

Table 5.3. Interpretation of Acid/Base Imbalance[2]

Acid/base disturbance	pH	pCO2	HC03-	Urine pH
Respiratory acidosis	⇩	⇧	Nl or ⇧	⇩
Respiratory alkalosis	⇧	⇩	Nl or ⇩	⇧
Metabolic acidosis	⇩	Nl or ⇩	⇩	⇩
Metabolic alkalosis	⇧	⇧	⇧	⇧

Nl = normal

Table 5.4. Characteristics of Plasma Proteins[3]

Parameter	Molecular weight (kd)	Half-life
Retinol-binding protein	21,000	12 hr
Prealbumin	54,980	2 d
Transferrin	76,000	8 d
Albumin	65,000	20 d

ferase (ALT), and alkaline phosphatase may be elevated, sometimes markedly, in PN-induced liver disease.[9] The direct bilirubin level is recommended as the most sensitive indicator of the onset and resolution of hepatic cholestasis related to PN.[10] Discontinuing PN is generally necessary for the return of liver function tests to normal ranges. Small volumes of enteral feedings have been shown to lessen the cholestatic effects of PN.[11, 12]

Alkaline phosphatase is an enzyme that originates mainly in liver and bone. It may be elevated in normal growth, liver disease, and/or bone disease.[13] Mild elevations in alkaline phosphatase (< 800 U/L) in infants is indicative of normal growth and osteoblast activity.[13] In liver disease, levels of alkaline phosphatase rise due to impaired biliary excretion of the enzyme. In metabolic bone disease, alkaline phosphatase levels rise due to osteocyte production and calcium dep-

Table 5.5. Normal Blood Chemistry Values

Constituent	Normal range Preterm	Term	Source
Sodium (mEq/L)	136-143	136-143	15
Potassium (mEq/L)	4.1-5.6	4.1-5.6	15
Chloride (mEq/L)	97-104	97-104	15
Glucose (mg/dL)			
newborn	20-80	20-80	15
> 1 mo	60-105	60-105	
Blood urea nitrogen (mg/dL)			
≤ 1 wk	3-25	3-12	16
> 1 mo		5-18	
Creatinine (mg/dL)	< 1.3	0.2-1.0	15,17
Prealbumin (g/dL)			
≤ 1 wk	0.7-1.8	0.7-1.7	7
1 mo	0.7-2.2	1.1-2.8	
3 mo	0.9-3.3	1.1-3.4	
Transferrin (g/L)			
newborn	1.2-2.8	1.5-2.9	7
1 mo	0.9-3.1	1.4-2.8	
3 mo	1.4-3.7	2.0-3.7	
Transferrin saturation	> 16%	> 16%	14
Total protein (g/dL)			
≤ 1 wk		4.6-7.4	15
4 mo	4.7-6.2		
1 yr	5.8-7.1	6.1-6.7	
Albumin (g/dL)			
≤ 1 wk	2.4-4.2	2.8-4.3	7
1 mo	2.3-4.1	3.0-4.0	7
3 mo	3.1-4.6	3.4-4.5	7
1 yr	3.2-4.5	4.1-5.0	15
Retinol binding			
Protein (g/dL)			
≤ 1 wk	0.1-0.3	0.1-0.3	7
1 mo	0.1-0.3	0.2-0.6	
3 mo	0.1-0.5	0.2-0.6	
Calcium (mg/dL)			
< 1 wk	6-10	7-12	17
3-7 wk	8-11		
3 mo-1 yr		9-12	
Phosphorus (mg/dL)			
< 1 wk	6.1-11.7	4.9-8.9	17
3-7 wk	5.3-8.3		
1 mo		5.0-9.5	

Table 5.5. Normal Blood Chemistry Values (continued)

Constituent	Normal range Preterm	Term	Source
Magnesium (mEq/L)	1.5-2.3	1.5-2.3	15,17
Alkaline phosphatase (U/L) 1 mo-1 yr	≤ 5 x adult norms	95-368 146-477	18
Serum glutamic oxaloacetic transaminase (SGOT)/asparate amino transferase (AST)		16-74	15
Serum glutamic pyruvate transaminase (SGPT)/alanine amino transferase (ALT)		1-25	15
Bilirubin (mg/dL)			
Total	< 2.0	< 2.0	16
Direct	< 0.2	< 0.2	16
Triglycerides (mg/dL)	≤ 250	10-140	19
Triene: Tetraene Ratio		< 0.4	20
Carnitine (uMol/L)		20-45	15
Hemoglobin (g/dL)			
1 mo	11-17	11-17	15
1 yr	11-15	11-15	
Hematocrit (g/dL)			
1 mo	35-49%	35-49%	15,17
1 yr	30-40%	30-40%	
Iron			
Reticulocytes			
1 mo	0-0.5%	0-0.5%	15
3 mo	0.5-4%	0.5-4%	
1 yr	0.4-1.8%	0.4-1.8%	
Platelets (#/mcL)			
≤ 1 mo	350,000	350,000	15
3 mo	260,000	260,000	
Zinc (µg/dL)	74-146	74-146	14
Ceruloplasmin (mg/dL) 6 mo-1 yr		15-50	16
Copper (µg/dL)			
newborn		1.4-7.2	14
1 yr		12.6-23.6	
Selenium (µg/dL)		5.7-9.4	16
Thyroxine (T_4)(µg/dL)			
newborn	9-18	9-18	16
infant	7-15	7-15	

Table 5.6. Laboratory Tests and Normal Serum Values of
Selected Vitamins

Constituent	Test	Normal serum value	Reference
Vitamin A (μg/dL)	Plasma retinol	20-43	14
Vitamin D (ng/dL)	Serum 1,25 di-hydoxy vitamin D	12-60	14
Vitamin E (mg/dL)	Serum tocopherol	0.5-3.5 preterm 1.0-6.0 term 2.0-6.0 2-5 mo 3.5-8.0 1 yr	14
	Hydrogen peroxide hemolysis	< 10%	14
Vitamin C (mg/dL)	Serum ascorbic acid	> 0.2	14
Folacin (ng/dL)	Serum folate	> 6.0	14
	Red cell folate	≥ 160	14
Vitamin B_{12} (pg/mL)	Serum B_{12}	> 100	14

osition in bones. Two different isoenzymes of alkaline phosphatase are formed by the liver and bone, respectively. When alkaline phosphatase is elevated, isoenzyme tests may be helpful in distinguishing between liver and bone disease. If liver disease is present, discontinuing PN should be considered. If metabolic bone disease (osteopenia of prematurity) is implicated, attention should be given to providing adequate substrate (calcium, phosphorus, vitamin D) for bone formation (see Chapter 29.)

Premature infants are at risk for developing anemias from deficiencies of iron, vitamin B_{12}, folate, vitamin E, and copper.[14] Hemoglobin and hematocrit concentrations are helpful in diagnosing iron deficiency anemia. A hypochromic anemia that is unresponsive to iron therapy may indicate copper deficiency. A deficiency in vitamin B_{12}, and/or folate will result in megaloblastic anemia. Hemolytic anemia occurs in vitamin E deficiency. Laboratory tests used for diagnosis of vitamin deficiency are costly and should be reserved for infants who are at higher risk of developing a deficiency, e.g., malabsorptive diseases and long-term PN. Most hospital laboratories are able to perform a wide variety of blood tests and have developed their own standards, or use published standards for normal values (see Tables 5.5-5.6).

References

1. Moyer-Mileur LJ. Nutrition guidelines for the high-risk infant. Policy/Procedure manual, University Hospital Newborn Intensive Care Center, University of Utah, Salt Lake City, UT, 1997.
2. Shapiro BA, Harrison RA, Cane RD, et al. Clinical applications of blood gases. 4th ed. Chicago: Year Book Medical, 1989.
3. Winkler MF, Gerrior SA, Pomp A, et al. Use of retinol-binding protein and prealbumin as indicators of the response to nutrition therapy. J Am Diet Assoc 89:684, 1989.
4. Giacoia GP, Watson S, West K. Rapid turnover transport proteins, plasma albumin, and growth in low birthweight infants. J Parent Ent Nutr 8:367, 1984.
5. Sasanow SR, Spitzer AR, Pereira GR, et al. Effect of gestational age upon prealbumin and retinol binding protein in preterm and term infants. J Pediatr Gastroenterol Nutr 5:111, 1986.
6. Georgieff MK, Sasanow SR, Pereira GR. Serum transthyretin levels and protein intake as predictors of weight gain velocity in premature infants. J Pediatr Gastroenterol Nutr 6:775, 1987.
7. Kanakoudi F, Drossou V, Tzimouli V, et al. Serum concentrations of 10 acute-phase proteins in healthy term and preterm infants from birth to 6 months. Clin Chem 41:605, 1995.
8. Vahlquist A, Rack L, Peterson PA, et al. The concentrations of retinol-binding protein, prealbumin, and transferrin in the sera of newly delivered mothers and children of various ages. Scand J Clin Lab Invest 35:569, 1975.
9. Pereira GR, Sherman MS, DiGiacomo J, et al. Hyperalimentation-induced cholestasis. Am J Dis Child 135:842, 1981.
10. Beale EF, Nelson RM, Bucciarelli RL, et al. Intrahepatic cholestasis associated with parenteral nutrition in premature infants. Pediatrics 64:342, 1979.
11. Mileur LM, Chan GM, Kimura RE. Effect of early, low volume feedings on very low birthweight (VLBW) infants. Pediatr Res 29:373A, 1991.
12. Dunn L, Hulman S, Weiner J, et al. Beneficial effects of early hypocaloric enteral feeding on neonatal gastrointestinal function: Preliminary report of a randomized trial. J Pediatr 112:622, 1988.
13. Schiele F, Henny J, Hitz J, et al. Total bone and liver alkaline phosphatases in plasma: Biological variations and reference limits. Clin Chem 29:634, 1983.
14. Gross S. Hematologic problems. In: Klaus MH, Fanaroff AA, eds. Care of the High Risk Neonate. 3d ed. Philadelphia: Saunders, 1986; 350-51, 122.
15. Hammond KB. Interpretation of biochemical values. In: Hathaway WE, Groothius JR, Hay WW, et al., eds. Current Pediatric Diagnosis and Treatment. Los Altos, Calif.: Lange Medical Publishers, 1991; 1099-1107.
16. Mabry CC, Tietz NW. Reference ranges for laboratory tests. In: Behrman RE, Kliegman RM, eds. Nelson Textbook of Pediatrics. Philadelphia: Saunders, 1992; 1827-60.
17. Meites S, ed. Pediatric Clinical Chemistry: Reference (Normal) Values. 3d ed. Washington, D.C.: AACC Press, 1989; 190-298.

18. Kovar I, Wayne P, Barltrop D. Plasma alkaline phosphatase activity: A screening test for rickets in preterm neonates. Lancet 1(8267):308, 1982.
19. Adamkin DH, Gelke KN, Andrews BF. Fat emulsions and hypertriglyceridemia. J Parent Ent Nutr 8:563, 1984.
20. Holman RT. The ratio of trienoic:tetraenoic acids in tissue lipids as a measure of fatty acid requirement. J Nutr 70:405, 1960.

Bibliography

Alvarez F, Cresteil D, Lemonnier F, et al. Plasma vitamin E levels in children with cholestasis. J Pediatr Gastroenterol Nutr 3:390, 1984.

Freeman I, Pettifor JM, Woodley GM. Serum phosphorus in protein energy malnutrition. J Pediatr Gastroenterol Nutr 1:547, 1982.

Glass EJ, Hume R, Hendry GMA, et al. Plasma alkaline phosphatase activity in rickets of prematurity. Arch Dis Child 57:373, 1982.

Hillman LS. Serial serum copper concentrations in premature and small for gestational age infants during the first three months of life. J Pediatr 98:305, 1981.

Rassin, DK. Protein requirements in the neonate. In: Lebenthal E, ed. Textbook of Gastroenterology and Nutrition in Infancy, 2d ed. New York: Raven Press, 1989; 281-92.

Shenai JP, Chytil R, Jhaveria A, et al. Plasma vitamin A and retinal-binding protein in premature and term neonates. J Pediatr 99:302, 1981.

Smith AM, Chan GM, Moyer-Mileur LJ, et al. Selenium status of preterm infants fed human milk, preterm formula, or selenium-supplemented preterm formula. J Pediatr 119:429, 1991.

Nutritional Care for High-Risk Newborns (Rev. 3d. Ed.)
S. Groh-Wargo, M. Thompson, J. Cox, editors
© 2000, Precept Press, Inc., Chicago

6

COMPUTER USE IN NEONATAL NUTRITION INFORMATION MANAGEMENT

Melody Thompson, MS, RD, LD
and Janine M. Bamberger, MS, RD, CD, CSP

COMPUTERS ARE UBIQUITOUS in most current neonatal intensive care units (NICUs). They are repositories of patient information, communication tools between the NICU and other departments, word processors, sophisticated calculators, and the source of a wide variety of information. Some NICUs and hospitals have evolved to use only computerized nursing notes and medical records. Computer technology is even being used to automatically adjust ventilator settings for neonates.[1,2] This chapter will focus on the use of computers to manage and share neonatal nutrition information.

Managing Neonatal Nutrition Information

The computer entered the NICU at about the same time as parenteral nutrition (PN). In fact, the first NICU programs were designed to perform PN calculations for busy clinicians. Many people developed their own software programs to calculate PN and even some enteral intakes.[3-10]

In many NICUs, day-to-day nutrition calculations are performed using conventional hand-held calculators. In a study of computerized versus hand calculations among house officers, the error rate with hand calculations was up to 20%.[11] An average of three calculations was made for each infant, and only the most critically ill infants were assessed. The same house staff, using a computer, averaged seven calculations per patient per day with a 5% error rate (related to improper keystrokes and incorrect data entry). In a similar study, surgical house staff doing hand calculations were found to be more likely to make errors in fluid and nutrition calculations for infants weighing < 2 kg (i.e., those at highest nutritional risk) as compared to larger infants.[12] Indeed, house officers early in their training years are more likely to make multiple hand calculation errors, some even 10-fold errors.[13] Gale et al. reported that their computer program reduced calculation time from 30-45 minutes to 4-5 minutes per patient per day, at the same time eliminating the risk in human error.[14] In addition to time savings, Puangco et al. found significant improvements in nutrient composition of the PN solution and earlier achievement of calorie and protein goals when computer ordering was used.[15] Calcium and phosphorus content of PN solutions can also be optimized by using computer technology.[16] Clearly, the use of computers in nutrition calculations saves time, reduces errors, increases calculated data output, and may aid in achievement of nutritional goals.

Current computer software programs can be sophisticated enough to assist in answering some of the questions commonly asked on rounds in the NICU. For example:

- What is the nutrient composition of preterm compared to standard formula?
- Which formula is highest (or lowest) in calcium content?
- How well is this baby growing?
- How much potassium is this baby receiving from PN, formula, and supplements?
- Does caloric intake correlate with weight changes?
- Is weight gain related to decreased urine output?
- How has weight gain been affected by the use of steroids?
- What is the difference in nutrient composition between 27 kcal/oz concentrated formula and 20 kcal/oz formula with added glucose polymers and oil?
- How many of our patients of < 1,000 g birth weight develop osteopenia of prematurity?
- What is the nutrient composition of this 4-oz bottle of soy formula?
- How does nutrient composition change with varying proportions of human milk fortifier added to mother's milk?

Most of these questions can be answered on the spot in a general way. But it is often helpful to follow up with some written, quantitative data (i.e., computer printout). In addition to mathematical calculations, analytical and database management functions including graphical presentations may be desirable. Examples of these functions include the ability to:

- Compare patients' intakes with standard reference(s)
- Organize and store nutrition assessment data
- Allow prospective planning to meet nutrient needs
- Store retrospective actual intake data
- Compare formulas to one another
- Compare reference data sets to one another
- Express nutrient intake in absolute quantities, amount per kilogram, or amount per 100 calories, as desired
- Sort data in various categories
- Display and print data as tables or graphs
- Plot growth curves
- Organize and summarize information for reports
- Prepare educational materials for house staff
- Allow research applications (storing, extracting, and transporting data to other programs)
- Share research data among multiple sites

Selecting a Computer Program

When selecting a computer program, software should always be chosen before hardware.[17] It is, however, important to know what, if any, hardware limitations may exist in your setting prior to committing to the acquisition of computer software. Software selection should be based on the needs and resources of the institution as a whole, as well as the needs of the user(s). Although most hospitals depend on some sort of mainframe computer to manage patient data, more and more institutions are also tapping into the power of individual or networked personal computers (PCs). One's hospital-based information services (IS) department can be an invaluable resource in selecting, installing, and maintaining software and hardware. Readers interested in any of the software described on the following pages are advised to contact the developer/distributor for current information on cost and availability.

Home-Grown Institution-Based Software

Some institutions choose to develop their own software. This requires a detailed vision of what is desired from the software, an ability to communicate this vision clearly to computer programmers, and lots of patience (to work through and revise prototype versions). Such a software program can work very well at a specific institution, but it can be unacceptable at another.

Using software developed for another institution may be a viable alternative if one's needs do not go beyond those of the original developer, including their methods and formulas for calculations.

Factors that limit the usefulness of home-grown software packages to other institutions include:

- A fixed (unalterable) formula data base (with limited enteral and parenteral products)
- Inflexible nutrient units (i.e., mEq, mg, or mM)
- Preset limits or guidelines that may be hard-coded permanently in the program
- Inflexible, tedious data-entry sequences
- Specific hardware requirements (hardware may become difficult or impossible to obtain or maintain over time)

An example of home-grown software which has become more and more sophisticated over time is the Cedars-Sinai Medical Center (CSMC) NICU Computer-Assisted Parenteral Nutrition Program. This program, which has been in use by NICU housestaff, attending physicians, and nurse practitioners since 1978, was designed to produce a timely and accurate parenteral nutrition order based on relevant information. It was also intended to allow the user to analyze the baby's current intake, develop nutritional goals, and aid in the standardization of care. A valuable feature of the program is that it drives the parenteral nutrition components towards nutritional goals over a period of days or weeks. (See Table 6.1.) For further information, visit http://www.neonatology.org/cin/apps/tpn/default.html on the web.

Commercially Distributed Institution-Based Software

Some institution-based software has proven to be flexible enough to be useful to other institutions and is sold commercially. An example of this is the program developed by Children's Medical Center, Oakland, Calif. This package (Nutritional Analysis for your Intensive Care Nursery) stores and retrieves patient nutrition data and calculates intakes (fluids, calories, carbohydrate, protein, fat, sodium, potassium) from I.V. and enteral sources. It also calculates output and weight gain/loss. Growth can be plotted on preterm infant curves. This software was designed for planning the nutritional care of infants in the intensive care nursery, but is flexible enough to be useful for pediatric and adult patients as well.

MacNICU DataBase is another example of a commercially distributed institution-based software program currently in use. (See Table 6.1.) MacNICU tracks patient demographics and features a complete fluid and nutritional analysis. Intake and output entry is incorporated into the nursing function. The program sums parenteral and enteral calories, protein, carbohydrate, and fat.

Commercial Off-the-Shelf Software

The following software available from commercial sources is listed in increasing order of power and sophistication as related to nutritional features.

Nutrition packages available for patient bedside monitors—These computer software packages are usually limited to assessing patient fluid intake and output (I/O) and sometimes calorie intake. The formula database may be quite limited (< 20 product choices) and restricted to a predefined list that may not be applicable to, or flexible enough for, one's needs. Specially designed hand-held calculators sometimes fit into this category. Tools for adult nutrition may be adapted for use in neonatal/infant nutrition analysis on a limited basis.

Nutrition section included as part of package for design of parenteral nutrition solutions—These sections vary in their level of nutritional sophistication. Most include basic nutritional analysis of parenteral fluids, calories, protein, carbohydrate, and fat. Some, such as NeoFax-pc, also offer the option to include enteral products.

Nutrition sections in comprehensive perinatal database systems— These sections may have larger, more flexible formula databases than those in bedside monitors, but still have limited output, often calculating less than six nutrients (volume, calories, protein, carbohydrate, fat). The data entry sequence may be awkward and inflexible; intermediate calculations may be required between data collection and entry. NeoKnowledge from Medical Data Systems (MDS), known as the most widely used neonatal clinical information system in the US, allows users to monitor nutritional support and growth (see Table 6.1). This feature, however, is only part of a very large, comprehensive, and costly program, prohibiting its use by dietitians who do not have access to NeoKnowledge.

Comprehensive neonatal nutrition information management— Ross Products Division of Abbott Laboratories (Columbus) has developed a comprehensive and powerful, yet flexible software program (Neonova Nutrition Optimizer) for neonatal nutrition information management (see Table 6.1). The Neonova program stores and retrieves patient data, includes an expandable formula database (> 100 parenteral and enteral products made by many manufacturers), calculates intake analyses for > 40 nutrients, allows comparison to reference standards, and prints custom reports for clinical, administrative, and research purposes. Graphic and statistical analyses are available. The Neonova program is capable of performing all of the functions mentioned in this chapter and is a practical data management system with many potential applications in the NICU. Neonova's popularity stems from its ease of use (menu-driven [optional], context-sensitive help screens) and institutional customization features that allow many aspects of the program to be individualized to the conventions of the particular

Table 6.1.   Neonatal Nutrition Software: Questions to ponder during selection

Program title:	Cedars-Sinai	MacNICU Database	Children's Hosp Oakland	Neonova Nutr Optimizer	NeoKnowledge	NeoHal NeoNotes 2000
Operating system	M	M	W	W	W	W
Nutrient Intake						
Analyzes past intake	Y	Y	Y	Y	Y	Y
Allows for analysis of future intake	Y	N	?	Y	Y	Y
Generates PN order	Y	N	N	Y	Y	Y
Nutrients included in analysis may be selected by user	Y	N	N	Y	Y	Y
No. nutrients analyzed	12+	3	7	40	5-7	?
No. nutrients analyzed may be expanded by user	N	N	N	Y	N	?
Formula Database						
No. intravenous solutions in database	†	20	?	U	U	U
No. enteral products in database	15	20	?	U	U	21
Formula database may be customized by user	N	Y	?	Y	Y	Y
Laboratory Data						
Allows user input of laboratory data	Y	Y	N	Y	Y	Y
Laboratory data may be compared with normal values	Y	Y	n/a	Y	N	N
Laboratory normal values may be added/modified by user	N	N	n/a	Y	N	N
Growth						
Allows user input of anthropometric data	Y	Y	Y	Y	Y	Y
Anthropometric variables may be added/modified	N	N	N	Y	Y	N
Anthropometric variables may be plotted on standard curves	Y	Y	Y	Y	N	N
Growth curves may be added	N	Y	N	Y	N	Y
Assessment/Documentation Cpabilities						
Intake data may be compared to standard recommendations*	Y	N	N	Y	N	N
Intake recommendations may be added/modified	Y	n/a	n/a	Y	n/a	n/a
Allows user input of diagnoses	N	Y	N	Y	Y	Y
Permits sorting of database variables	N	Y	N	Y	Y	Y
Decision support information included in program	Y	N	N	Y	Y	Y
Narrative notes allowed	N	Y	?	Y	Y	Y
Includes nutrition care plan tool	N	N	?	Y	Y	Y

KEY

W = Windows   M = Macintosh   Y = Yes   N = No   U = Unlimited
† = All custom solutions   * = Within program   n/a = Not available

Complete program title and contact:
1. Cedars-Sinai NICU Computer-Assisted Parenteral Nutrition Program: Ray Duncan, MD *See text for contact info*
2. MacNICU DataBase: Robert Stavis, MD, 610/526-4618
3. Nutritional Analysis for your Intensive Care: Linda Lefrak, RD, 510/428-3000
4. Neonova Nutrition Optimizer: Ross, *Contact local Ross representative*
5. NeoKnowledge: Medical Data Systems, 610/975-9300
6. NEOHAL/NeoNotes 2000: Andrew B. Kairalla, MD, 305/663-8469

nursery. Ross has provided hands-on workshops to demonstrate its use, a comprehensive user's manual, and telephone support. Neonova has been made available by Ross to selected hospitals.

Data Entry Considerations

The amount of data to be collected and entered into the computer each day, along with the location of the computer, will be the main determinants of a successful data entry strategy. Data collection and entry can be time-consuming and tedious. If only limited data on a limited number of patients are needed daily, then the clinician alone may efficiently collect and enter the data. If more data for additional patients are collected daily, then the assistance of a technician may be helpful. If the computer is not located near the data, data collection forms designed to flow along data entry sequences may be developed to assist in thorough data capture. The use of a computer that can be easily transported to patients' bedsides eliminates the data collection step by allowing direct data entry into the program. The time invested in data collection/entry can be a trade-off. More comprehensive nutrition assessments can be completed over time with more thorough data collection and entry. Fewer available data may result in "snapshot" one-day assessments.

Caveats for Computer Use in Neonatal Nutrition

1. *Beware of computer worshipers.* Some people are overly impressed by data that comes from a computer. In fact, they can be so impressed that they blindly accept information that reasoning would tell them is wrong. Always critically analyze computer output. If errors are found in output, almost always an error has been made in input (wrong I.V. solution, wrong volume, decimal point error). Occasionally, however, the database in the program is in error, or the program may be processing the information incorrectly (contains a "bug"). If a bug is found in any program (i.e., data input or operator error has been ruled out as the source of the problem), the programmer should be notified immediately so that a correction can be made.

2. *Know neonatal nutrition principles and practice.* There is no substitute for education and experience in neonatal nutrition. A case example may serve to illustrate this point. Baby girl Brown weighed 1,000 g and was receiving 100 kcal/kg/day of 20 kcal/oz premature infant formula. The nurse told the intern that the baby's serum albumin level was low. The intern went to the computer for consultation, came back and ordered a 20 kcal/oz soy formula with an added protein module. The intern then told the neonatal nutritionist, "The

baby's albumin was low so I looked for a higher protein formula on the computer. This soy formula contains more protein per unit volume than her preterm formula did and I also selected a concentrated protein module to be added." The neonatal nutritionist explained that the baby needed: (1) a balance of protein/fat/carbohydrate; (2) adequate calorie as well as protein intake to avoid using protein as an energy source; and (3) a preterm formula, since use of soy formula is associated with osteopenia of prematurity in babies this small. The computer output was correct, but the intern's knowledge base was inadequate and thus the care plan was flawed.

3. *Initially, maintain the "old system" in parallel with the computerized system.* Until users are sure that the new computer system will reliably replace the old system, the old method of doing calculations and keeping records should be retained. Experts recommend running both systems in parallel for at least three months.[17,18] This will allow time for users to learn the new system and work out the kinks in its implementation without risking loss of any valuable data.

4. *Enjoy using the computer.* Computer use should be a joy. If it's a chore, reevaluate what you're doing. The computer serves the user, not the reverse. Perhaps other data collection and entry options need to be explored. Is replacing handwritten records completely with computerized records the objective? Maybe it's "too much, too soon," or maybe a compromise between part handwritten, part computer records will work out best in some settings. Maybe the software and/or hardware are outdated and need to be replaced. Pinpointing and resolving the problem can make computer use enjoyable again.

Sharing Neonatal Nutrition Information

In this era of the Internet, more and more clinicians are connecting with information and with each other instantly through cyberspace. The Internet and the World Wide Web (WWW or the Web) have introduced a wealth of new abbreviations and jargon into popular culture (see Figure 6.1).[19] And the Internet is changing our concepts of education, publication, and communication as no medium has before. A brief overview of the impact of the Internet and the Web will be presented here. The reader is referred to a series of papers on the Web, communication trends, and children's health for more in-depth reading.[20-24]

Medical schools are using the Web to deliver computer-assisted instruction.[25-27] Multimedia instructional materials can be uploaded to Web sites in much less time than it takes to publish traditional classroom materials. Digitized Web images do not degrade or fade over time like slides, photographs or actual tissue specimens do. And students can access Web-based instruction from home 24 hours a day. This may be especially beneficial if family obligations, campus safe-

Figure 6.1. Internet jargon.

(adapted from Net Jargon. *Lancet* 351:S18, 1998)

Bookmark	A saved link to a Web page that allows the user to return to it later
Browser	A program that accesses the Web and reads hypertext (see *client*)
Bulletin board	The Internet equivalent of a notice board, where messages can be posted and read by anyone
Client	A computer (or, more specifically, a software application—e.g. a *browser*) that uses the resources provided by another computer (the *server*)
Domain	The naming hierarchy of the Internet is based on domains (e.g., a university department), within which each computer has a unique name
E-mail	Electronic mail; a means of exchanging messages that may include enclosed files and graphics, depending on the sophistication of the system
Firewall	Software and hardware that limits access to a Web site and provides a degree of security
Home page	The starting page for access to the Web, or, alternatively, a personal page of information
HTML	HyperText Markup Language; the coding syntax used to write Web pages, which are read by *browsers*
HTTP	HyperText Transfer Protocol; the *WWW* protocol that performs the request and retrieve functions of a *server*.
Hypertext	The basic concept behind the Web, whereby one resource can be linked to any other information elsewhere on the Web.
Icon	A graphical image used on a Web page; often with a hyperlink to another page
Internet	The Worldwide distributed network of computers connected using *TCP/IP* or similar protocols
Internet service provider (ISP)	A commercial company that sells Internet connection facilities
LAN	Local Area Network
Listserv	A program that sends mailing lists to subscribers by *e-mail*
Modem	Modulator/Demodulator; hardware that translates digital computer signals into sounds that can be transmitted over a telephone line
Netiquette	Internet etiquette; unwritten rules of conduct governing communications over the Internet
Server	A computer, or a program on the computer, acting as an Internet site whose data are available to the *client*
Site	A collective term covering all the Internet facilities offered by one organization
TCP/IP	Transmission Control Protocol/Internet Protocol; the communications program common to most connected Internet computers
URL	Uniform Resource Locator; an address that specifies the location of a file on the Internet (e.g., http://thelancet.com), usually used for the Web
Web site	A collection of Web documents on a *server*
WWW	World Wide Web (or just 'the Web'); a hypertext-based Internet service providing information and resources

Table 6.2.   Nutrition Web Sites Useful in Neonatal Care, Education, and Research

Title of site	World Wide Web address
American Dietetic Association	http://www.eatright.org/
American Journal of Clinical Nutrition Home Page	http://www.faseb.org/ajcn/
CDC Search	http://www.cdc.gov/search.htm
Computers in the NICU	http://www.neonatology.org/cin/survey/cin.html
Computers in the NICU—Computer Assisted PN	http://www.neonatology.org/cin/apps/tpn/default.html
CSMC: Neonatology Teaching Files	http://www.csmc.edu/neonatology/syllabus.html
Food and Drug Administration	http://www.fda.gov/
Healthcare Financing Administration	http://www.hcfa.gov/
Health Statistics Bibliography	http://www.lib.umich.edu/libhome/PubHealth.lib/bib.statistics.html#Anchor96189
MedConnect: Infomation Services for the Medical Community	http://www.medconnect.com/
Medical Data Systems (NeoKnowledge)	http://www.mdsinfo.com
National Institutes of Health	http://www.nih.gov/
Neofax-pc, Inc. On-line Demo	http://www.neofax.com/demomenu.htm
Neonatal Journal Abstracts	http://www.acenet.com.au/~callande/journals.html
Neonatology on the Web: Parenteral Nutrition for Neonates	http://www.neonatology.org/syllabus/parenteral.nutrition.html
NeoNotes Home Page (NeoHal)	http://www.neonotes.com/
Pediatrics electronic pages	http://www.pediatrics.org/
Pedlinks—Links to pediatric journals	http://www.angelfire.com/in/pedscapes/index.html
SI Units: a refresher tool	http://physics.nist.gov/Documents/sp811.pdf
The National Center for Health Statistics Home Page	http://cdc.gov/nchswww/
Tufts University Nutrition Navigator	http://www.navigator.tufts.edu/
United States Department of Agriculture	http://www.usda.gov/
World Health Organization	http://www.who.ch/Welcome.htm

ty, or campus computer resources pose limitations. Web-based teaching may even improve students' scores on standardized exams.[27]

Electronic publishing may change the future of pediatric literature review. The well-established, respected journal *Pediatrics* has begun publishing peer-reviewed research papers electronically, including only the abstracts in its printed edition. Traditional publishing is expensive, slow, and inefficient compared to electronic publishing.[28,29] However, since anyone can "publish" electronically, there is concern about the quality of studies posted without rigorous peer review.

Physicians are starting to use e-mail as a method to communicate with patients, especially about routine, nonemergent topics. However, experts recommend that patient confidentiality and medicolegal issues should be addressed before physician-to-patient e-mail communication is implemented.[30,31]

Increasingly, the lay public is using the Internet for information on medical topics.[32] Since the Internet is owned and monitored by no one, there is a wide range in the quality of information posted in terms of accuracy, currency, and aesthetics. A recent survey of Internet recommendations for treatment of childhood diarrhea showed that only 20% conformed to current American Academy of Pediatrics (AAP) recommendations.[33] Even recommendations from major academic medical centers did not necessarily comply with AAP guidelines. The authors call for more careful monitoring and quality control by major medical institutions of their Internet site content. They also suggest warning patients about the voluminous misinformation available on medical topics on the Internet.[33,34]

Although the Internet is unregulated, the World Health Organization convened an ad hoc working group to develop recommendations to help curb the escalating use of the Internet by perpetrators of health fraud and marketers of illegal drugs.[35] The U.S. Food and Drug Administration (FDA) has also called for discussions on regulation of clinical software programs as medical devices, specifically those posing highest clinical risk.[36]

Web sites come and go, but some are consistently good sources of information. Web sites that may be of interest to the neonatal nutritionist and colleagues are listed in Table 6.2. These sites were active at the time that this chapter was written. Given the dynamic nature of the Internet, some sites may no longer exist or may have been renamed by the time that the reader attempts to access them.

Neonatal nutritionists may also be interested in subscribing to some list servers (listservs).[37] A listserv is generally an unmoderated exchange of ideas—analagous to sitting down for an informal discussion with colleagues around the world. Messages sent to a listserv's e-mail address are automatically forwarded to all members of the mailing list. Any member can choose to initiate or respond to messages publicly to the listserv or privately to another member's e-mail address. Active listservs can overwhelm members with e-mail. Most offer the option of receiving a "digest," or one e-mail posting daily containing all of the day's postings in chronological order. Although listservs also carry legal implications, many professionals benefit from membership.[38] Two listservs that have had some neonatal nutrition content include:

Pedi-RD

The listserv Pedi-RD is an electronic forum for discussion of neonatal/perinatal and pediatric nutrition issues. Free membership is by subscription only for dietitians and other health care providers. The purpose of Pedi-RD is to allow members to share ideas and strategies for management of nutritional problems or concerns of infants and children. Topics of discussion may include:

- General concerns in pediatric and neonatal nutrition
- Dilemmas in nutritional assessment, management, ethics
- Enteral and parenteral nutrition support
- Current nutrition research/publications
- Informal surveys of nutrition practices.

To subscribe: Send an e-mail message to Pedi-RD-request@list.uiowa.edu
On the first line, type: subscribe
On the second line, type: end

NICU-Net

The listserv NICU-Net is an electronic forum for open discussion of neonatal intensive care issues.[39] Free membership is by subscription only and is open to health care providers (primarily MDs, but also including RNs, RDs, RPhs, RRTs, OTs, PTs, and others). The stated purpose of NICU-Net is discussion of such neonatal issues as:

- Dilemmas in diagnosis, management and ethics
- Recently published clinical trials or recommendations
- Proposed or ongoing multicenter trials
- Effects of health care reform on neonatology
- Role of computers in neonatal practice
- Informal surveys of clinical practice.

To subscribe: Send an e-mail message to listproc@u.washington.edu with a one-line message: Subscribe NICU-Net [your name here]

In summary, whether used for communication, education, publication, information, or calculations, computers are here to stay in the NICU. With the advent of the Internet and the Web, we are on the brink of a dramatic change in worldwide interactions that will change the face of relationships everywhere.

References

1. Sun Y, Kohane IS, Stark AR. Computer-assisted adjustment of inspired oxygen concentration improves control of oxygen saturation in newborn infants requiring mechanical ventilation. J Pediatr 131:754, 1997.
2. Claure N, Gerhardt T, Hummler H, et al. Computer-controlled minute ventilation in preterm infants undergoing mechanical ventilation. J Pediatr 131:910, 1997.
3. Picart D, Guillois B, Nevo L, et al. A program for parenteral and combined parenteral and enteral nutrition of neonates and children in an intensive care unit. Intensive Care Med 15:279, 1989.
4. Yamamoto LG, Gainsley GJ, Witek JE. Pediatric parenteral nutrition management using a comprehensive user-friendly computer program designed for personal computers. J Parent Ent Nutr 10:535, 1986.
5. Harper RG, Carrera E, Weiss S, et al. A complete computerized program for nutritional management in the neonatal intensive care nursery. Am J Perinatol 2:161, 1985.
6. Ball PA, Candy DC, Puntis JW, et al. Portable bedside microcomputer system for management of parenteral nutrition in all age groups. Arch Dis Child 60:435, 1985.

7. MacMahon P. Prescribing and formulating neonatal intravenous feeding solutions by microcomputer. Arch Dis Child 59:548, 1984.

8. Wilson FE, Yu VY, Hawgood S, et al. Computerised nutritional data management in neonatal intensive care. Arch Dis Child 58:732, 1983.

9. Thorp JW, Robbins S. Diet analysis for intensive care nursery patients with a programmable calculator. J Pediatr Gastroenterol Nutr 2:268, 1983.

10. Ochoa-Sangrador C, Brezmes-Valdivieso MF, Gil-Valino C. Pediatric parenteral nutrition mixtures design program: Validity and stability study. Comput Biomed Res 28:271, 1995.

11. Hermansen MC, Kahler R, Kahler B. Data entry errors in computerized nutritional calculations. J Pediatr 109:91, 1986.

12. Tepas JJ, Mollitt DL, String DL, et al. Error in fluid and calorie calculation in the surgical neonate. J Pediatr Surg 26:132, 1991.

13. Rowe C, Koren T, Koren G. Errors by paediatric residents in calculating drug doses. Arch Dis Child 79:56, 1998.

14. Gale R, Gale J, Granski D, et al. An interactive microcomputer program for calculation of combined parenteral and enteral nutrition for neonates. J Pediatr Gastroenterol Nutr 2:653, 1983.

15. Puangco MA, Nguyen HL, Sheridan MJ. Computerized PN ordering optimizes timely nutrition therapy in a neonatal intensive care unit. J Am Diet Assoc 97:258, 1997.

16. Porcelli PJ, Block SM. Increased parenteral nutrition calcium and phosphorus for very-low-birthweight-infants using computer software assisted ordering. J Am Coll Nutr 16:283, 1997.

17. Bear J. Computer wimp. Berkeley, Calif.: Ten Speed Press, 1983; 35, 116.

18. Calmus L. The business guide to small computers. New York: McGraw-Hill, 1983; 167.

19. Net jargon. Lancet 351 (suppl 1):8, 1998.

20. Izenberg N, Lieberman DA. The web, communication trends, and children's health. Part 1: Development and technology of the internet and web. Clin Pediatr 37:153, 1998.

21. Izenberg N, Lieberman DA. The web, communication trends, and children's health. Part 2: The web and the practice of pediatrics. Clin Pediatr 37:215, 1998.

22. Izenberg N, Lieberman DA. The web, communication trends, and children's health. Part 3: The web and health consumers. Clin Pediatr 37:275, 1998.

23. Izenberg N, Lieberman DA. The web, communication trends, and children's health. Part 4: How children use the web. Clin Pediatr 37:335, 1998.

24. Izenberg N, Lieberman DA. The web, communication trends, and children's health. Part 5: Encouraging positive and safe internet use. Clin Pediatr 37:397, 1998.

25. Dev P. To reach and teach with the internet. JAMA 278:1789, 1997.

26. Lehmann HP, Lehmann CU, Freedman JA. The use of simulations in computer-aided learning over the world wide web. JAMA 278:1788, 1997.

27. Klatt EC. Web-based teaching in pathology. JAMA 278:1787, 1997.

28. Anderson K, Lucey JF. Pediatrics electronic pages: Looking back and looking ahead. Pediatrics 102:124, 1998.

29. Delamothe T. The electronic future of scientific articles. Lancet 351 (suppl 1):5, 1998.

30. Kane B, Sands DZ, for the AMIA Internet Working Group, TaskForce on Guidelines for the use of Clinic-Patient Electronic Mail. White paper: Guidelines for the clinical use of electronic mail with patients. J Am Med Inform Assoc 5:104, 1998.

31. Committee on Maintaining Privacy and Security in Health Care Applications of the National Information Infrastructure. For the record: Protecting electronic health information. Computer Science and Telecommunications Board Commission on Physical Sciences, Mathematics, and Applications. National Research Council. Washington, DC: National Academy Press, 1997.

32. Bader SA, Baude RM. Patient informatics: Creating new partnerships in medical decision making. Acad Med 73:408, 1998.

33. McClung HJ, Murray RD, Heitlinger LA. The internet as a souce for current patient information. Pediatrics 101:E2, 1998.

34. Vozenilek G. The wheat from the chaff: Sorting out nutrition information on the Internet. J Am Diet Assoc 98:1270, 1998.

35. Skolnick AA. WHO considers regulating ads, sale of medical products on internet. JAMA 278:1723, 1997.

36. Miller FA, Gardner RM. Recommendations for responsible monitoring and regulation of clinical software systems. J Am Med Inform Assoc 4:442, 1997.

37. Cappellano KL. More food and nutrition internet resources. Mailing lists and electronic newsletters. Nutr Today 33:94, 1998.

38. Elliot SJ, Elliot RG. Internet list servers and pediatrics: Newly emerging legal and clinical practice issues. Pediatrics 97:399, 1996.

39. Tarczy-Hornoch P. NICU-Net: An electronic forum for neonatology. Pediatrics 97:398, 1996.

Nutritional Care for High-Risk Newborns (Rev. 3d. Ed.)
S. Groh-Wargo, M. Thompson, J. Cox, editors
© 2000, Precept Press, Inc., Chicago

7

COLLABORATIVE CARE

Elaine Poole Napp MS, RD, LD, and
Mary Jo Fink MEd, RD, LD

The delivery of health care is entering a new era. Ethical standards continue to demand that disease and disability be eliminated or minimized. Cost containment and quality of life issues demand that the processes by which these goals are attained be reevaluated and streamlined to eliminate those that are ineffective or superfluous within systems.[1] Health care often requires the expertise of providers from various disciplines. Communication and collaboration are needed to coordinate and focus resources on achieving identified outcomes efficiently. Collaborative care is a term that is used to identify a system of health care delivery that accomplishes this goal.[2] A collaborative care system uses a case manager or coordinator to integrate the plans of care from various providers into one plan. Patient problems, expected intermediate and final outcomes, and the interventions needed to achieve those outcomes are identified and documented.[1]

Unquestionably, a healthy, well-nourished, and toxin-free uterus is the best environment for the developing fetus until approximately 40 weeks' gestation. Even under the normal circumstances the newborn infant is vulnerable and quite dependent on others for survival. When birth occurs prematurely or is associated with other health problems, complex therapeutic and supportive care measures must be taken to sustain life, resolve disease, and promote normal growth and development.[3] The neonatal intensive care unit (NICU) is equipped and staffed to provide this complex care, but it is also one of the most costly and highest resource-consuming areas of the hospital. Length of hospitalization may be two to three months or longer, depending upon gestational age at birth and diagnoses. Control of health care costs in the NICU is imperative.[2] Screening, standards of care, clinical pathways and outcomes studies are all tools that can be used as part of a more cost-effective collaborative care system. The purpose of this chapter is to describe these tools as they relate to nutrition and the high-risk newborn.

Nutrition Screening

Nutrition screening is the process of identifying patients who present with characteristics known to be associated with poor nutritional status or high risk of developing nutrition-related problems. The Joint Commission on Accreditation of Health Care Organizations (JCAHO) guidelines require that all patients be screened to determine their nutritional risk status within 24 hours of hospital admission.[4] JCAHO guidelines do not specify that a registered dietitian do the initial screening, but the screening policy should be developed or approved by a registered dietitian. Each health care organization may determine who does the initial screening, the specific components of the screening (reflecting the needs of the population served), and criteria for nutrition assessment and follow-up. Screening patients for nutritional risk is a low-cost means of identifying patients who may benefit from a modified course of nutritional treatment to maximize outcome.[5] Since many NICU patients have lengthy stays, rescreening at regular intervals may also be needed to identify changes in nutritional risk status. Screening guidelines or policies and procedures need to be validated to confirm that the criteria established do in fact identify patients who are at nutritional risk.

The initial screening tool may take many forms. Nutritional care is an interdisciplinary process, integrating with other aspects of the patient's care, and screening policies often reflect this. An example of a screening tool is given in Figure 7.1. In this example, the nursing staff completes the database, including the nutrition screen, when the patient is admitted to the NICU. Nutrition-related information about mother's intent to breast-feed, anthropometric and diagnostic data initially identified may engage specific components of medical, nursing, and nutritional care. For example, if an infant is of < 32 weeks' gestation and weighs < 1.5 kg at birth, the feeding protocol indicated for this infant may be different from that for an infant of > 32 weeks' gestation who weighs > 1.5 kg at birth, based on differences in nutrient stores and organ maturity. Another example is an infant who is large for gestational age. This infant may require immediate assessment of serum glucose levels and intravenous administration of glucose by medical or nursing staff. Subsequently, this infant may require an evaluation of weight-for-length status to

Table 7.1.   Examples of NICU Admission
              Nutrition Screening Criteria*

Criteria based on anthropometric measures†

Birth weight ≤ 1,000 g
Birth weight ≤ 1,500 g
Small for gestational age (SGA)
Large for gestational age (LGA)
Disproportional growth (weight for length < 10th percentile or > 90th percentile)

Criteria based on diagnosis (or suspected diagnosis)

Congenital heart disease
Cystic fibrosis
Extreme prematurity (< 28 wk gestation)
Gastrointestinal tract anomaly
Metabolic disorder
Syndrome or condition that affects growth or oral motor development
      (such as Down, Prader-Willi, spina bifida, severe asphyxia, etc.)

* Examples are given. Criteria used by a specific NICU varies based on population served.
† See growth charts in Appendix D.

determine appropriate goals for intake that may vary from standard guidelines.

Nutrition screens used at various hospitals may be quite diverse, but they often include criteria such as those listed in Table 7.1. Initial screening criteria may be used to indicate a specific course of nutrition intervention and/or referral to a registered dietitian if one is available. Rescreening may occur at regular intervals throughout the hospitalization using various growth charts, laboratory assessments, or indications such as a change in clinical condition or diagnosis.[6,7] Table 7.2 lists frequently used criteria. Figure 7.2 is a sample screening policy, and Appendix D provides growth graphs used.

Nutrition Assessment

Nutrition assessment is defined as a comprehensive process for defining nutritional status by integrating information from different sources: the individual's medical, nutritional and medication histories; physical examination, anthropometric measurements; laboratory data; and parent interview to identify the nutritional needs of the patient and ability/resources of the parents to eventually meet these

Figure 7.1. Sample Screeing Tool—Newborn intensive care patient database

(used with permission of Promedia)

Children's
MEDICAL CENTER OF NORTHWEST OHIO
NEWBORN INTENSIVE CARE
PATIENT DATA BASE

Addressograph Stamp

DEMOGRAPHICS
Patient Name _____ Identification Band # _____
Phone Number _____ Other Phone Number _____
Whate is your main language ? English   Spanish Other _____
Family Members and Address:
Mother's Name _____ Education _____
Address _____
Distance from NICU _____ County _____
Father/Significant Others Name _____ Age _____
Address _____ Education _____
Married / Single / Divorced_____ General Health _____
Other Children Names and ages: _____
_____
Other Significant History: _____
_____

MATERNAL HISTORY
Age _____ OB Physician _____
EDC _____ Gravida _____ Para _____ ABS _____
Living _____ ROM _____ Blood Type _____
Type of Delivery _____
Significant History / Complications: _____
_____
_____
_____

NEWBORN HISTORY
Date of Birth _____ Time _____
Weight _____lbs. _____gms.
Apgars _____ Gestation _____
Head _____ Chest _____ Length _____
Resucitation Type _____
_____
Pediatrician _____
Baptism _____ Footprints _____

FEEDING ARRANGEMENTS   Breast _____ Bottle _____
Breast feeding experience ☐ Yes ☐ No Concerns_____
General feeding concerns _____
Dietitian Consult: ☐ Yes ☐ No   If Yes date:_____ *Criteria 24° of admission: SGA, GI/Cardiac anomaly, renal dysfunction, metabolic disorder (suspected) birthweight ≤ 1500 gms, breast fed infant, CF, feeding problems, poor weight gain since discharge.*

FAMILY ASSESSMENT
Direct Donor   ☐ Yes ☐ No
Religious / Cultural Practices   ☐ Yes ☐ No If yes: _____
Who else will be visiting _____
Special arrangements / visitors _____
Any barriers _____
Previous babu care experience?   ☐ Yes ☐ No   NICU experience   ☐ Yes ☐ No
Families readiness to participate in baby care   ☐ Yes ☐ No   Financial concerns ☐ Yes ☐ No
Home environment preparation for baby _____
Concerns of major crises / stressors: ☐ Yes ☐ No If yes _____
Insurance _____
Employment: Mother _____ Father / S.O. _____
Return to Work ☐ Yes ☐ No   Social Service Referral: Needed _____ Done _____

CMC-460 7/97   Approved Medical Executive Committee 7/97   PAGE 1 OF

Figure 7.1. Sample Screeing Tool—Newborn intensive
care patient database (continued)

INTERDISCIPLINARY PLAN OF CARE / INTERVENTIONS

Addressograph Stamp

Baby / Family Need   Date   Consult Discipline / Name

_____
_____
_____
_____
_____
_____
_____
_____

DIAGNOSIS: Resolved ☐ Yes ☐ No

_____
_____
_____
_____
_____

NIDCAP _____
ATTENDING: _____
MD / NNP_____
SPECIAL TESTING / PROCEDURES: (list, date and outcome)
1. _____   2. _____
3. _____   4. _____
5. _____   6. _____
METABOLIC SCREENINGS:
#1 _____ Date _____   #2 _____ Date _____
IMMUNIZATIONS:
Hepatitis B _____   Date _____   Other _____
Immunizations consent signed ☐ Yes ☐ No
DISCHARGE
Discharge Date _____ Weight _____ Length _____ Head _____
Pneumogram: ☐ Yes ☐ No   HOME O2 IF NEEDED--TOUR PEDS ☐ Yes ☐ No
Eye Screening ☐ Yes ☐ No Date _____ Follow-up checks if needed
Hearing Screening ☐ Yes ☐ No Date _____
Nutrition Teaching ☐ Yes ☐ No   WIC papers given ☐ Yes ☐ No
Special Care Clinic _____ Date _____
CAR SEAT / CAR SEAT SCREENING FOR PREMIES ☐ Yes ☐ No Date _____
Circumcision ☐ Yes ☐ No   Consent signed ☐ Yes ☐ No
MEDICATION TEACHING

_____
DATE _____
24 Hour Care _____ Date _____
CPR classes ☐ Yes ☐ No Date _____
Other Special Needs / Infant Monitoring Program / Home Health Care _____

Pictures / Video   ☐ Yes ☐ No   Consent signed ☐ Yes ☐ No   Footprints ☐ Yes ☐ No

Figure 7.2.   Policy and Procedures for Nutrition Screening of Neonates Admitted to NICU

PURPOSE: To describe the nutrition screening procedure for patients in the NICU to identify patients that may benefit from a comprehensive nutrition assessment.

PROCEDURE: Significant nutrition risk in neonates may be identified as outlined below. Neonates at significant nutrition risk are evaluated by the dietitian within 48 hours of referral.

A.   The initial nutrition screen is found on the "Newborn Intensive Care Patient Data Base".
   1.   Gestational age is assessed and recorded. Weight, length, and head circumference are measured and plotted on the Lubchenco Intrauterine Growth Chart and the Oregon Growth Record for infants within 24 hours of admission. Infants ≤ 1000 grams birthweight are referred to the registered dietitian.
   2.   Small for gestational age (SGA) infants whose weight, length or head circumference fall below the 10th percentile on the Lubchenco Intrauterine Growth Chart or below - 2 standard deviations (S.D.) below the mean on the Oregon Growth Record for Infants are referred to the registered dietitian.
   3.   Diagnoses related to high nutritional risk are identified and the patient is referred to the registered dietitian: cardiac, gastrointestinal tract or renal anomaly; inborn error of metabolism (suspected or known); cystic fibrosis (suspected or known); readmission (< 28 days) with poor weight gain (< 20 gm/d) or poor feeding; neurological dysfunction affecting growth or feeding
B.   Rescreening during hospitalization occurs as follows:
   1.   Weight is measured, recorded and plotted on the Shaffer-Hall-Wright Postnatal Growth Chart daily until term, then weekly thereafter. This growth chart allows identification of patients who are at nutritional risk due to:
     a.   initial weight loss > 15% of birth weight
     b.   birth weight not regained by day 15
     c.   subsequent weight gain < 10 grams/kg/d for > 5 days (< 38 weeks' gestation)
     d.   subsequent weight gain < 20 grams/day for ≥ 7 days (> 38 weeks' gestation)
   2.   Weight, length and head circumference are measured, recorded and plotted on the Oregon Growth Record for Infants weekly until term and monthly thereafter. This chart demonstrates nutritional risk when length or head circumference falls below - 2 S.D. from the mean.
   3.   The first Outcome on the weekly Patient Care Progress Record is "Consistent weekly growth per Shaffer-Hall-Wright Postnatal Growth Chart and Oregon Growth Record for Infants."
     a.   On day 7, if growth is within the normal limits on the Shaffer-Hall-Wright and Oregon charts, the goal is recorded as "achieved".
     b.   On day 7, if growth is below the normal limits on the Shaffer-Hall-Wright and Oregon charts; the goal is recorded as "not achieved"; a note including a referral to the dietitian is documented in the Progress Notes.
   4.   Intake data is recorded daily for all patients. Clinical pathways indicate the need for dietitian consultation when nutrition risk is present as follows:
     a.   Parenteral nutrition is required beyond 3 weeks without significant enteral or oral feedings.
     b.   Tube feeding is required beyond 38 weeks' gestation.
     c.   Infant demonstrates intolerance to premature infant formula or human milk fortifier.
     d.   Infant requires feeding additives or supplements other than standard multivitamin or iron.
   5.   Clinical pathways indicate laboratory assessment when needed. Indices of nutritional risk include:
     a.   Prealbumin < 7 mg/dL or albumin < 2.5 gm/dL
     b.   Direct bilirubin > 2 mg/dL
     c.   Triglyceride > 250 mg/dL
     d.   Serum phosphorus < 4 mg/dL or alkaline phosphatase > 600 U/L
   6.   Patients with diagnoses associated with nutritional risk including but not limited to: bron chopulmonary dysplasia, cholestasis, cystic fibrosis, inborn error of metabolism, osteopenia, and short bowel syndrome are referred to the registered dietitian at Multidisciplinary Patient Care Rounds.

Approved: _____   Date _____
Reviewed: _____   Date _____

Figure 7.3.   Policy for nutrition assessment of neonatal intensive care unit (NICU) patients by a registered dietitian

PURPOSE: To provide nutrition assessment of NICU patients who have been identified through nutrition screening to be at significant nutritional risk, that is, have nutritional needs that are not met by standard nutritional care.

PROCEDURE: Nutrition assessment of NICU patients is completed within 48 hours of referral as outlined below and documented using SOAP format. A plan of care is established in concert with the interdisciplinary team. Patients' progress is periodically evaluated and documented as outlined below.

A.   Subjective information may include the following:
   1.   Parents' intent to breastfeed
   2.   Parents' intent to participate in food supplemental WIC program
   3.   Patients' tolerance to feeding

B.   Objective information may include the following:
   1.   Growth parameters: weight, length, head circumference and comparison to Shaffer-Hall-Wright Postnatal Growth Chart, Oregon Growth Record for Infants or National Center for Health Statistics Growth Chart
   2.   Rate of weight gain, linear growth or head growth and comparison to norms
   3.   Recorded intake of parenteral, enteral, and oral nutrition
   4.   Recorded output of urine and/or feces; urinary electrolyte and/or ketone excretion; fecal excretion of reducing substances, fat, sugars, and/or fecal pH.
   5.   Serum laboratory values of electrolytes, albumin, prealbumin, minerals, vitamins, triglycerides, cholesterol, or others as available or indicated by clinical condition.
   6.   Medications that may affect nutrition status are noted.

C.   Assessment may include the following:
   1.   Growth as a measure of "nutrition outcome"
   2.   Actual and prescribed intake compared to current recommendations (Diet Manual) and individual needs
   3.   Parents' understanding and/or ability to meet patient's nutritional needs after discharge

D.   Plan of nutritional care may include the following:
   1.   Continue present nutritional care
   2.   Recommendations to change nutritional care should include the following:
      a. what the changes will accomplish
      b. short term goals and long term goals if applicable
      c. specific information needed to facilitate change in plan (eg. recipes, how to procure specific product(s) needed, rates of delivery or feeding schedules, etc.)
   3.   Schedule of follow-up planned to measure compliance with recommendations and achievement of short term and long term goals
   4.   Education/information that parents need prior to discharge
   5.   When collaborative care plan prevents nutritional needs from being met, this plan is documented and justified in medical record.

Approved: _____   Date:_____

Reviewed: _____   Date:_____

needs.[8] JCAHO requires that an assessment policy be written to define the scope of assessment performed within each discipline.[4] This policy can be used to help prioritize and plan nutritional care. An example policy that outlines nutritional assessment is given in Figure 7.3. (Also, see Chapters 1-5 for detailed guidelines for assessment.)

From the assessment, nutritional problems can be identified and a plan of care established with specific goals. Nutrition care plans for neonates identify expected outcomes for growth, nutrient intake, and clinical or laboratory indexes. Recommendations may include nutrient supplementation, formula, or parenteral nutrient solution changes; alternative forms of nutrition support when needed; suggestions for obtaining laboratory or radiographic data to better identify nutrition related problems; and parental education. The nutrition care plan also identifies how progress toward achieving desired outcomes will be monitored and when follow-up will occur. Discharge planning is interdisciplinary, ongoing, and should include referral for additional nutrition interventions and community based services when needed.[9]

Standards of Care

Standards of care are specific desirable and achievable levels of performance by a health care provider.[10] They are not idealistic prescriptions or requirements for care. They are realistic guidelines for delivering patient care for a specific diagnosis or intervention and are used to ensure that routine care is consistent and adequate. The comprehensive interdisciplinary or collaborative care plan may include standards of care from several disciplines. Defined standards enhance accountability, consistency, prioritization and organization of care delivery of all team members.

Nutritional care includes screening, assessment and reassessment of nutritional needs, development of a nutrition care plan or intervention when indicated, prescribing or ordering of food and other nutrients, and monitoring the patient's response to nutritional care or interventions. The registered dietitian develops standards for the nutritional care of the population served, validating these standards through review by other dietitians or health care professionals knowledgeable in neonatal nutrition. Standards of care for nutrition in the NICU most often include general standards for very low birth weight infants, low-birth-weight infants, infants with bronchopulmonary dysplasia, necrotizing enterocolitis, and osteopenia of prematurity. These are published elsewhere.[11] Other standards of care may be adapted from these as needed. Neonatal nutrition is a rapidly changing body of knowledge. Guidelines based on current

Table 7.2.   Examples of NICU Nutrition Rescreening Criteria Indicating Need for Nutrition Assessment*

Criteria based on anthropometric measures†

Poor weight gain ≥ 5 days using a portnatal growth chart
Weight or length -2 S.D. from the mean on the Oregon Growth Record
Dysproportional growth (weight for length < 10th percentile or > 90th percentile)

Criteria based on laboratory assessment

Serum prealbumin < 7 µg/ml or albumin < 2.5 g/dl
Serum phosphorus < 4.5 mg/dl
Serum direct bilirubin > 2 mg/dl
Serum alkaline phosphatase > 5 times adult reference standard or > 600 IU/L
Stool pH < 6
Stool reducing substances > 1%

Criteria based on clinical assessment

Feeding problems or multiple feeding trial intolerence
Diarrhea or constipation > 1 week duration
Frequent vomiting or gastroesophageal reflux

Criteria based on diagnosis

Bronchopulmonary dysplasia	Malabsorption
Cholestatic jaundice	Neurological condition that impairs feeding skill development
Cyanotic heart disease	Renal insufficiency
Cystic fibrosis	Short bowel syndrome
Inborn errors of metabolism	

Criteria based on presence of other therapies/medications

Tube feeding required to achieve adequate nutritional intake at > 37 weeks' gestation
Prolonged need for parenteral nutrition (> 3 weeks)
Prolonged need for steroids, diuretics, antibiotics, anticonvulsants, or other medications that
    affect nutrition (> 3 weeks)

* Examples are given. Criteria used by a specific NICU varies based on population served.
† See growth charts in Appendix D.

knowledge can become obsolete fairly quickly, so timely review is recommended.

There are many ways to develop a standard of care, but the basic components are generally similar. Each standard usually identifies

Figure 7.4A. Clinical Pathway: Prematurity 28-31 Weeks' Gestational Age

Adapted with permission to include primarily nutrition-related items from Clinical Pathway: Prematurity, 28-31 Weeks. © The Children's Hospital at Bronson, Bronson Methodist Hospital, Kalamazoo, Mich., 2000.

Name _____ Hospital # _____ Code status: Full Modified NoCode

DOB _____ Adm _____ EGA _____ wks Birth weight _____ Referring doctor/midwife _____

Adm from _____ gms Adm weight _____ gms Adm diagnosis _____

Expected Outcomes: Medically stable and able to be back transferred to community hospital (optional)

1. Weight follows postnatal growth grid
2. Parent reports/demonstrates:
   a. ability to feed infant (cues, method, amount, frequency)
   b. correct formula preparation and administration of feeding supplements
   c. recognition of infant's signals during handling and responds appropriately
3. Free from signs and symptoms of respiratory distress, apnea of prematurity and sepsis
4. Home assessment completed (if needed)
5. Parent education completed

DATE / WEEK	28 WEEKS	29 WEEKS	30 WEEKS	31 WEEKS
DIET	If new admit: NPO until medically stable			
	Peripheral IV (decrease as feedings increased)			
	Parenteral nutrition: If NPO > 24 to 48 hours or if full enteral feedings not expected within 5 to 7 days			
	Trophic feedings: Colostrum or 20 Cal/oz premature formula	↑	↑	↑
	Advance feeding volume as tolerated: Protocol	↑	↑	↑
	Advance feeding concentration: Add human milk fortifier to breast milk: After day 14 and If parenteral nutrition < 25% intake Increase to 24 Cal/oz premature formula:	↑	↑	↑
	Inadequate weight gain/fluid restriction Promote Kangaroo Care	↑	↑	↑
		Offer pacifier	↑	↑
				For breastfeeding, assess non-nutritive suckling at breast

BM/Formula: _____

Amount: _____

Continuous q2 q3 q4 q6

Times: OG OJ NG NJ

Additives:
[ ] NaCl _____ meq/100 cc
[ ] KCl _____ meq/100 cc
[ ] Natural Care 1:1
[ ] HMF 1 pkg per _____ cc
[ ]
[ ]

PICC location: Central Peripheral   Hep Lock: Site _____ Irrigate q2–3 hours _____ cc (_____ times)

PIV PICC HL IV solution: _____

Change OG/OJ/NG/NJ q wk: _____ (day)   Change chamber: q4 q8 qd   Fill chamber: q4 q8 q12   Rate _____ cc/hour

| **MEDICATIONS** | Iron supplement 2 to 4 mg/kg/day if on breast milk | ↑ | ↑ | ↑ |

[ ] Vit K [ ] Eye drops

(continued)

Figure 7.4A. Clinical Pathway: Prematurity 28-31 Weeks' Gestational Age (continued)

Name _____   Hospital # _____

	28 WEEKS	29 WEEKS	30 WEEKS	31 WEEKS
DIAGNOSTIC TESTS Newborn screen: Day 2 ___ ; ___ ; Day 9 ___ ; ___ ; Hematocrit qod: odd even	**If new admit:** Na, K, Cl Day 2 ___, Day 3 ___ ; Ca Day 2 ___ Parenteral nutrition labs: Na, K, Cl qd x 3 ___, ___, ___ ; then QOD x 3 ___, ___, ___ ; then x2/wk ___ / Triglyceride Day 3 ___ ; then q week ___ ; then q 2 weeks ___ or as ordered Alkaline phosphatase, Ca, Phos, Bili T/D			
ASSESSMENTS Temp q ___ PR q ___ Breath sounds q ___ BP q ___ Blood glucose ___ Mulitstik q ___ Weight/Chart QD ___ WT/L/HC Chart on Oregon ___	**If new admit:** Adm. hx/Asses. Completed ___ Printed ___ ; Nutrition screen done ___ ; Rehab screen done ___ ; Discharge screen done ___ Vital signs per NICU routine Physical assessment per protocol Signs of fatigue: continuous monitoring Signs of sensory overload: continuous monitoring Comfort level: Q shift and prn	→	→	→
CONSULTS [ ] Dietitian ___ (date) [ ] Lactation ___ (date) [ ] Developmentalist ___ (date)	Consult dietitian if: [ ] SGA or LGA (new admit) [ ] Weight gain does not follow postnatal growth grid for 5 or more days [ ] Does not tolerate human milk fortifier or premature infant formula > 3 weeks of age	→	→	→

Clinical pathways do not represent a standard of care, nor do they constitute or take the place of physician orders. The purpose of the Clinical Pathway is to provide multidisciplinary guidelines to assist the patient care team. These guidelines may be modified according to the individual patient's needs.

which component of nutritional care must take place and when it must do so. Most nutrition interventions require a "focus" on nutritional assessment, a short-term plan and a long-term plan of care. The short-term plan may include recommendations for changes in diet or obtaining laboratory assessments. The long-term plan may include recommendations for monitoring and future reassessment, education of parents, discharge planning, and referrals after discharge. The components of assessment and interventions that are recommended and when these interventions occur may vary depending upon the birth weight, age, or diagnosis.

Process standards incorporate what is to be done for the patient, and how and when it is to be done, including assessment parameters and plan of care. Outcome standards describe changes that should occur as a result of interventions and delineate the expected condition of the patient at discharge or at outpatient follow-up. Specific indicators of successful outcome provide direction for the development of process standards.[12] These guidelines are often implemented by incorporating them into clinical pathways.

Clinical Pathways

Clinical pathways, collaborative care paths, and care maps are essentially synonymous. They are documents that provide a clear and concise outline of care usually indicated for patients with a specific diagnosis or clinical condition, including treatments, assessments, referrals, and interdisciplinary team member contributions. Clinical pathways have been developed and used in managed care programs to help standardize care and control costs by monitoring resource utilization and facilitating progress toward discharge, ultimately decreasing length of hospitalization.[2] Although written for a specific population group or diagnosis, each pathway must also accommodate the unique needs of the patient. Expected outcomes should encompass the patient's total care needs and promote achievement of these outcomes in a prospective and progressive manner.[13]

As a first step in developing a clinical pathway, the interdisciplinary team identifies the population group for whom a pathway will be used. Second, a format is established to include a collaborative prospective problem list and the interventions, intermediate outcomes, and discharge outcomes from each discipline. The team then incorporates its contributions into one document and organizes the planned interventions progressively so that outcomes can be met within a projected timeframe. Table 7.3 provides examples of nutrition interventions and outcomes that may be incorporated into various clinical pathways that are used in the NICU.

Figure 7.4B. Sample clinical pathway and progress record

Adapted with permission from Progress Notes 28 to 29 Weeks. © The Children's Hospital at Bronson, Bronson Methodist Hospital, Kalamazoo, Mich., 2000.

PROGRESS NOTES PATIENT NAME/HOSPITAL#

✓ Achieved   * Not achieved, note below
→ Not achieved, same status and plan

Prematurity Outcomes Date:								
Week: 28 29	Day:	1	2	3	4	5	6	7
1. Weight follows postnatal growth grid.								
2. Tolerates advancement of feedings.								
3. Maintains periods of deep sleep AEB, regular breathing, no eye movements under closed lids, relaxed face, only activity is isolated startles.								
4. Maintains autonomic stability in supportive flexion.								
5. Tolerates a minimum of 30-60 minutes of Kangaroo holding or non-stressful holding.								
6. Parents able to verbalize accurate understanding of infant status.								
7. Parents recognize and respond appropriately to infant's status.								
8. Family is aware of case manager role, resources, referrals (new admit).								
9. General information section of education record completed (new admit).								
10. Develomental information section of teaching record completed.								
11. Progressing in completion of teaching record.								
12. Parents identify and accomplish weekly goal.								

Initials/Name	Initials/Name	Initials/Name	Initials/Name

Outcome number	Title	Date/ Time	Progress Notes

Although pathways may vary considerably in content, the format and method for documentation should be consistent in order to facilitate their use. Care paths developed for use in the NICU are often organized by gestational age or weight classification. Documentation is often limited to a check mark indicating that an intervention has been implemented or an outcome met, along with the date and interventionist's initials. Figures 7.4A and 7.4B provide an example of a clinical pathway and progress record that may be used in the NICU.

Because an expected outcome is that parents will be able to care for their infant at home, discharge planning is a major consideration in developing a clinical pathway. Each member of the health care team needs to be able to document that outcomes relating to their discipline have been met in preparing each infant and family for discharge. Criteria for discharge that are related to nutrition often include the infant's proficiency at oral feedings and adequate weight gain; parents' proficiency in feeding; parents' ability to procure and accurately prepare formula for nonbreast-feeding families; and referral to community programs for follow-up.

Quality Assurance and Improvement

Quality assurance is a process aimed at achieving guaranteed levels of excellence. It is an ongoing process for collecting data that relate the process of clinical care to predicted and desirable outcomes.[12] In 1986, JCAHO began an initiative called "Agenda for Change." The goal of this initiative is to create a more sophisticated accreditation format that includes development of an outcome oriented monitoring and evaluation process to assist health care organizations not only to assure quality but to improve the quality of care they provide.[14] The focus moves from the individual's performance to the overall performance of the organization. Do the interdisciplinary systems and processes of an organization produce acceptable outcomes? Do outcomes continue to improve?

Monitoring the effectiveness of the nutrition component of clinical pathways, nutrition interventions, and nutrition education is an integral part of establishing a quality improvement program. This may be accomplished through chart review, family satisfaction surveys, or staff utilization data, but ultimately requires a definition of expected or acceptable outcomes. A sample chart audit is given in Figure 7.5. Quality may be defined not only by the caregivers, but also by the consumer. Well-developed standards of care, clearly documented and using clinical pathways, give assurance to consumers that a level of quality will be maintained and improved whenever possible.[12,15]

Figure 7.5.   Nutrition Services Chart Audit (NICU)

Patient # _____   Diagnosis _____

Author _____   Date _____

Y = yes
N = no
N/A = does not apply

Process Criteria		Comments
1. Weight, length and head circumference are recorded within 24 hours of admission.	Y N N/A	
2. Weight is measured daily and plotted on the Shaffer/Wright Postnatal Growth Chart.	Y N N/A	
3. Nutrition intake is recorded daily.	Y N N/A	
4. Patient on all enteral feeds receives at least 120 kcal/kg/d or dietitians recommendations. (> 7 days of age)	Y N N/A	
5. If weight gain is inadequate > 5 days, patient is referred to dietitian.	Y N N/A	
6. Nutrition assessment completed within 48 hours of referral.	Y N N/A	
7. Response to nutrition plan is monitored at regular intervals.	Y N N/A	
8. Human milk fortifier is started at day 14 or when infant is on at least 100cc/kg breast milk. (Infants < 1850 grams birth weight).	Y N N/A	
Outcomes		
9. Desired outcome(s) are clearly documented on the Patient Care Progress Record.	Y N N/A	
10. Birth weight is regained before 21 days of age.	Y N N/A	
11. Weight gain is consistent with Shaffer/Wright postnatal growth chart.	Y N N/A	
12. Serum phosphorus does not fall below 4.2 mg/dL.	Y N N/A	

Outcomes

The ultimate outcome or end result of care provided may be examined from several perspectives. Clinical outcomes measure parameters of health or absence of disease. Functional outcomes measure physical, mental, and psychological ability. Patient (or par-

Table 7.3.   Examples of nutrition interventions and outcomes used in NICU critical paths*

Nutrition outcome	Critical time
Infant maintains growth pattern that parallels or exceeds the Shaffer/Wright growth chart and/or Oregon Growth Record	Weekly assessment, birth to discharge
Infant does not lose more that 15% of birth weight	Birth to day 8
Infant gains at least 10 g/kg/d	Days 8 to 21
Infant regains birth weight	Day 21
Infant gains at least 15 g/kg/d	Day 21 to 2 kg
Infant gains at least 25 g/d	> 2 kg

Nutrition intervention	Critical time
If birth weight < 2 kg, breast-fed infant receives human milk fortifier	Day 14 if enteral or oral feedings > 100 ml/kg/d
If birth weight < 2 kg, breast-fed infant receives multivitamin supplement	Day 14 if enteral or oral feedings > 100 mL/kg/d
If birth weight < 2.5 kg, breast-fed infant receives iron supplement	Day 60 or prior to discharge
Birth weight < 1.85 kg and infant requires alternate feeding (feedings other than premature formula or breast milk with human milk fortifier) generates nutrition consult	> 3 wk
Serum phosphorus < 4.0 mg/dl or alkaline phosphatase > 600 IU/L generates nutrition consult	Day 21; routine lab draws on TPN or alternate feeding
Serum prealbumin < 7 mg/dl or albumin < 2.5 mg/dl generates nutrition consult	Day 21; routine lab draws on TPN or alternate feeding
No consistent tolerance to gut feeds generates nutrition consult	Day 21
LGA or SGA classification generates nutrition consult	Birth
Weight gain outcomes failed generates nutrition consult	Birth to discharge
Tube feeding needed beyond 37 weeks' gestation generates nutrition consult or request for nutrition education prior to discharge	≥ 37 weeks' gestation; prior to discharge
WIC referral completed	Prior to discharge

* These are examples of interventions and outcomes that are generally consistent with recommendations in the literature, but exact criteria or critical times may vary depending upon the population served and the philosophy of care in the individual NICU. This list does not include all possible examples, and some items may be included in place of others.

ent) satisfaction outcomes measure how well an intervention meets their expectations. Economic outcomes include how the costs are borne by the patient and health care system.[6] Nutritional outcomes may include anthropometric or physiologic measures or indicators, such as those listed in Table 7.4.[4,6] Documented outcomes based on an organization's operations may be compared with others that have documented "best" outcomes or clinical benchmarks.[16] This may help the organization identify specific differences that yield optimal outcomes and provide a catalyst for change in operations.

Most of the outcomes research done with neonates has been related to neurodevelopmental progress and growth (see Chapter 34).[17-20] These studies reflect the interests of investigators, who are often neurologists or developmental psychologists. Morbidity and mortality have been examined and reported.[20-23] However, there has been some concern recently regarding whether or not these outcome studies provide useful information for clinical decisionmaking or planning of health care services for neonates.[24] Further studies have many significant variations in clinical outcomes in different NICUs, variations that cannot be explained simply by different degrees of prematurity or illness but may reflect differences in medical practice.[23-25]

Growth has often been used as an outcome measure, but it has not always been related to specific nutritional processes or practices. When related to specific medical nutrition therapies, growth is probably the best measure of positive nutritional outcome in this population.[26,27] Nutrition-related outcomes may reflect variations in nutrition personnel and feeding practices (see Appendix A).[26-33] Other clinical outcomes, such as necrotizing enterocolitis, nosocomial infection, poor weight gain, and chronic lung disease, have also been related to specific nutritional practices, as outlined in Table 7.4.[34,35]

Measurement, documentation, and evaluation of outcomes may indicate that changes in current care practices are needed to improve clinical, functional, patient/parent satisfaction, or economic outcomes. Several nationwide database systems are available to provide benchmarks, and many of the NICUs in the United States use such a system. Examples of national databases include the National Institutes of Health Database, Vermont-Oxford Neonatal Network, Burroughs-Wellcome Company Database, the Neonatal Research Network, National Neo-Knowledge (Medical Data Systems Company), and the Ross Products Division of Abbott Laboratories Database.[19,36] These databases provide many opportunities for clinical trials, outcome research and quality improvement projects.[36,37]

At first glance, collection and management of data can seem overwhelming. Outcome research requires both time and money, but clinicians must be accountable for the quality of care they provide, and evaluating outcomes can lead to improvements in care and cost containment.[15] Outcome research requires prioritization and selection of topics to be studied, documentation of intervention, and measure-

Table 7.4.   Examples of Nutrition Related Indicators
             for Outcome Studies*

Nutrition practice	Examples of corresponding indicators or measures of outcome
Day parenteral nutrition (PN) initiated Days to reach adequate PN to support growth Day enteral feeding started (trophic feeding) Days to reach adequate feeding to support growth	% birth weight lost Days to regain birth weight Subsequent growth percentile achievement Average weekly weight gain
Fluid balance during first 2 wk of life	Incidence of congestive heart failure Incidence of chronic lung disease
Provision of adequate energy and protein intake, e.g. number of days intake meets goals	Late onset sepsis/infection (beyond initial 2 wk) Growth in weight gain (g/kg/d or g/d)
Number of days on iron-fortified formula or receiving iron supplement	Number of transfusions needed Incidence/severity of anemia
Progression of feeding in daily volume increments	Incidence of necrotizing enterocolitis
Postpartum day mother begins to express milk with electric pump	Availability of mother's milk for initial feedings Milk supply adequacy at 1 mo postpartum
Date to start human milk fortification	Incidence of osteopenia in breast-fed infants Linear growth in cm/wk
Daily weight gain and nippled intake during week prior to discharge	Rates of readmission for nutrition related problems Growth in g/day at 2 wk postdischarge
Number of days of PN without trophic feedings	Incidence of cholestatic jaundice Date full enteral feedings achieved

* Examples are given. Criteria used by a specific NICU varies based on population served.

ment of the end results of intervention. When outcomes must be improved, interventions and standards of care are analyzed to identify changes needed. Once changes have been implemented, outcomes are reevaluated to measure improvement.

In summary, nutritional care includes screeening, rescreening, assessment and reassessment of nutritional needs, development of a plan of care for intervention when indicated, prescribing the appropriate feeding regimen, and monitoring the patient's response to nutrition intervention. Policies written to guide nutrition intervention and documentation tools used in the NICU should encompass these components. Measurement of outcomes, when compared with outcomes identified in a broadly based system, provides an opportunity for improvement in care. Well-defined outcomes offer registered dietitians the opportunity to evaluate the effectiveness of nutrition services in the NICU and high-risk newborn follow-up setting.[26,27,37-39]

References

1. Etheredge M, ed. Center for Nursing Case Management. New England Medical Center Hospitals. American Hospital Publishing, 1989.
2. Vecchi C and Vasquez L. Neonatal individualized predictive pathways: A discharge planning tool for parents. Neonatal Network 15:4, 1996.
3. Cox, JH, ed. Nutrition manual for at-risk infants and toddlers. Chicago: Precept Press, 1997; ix.
4. Joint Commission on Accreditation of Health Care Organizations. Comprehensive accreditation manual for hospitals, 1996. Oakbrook Terrace, Ill: Joint Commission on Accreditation of Health Care Organizations, 1996.
5. Smith PE and Smith AE. Superior nutritional care cuts hospital costs. Tucker, Ga.: Nutritional Care Management Institute, 1988.
6. Ross Products Division, Abbott Laboratories. Nutrition intervention and patient outcomes: A self study manual, Columbus, Ohio: Ross, 1995.
7. Bamberger JM. Nutrition screening in the neonatal intensive care unit. Pediatr Nutr Pract Group Newsletter, Summer 1997.
8. Charles E. Charting by exception: A solution to the challenge of the 1996 Joint Commission on Accreditation of Health Care Organizations nutrition care standards. Future Dimen Clin Manage. 15:2, April 1996.
9. Kotogal U, Pelstein P, Gambian V, et al. Description and evaluation of a program for the early discharge of infants from a neonatal intensive care unit. J Pediatr 127:285, 1995.
10. American Dietetic Association standards of professional practice for dietetic professionals. J Am Diet Assoc 98:83, 1998.
11. American Dietetic Association Quality Assurance Committee. Standards of practice: A practitioner's guide to implementation. Chicago: American Dietetic Association, 1986.
12. Suhayda R, Fredricks J. Linking neonatal documentation with standards of care and quality improvement. J Perinatal Neonatal Nurs 7:64, 1993.
13. Malnight M, Wahl J. An alternative approach for neonatal clinical pathways. Neonatal Network 16:4, 1997.
14. Kusher R, Avello E. National Coordinating Committee: Clinical indicators of nutrition care. J Am Diet Assoc 94:10, 1994.
15. Grossman RG. Quality improvement: An overview. J Perinatal Neonatal Nurs 12:42, 1998.
16. Fitzgerald K. Clinical benchmarking: Implications for perinatal nursing. J Perinatal Neonatal Nurs 12:23, 1998.
17. The Infant Health and Development Program. Enhancing the outcomes of low-birth-weight, premature infants. JAMA 263:3035, 1990.

18. Chaplain MD, Mayes LC, eds. Outcomes of low birthweight premature infants. Semin Perinatol 21:161, 1997.

19. Hack M and Fanaroff AA. Outcomes of children of extremely low birthweight and gestational age in the 1990's. Early Hum Develop 53:193, 1999.

20. Lee K, Keim B, Khoshnood B, et al. Outcome of very low birth weight infants in industrialized countries 1947-1987. Amer J Epidemiology 141:1188, 1995.

21. Phibbs CS, Bronstein JM, Buxton E, et al. The effects of patient volume and level of care at the hospital of birth on neonatal mortality. JAMA 276:1054, 1996.

22. Schoendorf KD, Kiely JL. Birth weight and age specific analysis of the 1990 US infant mortality drop: Was it sufficient? Pediatr Adolesc Med 151:129, 1997.

23. Svenningsen MW, Bjorklund L, Lindroth M. Changing trends in perinatal management and outcome of extremely low birth weight (ELBW) infants. Acta Paediatr Suppl 422:89, 1997.

24. McCormick MC. The outcomes of very low birthweight infants: Are we asking the right questions? Pediatr 98:869, 1997.

25. Harding JE, Morton SM. Outcome of neonates transported between level III centers depends upon center of care. J Paediatr Child Health 30:389, 1994.

26. Carlson SJ, Redlin J. Use of nutrition outcomes monitors in the intensive care nurseries. J Am Diet Assoc 97:A-102, 1997.

27. Bryson SR, Theriot L, Ryan NJ, et al. Primary follow-up care in a multidisciplinary setting enhances catch-up growth of very-low-birth-weight infants. J Amer Dietet Assoc 97:386, 1997.

28. Olsen I, Awnetwant E, Cardi G, et al. Variations in nutrition personnel and practice among 7 neonatal intensive care units. J Am Diet Assoc 97:A30, 1997.

29. Rubin LP, Richardson DK, Bednarek FJ, et al. Longitudinal growth in hospitalized VLBW infants: Identification of patient characteristics and inter-nicu differences. Pediatr Res 41:239A, 1997.

30. Valentine C, Schanler RJ. Neonatal nutritionist intervention improves nutritional support and promotes cost containment in the management of low birth weight (LBW) infants. Aspen 17th Clinical Congress Nutrition Practice Poster 46, Feb 14-17, 1993.

31. Lair C, Albrecht J, Kennedy KA. Randomized controlled trial of neonatal nutrition support team (NNST) services. Pediatr Res 43:177A, 1998.

32. Elsaesser KR. Dietitian intervention in neonatal intensive care reduces errors and improves clinical outcomes. J Am Diet Assoc 98:A22, 1998.

33. Carlson SJ, Ziegler EE. Nutrient intakes and growth of very low birth weight infants. J Perinatol 18:252, 1998.

34. Unger A et al. Nutrition practices and outcomes of extremely premature infants. Am J Dis Child 141:1027, 1988.

35. Schanler RJ, Shulman RJ, Lau C. Feeding strategies for premature infants: Beneficial outcomes of feeding fortified human milk versus preterm formula. Pediatr 103:1150, 1999.

36. Horbar JD. The Vermont-Oxford Neonatal Network: Integrating research and clinical practice to improve the quality of medical care. Semin Perinatol 19:124, 1995.

37. Wirtschaften D, Jones KR, Thomas JT. Using health care outcomes to improve patient care in nicu. J Qual Improv 20:57, 1997.

38. Weddle DO, Tu Natalie S, Guzik CJ, et al. Positive association between dietetics recommendations and achievement of enteral nutrition outcomes of care. J Am Diet Assoc 95:753, 1995.
39. Baggs JG. Development of an instrument to measure collaboration and satisfaction about care. J Advanc Nurs 20:176, 1990.

SECTION II

PARENTERAL NUTRITION

Nutritional Care for High-Risk Newborns (Rev. 3d. Ed.)
S. Groh-Wargo, M. Thompson, J. Cox, editors
© 2000, Precept Press, Inc., Chicago

8

PARENTERAL NUTRITION: ADMINISTRATION AND MONITORING

Pamela T Price, PhD, RD, CNSD

PARENTERAL NUTRITION (PN) IS the intravenous provision of nutrients for both repletion of tissue losses and tissue accretion for rapid growth during the postnatal period if enteral feedings are inadequate or impossible. Total parenteral nutrition (TPN) is the provision of all nutrients I.V.; partial parenteral nutrition (PPN) is the provision of I.V. nutrition in conjunction with some enteral feedings. The term parenteral nutrition is used in this chapter to encompass both terms.

The initial goal of PN is to provide sufficient calories and amino acids to prevent negative energy and nitrogen balance; this may be achieved with a minimum intake of 60 nonprotein kcal/kg/day and 2.5 g of amino acids/kg/day.[1,2] Subsequently, the goal is to promote weight gain and growth, which is usually achieved by providing 70-90 nonprotein kcal/kg/day and 2.5-3.0 g of amino acids/kg/day, until enteral feedings are established.[3,4]

Indications for parenteral nutrition are:

- Functional immaturity of G.I. tract
- Surgical G.I. disorders (i.e., gastroschisis, omphalocele, malrotation and volvulus, diaphragmatic hernia, obstruction, tracheoesophageal fistula, G.I. fistulas, intestinal atresias)
- Short bowel syndrome
- Inadequate enteral nutrient intake
- Intractable diarrhea of infancy
- Necrotizing enterocolitis
- Meconium ileus

Heird[5] estimated that energy reserves of very low birth weight (VLBW) infants would become depleted in 8-12 days even if given 30 kcal/kg/day of a dextrose-containing I.V. fluid, with additional energy being drawn primarily from catabolism of endogenous protein (probably skeletal muscle) as opposed to fat stores.[6] Thus, insufficient exogenous calories and protein may be life-threatening to the sick, preterm infant.

PN is not indicated in infants with adequate intestinal function who may be maintained by oral, tube, or gastrostomy feedings or infants who will be receiving parenteral nutrition for less than three days. An infant whose death is imminent due to the underlying disease is not a candidate for PN.[3]

Initiating Parenteral Nutrition

Intravenous access is established during the first hours of life, and I.V. fluids are started at about 80-100 ml/kg/day, providing 5-7 mg glucose/kg/min and 27-34 kcal/kg/day. If nutritional needs cannot be met by enteral feedings within five to seven days, the addition of amino acids, vitamins, and minerals to the PN solution should begin no later than the third day of life and preferably earlier.[7-9,52] It has been demonstrated that when VLBW infants were given 1.15 g/kg/d protein on the first day of life, average nitrogen retention improved even when energy intake was < 30 kcal/kg/d.[9,53] For sick ELBW infants < 750 g, I.V. fat should be delayed until 3-4 days of life due to a report of increased mortality and pulmonary hemorrhage in 600-800 g infants receiving early I.V. fat infusions.[10] A 20% I.V. fat emulsion, 0.5 g/kg/d, is usually initiated at the same time the amino acid-glucose solution is started or the following day, since the risk of essential fatty acid deficiency is accelerated by the anabolic effects of amino acid administration.[1,10,11] Due to the potential for the formation of lipid hydroperoxides, which are cytotoxic and may cause vascular damage, some recommend wrapping tubing and syringes containing lipid emulsion in aluminum foil to shield the fluid from both ambient and phototherapy lights.[12,54]

Peripheral Versus Central Venous Access

In most clinical conditions, PN delivered through a peripheral vein is preferred and will provide adequate nutrition support.[4] A PN solution of 12.5% dextrose and 2.0% amino acids at a rate of 130-135 ml/kg/day used in conjunction with a 20% I.V. fat emulsion at 2.0-3.0 g lipid/kg/day (10-15 ml/kg/day) will provide 90-100 kcal/kg/day and 2.7 g protein/kg/day in 140-150 ml fluid/kg/day. Dextrose concentration is limited to 12.5% in a peripheral vein, since concentrations above this are associated with an increased incidence of phlebitis and skin sloughing due to the high osmolality of the solution.[13]

Umbilical catheters have been used for infusion of PN solutions in the sick neonate requiring arterial access for blood gas analysis. Of 117 NICUs responding to a survey, 36% routinely administered PN through the umbilical arterial catheter (UAC), 26% administered PN sometimes through the UAC, and 35% never used the UAC for PN infusion.[14] Few articles have addressed the safety of the use of the UAC and umbilical venous catheter (UVC) for PN infusion.[15-18] Complications include thromboses, tricuspid valve vegetation,[16] transient episodes of hyperglycemia,[18] and glucosuria with dehydration.[15]

Central venous access may be required in infants (1) who are fluid restricted, necessitating a hypertonic PN solution to provide adequate nutrition; (2) who have limited peripheral vascular access; or (3) for whom prolonged PN is anticipated (usually greater than two to three weeks). Placement of the central venous catheter is either by a percutaneous method or by a cut-down technique.[3] Catheter tip placement is often at the junction of the superior vena cava and the right atrium, although placement may vary. Correct position of the central line should be verified radiologically at the time of placement. A line whose tip is not placed in the area of large blood flow must be treated as a peripheral line for PN administration with the maximum dextrose concentration no greater than 12.5%. A discussion of proper catheter placement has been written by Jewett.[19]

The concentration of each of the nutrients in the PN solution is determined by the route of venous access, the compatibility of various nutrients in the solution, the simultaneous administration of enteral feedings, and the age, weight, fluid tolerance, and clinical condition of the infant. I.V. fat emulsion may be administered simultaneously through a separate line attached to the PN tubing via a "Y" connector below the filter and should be infused over a 24-hour period for best tolerance (see Chapter 10).

Standard PN solutions are designed with a combination of nutrients that, when given near maintenance fluid requirements, will provide safe and adequate initial nutrition intake for most neonatal patients. Standard PN orders should allow for individual dosing of vitamins and trace minerals according to the weight of the infant. The use of standard PN solutions has the advantages of decreasing errors in ordering, expediting the ordering process, and reducing costs as a result of decreased preparation time in the pharmacy. Obviously, individually designed PN solutions will be necessary for some infants. A well-drafted order form will assist the clinician in developing these specialized formulations. A sample order form is shown in Figure 8.1. Additional examples can be found in reference 20.

Figure 8.1. Sample parenteral nutrition order form.

Reprinted with permission from MetroHealth Medical Center, Cleveland, Ohio.

MetroHealth Medical Center
PEDIATRIC PARENTERAL NUTRITION PHYSICIAN ORDER SHEET
1) **Each order is for one bag. Order should be written to provide a 24-hr supply.**
2) Order must be received in Pharmacy by **NOON** for same day delivery.
3) Any change after pharmacy receives the order sheet should be called to ext. 85396 and written on a physician order sheet.

Date: _____ **Dosing Weight:** _____ **kg**
☐ **CENTRAL LINE** ☐ **PERIPHERAL LINE**

☐ Standard Amino Acids
☐ Pediatric Amino Acids (e.g. TrophAmine®)
 (Includes cysteine; **For pharmacy use only:** _____ g protein/L X 30 mg cysteine = ____ mg cysteine/L)
 (RESTRICTED to use in infants ≤ 1 kg at birth or on TPN > 2 weeks)

BASE SOLUTION
☐ Pediatric Solution I Amino Acids 1.5% and Dextrose 10% (15 gm protein and 400 Kcal/liter)
☐ Pediatric Solution II Amino Acids 2% and Dextrose 12% (20 gm protein and 488 Kcal/liter)
☐ Pediatric Solution III Amino Acids 2.5% and Dextrose 15% (25 gm protein and 610 Kcal/liter)
☐ Pediatric Solution IV Amino Acids 3% and Dextrose 20% (30 gm protein and 800 Kcal/liter)
☐ Tailored Solution Amino Acids _____% and Dextrose _____% (_____ gm protein/liter)

ELECTROLYTES AND MINERALS:

		Usual Pediatric Range			
		Neonates	1mo–1yr	1-11 yrs	≥12 yrs
Sodium	____mEq/kg/day	(2-5)	(3-4)	(2-4)	(1-3)
Potassium	____mEq/kg/day	(2-3)	(2-3)	(2-3)	(1-3)
Magnesium (as Sulfate)	____mEq/kg/day	(0.4-0.6)	(0.3-0.6)	(0.2-0.5)	(0.25)
Chloride* ☐none ☐1/3 ☐1/2 ☐2/3 ☐all		(1/3)	(1/3)	(1/3)	(1/2)
*remaining anions will be given as acetate					
Phosphate	____mmol/kg/day	(1-2)	(1-1.5)	(0.5)	(0.5)

OR ☐ phosphate per NICU guidelines

Calcium (as Gluconate)	____mg/kg/day	(500-700)	(400-600)	(100-200)	(50)

_____ mg/kg/day Ca (as Gluconate) X 0.0046 = ____ mEq/kg/day Ca (elemental)

OR ☐ calcium per NICU guidelines

VITAMINS AND TRACE ELEMENTS: *(Dose changes and additional items must be handwritten on the lines below.)*

Multiple Vitamins	accept guidelines	☐Yes or ☐No
Multiple Trace Elements (delete if direct bili > 2 mg/dl)	accept guidelines	☐Yes or ☐No
Zinc (indicated when multiple trace elements are deleted)	age appropriate	☐Yes or ☐No
Selenium (indicated for parenteral nutrition > 2 weeks)	2 mcg/kg/day (max 40mcg)	☐Yes or ☐No
Vitamin K (for children > 11 years old)	5 mg every Monday	☐Yes or ☐No

MISCELLANEOUS ADDITIVES: *(Dose changes and additional items must be handwritten on the lines below.)*

Heparin (deletion requires attending approval)	1 unit/ml	☐Yes or ☐No
Ranitidine (only if indicated)	3 mg/kg/day	☐Yes or ☐No
Carnitine (indicated for NICU TPN > 2 weeks)	10 mg/kg/day	☐Yes or ☐No

_____ _____
_____ _____
_____ _____

TOTAL VOLUME (without lipids)   **20% LIPIDS**
_____ml (24 hour supply)   _____ gm/kg/day = _____ ml to infuse over _____ hours

Physician Signature_____ **Beeper**_____ **Date**_____

Nurse Signature _____ **Date** _____ **Time** _____
Forward TPN questions to: Pharmacy, ext. 85396; Neonatal Dietitian, ext. 85918; Pediatric Dietitian, ext. 85316

Figure 8.1.   Sample parenteral nutrition order form (continued).

NICU CALCIUM/PHOSPHATE GUIDELINES

Standard Amino Acids

	1.5%	2%	2.5%	3%
Ca (mEq/L)	14	22	24	26
P (mmol/L)	7	11	12	13

Pediatric Amino Acids

	1.5%	2%	2.5%	3%
Ca (mEq/L)	22	24	26	30
P(mmol/L)	11	12	13	15

- Maximum Calcium = 4 mEq/kg/day
- Maximum Phosphate = 2 mmol/kg/day
- If the amino acid concentration falls between two listed on the table, the lower concentration will be used to calculate the calcium and phosphate doses.

DOSING WEIGHT

- Defined as the weight used for parenteral nutrition calculation.
- Usually the current weight; As appropriate, could be
  - Birthweight (ex. Newborns)
  - Estimated "dry" weight (ex. Edema)
  - Ideal body weight (ex. Obesity)

TRACE ELEMENT GUIDELINES

	<3kg	3kg-5yr	>5yr
Zn	400 mcg/kg/day	200 mcg/kg/day	5 mg/day
Cu	40 mcg/kg/day	20 mcg/kg/day	1 mg/day
Mn	10 mcg/kg/day	5 mcg/kg/day	0.5 mg/day
Cr	0.4 mcg/kg/day	0.2 mcg/kg/day	10 mcg/day

MULTIVITAMIN GUIDELINES (DOSE/DAY)**

	<1kg	1-3kg	>3kg-11yrs	>11yrs
Dose	1.5ml peds	3.25ml peds	5ml peds	10ml adult
Vit A	690 IU	1495 IU	2300 IU	1 mg
Vit D	120 IU	260 IU	400 IU	5 mcg
Vit E	2.1 IU	4.55 IU	7 IU	10 mg
Vit K	60 mcg	130 mcg	200 mcg	*note
Vit C	24 mg	52 mg	80 mg	100mg
Vit B1	0.36 mg	0.78 mg	1.2 mg	3 mg
Vit B2	0.45 mg	0.91 mg	1.4 mg	3.6 mg
Vit B6	0.3 mg	0.65 mg	1mg	4 mg
Vit B12	0.3 mcg	0.65 mcg	1 mcg	5 mcg
Folate	42 mcg	91 mcg	140 mcg	400 mcg
Niacin	5.1 mg	11 mg	17 mg	40 mg
Biotin	6 mcg	13 mcg	20 mcg	60 mcg
Pantothenic Acid	1.5 mg	3.25 mg	5 mg	15 mg

* > 11yrs receive 5mg vitamin K every Monday if ordered.
** If necessary because of volume or osmolality (peripheral line) limitations, the multivitamin dose may be decreased or eliminated.

RECOMMENDED LAB MONITORING

- **Day 1:** prealbumin, LFTs, Triglyceride, Chem 7, Ca, Mg, Phos
- **Weekly:** prealbumin, Chem 7, Ca, Mg, Phos
- **Biweekly**: LFTs
- Check labs after making a change to the solution. (ex. dextrose, protein, lipids, electrolytes)

Place Label Here

SOLUTION INDICATIONS

A. Pediatric Solution I: Designed as the initial neonatal solution, it provides glucose and protein in amounts generally tolerated in the first few days of life. Some tiny infants, especially those receiving large fluid volumes, may require lower concentrations of protein and/or dextrose than those found in this solution. Provision of ≈ 1.5 g/kg/day of protein replaces urinary nitrogen (N) losses and may maintain N balance in newborns.

B. Pediatric Solution II: This solution is designed for older infants who have documented glucose tolerance to Pediatric Solution I. Care should be taken that adequate non-protein calories are provided. This can be accomplished by giving about 1-3 g/kg/day of intravenous fat. Provision of 2.7-3.5 g/kg/day of protein promotes positive N balance

C. Pediatric Solution III and IV: These solutions are intended solely for the infant or child with a central line in place. They are designed for those who require prolonged parenteral support, who have increased nutritional requirements, or who are fluid restricted. Non-protein calories should come from both carbohydrate and fat in an approximate ratio of 60:40. Provision of > 3.5 g/kg/day of protein is not recommended.

D. Intravenous Fat Emulsion (IFE): A dose of 0.5-1 g/kg/day delivers sufficient fat to meet essential fatty acid requirements. Higher doses up to 3 g/kg/day will provide energy as well. Incremental increases by 0.5 g/kg/day are recommended. The stated maximum pediatric dose on product literature is 4 gm/kg/day. Infusion time should be over as many hours as possible. An infusion rate of < 0.15 g/kg/hour, especially for premature and SGA infants, is recommended. IFE should be used cautiously in infants with documented sepsis or pulmonary hypertension, and in extremely low birthweight infants less than 4 days old.

Place Label Here

Total Nutrient Admixture

Some centers are using a three-in-one solution (also called total nutrient admixture), whereby the lipid emulsion is mixed with the amino acid-dextrose solution and administered through a single line. This method of delivery has certain advantages. It simplifies administration, which may prove to be a cost savings;[21,22] requires less manipulation of the delivery system, resulting in reduced opportunity for contamination;[21] reduces the loss of vitamin A;[23] and provides continuous administration of all nutrients.[21] However, this system does have some disadvantages. If changes in solution are required more often than once every 24 hours due to hyperlipidemia, the resultant waste increases costs. The addition of the I.V. lipid emulsion to the amino acid-dextrose solution increases the pH of the solution, which may result in a decrease in solubility of calcium and phosphorus and, therefore, a lower concentration of these nutrients available to the infant.[24] Due to the opacity of the fat emulsion, visual inspection for particulate matter (i.e., calcium-phosphorus precipitate) is difficult; thus, there is an increased risk of adverse reactions associated with the infusion of precipitate. Three-in-one solutions can be filtered if the pore size is $\geq 1.2\mu$, resulting in the removal of some of the particulates (see Chapter 12).

Cyclic TPN

Some long-term, stable central PN patients may benefit from cyclic TPN, infusion of TPN over approximately 18 hours as opposed to a continuous 24-hour infusion. Because constant infusion of a hypertonic dextrose solution results in high circulating insulin levels, lipogenesis (conversion of dextrose to fat in the liver) is enhanced, and release of free fatty acids from adipose tissue is depressed. Constant lipogenesis and excessive glycogen deposition engorge hepatocytes with fat and glycogen, resulting in hepatomegaly, fatty infiltration of the liver, and increased risk of hepatic dysfunction. Cyclic TPN gives the opportunity to interrupt the flow of glucose and thus decrease circulating insulin levels for a short period to facilitate the mobilization of fat and glycogen stores.[25] Additionally, cyclic TPN allows more time for physical activity, opportunity to establish enteral feedings, and may help maintain the normal circadian rhythm of the body.[26] (See reference 27 for a detailed administration schedule.) Cyclic TPN is rarely used in young infants due to the risk of hypoglycemia and hyperglycemia in these metabolically fragile patients. However, for metabolically stable, growing infants who have central venous access and who require long-term TPN, cyclic TPN has been used successfully.[27,28] Besides careful monitoring of blood glucose and electrolytes during cyclic

(TEXT CONTINUED ON PAGE 101)

Table 8.1   Metabolic Complications of Parenteral Nutrition

Metabolic complications	Possible cause	Management
Glucose Metabolism		
Hyperglycemia with glucosuria, osmotic diuresis, hyperosmolar dehydration, intracranial hemorrhage, or coma	Excessive rate or amount of glucose infusion, inadequate endogenous insulin, glucocorticoids, sepsis, malnutrition, renal disease, thiazide diuretics	Dilute the infusate or slow the rate of infusion, correct fluid and electrolyte deficits by peripheral vein. Monitor serum glucose. Evaluate for sepsis and treat, if necessary. Consider insulin only if additional calories are needed and cannot be provided with fat emulsion
Hypoglycemia (postinfusion)	Increased insulin production, hepatic glycogenic enzyme immaturity, interrupted or too-rapid weaning of dextrose solution	Carefully taper infusion rate; if central parenteral nutrition is interrupted, infuse $D_{10}W$ peripherally. Monitor serum glucose
Amino Acid Metabolism		
Hyperammonemia	Liver disease or hepatic immaturity. Too high parenteral intake of amino acids (in excess of 3.5 g/kg/d), inborn errors of protein metabolism	Lower protein intake Monitor serum ammonia, serum proteins and albumin
Prerenal azotemia	Excessive nitrogen infusion, especially in LBW infants when protein in excess of 3 g/kg/d or inappropriate calorie/nitrogen ratio, intravascular volume depletion, catabolism	Lower protein intake; achieve calorie:nitrogen ratio between 150:1 to 250:1; provide adequate caloric intake Monitor BUN, serum proteins and albumin
Lipid metabolism		
Essential fatty acid deficiency	Inadequate EFA (linoleic acid) administration, long-term fat-free TPN	Requirements can be met by providing 0.5 g lipid/kg/d

Table 8.1   Metabolic Complications of Parenteral Nutrition (continued)

Metabolic complications	Possible cause	Management
Lipid metabolism (continued)		
Hypertriglyceridemia and high levels of free fatty acids	Rapid infusion of fat emulsion, malnutrition, stress, infection, prematurity, excessive glucose intake	Slow administration of fat emulsion; in premature infants infuse over 24 hr
		Monitor serum triglycerides. Heparin in parenteral nutrition solution may be beneficial
Hyperbilirubinemia	Potential displacement of bilirubin from albumin binding sites by high serum free fatty acid levels	Limit lipid infusion to 0.5-1.0 g/kg/d Monitor serum bilirubin and triglycerides, maintaining triglycerides at < 150 mg/dl
Hepatic dysfunction and hepatic failure	The glucose, protein, and vitamin components have been implicated but studies are inconclusive. May be due to sepsis, prematurity, ischemia, or postoperative status. Lack of enteral feeding resulting in decreased bile flow; rarely occurs when both enteral and parenteral nutrition are provided	If there is no other means of nutritional support, continue parenteral nutrition, adjusting solution on an individual basis; avoid excessive calories and protein intake; limit I.V. protein intake to ≤ 2.5 g/kg/d. If standard crystalline amino acid (CAA) solution is being infused, change to a pediatric CAA solution
		Shield TPN from light. Cycle TPN for older infants.
		Start enteral feedings as soon as possible.
		If cholestatic, remove manganese and copper from the solution. Rule out infectious and other causes of hepatic dysfunction. Monitor liver function weekly and serum copper bimonthly

Table 8.1 Metabolic Complications of Parenteral Nutrition (continued)

Metabolic complications	Possible cause	Management
Mineral and Electrolyte Metabolism		
Electrolyte imbalances	Sodium, potassium, and chloride imbalances are usually secondary to increased losses from diarrhea, renal disease, or drug therapy	Electrolyte losses should be measured and replaced with a separate I.V. solution; once stable, appropriate changes in the TPN may be made
Hyperphosphatemia	Excessive intake, decreased renal function or PTH deficiency	Decrease phosphorus intake. Monitor calcium and phosphorus
Hypophospatemia	High glucose infusions, inadequate phosphorus administration, malnutrition, rapid refeeding, rapid growth	Increase phosphorus content of solution. Monitor serum phosphorus and calcium
Hypocalcemia	Inadequate intake may follow a previous increase in phosphorus intake, diuretic administration (Lasix), PTH deficiency, inadequate magnesium intake	May begin calcium replacement using separate I.V. line (not mixing with TPN to avoid precipitation), then increase calcium content of solution
		Monitor serum phosphorus and calcium
Hypercalcemia	Excessive calcium load perhaps due to high fluid intake given as TPN	Investigate etiology and institute appropriate medical management. If needed, decrease calcium content of solution
		Monitor serum calcium, phosphorus and alkaline phosphatase
Hypomagnesemia	Inadequate magnesium administration relative to increased requirements for protein anabolism and glucose metabolism, chronic diarrhea, amphotericin B	Increase magnesium content of solution
		Monitor serum magnesium, calcium, and phosphorus
Hypermagnesemia	Excessive magnesium administration, renal decompensation, tocolysis	Decrease magnesium content of solution Monitor serum magnesium, calcium, and phosphorus

Table 8.1   Metabolic Complications of Parenteral Nutrition (continued)

Metabolic complications	Possible cause	Management
Mineral and Electrolyte Metabolism (continued)		
Hypokalemia	Inadequate potassium administration relative to increased requirements for protein anabolism, diuresis, amphotericin B	Increase potassium content of solution Monitor serum potassium
Hyperkalemia	Excessive potassium administration, metabolic acidosis, renal decompensation, spironolactone	Decrease potassium content of solution Monitor serum potassium
Hypochloremic alkalosis	Too much acetate and too little chloride in solution, diuretics	Increase chloride content and decrease the acetate content of solution Monitor serum chloride and bicarbonate
Hyperchloremic acidosis	Excessive chloride content of solution and/or flushes	Decrease chloride content and increase the acetate content of solution Monitor serum chloride and bicarbonate

Adapted from Hendricks KM, Walker WA. Manual of pediatric nutrition. 2d ed. Philadelphia: Decker, 1990; 121.

Table 8.2.   Sample Monitoring Schedule for Infants on Parenteral Nutrition

Parameter	Initial	Daily	Weekly	As needed
Anthropometric				
Weight	x	x		
Length	x		x*	
Head circumference	x		x*	
Metabolic (blood or plasma)				
Sodium/potassium/chloride	x		x†	
Bicarbonate	x		x†	
Glucose	x		x†	
BUN/creatinine	x		x†	
Calcium/phosphorus	x		x†	
Magnesium	x		x	
Triglycerides	x		x‡	
Albumin/total protein	x		x	
Liver function studies (incl SGPT & alk phos)	x		x	
Bilirubin (total and direct)	x		x	
Hgb/Hct	x		x	
Platelets, PT, PTT	x			x
WBC count and differential				x
Prealbumin				x
Copper/zinc				x
Iron studies				x
Ammonia				x
Vitamin E				x
pH				x
Cultures				x
Urine				
Glucose	x	x		x
Ketones	x	x		x

* Until 3 mos corrected age, then monthly thereafter
† Daily until stable, then twice weekly
‡ Initially and before each I.V.lipid increase. Once I.V.lipids are maximized, weekly determinations are adequate. If an infant becomes septic, a triglyceride level should be assessed, since lipid intolerance is often present during sepsis.

PN, the infants must be monitored for symptoms of nausea and vomiting, which have been reported as a side effect of cyclic TPN in infants and young children.[29]

Home Parenteral Nutrition

Occasionally, infants may require TPN after discharge (i.e., short bowel syndrome). This requires multidisciplinary discharge planning and coordination with a home health care service to provide PN equipment, solution, and home monitoring services. Before discharge, the solution to be used should be initiated to monitor tolerance while the infant is still in the hospital. An intensive education program with the primary care-giver(s) is imperative (see Chapter 13).

Discontinuing TPN

Discontinuation of PN should be gradual as more daily fluid allowance is provided enterally. This should be done in a manner to provide adequate calories to prevent weight loss. Caloric intake should be closely monitored, because weight often plateaus or actually drops during this transition period.[30] Weight loss is often seen in infants who have received central TPN due to reduced caloric intake and a significant fluid loss.

Careful monitoring of other nutrients, especially electrolytes, minerals, vitamins, and protein, is necessary to prevent inadequate or excessive nutrient intake as enteral feedings are advanced. For example, continued concentration of parenteral protein as enteral feedings are advanced may result in excessive nitrogen intake and azotemia. PN should be continued for the preterm infant until about 75% of energy needs (90-100 kcal/kg/day) are being met by enteral feedings.

Monitoring and Complications

Although parenteral nutrition can prove to be a life-saving therapy, this technique of nutrient delivery should not be undertaken without knowledge and respect for potential complications (see Table 8.1). Goals for nutrient intake should be set and actual intake calculated daily (see Chapters 9-11 for specific recommendations for each nutrient). Infants on PN must be monitored regularly to assure adequacy of intake, to assess tolerance to the solutions, and to prevent complications (see Table 8.2); infants on long-term TPN with stable laboratory values may be monitored on a less frequent basis.

Anthropometric assessments, including daily weights and weekly lengths and head circumferences, should be plotted on appropriate growth charts and average daily weight gain over a one-week period determined (see Chapter 2).

The potential metabolic and catheter-related complications of PN are numerous.[3,31-36,55] Additionally, a number of deficiency states have been described in patients on PN, usually when this is the sole source of nutrition for more than four weeks or when mineral losses are excessive, such as in patients with ileostomies or chronic diarrhea.[37-45] See Table 8.3 for a list of the most common deficiencies, their manifestation, and treatment.

Table 8.3. Potential Nutrient Deficiency States

Deficiency	Manifestation	Treatment*
Essential fatty acid	Desquamating skin rash Reduced growth rate Thrombocytopenia Hemolytic anemia	Preventable by providing at least 4-8% of total caloric needs as fat emulsion or 0.5-1.0 g lipid/kg/d[50,51]
Calcium, phosphorus, and/or vitamin D	Early biochemical findings include decreased phosphorus and increased alkaline phosphatase with osteopenia. Later, radiologic evidence of rickets is seen	Primarily seen in preterm infants on prolonged parenteral nutrition alone, especially in the presence of cholestasis. Treat by maximizing calcium and phosphorus in the parenteral nutrition solution, and if necessary, by supplemental PO or I.V. calcium, vitamin D, and phosphorus
Iron	Microcytic anemia Poor growth Low serum iron and TIBC	Iron is not routinely provided in the parenteral nutrition solution. It may be given as iron dextran 2-3 days/mo
Copper	Osteopenia or rickets Neutropenia Depigmentation of skin Hemolytic anemia Low serum copper	Document level of intake; alter dosage as required
Chromium	Glucose intolerance Low serum chromium	Document level of intake; alter dosage as required
Selenium	Cardiomyopathy	Only rare case reports. Add selenium to infusate if sole source of nutrition for >1 mo
Zinc	Diarrhea Poor growth Alopecia Desquamating rash Low serum zinc Low alkaline phosphatase	Document level of intake; alter dosage as required
Carnitine	Cardiomyopathy Encephalopathy Nonketotic hypoglycemia Hypotonia Poor growth Frequent infections	Supplement with parenteral levocarnitine if documented deficiency exists.

* Consult clinical pharmacist for assistance in determining method of delivery; see following chapters for guidance in determining appropriate dosage levels.

Most complications can be avoided. Careful biochemical monitoring and prompt intervention when appropriate is imperative. Solution mixing errors are a frequent cause of sudden changes in glucose and electrolyte levels. Complication rates are minimized when PN is administered with strict adherence to established protocols.[46] PN should be administered and monitored by health care professionals who have been specifically trained in this delivery method. At minimum, a nurse, a clinical dietitian, and a clinical pharmacist working under the supervision of a physician, should routinely monitor the quality of the PN solution and the infant's catheter insertion site, I.V. line, nutrient intake, metabolic tolerance, and growth parameters. An occupational or physical therapist can provide innovative ways to allow normal positioning and activities for the infant to promote normal development despite the restrictions often imposed by this therapy. The development of nutrition support teams has been described elsewhere.[47-49] Chapters 9 through 13 of this book describe specific considerations for the dosage and delivery of nutrients parenterally to the high-risk neonate

References

1. Anderson TL, Muttart CR, Bieber, MA, et al. A controlled trial of glucose versus glucose and amino acids in premature infants. J Pediatr 94:947, 1979.
2. Rubecz I, Mestyan J, Varga P, et al. Energy metabolism, substrate utilization, and nitrogen balance in parenterally fed postoperative neonates and infants. J Pediatr 98:42, 1981.
3. Kerner JA Jr. Parenteral nutrition. In: Walker WA, Durie PR, Hamilton JR, et al., eds. Pediatric gastrointestinal disease: Pathophysiology, diagnosis, management. vol. 2. Philadelphia: Decker, 1991; 1645.
4. Zlotkin SH, Bryan MH, Anderson GH. Intravenous nitrogen and energy intakes required to duplicate in utero nitrogen accretion in prematurely born human infants. J Pediatr 99:115, 1981.
5. Heird WC, Greene HL. Panel report on nutritional support of pediatric patients. Am J Clin Nutr 34:1223, 1981.
6. Mayfield SR. Energy expenditure and body composition in vlbw mechanically vetilated infants during the first 3 days of life. Pediatr Res 23:487A, 1988.
7. Saini J, MacMahon P, Morgan JB, et al. Early parenteral feeding of amino acids. Arch Dis Child 64:1362, 1989.
8. Rivera Sr A, Bell EF, Bier DMh. Effect of intravenous amino acids on protein metabolism of preterm infants during the first three days of life. Pediatr Res 33:106, 1993.
9. Van Goudoever JB, Colen T, Wattimena JLD, et al. Immediate commencement of amino acid supplementation in preterm infants: effect on serum amino acid concentrations and protein kineticson the first day of life. J. Pediatr 126:785, 1995.

10. Sosenko IRS, Rodrigez-Peirce MP, Bancalare E. Effect of early initiation of intravenous lipid administration on the incidence and severity of chronic lung disease in premature infants. J Pediatr 123:975, 1993.

11. Salas-Salvado J, Molina J, Figueras J, et al. Effect of the quality of infused energy on substrate utilization in the newborn receiving total parenteral nutrition. Pediatr Res 33:112, 1993.

12. Neuzil J, Darlow BA, Inder TE. Oxidation of parenteral lipid emulsion by ambient and phototherapy lights: potential toxicity of routine parenteral feeding. J Pediatr 126:785, 1995.

13. Cochran EB, Phelps SJ, Helms RA. Parenteral nutrition in pediatric patients. Clin Pharm 7:351, 1988.

14. Gilhooly J, Lindenberg J, Reynolds JW. Survey of umbilical artery catheter practices. Clin Care Med 18:247, 1990. 15. Kerner JA. The use of umbilical catheters for parenteral nutrition. In: Manual GR, Lim BK, Ing C, Medeiros HF. Umbilical vs peripheral vein catheterization for parenteral nutrition in sick premature neonates. Yonsei Med J 33:224, 1992.

15. Kerner JA. The use of umbilical catheters for parenteral nutrition. In: Manual of Pediatric Parenteral Nutrition. Kerner JA (ed). New York: John Wiley & Sons, 1983; 303-306.

16. Kanarek KS, Kuznicki MB, Blair RC. Infusion of total parenteral nutrition via the umbilical artery. J Parenter Enter Nutr 15:71, 1991.

17. Rejjal AR, Galal MO, Nazar HM, et al. Complications of parenteral nutrition via an umbilical vein catheter. Eur J Pediatr 152:624, 1993.

18. Pereira GR, Lim BK, Ing C, medeiros HF. Umbilical vs peripheral vein catheterization for parenteral nutrition in sick premature neonates. Yonsei Med J 33:224, 1992.

19. Jewett TC Jr. Techniques with catheters and complications of total parenteral nutrition. In: Lebenthal E, ed. Total parenteral nutrition: Indications, utilization, complications, and pathophysiological considerations. New York: Raven Press, 1986; 185.

20. Storm HM, Young SL, Shandler RH. Development of pediatric and neonatal parenteral nutrition order forms. Nutr Clin Prac 10:54; 1995.

21. Eskew JA. Fiscal impact of a total nutrient admixture program at a pediatric hospital. Am J Hosp Pharm 44:111, 1987.

22. Rollins CJ, Elsberry VA, Pollack KA. Three-in-one parenteral nutrition: A safe and economical method of nutritional support for infants. J Parenter Enter Nutr 14:290, 1990.

23. Smith JL, Canham JE, Kirkland WD, et al. Effect of Intralipid, amino acids, container, temperature, and duration of storage on vitamin stability in total parenteral nutrition admixtures. J Parenter Enter Nutr 12:478, 1988.

24. Bullock L, Fitzgerald JF, Walter WV. Emulsion stability in total nutrient admixtures containing a pediatric amino acid formulation. J Parenter Enter Nutr 16:64, 1992.

25. Friel C and Bistrian B. Cycled total parenteral nutrition: is it more effective? Am J Clin Nutr 65:1078, 1997.

26. Morimoto T, Tsujinala T, Ogawa A, et al. Effects of cyclic and continuous parenteral nutrition on albumin gene transcription in rat liver. Am J Clin Nutr 65:994, 1997.

27. Collier S, Crouch J, Hendricks K, Caballer B. Use of cyclic parenteral nutrition in infants less than 6 months of age. Nutr Clin Pract, 9:65, 1994.

28. Takehara H, Hino M, Kameoka K, et al. A new method of total parenteral nutrition for surgical neonates: is it possible that cyclic tpn prevents intrahepatic vholestasis? Tokushima J Exp Med 37:97, 1990.

29. Nicol JJ, Hoaglan RL, Heitlinger LA. The prevalence of nausea and vomiting in pediatric patients receiving home parenteral nutrition. Nutr Clin Pract 10:189, 1995.

30. Price PT, Garde KA, Flammang MA, et al. Identifying priorities for a nutrition support team in a neonatal intensive care unit. American Society for Parenteral and Enteral Nutrition, 14th Clin Cong abstr, 1990; 438.

31. Agarwal KC, Khan MAA, Falla A, et al. Cardiac perforation from central venous catheters: Survival after cardiac tamponade in an infant. Pediatrics 73:333, 1984.

32. Leibovitz E, Ashkenazi A, Levin S, et al. Fatal cardiac tamponade complicating total parenteral nutrition via a Silastic central vein catheter (ltr). J Pediatr Gastroenterol Nutr 7:306, 1988.

33. Hofmann AF. Defective biliary secretion during total parenteral nutrition: probable mechanisms and possible solutions. J Pediatr Gastroenterol Nutr 20:376, 1995.

34. Roslyn JJ, Berquist WE, Pitt HA, et al. Increased risk of gallstones in children receiving total parenteral nutrition. Pediatrics 71:784, 1983.

35. Gutcher G, Cutz E. Complications of parenteral nutrition. Semin Perinatol 10:196, 1986.

36. Mactier H, Alroomi LG, Young DG, et al. Central venous catheterisation in very low birthweight infants. Arch Dis Child 61:449, 1986.

37. Kien CL, Ganther HE. Manifestations of chronic selenium deficiency in a child receiving total parenteral nutrition. Am J Clin Nutr 37:319, 1983.

38. Hambidge KM. Zinc deficiency in the premature infant. Pediatr Rev 6:209, 1985.

39. Arakawa T, Tamura T, Igarashi Y, et al. Zinc deficiency in two infants during total parenteral alimentation for diarrhea. Am J Clin Nutr 29:197, 1976.

40. Lockitch G, Jacobson B, Quigley G, et al. Selenium deficiency in low birth weight neonates: An unrecognized problem. J Pediatr 114:865, 1989.

41. Heller RM, Kirchner SG, O'Neill JA Jr, et al. Skeletal changes of copper deficiency in infants receiving prolonged total parenteral nutrition. J Pediatr 92:947, 1978.

42. Abumrad NN, Schneider AJ, Steel D, et al. Amino acid intolerance during prolonged total parenteral nutrition reversed by molybdate therapy. Am J Clin Nutr 34:2551, 1981.

43. Oski FA, Barness LA. Vitamin E deficiency: A previously unrecognized cause of hemolytic anemia in the premature infant. J Pediatr 70:211, 1967.

44. Sutton AM, Harvie A, Cockburn F, et al. Copper deficiency in the preterm infant of very low birth weight. Arch Dis Child 60:644, 1985.

45. Shulman RJ, DeStefano-Laine L, Petitt R, et al. Protein deficiency in premature in-fants receiving parenteral nutrition. Am J Clin Nutr 44:610, 1986.

46. Nehme AE. Nutritional support of the hospitalized patient: The team concept. JAMA 243:1906, 1980.

47. Mayfield SR, Albrecht J, Roberts L, et al. The role of the nutritional support team in neonatal intensive care. Semin Perinatol 13:88, 1989.
48. Poole RL, Kerner JA Jr. The nutrition support team. In: Kerner JA Jr, ed. Manual of pediatric parenteral nutrition. New York: John Wiley & Sons, 1983; 281.
49. Suskind RM. The nutrition support service: An organized approach to the nutritional care of the hospitalized and ambulatory pediatric patient. In: Suskind RM, ed. Textbook of pediatric nutrition. New York: Raven Press, 1981; 375.
50. Uauy R, Treen M, Hoffman DR. Essential fatty acid metabolism and requirements during development. Semin Perinatol 13:118, 1989.
51. American Academy of Pediatrics Committee on Nutrition. Use of intravenous fat emulsions in pediatric patients. Pediatrics 68:738, 1981.
52. Thureen PJ, Hay WW. Intravenous nutrition and postnatal growth of the micropremie. Clin Perinatol 27 (1):197, 2000.
53. Hay WW, Lucas A, Heird WC, et al. Workshop Summary: Nutrition of the extremely low birth weight infant. Pediatrics 104 (6):1360, 1999.
54. Putet G. Lipid metabolism of the micropremie. Clin Perinatol 27 (1):57, 2000.
55. Moss RL, Haynes AL, Pastuszyn A, Glew RH. Methionine infusion reproduces liver injury of parenteral nutrition cholestasis. Pediatr Res 45:664, 1999.

Nutritional Care for High-Risk Newborns (Rev. 3d. Ed.)
S. Groh-Wargo, M. Thompson, J. Cox, editors
© 2000, Precept Press, Inc., Chicago

9

PARENTERAL NUTRITION: FLUID AND ELECTROLYTES

Diane M. Anderson, PhD, RD, CSP, FADA

NEONATES REQUIRE WATER AND electrolytes to replace losses and to provide substrate for growth. Fluid is lost via the skin, lungs, stool, and urine, and electrolytes are lost via the skin, stool, and urine.[1] The goal for hydration status is to maintain normal volume and tonicity of body fluids and to prevent clinical and biochemical signs of dehydration or water intoxication.[2] Fluid and electrolyte guidelines for the premature neonate can serve only as a rough estimate because of the many variables that alter insensible water loss (IWL) or renal excretion.[3] Fluid and electrolyte homeostasis in the preterm neonate differs from that of the full-term newborn due to differences in body composition, clinical condition, neuroendocrine control of fluid, and renal function immaturity.[4]

Components of Neonatal Fluid and Electrolyte Balance

Body fluid composition changes throughout gestation and rapidly after birth (see Chapter 2, Figure 2.1).[4] With the length of gestation, the fetus's total body water and extracellular water (ECW) decrease, and intracellular water increases.[4] Total body water and ECW continue to decrease after birth, with the greatest percentage of change occurring with the tiniest infants.[4,5]

Provision of fluids and electrolytes during the first few days of life must allow for the normal transition of body fluid from fetal to neonatal status.[4] Fluid overload during the first weeks of life has been reported to be associated with the development of congestive heart failure-patent ductus arteriosus,[6,7] necrotizing enterocolitis,[8] bronchopulmonary dysplasia,[9,10] and intraventricular hemorrhage.[11,12] Lorenz et al. report that by controlling the percentage of fluid loss, these complications do not occur.[13] They allow for a daily decrease in body weight of 1-2% or 3-5% for a total of 8-15% loss from birth weight.[13] Neonates generally lose 5-15% of their birth weight during the first week of life.[14] The extremely low birth weight infant may lose up to 20% of birth weight without complications.[15]

Preterm neonates have an increased IWL due to the immaturity of their skin.[14,16] The epidermis is thin, has a high water content, and has increased permeability.[14] The large body-surface-area-to-weight ratio in the premature infant further enhances IWL.[14] Respiratory insensible water losses are one third of total IWL.[4] The use of humidified inspired air can greatly decrease these losses.[4]

Neonatal renal function is immature, especially in the infant of < 34 weeks' gestation.[17] Glomerular filtration rate and the distal and proximal tubular functions are decreased.[17] These functions mature with increasing postnatal age.[4] The premature infant has a limited ability to concentrate urine.[4] Premature infants concentrate urine up to 500-700 mOsm/L, term infants up to 800 mOsm/L, and adults up to 1,200 mOsm/L.[14] At the same time, fluid loads are not handled rapidly by the premature neonate, which may lead to overhydration.[4,5] Several recent reports provide an overview of the hormonal control of renal function.[4,5,17-19]

The extremely low birth weight infant is prone to hyperkalemia during the first few days of life.[3,20] This electrolyte abnormality reflects the shift of potassium from the intracellular to the extracellular fluid compartment and the infant's immature renal function. The infant's decreased glomerular filtration rate and fractional excretion of sodium limits renal potassium secretion.[20] This prediuretic phase (in which renal excretion of fluid and electrolytes is minimal) represents the newborn infant's transition period. As the infant progresses to the diuretic phase, fluid, electrolyte, and weight loss occurs. Hypokalemia is a risk unless adequate potassium is provided.[21] Improved homeostasis of fluid and electrolytes occurs within the first week of life in the postdiuretic phase.[3]

Suggested Guidelines for Fluid and Electrolyte Administration

Fluid administration guidelines reflect only an estimate of fluid needs. The steps in fluid and electrolyte management consist of estimating standard needs, adjusting these estimates by factors influ-

Table 9.1. Fluid and Electrolyte Guidelines

Nutrient	Day of life	Beginning quantity	Goal
Fluid* (ml/kg/d)	1	80-140† 60-100‡	120-160
Sodium chloride (mEq/kg/d)	2-5	1-3	2-5
Potassium (mEq/kg/d)	2	1-3	2-3

* Small infants often will require higher fluid volumes due to increased insensible water losses. Total fluids can be advanced by 10-20 ml/kg/d as indicated by fluid and electrolyte assessment.
† Fluid guidelines for the infant nursed under a radiant warmer or dry incubator.
‡ Fluid guidelines for the infant nursed in a humidified incubator or under a radiant warmer with a plastic blanket.

Table 9.2. Electrolyte Content of Body Fluids (mEq/L)*

Fluid source	Na+	K+	Cl-
Stomach	20-80	5-20	100-150
Small intestine	100-140	5-15	90-120
Bile	120-140	5-15	90-120
Ileostomy	45-135	3-15	20-120
Diarrheal stool	10-90	10-80	10-110
Cerebrospinal fluid	130-150	2-5	110-130

* Adapted with permission from Bell EF, Oh W. Fluid and electrolyte management. In: Avery GB, Fletcher MA, MacDonald MG, eds. Neonatology: Pathophysiology and Management of the Newborn. 4th ed. Philadelphia: Lippincott, 1994; 312.

encing needs, continuous monitoring of fluid and electrolyte balance, and adjusting administration as indicated.[3,4,14]

For the term newborn, fluid need on the first day of life may be as low as 60 ml/kg/day.[4] This baseline value is represented by an IWL of 20 ml/kg/day and renal losses of 40-50 ml/kg/day.[4] As the infant matures, fluid needs will increase to 120-150 ml/kg/day to allow for increases in renal solute load, stool water output, and infant growth.[14] Increased intake of protein and electrolytes for growth will necessitate increased renal water needs. Stool water losses are 5-10 ml/kg/day for term and preterm infants.[4,22] Water comprises 70% of tissue growth, so a weight gain of 25-30 g/kg/day would demand 20-25 ml water per kilogram daily.[14] For the preterm infant, baseline fluid needs are approximately 80 ml/kg/day on day of life one.[4] This 80 ml is represented by 60 ml for IWL, 40 ml for urine production, and a negative 20 ml for the desired negative water balance.[4] IWL is highly variable in the preterm infant, dictating a minimum of daily fluid and electrolyte assessment during the first week of life.[4,14] Suggested guidelines for fluid and electrolytes are given in Table 9.1.[14,15,23]

Electrolytes are generally not administered on the first day of life.[14,17] Sodium is added once diuresis begins and potassium after urinary flow is established.[16] Generally, requirements are the same for preterm and full-term newborns. Greater electrolyte intake may be indicated with vomiting, diarrhea, or ileostomy drainage.[4] Fluid output can be analyzed for the actual electrolyte concentrations, or electrolyte content of body fluids can be estimated using Table 9.2. To correct for hyponatremia, fluid restriction is usually the treatment of choice, since fluid overload is frequently the cause.[17,19] Sodium supplementation is indicated when the infant has not received adequate sodium or is losing excessive sodium.[12] The equation used to correct for hyponatremia is: sodium intake required (mEq/day) equals plasma sodium desired (mEq/L) minus present plasma sodium level (mEq/L) times total body fluid (0.6 L/kg).[17] This equation is used as a tool to estimate sodium replacement. Often half of the replacement will be given over a 24-hour period, and then the patient will be reevaluated for additional supplementation.

Factors that Alter Fluid and Electrolyte Requirements

Various factors will change fluid and electrolyte needs. They are summarized below.[4,12,14-16,24-39] These elements should be addressed when deciding the fluid volume and electrolyte levels to be provided. Medications that alter electrolyte status are listed in Appendix E.

Factors That Increase Insensible Water Loss

- Increased activity (motor, crying, etc.)
- Respiratory distress
- Low relative humidity
- High ambient temperature
- Fever
- Extremely low birth weight
- Inverse relation to gestational age
- Metabolic acidosis (increased respiratory loss)
- Cardiac disease (increased respiratory loss)
- Skin breakdown, injury, or congenital defects
- Phototherapy (increases IWL 30-50% except in a thermally stable environment)
- Radiant warmer (increases IWL 40-50%)

- Radiant warmer and phototherapy together have a further 44% increase over radiant warmer by itself

Factors That Decrease Insensible Water Loss

- Humidified incubator (decreases IWL 30-75%)
- Plastic heat shield with incubator (decreases IWL 10-30%)
- Plastic blanket with radiant warmer (decreases IWL 30-70%)
- Humidifying inspired gas
- Double-wall incubator
- Semipermeable polyurethane membrane
- Topical agents

Miscellaneous Fluid Losses

- Chest tube drainage
- Ileostomy drainage
- Gastric suction
- Vomiting
- Third space loss
- External ventriculostomy
- Diarrhea
- Phototherapy (increases stool water losses)
- Glycosuria (increases urinary water losses)
- High renal solute load (increases urine fluid loss)

Conditions Indicating Need for Fluid Restriction

- Renal failure
- Congestive heart failure, significant patent ductus arteriosus
- Postoperative status-inappropriate antidiuretic hormone secretion with decreased urine output
- Meningitis

Early Neonatal Hypocalcemia

Hypocalcemia is defined as a total serum calcium of less than 8.0 mg/dL (2.0 mmol/L) for the term infant and less than 7.0 mg/dL for the preterm infant.[40] Often, less than 7.0 mg/dL is used for all neonates.[40] A range of ionized calcium levels (less than 4.8-2.5 mg/dL [1.2-0.62 mmol/L]) has been reported.[40] Quantified levels of ionized calcium will vary by the type of instrument employed to quantify ionized calcium levels.[40] In addition, ionized calcium levels will decrease in the presence of high serum albumin, phosphorus, and magnesium levels, as well as a high blood pH concentration.[40] Clinical signs of hypocalcemia are neuromuscular hypersensitivity, muscle twitching, or convulsions.[41] These clinical signs may also be seen with asphyxia, central nervous system injury or malformation, sepsis, hypoglycemia, hypomagnesemia, and narcotic withdrawal.[41]

After birth, serum calcium levels fall because of the sudden cessation of placental calcium flow, decreased release of parathyroid hormone, and elevated calcitonin levels.[4] Serum calcium levels will be normal by 24-48 hours in the healthy, term infant.[40] Infants at risk for hypocalcemia are those who (1) are premature, (2) were asphyxiated at birth, (3) have mothers with diabetes, (4) have hypoparathyroidism secondary to maternal hyperparathyroidism, (5) undergo phototherapy, or (6) were exposed to anticonvulsants in utero.[41] Serum calcium levels should be monitored daily until stable for these high-risk neonates.[40]

Most infants will be asymptomatic, and their serum calcium levels will increase without calcium supplementation.[41] Because the infant is often asymptomatic, routine supplementation is controversial.[41,43] However, the practice of initiating parenteral nutrition within the first 24 hours of life may aid in calcium homeostasis. Potential complications from I.V. supplementation include bradycardia, cardiac arrest, and skin sloughing from I.V.. line infiltration.[44] Oral supplementation has been associated with gastric irritation, diarrhea, and necrotizing enterocolitis.[44]

Preventive or treatment therapy consists of a dosage of 25-75 mg/kg/day of I.V. elemental calcium.[41,42] A 10% calcium gluconate I.V.. solution can be used parenterally or enterally.[41] Intravenously, the dosage should be given over a 24-hour period and can be administered in the parenteral nutrition solution. Enterally, the calcium supplement of 75-110 mg/kg/day should be divided into every 4- or 6-hour dosages.[42]

Additional laboratory evaluation with persistent hypocalcemia may include serum phosphorus, magnesium, vitamin D, parathyroid, and calcitonin levels.[40,42] Hypomagnesemia can be a cause of early onset hypocalcemia; it is often found in infants of diabetic mothers.[42] Hypomagnesemia may be associated with decreased release of parathyroid hormone, decreased intestinal calcium absorption, decreased renal calcium reabsorption, and decreased bone calcium release. Restoring magnesium levels will usually correct the hypocalcemia as well. Additional reviews elaborate on the pathology of neonatal hypocalcemia.[40-43]

Monitoring

Hydration may be monitored by daily assessment of the following: (1) intake of fluids and electrolytes; (2) volume of urine output; (3) serum electrolytes; (4) blood urea nitrogen (BUN); (5) serum creatinine; (6) urine specific gravity and/or osmolality; (7) electrolyte output; (8) clinical assessment by physical exam; and (9) daily or twice daily weighing.[4,14] Caloric, electrolyte and fluid intake, urine output, and weight changes are assessed together to differentiate between tissue gain or hydration alterations.

Clinical signs of dehydration include dry skin, dry mucous membranes, and sunken fontanel and eyes.[4] These signs are often difficult to assess with the extremely low birth weight infant since many clinical therapies themselves have a drying effect on the skin and mucous membranes.[4,5] Additional signs of dehydration are hypotension, tachycardia, mottled skin, hypothermia, and metabolic acidosis.[4] Serum sodium is elevated, urine output decreases, urine specific gravity increases, and weight loss occurs.[3,4] Overhydration can be demonstrated by edema, weight gain, dilute urine, and low serum sodium; pulmonary edema and congestive heart failure may result.[4]

Urine output should be 1-3 ml/kg/hour.[4] During diuresis, urine output may increase to 5-7 ml/kg/hour.[5] Urine specific gravity should be 1.005-1.015 and urine osmolarity should be kept under 300 mOsm/L.[4] Urine specific gravity can accurately estimate urine osmolarity except when glycosuria or proteinuria are present.[5]

In summary, fluid balance assessment is a continuous process with the preterm newborn. These infants must be constantly assessed due to the great variations in fluid requirements by gestational age, postnatal age, environmental factors, and clinical condition. An estimate of fluid needs should be decided, provided, and then evaluated daily.

References

1. Fomon SJ, Ziegler EE. Water and renal solute load. In: Fomon SJ, ed. Nutrition of Normal Infants. St. Louis: Mosby, 1993; 91.
2. Fanaroff AA, Hack M. Water. In: Sunshine P, ed. Feeding the neonate weighing less than 1500 grams. Nutrition and beyond. Columbus: Ross Laboratories, 1980; 3.
3. Lorenz JM, Kleinman LI, Ahmed G, et al. Phases of fluid and electrolyte homeostasis in the extremely low birth weight infant. Pediatrics 96:484, 1995.
4. Bell EF, Oh W. Fluid and electrolyte management. In: Avery GB, Fletcher MA, MacDonald MG, eds. Neonatology: Pathophysiology and Management of the Newborn. 4th ed. Philadelphia: Lippincott, 1994; 312.
5. Shaffer SG, Weismann DN. Fluid requirements in the preterm infant. Clin Perinatol 19:233, 1992.
6. Stevenson JG. Fluid administration in the association of patent ductus arteriosus complicating respiratory distress syndrome. J Pediatr 90:257, 1977.

7. Bell EF, Warburton D, Stonestreet BS, et al. Effect of fluid administration on the development of symptomatic patent ductus arteriosus and congestive heart failure in premature infants. N Engl J Med 302:598, 1980.

8. Bell EF, Warburton D, Stonestreet BS, et al. High-volume fluid intake predisposes premature infants to necrotising enterocolitis. Lancet 2:90, 1979.

9. Brown ER, Stark A, Sosenko I, et al. Bronchopulmonary dysplasia: Possible relationship to pulmonary edema. J Pediatr 92:982, 1978.

10. Van Marter LJ, Leviton A, Allred EN, et al. Hydration during the first days of life and the risk of bronchopulmonary dysplasia in low birth weight infants. J Pediatr 116:942, 1990.

11. Goldberg RN, Chung D, Goldman SL, et al. The association of rapid volume expansion and intraventricular hemorrhage in the preterm infant. J Pediatr 96:1060, 1980.

12. Costarino AT, Baumgart S. Neonatal water and elctrolyte metabolism. In: Cowett RM, ed. Principles of Perinatal-Neonatal Metabolism. 2nd ed. New York: Springer, 1998; 1045.

13. Lorenz JM, Kleinman LI, Kotagal UR, et al. Water balance in very low birth weight infants: Relationship to water and sodium and effect on outcome. J Pediatr 101:423, 1982.

14. Oh W. Fluid, electrolytes, and acid-base homeostasis. In: Fanaroff AA, Martin RJ, eds. Neonatal-Perinatal Medicine. Diseases of the Fetus and Infant, vol 1, 6th ed. St. Louis: Mosby, 1997; 622.

15. Costarino AT, Baumgart S. Water as nutrition. In: Tsang RC, Lucas A, Uauy R, Zlotkin S, eds. Nutritional Needs of the Preterm Infant. Baltimore: Williams & Wilkins, 1993; 1.

16. Fanaroff AA, Wald M, Gruber HS, et al. Insensible water loss in low birth weight infants. Pediatrics 50:236, 1972.

17. Seri I, Evans J. Acid-base, fluid, and electrolyte management. In: Taeusch HW, Ballard RA, eds. Avery's Diseases of the Newborn. 7th ed. Philadelphia: Saunders, 1998; 372.

18. Arant BS. Sodium, chloride, and potassium. In: Tsang RC, Lucas A, Uauy R, Zlotkin S, eds. Nutritional Needs of the Preterm Infant. Baltimore: Williams & Wilkins, 1993; 157.

19. Modi N. Hyponatraemia in the newborn. Arch Dis Child Fetal Neonatol Ed 78:F81, 1998.

20. Lorenz JM, Kleinman LI, Markarian K. Potassium metabolism in extremely low birth weight infants in the first week of life. J Pediatr 131:81, 1997.

21. Sato K, Kondo T, Iwao H, et al. Internal potassium shift in premature infants: Cause of nonoliguric hyperkalemia. J Pediatr 126:109, 1995.

22. Patrick CH, Pittard WB. Stool water loss in very-low-birth-weight neonates. Clinical Pediatr 27:144, 1988.

23. Hansen JW. Consensus recommendations. In: Tsang RC, Lucas A, Uauy R, Zlotkin S, eds. Nutritional Needs of the Preterm Infant. Baltimore: Williams & Wilkins, 1993; 287.

24. Agren J, Sjors G, Sedin G. Transepidermal water loss in infants born at 24 and 25 weeks of gestation. Acta Paediatr 87:1185, 1998.

25. Kjartansson S, Hammarlund K, Sedin G. Insensible water loss from the skin during phototherapy in term and preterm infants. Acta Paediatr 81:764, 1992.

26. Kjartansson S, Hammarlund K, Riesenfeld T, et al. Respiratory water loss and oxygen consumption in newborn infants during phototherapy. Acta Paediatr 81:769, 1992.

27. Kjartansson S, Arsan S, Hammarlund K, et al. Water loss from the skin of term and preterm infants nursed under a radiant heater. Pediatr Res 37:233, 1995.

28. Marks KH, Friedman Z, Maisels MJ. A simple device for reducing insensible water loss in low-birth-weight infants. Pediatrics 60:223, 1977.

29. Baumgart S. Reduction of oxygen consumption, insensible water loss, and radiant heat demand with use of a plastic blanket for low-birth-weight infants under radiant warmers. Pediatrics 74:1022, 1984.

30. Sosulski R, Polin RA, Baumgart S. Respiratory water loss and heat balance in intubated infants receiving humidified air. J Pediatr 103:307, 1983.

31. Yeh TF, Voora S, Lilien LD, et al. Oxygen consumption and insensible water loss in single- versus double-walled incubator. J Pediatr 97:967, 1980.

32. Bell EF, Neidich GA, Cashore WJ, et al. Combined effect of radiant warmer and phototherapy on insensible water loss in low-birth-weight infants. J Pediatr 94:810, 1979.

33. Nopper AJ, Horii KA, Sookdeo-Drost S, et al. Topical ointment therapy benefits premature infants. J Pediatr 128:660, 1996.

34. Vernon HJ, Lane AT, Wischerath LJ, et al. Semipermeable dressing and transepidermal water loss in premature infants. Pediatrics 86:377, 1990.

35. Knauth A, Gordin M, McNelis W, et al. Semipermeable polyurethane membrane as an artificial skin for the premature neonate. Pediatrics 83:945, 1989.

36. Cartlidge PHT, Rutter N. Skin barrier function. In: Polin RA, Fox WW, eds. Fetal and Neonatal Physiology, vol 1. 2nd ed. Philadelphia: Saunders, 1998; 771.

37. Bell EF, Gray JC, Weinstein MR, et al. The effects of thermal environment on heat balance and insensible water loss in low-birth-weight infants. J Pediatr 96:452, 1980.

38. Reynolds DW, Dweck HS, Cassady G. Inappropriate antidiuretic hormone secretion in a neonate with meningitis. Am J Dis Child 123:251; 1972.

39. Denne SC, Clark SE, Poindexter BB, et al. Nutrition and metabolism in the high-risk neonate. In: Fanaroff AA, Martin RJ, eds. Neonatal-Perinatal Medicine. Diseases of the Fetus and Infant, vol 1. 6th ed. St. Louis: Mosby, 1997; 562.

40. Mimouni F, Tsang RC. Pathophysiology of neonatal hypocalcemia. In: Polin RA, Fox WW, eds. Fetal and Neonatal Physiology, vol 2, 2nd ed. Philadelphia: Saunders, 1998; 2329.

41. Demarini S, Mimouni FB, Tsang RC. Metabolic and endocrine disorders, Pt 2: Disorders of calcium, phosphorus, and magnesium metabolism. In: Fanaroff AA, Martin RJ, eds. Neonatal-Perinatal Medicine. Diseases of the Fetus and Infant, vol 2. 6th ed. St. Louis: Mosby, 1997; 1463.

42. Kliegman RM. Problems in metabolic adaptation: Glucose, calcium, and magnesium. In: Klaus MH, Fanaroff AA. eds. Care of the High Risk Neonate. 4th ed. Philadelphia: Saunders, 1993; 282.

43.   Greer FR. Disorders of calcium homeostasis. In: Spitzer AR, ed. Intensive Care of the Fetus and Neonate. St. Louis: Mosby, 1996; 993.
44.   Young TE, Mangum OB. Neofax: A Manual of Drugs Used in Neonatal Care. 10th ed. Raleigh, N.C.: Acorn Publishing, 1997.

Nutritional Care for High-Risk Newborns (Rev. 3d. Ed.)
S. Groh-Wargo, M. Thompson, J. Cox, editors
© 2000, Precept Press, Inc., Chicago

10

PARENTERAL NUTRITION: ENERGY, CARBOHYDRATE, PROTEIN, AND FAT

Amy L. Sapsford, RD, CSP, LD

Energy

ENERGY IS REQUIRED FOR all vital functions of the body. It is required to meet demands of the circulatory, respiratory, neurological, and muscular systems. At the cellular level, energy is required for the continuous catabolism and anabolism cycles of body tissue turnover, transport systems, and for the regulation of body temperature.[1] Parenteral energy needs are based on basal metabolic rates, thermal stresses, physical activity, and growth allowances.[1-4] Energy requirements in parenterally fed newborns are lower than in those enterally fed because there are no energy requirements of digestion or fecal losses due to incomplete absorption.

Sick, premature infants given 60 kcal/kg/day in a solution containing glucose alone or glucose and crystalline amino acids (CAA) may not gain weight.[5] However, infants who receive 2.5 g protein/kg/day as CAA may achieve slightly positive nitrogen (N) balance, whereas those who receive only glucose may be in negative N balance.[5] At a constant N intake, increasing energy intake from 50 to 80 kcal/kg/day may result in a significant increase in N retention and weight gain. When infants are given > 70 nonprotein kcal/kg/day and 2.7-3.5 g protein/kg/day, intrauterine N accretion and growth rates can be duplicated.[6] If protein needs are met, infants generally require at least 70 nonprotein kcal/kg/day parenterally to achieve growth. Many factors affect calorie needs, including infection and chronic lung disease.[7]

Table 10.1   Total Parenteral Nutrition Guidelines in the Newborn

Nutrient	Initial dose		Advancement[1]		Maximum		Recommended initiation and distribution[2,3]
Gestational Age:	*Premature*	*Term*	*Premature*	*Term*	*Premature*	*Term*	*Infants*
Glucose infusion mg/kg/min	5-7	7-9	1-2	1-2	Progress to achieve calorie goals, balanced solution, euglycemia, and growth	Peripheral: 11-12 Central: ≈ 14-16	60-70% of total **non-protein** calories or remainder of energy intake not supplied by lipid source
% Dextrose in water solution (3.4 kcal/g)	10% or less[4]	10%[4]	Depends on fluid volume infused. If fluid needs are extremely high, dextrose % may need to be decreased.		Peripheral: 12.5% Central: 20%[5]	Peripheral 12.5% Central: 25%[5]	Start immediately after birth on day 1
Protein g/kg/d (4.0 kcal/g)	1.0-1.5	1.0-1.5	1.0	1.0	2.5-3.5	2.5-3.5	Start day 1-2
Lipid g/kg/d (10 kcal/g for 20%)	0.5-1.0 Use of 20% recommended	0.5-1.0	0.25-0.5[6]	0.5[6]	3[7]	3-4[7]	May contribute 30-40% of total **non-protein** calories, but should not exceed 60%
Lipid g/kg/hr	0.02-0.04	0.02-0.04	Gradually increases with rate increases[6]		0.125	0.15 over 24 hr	Start day 2-3 over 24 hr
Non-protein energy kcal/kg/d	30-44	40-53	Gradually increases with rate increases		Peripheral: 90-120 Central: up to 130[8]		Monitor growth and adjust energy intake and protein as needed

Comments:
1. Gradual increases in all nutrients are usually well tolerated. Monitor tolerance.
2. Recommendation for initiation of therapy based on inability of infant to tolerate sufficient enteral feedings.
3. Non-protein calories: g nitrogen: To promote efficient protein utilization and to prevent its use as an energy source, range of 150-200 nonprotein calories: g N are required. One gram protein yields 0.16 g N.
4. If fluid needs are extremely high, dextrose % should be decreased. Ratio may be low in infants with glucose intolerance or limited lipid intake.
5. If clinical condition dictates, maximum dextrose infusion may be exceeded but is not recommended routinely. Example: Infusion of 200 ml/kg/day of dextrose 5% yields 7 mg/kg/min glucose.
6. May need to hold at 1 g/kg for up to 1 week in ELBW infants with respiratory compromise.
7. Lipids may need to be limited in certain clinical conditions such as sepsis or hyperbilirubinemia to 1-2 g/kg/day.
8. Maximum central calories are usually not required for optimal growth but may be required with increased needs such as wound healing, cardiac defect, sepsis, etc.

Studies have evaluated the appropriate composition, or fuel mix, of nonprotein calories. Infants with respiratory compromise present daily challenges for clinicians. Ventilator-dependent infants with mild bronchopulmonary dysplasia given moderate glucose loads of 14 g/kg/day and lower fat loads of < 1 g/kg/day appear to compensate for the increased carbon dioxide production when compared with infants given the same calories but increased lipid doses of 2 g/kg/day.[8] In the surgical neonate, positive N balance with glucose and amino acids may be unchanged when lipid is substituted for glucose as a non-protein energy source.[9] The addition of nonprotein calories as fat emulsion to the glucose and protein solutions in the surgical neonate may significantly decrease the protein contribution to energy expenditure and improve protein retention.[10] This is true in nonsurgical infants as well.[11]

Even though one energy source may not be better than another, the use of lipid is appropriate to avoid the metabolic consequences of excess glucose loads. For an intake of 60-80 nonprotein kcal/kg/day, glucose and fat provide equivalent nitrogen-sparing effects in the newborn.[12] When maintenance energy needs are met, the infant's clinical condition rather than the source of energy affects the participation of amino acids in energy metabolism. Infants on a constant protein intake and glucose as the only energy source may have higher protein turnover, breakdown, and amino acid oxidation rates than infants given both glucose and lipid as the source of nonprotein energy.[13] Most studies reinforce the need for a "balanced" total parenteral nutrition (TPN) solution containing both dextrose and lipid as nonprotein energy sources. Data on newborn infants suggest that optimal nitrogen retention results when nonprotein calories are provided as 60-70% carbohydrate and 30-40% fat.[14,15] Balancing the fuel mix may prevent excessive fat deposition.[16]

To promote efficient protein utilization and to prevent its use as an energy source, a nonprotein energy intake of 22 kcal/g of amino acid intake,[17] or about 150-200 nonprotein calories per gram of N are required.[2] For example, if the infant is receiving 100 nonprotein kcal/kg/day and 3 g protein/kg/day, the calculation of nonprotein calorie per gram N ratio is as follows:

$$100 \text{ kcal/kg} \div 0.48 \text{ g N} = 208 \text{ nonprotein kcal/g N}$$
$$1 \text{ g protein yields } 0.16 \text{ g N}$$

It is not possible to achieve this goal in initial TPN solutions when protein intake is low, or if glucose or lipid intake is restricted. Once the TPN is advanced to optimal levels of all nutrients, the goal can be achieved. (See Table 10.1 for recommended distribution of calories and quick reference for administration guidelines.)[2,4,18]

Indirect calorimetry, technically difficult in small babies, estimates daily energy expenditure of VLBW infants at 50-70 kcal/kg/d.[19,20] Indirect calorimetry measures oxygen consumption and carbon dioxide production. By using the volume of oxygen consumed and carbon dioxide produced, resting energy expenditure (REE) and respiratory quotient (RQ) can be calculated. Studies using flow-through indirect calorimetry with face mask, head hood and canopy breath sampling have been done.[21]

Factors affecting total energy expenditure and therefore energy needs include weight, gestational age, postnatal age, sex, environment, feeding regimen and composition, activity, and rate of growth and development.[22] Clinical conditions that increase caloric requirements include fever, cardiac failure, major surgery, burns, severe sepsis, long-term growth failure, protein-calorie malnutrition and bronchopulmonary dysplasia.[23-25] (see Chapter 21). Drugs such as theophylline act as a central nervous system (CNS) stimulant, which could affect energy needs.[26] Kangaroo care, or the practice of holding a premature infant against the parent's chest, has no adverse effects on energy expenditure.[27]

Specific documentation of energy needs using indirect calorimetry is not feasible in many centers. An equation has been developed to predict resting energy expenditure in surgical infants from birth to 5 months.[28] This may be a more practical approach. The equation is:

$$\text{REE (kcal/min)} =$$
$$-74.436 + (34.661 \times \text{weight in kg}) + (0.496 \times \text{heart rate in beats/min}) + (0.178 \times \text{age in days}).[28]$$

REE can be converted to kcal/kg/day by multiplying by 1.44 and dividing by weight in kg. Total energy requirements can be estimated as REE plus energy requirements for growth.[28] Energy requirements for growth are approximately 5 kcal/g of deposited tissue.[29] If an infant is gaining 10 g/kg/day, additional calorie needs would amount to 50 kcal/kg/day.[28] In reality, the goal of most clinicians is to maximize all components of TPN in high-risk infants within their ability to tolerate the substrates, while monitoring growth.

Carbohydrate

Glucose functions as an energy source for all cells, but it is essential for the CNS, erythrocytes, and other tissues such as the retina and renal medulla.[1] The brain uses as much as 90% of total glucose consumption.[30] Endogenous glucose production may provide only one third of the total glucose needed by preterm infants.[31] Dextrose (d-glucose) is the first and major source of nonprotein calories given to an infant requiring I.V. therapy to prevent hypoglycemia. Dextrose is commercially available in concentrations ranging from 2½ to 70% and can be diluted to any percentage required by the infant.[32] Because of the molecule of water incorporated into the monohydrate form of the dextrose molecule, the caloric value is 3.4 cal/g, rather than 4 cal/g assigned to enteral carbohydrates.

The osmolarity of the dextrose solution varies with concentration and with additives such as sodium chloride. Only a 5% dextrose in water solution is isotonic to serum. Most infants are managed with peripheral PN. Infusion of high concentrations of dextrose in peripheral lines is associated with an increased incidence of phlebitis, infiltration sequelae such as skin sloughing, and decreased life span of the line.[2,33] Infusion of ≤ 12.5% dextrose peripherally is usual clinical practice. Central lines are used for long-term I.V. access and for long-term nutrition in the extremely low birth weight (ELBW) infant or the surgical neonate. Central venous lines or percutaneous intravenous central catheters allow for infusion of greater concentrations of glucose and other nutrients such as calcium or sodium bicarbonate. They can also be used for drugs that irritate peripheral veins. A maximum concentration of 25% dextrose for central lines is the general rule.[34] This concentration is sometimes exceeded if fluids are restricted due to clinical conditions such as ECMO or renal failure.

Infants weighing < 1,000 g can generally tolerate initial glucose infusions of 6 mg/kg/min. Infants weighing > 1,000 g up to term newborns can tolerate infusions of 8 mg/kg/min initially.[35] To calculate glucose infusion, use the following equation:

$$g/kg/day \ dextrose \times 1,000 =$$
$$mg/kg/day \ dextrose \div 1,440 \ min/day =$$
$$mg/kg/min \ glucose$$

Infants with central lines generally tolerate gradual increases in glucose loads. A range of 10-30 g/kg of dextrose is recommended by the American Academy of Pediatrics (AAP).[36] Glucose loads of > 26 mg/kg/min may not be beneficial and may contribute to fatty infiltration of the liver.[36] Clinically, most infants will not require the maximum recommendation. A balanced solution with adequate calories > 100 kcal/kg/day will be achieved with a glucose infusion of < 20 mg/kg/min.

Example 10.A.

Patient weight	Fluid needs	Dextrose concentrations	Glucose infusion
0.5 kg	200 ml/kg	5.0 %	7.0 mg/kg/min
1.0 kg	80 ml/kg	10.0 %	5.5 mg/kg/min
1.5 kg	150 ml/kg	12.5 %	13.0 mg/kg/min
2.0 kg	120 ml/kg	20.0 %	16.6 mg/kg/min

Monitoring Tolerance of Carbohydrate Infusion

Regardless of the infusion rate, the infant on I.V. dextrose should be monitored closely, especially in the first 48 hours, or as the glucose infusion rate is increased.[2] Hypoglycemia can occur if the solution containing dextrose is abruptly stopped.[35,36] This may be the result of limited glycogen stores or high circulating levels of insulin when the glucose concentration is high.[35] Some other causes of hypoglycemia include: small for gestational age (SGA) infant, infant of diabetic mother (IDM), prematurity, and asphyxia. Symptoms of hypoglycemia include apnea, cyanosis, hypotonia, seizures, and tachypnea, among others.[37] Treatment of a parenterally fed infant with hypoglycemia is determined by the severity of the symptoms and may include increasing the glucose concentration and/or administering a bolus of dextrose. Some infants can tolerate a window in their parenteral nutrition therapy. This is most frequently done with home TPN. Their parenteral infusion may be tapered off by running the solution at half rate for one hour to prevent hypoglycemia[38] (see Chapter 8).

Hyperglycemia may be caused by decreased insulin production or insulin resistance, increased hepatic glucose production, excessive glucose infusion rates, or other causes.[2] When hyperglycemia and glycosuria occur, the infant may develop dehydration from osmotic diuresis, which may lead to calcium and sodium losses.[35] A decrease in the glucose infusion is indicated. If hyperglycemia occurs in an infant who was tolerating a stable infusion of glucose, the infant should be evaluated for sepsis.[2] Surgical stress can also affect the infant's ability to metabolize glucose.[39] Hyperglycemia can also occur with the use of steroids such as dexamethasone, which may be used in the treatment of very low birth weight (VLBW) infants with lung disease.[40,41] Close monitoring of blood and urine is essential. Some infants who receive infusions high in carbohydrate may tolerate them without signs of hyperglycemia but may have increased carbon dioxide production. This may result in carbon dioxide retention and respiratory acidosis in infants with pulmonary problems.[35] Long-term infusions of considerable amounts of I.V. dextrose will result in fatty infiltration of the liver.[42] Other disadvantages of using dextrose as the major or sole source of nonprotein energy include essential fatty acid deficiency; increased basal metabolism; and increased secretion of insulin, catecholamines, and cortisol.[1] Excess glucose loads may affect respiratory function by raising the respiratory quotient (RQ), resulting in increased CO_2 production.[43] Infusion of a combination of carbohydrate and fat in appropriate proportions should help avoid or resolve these problems.

Insulin

The use of insulin in the newborn is not routine. Continuous insulin infusion (CII) may improve tolerance of I.V. glucose in persistently hyperglycemic VLBW babies.[44] Insulin infusion may allow hyperglycemic infants to achieve energy intakes similar to normoglycemic infants.[45] In a controlled trial, increased energy intake and improved weight gain were documented with the use of insulin in the ELBW infant.[46] In a study of four ELBW infants on glucose alone, insulin produced no net protein anabolic effect. Euglycemic hyperinsulinemia was accompanied by a significant metabolic acidosis.[47] Specific guidelines are described for insulin infusion by piggyback into the infusion set for the PN fluids.[45] A method for infusion of insulin using a CII pump has also been described.[48] Insulin delivery varies with method of infusion. I.V. administration sets preflushed with insulin may deliver a more predictable amount of insulin[49] (see Chapter 12). The use of insulin may improve energy intake by allowing greater concentrations of dextrose to be used in hyperglycemic infants. Treatment varies with severity of hyperglycemia, but 1.0 mU/kg/min is an initial dose used in neonates.[37] This therapy must be used with caution and meticulous monitoring to prevent hypoglycemia and perhaps metabolic acidosis.[47] Amino acid administration soon after birth may stimulate endogenous insulin secretion and may prevent the need for insulin infusion.[18,19,50]

Protein

Protein is essential for cell maturation, remodeling, and growth as well as for functional activity of enzymes and transport proteins for all body organs.[51] Protein provides nitrogen and amino acids to the infant and must be given parenterally if the infant is unable to tolerate adequate enteral feedings. Low birthweight (LBW) infants starved during the first days after birth have protein losses of 1.0-1.2 g/kg/day.[18,19,52] The average well LBW infant receiving no exogenous protein source loses 1% of endogenous protein stores daily.[53] In the LBW infant, the generally accepted goals of protein administration are to promote "normal" plasma amino acid concentration, optimal weight gain without metabolic complications, and nitrogen retention at rates equivalent to those in utero.[54]

Amino acids essential for term infants are isoleucine, leucine, lysine, methionine, phenylalanine, threonine, tryptophan, valine, and histidine.[55] Arginine is considered semiessential for neonates because of decreased enzyme activity of arginine synthetase.[54] Tyrosine, cysteine, and taurine are considered to be essential for the premature, LBW infant due to metabolic immaturity.[52] Glutamine may be a conditionally essential amino acid for preterm babies.[56]

Table 10.2. Amino Acid Content of Selected Products: A Comparison of Estimated Amino Acid Requirements to a Protein Intake of 2.5 g/kg/day*

Amino acids	Estimated requirements (mg/kg/d)[1,2]	Aminosyn 10%[3] (mg/kg/d)	Aminosyn PF 10%[4] (mg/kg/d)	Travasol 10%[4] (mg/kg/d)	Trophamine 10%[5] (mg/kg/d)
Essential					
Term					
Isoleucine	180-200	180	190	150	205
Leucine	240-400	235	300	183	350
Lysine	120-168	180	169	145	205
Methionine	15-72	100	45	100	85
Phenylalanine	100-144	110	107	140	120
Threonine	60-144	130	128	105	105
Tryptophan	30 36	40	45	45	50
Valine	168-200	200	168	145	195
Histidine	50-58	75	78	120	120
Arginine	122-250	245	307	288	300
Considered Essential					
Preterm					
Cysteine†	72-85	0	0	0	< 4
Tyrosine	12.5-144	11	10	10	60
Taurine	-	0	18	0	6
Nonessential					
Alanine	100-144	320	174	517	135
Asparate	-	0	132	0	80
Glutamate	12.5-48	0	155	0	125
Glycine	100-396	230	96	258	95
Proline	50-192	215	203	170	170
Serine	100-166	105	124	125	95

* The amounts of amino acids listed for each product are the amounts the infant would receive on 2.5 g/kg/day of protein.

† Available as a separate additive: L-cysteine hydrochloride

1. Ghadimi H.[200]
2. Snyderman SE[201]
3. Abbott, North Chicago, Ill.
4. Clintec, Deerfield, Ill.
5. McGaw, Irvine, Calif.

Reviews on essential and nonessential amino acids have been published.[54] The content of amino acids varies with the various parenteral solutions available.[57] Standard and pediatric formulations contain levels of essential amino acids near the recommended range. Pediatric solutions contain taurine and tyrosine, and cysteine can be added separately. Estimates of requirements for these amino acids are based on fetal accretion rates and early studies in formula-fed infants.[58]

Protein hydrolysates were the first source of parenteral protein, but are no longer available.[32,59] Crystalline amino acid solutions (CAAs) have replaced protein hydrolysates and are regarded as more efficient sources of protein for physiologic usage. In the "new" formulations of CAAs, acetate is substituted for chloride in some amino acids. Thus, current formulations of CAAs are less likely to cause a metabolic acidosis than the original formulations.[32,36] CAAs are hypertonic solutions with concentrations varying from 3½ to 15% and can be diluted to any desired concentration. They are composed of a balance of essential and nonessential L-amino acids.[32] Products available include standard solutions and formulations designed to meet the specific needs of pediatric patients, patients under high metabolic stress, and those in hepatic or renal failure.[32]

Selected Amino Acid Review

Tyrosine is present in small amounts in most CAAs; however, it is insoluble in higher amounts in the L-tyrosine form. (See below for discussion of pediatric solutions.) Since tyrosine is a by-product of phenylalanine metabolism, administration of tyrosine has a sparing effect on the phenylalanine requirement. There are no recommendations for safe amounts, but excessive amounts should be avoided.[60] Transient tyrosinemia can occur due to the immature enzyme system of the newborn.[60]

Cysteine is not a component in CAAs, since it is unstable over time and will form an insoluble precipitate. It is commercially available as an additive for PN solutions.[32] Cystine and cysteine are interconvertible and their metabolic fates are identical.[60] This amino acid is synthesized from methionine in the adult, but the preterm infant lacks sufficient hepatic cystathionase to effect this conversion.[61] Cysteine is also a substrate for taurine production in children.[62] The activity of cystathionase increases with postnatal and, possibly, gestational age.[62]

Several studies have been published regarding the use of cysteine in newborns; however, its use remains controversial. Addition of cysteine to TPN given to weanling rats resulted in decreased hepatic steatosis and normalization of total plasma lipid, a common complication of TPN use in human infants.[63] Cysteine is a precursor to glutathione, which may prevent intestinal oxidative damage. Newborn premature rabbits fed a cysteine-free TPN solution had lower glutathione levels compared with those reared by their mothers or those given cysteine-containing TPN.[64] In human infants, supplementation with cysteine does not appear to improve N retention or growth, but may normalize plasma taurine concentrations.[62,65,66] Supplementation with cysteine along with histidine significantly increases urinary zinc excretion.[67]

Because addition of L-cysteine hydrochloride lowers the pH of the TPN solution, its effect on acid/base balance in the newborn was investigated.[68] With cysteine supplementation, neonates required additional acetate to prevent acidosis. The lower pH attained by using cysteine in the solution increases the solubility of supplemental calcium and phosphorus.[68] This positive effect on mineral solubility may be cysteine's most tangible benefit.

Taurine is absent from most CAAs, but is a component of the pediatric CAAs currently available.[32] Endogenous taurine synthesis occurs when the enzyme, cysteine sulphinic acid decarboxylase, converts cysteine to taurine; however, this enzyme activity may be low in the newborn.[54] Electroretinograms were abnormal in eight children on long-term taurine-free TPN solutions.[69-71] Premature and term newborns given enteral nutrition or TPN deficient in taurine have decreased plasma and urine taurine.[72] Taurine-free TPN solutions, along with the immature renal system, may result in taurine depletion in the first few weeks of life, which could have a detrimental effect on the developing brain and retina in infants.[73] No data are currently available to support the belief that taurine-containing TPN formulations will prevent TPN-induced cholestasis.[54] This hypothesis has been proposed, as infants on low intakes of taurine have altered bile salt production.[54,74]

Glutamine has generated interest in neonatal nutrition, although most studies have been done in animal models or adults. Glutamine has important functions as a fuel for intestinal epithelial cells and lymphocytes.[75] Current parenteral solutions do not contain glutamine due to solution stability issues. L-glutamine is available as L-alanyl-L-glutamine, and studies have documented its safety for use in humans.[76,77] Studies in infants demonstrate safety and suggest possible benefits when parenteral nutrition is supplemented with glutamine.[56,202] A large, multicenter trial is underway to study its effect on ELBW infants.

Composition Differences: Standard Versus Pediatric Solutions

Table 10.2 summarizes the content of four CAAs currently available and gives an estimated requirement range for each amino acid. It is important to note that the formulations may change; the reader should refer to product information from the manufacturer for the most current formulations. TrophAmine (McGaw, Irvine, Calif.) and Aminosyn PF (Abbott, North Chicago, Ill.) have been developed for use in infants. The formulation of TrophAmine uses a mathematical model intended to result in serum amino acids levels in the parenterally-fed infant similar to those of normally growing 30-day-old human milk-fed term infants. Aminosyn PF is modified from Aminosyn. The amino acid pattern of Neopham (Kabi-Vitrum, Sweden), not available in the United States, is similar to human milk protein.[53] The goal for developing the solutions for infants was to normalize plasma amino acid patterns, as well as to improve N retention and growth, and attenuate TPN-associated cholestasis seen in neonates receiving standard CAAs.

Pediatric solutions provide essential amino acids, including taurine and tyrosine.[32] TrophAmine has more tyrosine than Aminosyn PF, as the manufacturer of TyrophAmine uses a soluble form of tyrosine known as N-acetyl-L-tyrosine (NAT). Although NAT is retained by infants on TPN, the biologic availability of this source of tyrosine is uncertain.[54] Both solutions contain the nonessential amino acids glutamic acid and aspartic acid not found in other solutions. This results in lower amounts of glycine needed to balance the solutions and normalized plasma glycine concentrations in the baby.[54] The lower glycine levels in the pediatric solutions should be well tolerated, as hyperglycinemia and hyperammonemia can occur when excessive glycine is infused.[78]

Pediatric Solutions: Literature Review

Osteopenia is a possible complication in parenterally nourished VLBW newborns. As a result, calcium and phosphorus solubility in parenteral solutions has been investigated. Two studies conclude that the use of TrophAmine results in greater solubility of calcium (Ca) and phosphorus (P) compared with Aminosyn PF.[79,80] An adult formulation, Aminosyn may have increased Ca and P solubility over Aminosyn PF.[81] The addition of cysteine increases the solubility of these minerals by lowering the pH of the solution.[79] Solubility curves are published for FreAmine III (McGaw) and TrophAmine.[81,82]

Data from studies investigating the outcomes of VLBW newborns given pediatric amino acid solutions are more conflicting with regard to N retention, weight gain, and incidence of cholestasis than they are regarding mineral solubility. Several studies suggest better weight gain, improved nitrogen retention, normalized serum amino acid patterns and decreased incidence of cholestasis with the use of TrophAmine versus standard amino acid solutions intended for adults.[74,83-87] There are conflicting data,[88,89] however, and the conclusions from all of these investigations are confounded by small subject numbers, short study lengths, and inconsistent supplementation with cysteine. The equivalency of TrophAmine and Aminosyn PF is uncertain.[90,91] Despite these limitations in the literature, pediatric solutions are commonly used for VLBW infants and infants on TPN for more than a few weeks.

Other Amino Acid Solutions

The amino acid formulations for high metabolic stress and hepatic failure contain higher concentrations of the branched-chain amino acids isoleucine, leucine, and valine.[32] Formulations for patients in renal failure contain only the essential amino acids needed to promote urea reutilization.[32] The use of all of these specialized products in infants has not been studied, and their use is generally not recommended.

Protein Requirements

Parenteral protein is usually started on day of life 1-2 or as soon as serum electrolytes are stable.[18,19] If electrolytes or serum glucose concentrations are not stable, a portion of the total fluids can be written for TPN. Infants who do not receive amino acids during the first few days of life lose at least 1% of their endogenous protein stores, or ~ 1 g/kg/day.[92] Protein intakes of around 1.5 mg/kg/day started within the first few days of life in VLBW infants may be sufficient to establish positive nitrogen balance, prevent loss of protein mass, and appear to be safe.[18,19,93-97,203] Persistently low concentrations of plasma amino acids in TPN-fed newborns suggest that infused amino acids are used for protein synthesis or oxidized as energy sources.[94] Because sick preterm infants often receive only a fraction of their energy and protein needs during the first few days of life, the energy expended for metabolism is derived from body stores.[94] Minimizing the abrupt postnatal deprivation of amino acid infusion may prevent protein catabolism, glucose intolerance, and a drop in growth-regulating factors.[50]

A variety of clinical conditions affect protein metabolism in ELBW infants:

- Dexamethasone decreases growth by increasing protein breakdown.
- Insulin appears to have minimal effect on proteolysis in infants receiving only glucose.
- Exogenous growth hormone alone does not appear to be a significant anabolic agent.
- Narcotic use can enhance postoperative protein balance.[98]

Clinical conditions such as intrauterine growth retardation, sepsis, bronchopulmonary dysplasia, heart disease, and necrotizing enterocolitis and the surgery that often follows—all may increase the protein requirements of infants.[98-100]

Complications are rarely encountered with intakes of 2-3 g/kg/day for premature infants.[36] Recommendations vary, but they range from

2.0-4.0 g/kg/day for premature infants and 2.5 g/kg/day for infants up to a year.[2,18,101] Intakes of 2.7-3.5 g protein/kg/day and > 70 nonprotein kcal/kg/day result in duplication of intrauterine N accretion.[6]

Monitoring Tolerance of Protein

Protein deficiency identified by the flag sign or hair depigmentation was described in infants on a protein intake of 2.5 g/kg/day.[99] This study supports the recommendations for administration of up to 3.5 g protein/kg/day. Low serum albumin, lack of weight gain despite adequate calories, or rapid weight gain with edema may indicate inadequate intake of protein. Poor tolerance of protein may be revealed in the neonate by a rising blood urea nitrogen (BUN) level or rising serum ammonia level.[2] The liver's ability to convert ammonia to urea will determine which parameter will rise when there is impaired utilization. Prealbumin can be monitored weekly in infants on TPN.[102] Abnormal plasma aminograms, cholestatic jaundice, and hepatic dysfunction can also occur with long-term amino acid administration.[2,103] TPN-induced cholestasis is a diagnosis of exclusion; therefore, specific causes must be ruled out.[104,105]

Fat

Besides being a concentrated energy source, fat is essential for normal growth and development, including retinal development and function, brain development, and cell structure and function.[106,107] Biochemical evidence of essential fatty acid deficiency (EFAD) in premature infants has been reported during the first week of life and as early as the second day of life.[108] Therefore, if an infant is not able to tolerate enteral feedings as a source ot fat, provision of an I.V. fat emulsion (IFE) is necessary to provide essential fatty acids (EFA) as well as calories.

Composition

IFEs are prepared from either soybean oil or a combination of soybean and safflower oil (see Table 10.3). They provide a mixture of neutral triglycerides, predominantly unsaturated fatty acids.[32] The major fatty acids in the IFE are linoleic, oleic, palmitic, stearic, and linolenic acids. They also contain egg yolk phospholipids as an emulsifier and glycerol to make the emulsion isotonic to serum.[32] Although the fatty acid content varies, the caloric content of the various IFEs is the same. Fat contributes 9 kcal/g or 0.9 kcal/ml for 10% and 1.8 kcal/ml for 20%, with glycerol providing an additional 0.2 kcal/ml for both concentrations.[109] Thus, the caloric value for 10% and 20% IFEs is 1.1 and 2.0 kcal/ml, respectively. The emulsified fat

Table 10.3. A Comparison of Selected Intravenous Fat Emulsions

Product and distributor	Intralipid 10% and 20% (Clintec)	Liposyn II 10% and 20% (Abbott)	Liposyn III 10% and 20% (Abbott)
Oil base	Soybean	50% Soybean and 50% safflower	Soybean
Fatty acid content (%)			
Linoleic	50	65.8	54.5
Oleic	26	17.7	22.4
Palmitic	10	8.8	10.5
Linolenic	9	4.2	8.3
Stearic	3.5	3.4	4.2
Calories/ml			
10%	1.1	1.1	1.1
20%	2.0	2.0	2.0
Egg yolk phospholipids (%)	1.2	1.2	1.2
Glycerin (%)	2.25	2.5	2.5
Osmolarity mOsm/L			
10%	260	276	284
20%	260	258	292

Source: Drug facts and comparisons. 1998 ed. St. Louis: Wolters Kluwer Co.

---

particles are similar in size to naturally occurring chylomicrons. Clearance from the plasma is dependent on the activity of lipoprotein lipase in the capillary endothelial cells, primarily in muscle and adipose tissue.[2] The IFE is isotonic to serum and can be given peripherally or through a central line. There is a small amount of phosphorus in lipid emulsions, 4.68 mg/dl of 10% Intralipid (Clintec Nutrition, Deerfield, Ill.).[110] Precipitation or catheter occlusion may occur if an IFE is infused with a solution containing additional calcium and phosphorus that is near its precipitation curve.[81] There is a minimal amount of cholesterol in IFEs, < 3 mg/dl.[111]

Several manufacturers produce IFEs. The main difference between the soybean oil base and soybean-safflower oil base IFEs lies in the percentage of linoleic and alpha-linolenic acids contained in the emulsions. Linoleic acid is of primary concern as an essential fatty acid for humans. Metabolically, linoleic and linolenic acids are converted in part to arachidonic and docosahexaoic acids before incorporation into structural lipids in the central nervous system.[107] Liposyn I (Abbott), an IFE that is no longer available, was made with safflower oil only. It had 0.1% linolenic acid, compared with 6-9% in competing products based on soybean oil. A case of human linolenic acid deficiency was described in a child receiving an IFE low in linolenic acid.[112] Intralipid and Liposyn were compared, and hypertriglyceridemia during infusion of the safflower oil-based emulsion was documented.[113,114] Other studies reported adverse effects of the safflower oil emulsion on essential fatty acid status[115] and on triglyceride and free fatty acid levels.[116] Thus, the safflower-oil-only IFE was taken off the market. Liposyn II is an IFE-containing soybean and safflower oil. The linolenic acid content is about half of that in the soybean-only IFEs, Intralipid and Liposyn III. Studies in neonates comparing Liposyn II and Intralipid showed no difference in hypertriglyceridemia[117] and comparable plasma fatty acid profiles.[2,118,119]

Prevention of Essential Fatty Acid Deficiency

The use of IFEs for the prevention of EFAD and for a concentrated calorie source has been reviewed.[120-123] EFAD is defined by evaluating specific serum fatty acids. When a linoleic acid deficiency is present, the enzyme system that converts linoleic acid to arachidonic acid (a tetraene) acts on oleic acid to synthesize eicosatrienoic acid (a triene). Eicosatrienoic acid lacks the physiologic function of arachidonic acid.[2] EFAD is defined as a triene-to-tetraene ratio of ≥ 0.4.[2] This biochemical measure will precede clinical manifestations of EFAD, which include failure to thrive, scaly dermatitis, sparse hair growth, thrombocytopenia, increased susceptibility to infection, and impaired wound healing.[124] A study of 63 premature AGA infants who weighed < 2.0 kg indicated that by day 7, with no source of fat 67% of the infants had low plasma linoleic acid levels and 44% had a high triene-to-tetraene ratio, suggestive of EFAD.[125]

Recommended Intakes and Infusion Rates

To prevent EFAD, the AAP recommends providing 3% of the total enteral calories[126] or 2-4% of the nonprotein parenteral calories[123] as linoleic acid. This is equal to providing 4-8% of nonprotein calories as IFE. With a calorie intake of 120 kcal/kg/day, the dose would be about 0.5-1.0 g/kg/day. The AAP recommendation of 3% may be oversimplified.[127] Whereas the 3% figure is adequate to prevent clinical deficiency signs, it is insufficient to preserve functional and biochemical normalcy.[127] The neonatal EFA need is 4-5% of total calories, but up to 12% of total calories can be provided as EFA safely. This is equal to 0.6-0.8 g/kg/day and up to 1.5 g/kg/day.[127] The total fat intake, including EFA requirements, generally contributes 30-40% of the nonnitrogen calories in a balanced solution but should never be > 60%.[2,14] The rate should be gradually increased by 0.25-0.5 g/kg/day to a maximum of 3 g/kg/day in a small for gestational age (SGA) or premature infant or 4.0 g/kg/day in a term infant.[2,36] To avoid hyperlipemia, the rate of lipid infusion should not exceed 0.15 g/kg/hour.[4] Infusion of 3 g/kg/day over 24 hours would result in a rate of 0.125 g/kg/hour. In neonates, the maximal removal capacity was shown to be 0.3 g triglyceride/kg/hour.[128]

The AAP recommends that lipids be infused over 24 hours if possible; this results in a very low and well-tolerated infusion rate.[36] Other studies on infusion rates have been done.[129-132] No metabolic advantage to a rest period to allow lipid clearance from the plasma could be identified.[131,132]

Intravenous Lipid Emulsions: 10% Versus 20%

The infusion of 20% solutions allows adequate lipid intake in less volume. In comparative studies, the 20% solutions were found to be efficacious and as safe as the 10% solutions.[133,134] The 10% solution has a higher phospholipid/triglyceride weight ratio than the 20% solution—0.12 for 10% and 0.06 for 20%.[135] The higher ratio may affect the activity of lipoprotein lipase, the primary enzyme for lipid clearance, resulting in higher triglycerides and other plasma lipids in infants on 10% IFEs.[136] The 20% lipid emulsions are preferred in premature infants. A 10% lipid solution with the same phospholipid content as the 20% IFE may be well tolerated with no increase in triglycerides or serum cholesterol levels; however, this product is not on the market in the United States.[137]

Lipids and Heparin

Use of heparin has been suggested to enhance clearance of I.V. fat, and its safety has been reviewed.[120,138,139] Addition of heparin to the parenteral nutrition solution reduces the formation of a fibrin sheath around the catheter and may reduce phlebitis.[2,102] In addition to reducing the incidence of phlebitis, use of 1 unit heparin/ml of TPN increases the duration of catheter patency.[140] Heparin stimulates the release of lipoprotein lipase and may improve lipid clearance.[2,106] This activity, known as postheparin lipolytic activity, appears to be well developed in preterm infants.[106] Low doses of heparin do not prolong clotting times or cause generalized bleeding in preterm infants.[139,141] Although further studies are needed, 0.5-1.0 units heparin/ml of TPN solution is recommended[2,36] and used routinely in clinical practice.

Monitoring Tolerance of Lipids

Methods to monitor infants receiving IFE have been evaluated.[2,142-145] Recommendations include the following tests:

- Visual inspection of light-scattering index (LSI)[142,143]
- Free fatty acids[142]
- Triglycerides[2,142,144]
- Prothrombin time[2,144]
- Partial thromboplastin time[7]
- Cholesterol[2,144]
- Lipid-emulsion triglyceride levels using nephelometry or LSI[145]
- Platelet count[2]
- Free-fatty-acid-to-serum-albumin molar ratio (with hyperbilirubinemia)[2]

Serum triglyceride levels are commonly used to monitor IFE tolerance because of the availability of the test and the small amount of blood required. Levels should be checked initially, after each dose increase to ensure the infant tolerates the therapy, and weekly thereafter (see Chapter 8). Infants on steroid therapy may have elevated triglyceride levels.[146] Ideally triglyceride levels are kept below 150 mg/dl,[4,204] although many clinicians tolerate up to 200 mg/dl.

Lipids and Pulmonary Function

Although the value of IFEs is widely accepted, many cautions still surround their use. Pulmonary fat accumulation, altered pulmonary function, and hypoxemia have been reported in premature infants on IFE.[147-150] Deaths in preterm infants after infusion of IFE have been reported.[150,151] Autopsies revealed intravascular fat accumulation in the lungs, although lipid accumulation in the pulmonary capillaries of two infants who had never received lipids has also been reported.[133,152] Fat globules found in lungs of premature infants and thought to be fat embolism might have been postmortem artifacts.[153]

Studies have been done reviewing the effect of lipid infusion on pulmonary status.[154-160] Results are conflicting. Administration of small doses (~1 g/kg/day) of lipids on the first day of life, as compared with administration starting later in the first week, resulted in an increase in chronic lung disease (CLD) in one study,[159] but no difference in gas exchange or development of CLD in two others.[158,160] A meta-analysis of six randomized controlled trials of early (< 5 days) versus late (> 5 days) introduction of I.V. lipids in preterm, LBW infants revealed no effect on death or incidence of CLD.[161] The lipid preparation itself may contain toxic lipid peroxidation products, which may explain the lack of protective pulmonary effect of I.V. lipids sometimes seen.[162]

Recommendations for I.V. lipid infusions in this population vary. I.V. fat emulsions appear to be a safe source of calories for most seriously ill neonates, including those with pulmonary problems.[163] For infants < 750 g, initiation of lipids is usually delayed for 3-4 days, then started at 0.5 g/kg and advanced by 0.5 g/kg to a maximum dose of 3.0 g/kg/day.[162] For larger infants, lipids can begin sooner.[162] Many, including the AAP, recommend no more than 0.5-1.0 g/kg/day of fat emulsion during the first week of life.[2,36] The recommended rate of infusion is < 0.15 g/kg/hour.[4]

Lipids and Sepsis

The use of parenteral lipid emulsions in premature infants with septicemia is controversial, inasmuch as these infants have reduced clearance and utilization of lipids.[204] At a dose of 3 g/kg/day, septic infants may show significantly higher concentrations of triglycerides and free fatty acids (FFAs) than infants without sepsis.[164] LBW infants with septicemia should receive a maximum dose of 2 g/kg/day and careful monitoring of triglycerides.[163,164] If the infant develops hypertriglyceridemia, the lipid infusion should be reduced or discontinued until the problem is resolved.[204]

Five cases of Broviac catheter-related Malassezia furfur in infants receiving IFE have been described.[165,166] Various treatment methods include removal of the catheter along with use of either amphoteracin B[167] or miconazole.[168] Intravenous lipid emulsions may be a major determinant of coagulase-negative staphylococcal bacteremia in the VLBW infant.[169,170] Their importance relative to other factors such as intravenous catheter placement is controversial.[171-173]

Lipids and Hyperbilirubinemia

The effect of lipid on bilirubin binding has been examined.[174-178] As lipid emulsions are metabolized to FFAs and monoglycerides, the FFAs released by lipolysis compete with bilirubin for binding sites on serum albumin.[2,124] This could result in increased serum concentration of free bilirubin and theoretically increase the risk of kernicterus, although this has never been reported. One study found that infusion with Intralipid may enhance lumirubin formation, the principal bilirubin photoproduct excreted during phototherapy.[179] Thus, infusion of lipids may actually prove to be a useful adjunct to phototherapy.

IFEs are highly susceptible to oxidation. Exposure to ambient light and phototherapy light may increase the levels of oxidized lipids. There may be clinical significance, as lipid hydroperoxides are cytotoxic. This may be an additional source of morbidity in premature infants. Minimizing exposure of lipids to ambient and phototherapy light decreases the hydroperoxide levels.[180, 204] (See Chapter 12.)

The AAP recommends that infants with plasma bilirubin concentrations of > 8 to 10 mg/100 ml and an albumin concentration of 2.5-3.0 g/100 ml should not receive more than 0.5-1.0 g/kg/day of IFE.[122] Kerner recommends that the fatty-acid-to-serum-albumin ratio be kept below 4 in infants on IFE with elevated indirect bilirubin levels.[2]

Lipids and Thrombocytopenia

Thrombocytopenia is a possible side effect of lipid infusion in limited adult studies. No adverse effects on platelet concentrations were observed in premature infants on short- or long-term TPN.[181]

Lipids in Premature and SGA Infants: Carnitine

The infant of < 34 weeks' gestational age and the SGA infant often exhibit poor tolerance to parenteral lipids.[120] Their problem may be partially related to lack of exogenous carnitine along with altered synthesis and storage. Carnitine is essential for optimum oxidation of fatty acids in the mitochondria. Long-chain fatty acids can cross the mitochondria only in the form of acyl carnitine.[124] In the healthy adult or child, L-carnitine is synthesized in the liver and kidney from lysine and methionine.[182] Carnitine synthesis and storage are not well developed at birth. Premature infants of < 34 weeks' gestation receiving TPN develop carnitine deficiency 6-10 days after birth.[183] The age of transition from dependence on carnitine supplementation to independence from exogenous carnitine remains unclear.[184] VLBW infants requiring prolonged TPN may have carnitine deficiency with impaired ketogenesis. Supplemental carnitine alleviates this metabolic disturbance,[185] but may not improve growth or decrease hypoglycemia.[186] Other studies regarding carnitine deficiency and neonates on TPN have been published.[187-192]

Clinical symptoms of carnitine deficiency include cardiomyopathy, encephalopathy, nonketotic hypoglycemia, hypotonia, poor growth, and frequent infections.[193] Two types of carnitine deficiency have been identified. In the first type, the serum, hepatic, and extra-hepatic tissue levels of carnitine are depressed. In the second type, serum carnitine levels are normal and tissue levels are depressed. The latter type indicates a defect in carnitine uptake in tissue cells.[194] Premature infants on TPN suffer from the first type because they cannot synthesize carnitine and do not have an exogenous source. Infants able to tolerate human milk or carnitine-supplemented infant formula can avoid tissue depletion.[106] Carnitor (Sigma-Tau, Gaithersburg, MD) is available for intravenous supplementation. The dose should be individualized, but a safe, initial dose is 8-10 mg/kg/day (50.0-62.5 μmol/kg/d).[195,204] Blood levels should be closely monitored.

Many controversies surround the use of lipids in premature, high-risk newborns. Clinicians should use IFE with caution and carry out careful monitoring to prevent the major complications of hyperlipidemia, including impaired pulmonary function, diminished immune response, and displacement of albumin-bound bilirubin by FFAs in plasma.[2,19,204]

IFEs with Medium-Chain Triglyceride (MCT) and Olive Oil

Use of an IFE containing a portion of the fat as MCTs may be beneficial in infants with low carnitine stores and in icteric infants.[196,197] Infants may have significantly lower serum cholesterol concentrations and fewer effects on pulmonary hemodynamics when they receive the MCT/LCT emulsion than when they receive a LCT emulsion.[198] An IFE with a mixture of olive oil and soybean oil contains lower amounts of linoleic acid and more vitamin E than the soybean or the soybean/safflower oil IFEs. Preliminary data suggest that the olive oil emulsion is less sensitive to peroxidation and enhances production of metabolically important derivatives of linoleic acid.[204-206] Currently, neither the MCT nor the olive/soybean oil IFEs are available commercially in the United States. More studies are needed to confirm the advantages of these new products.[199,204]

References

1. Butte NF. Energy requirements during infancy. In: Tsang RC, Nichols BL, eds. Nutrition during infancy. Philadelphia: Hanley and Belfus, 1988; 86-99.
2. Kerner JA. Parenteral nutrition. In: Walker WA, Durie PR, Hamilton JR, Walker-Smith JA and Watkins JB, eds. Pediatric gastrointestinal disease: pathophysiology, diagnosis, management, vol 2. St. Louis: Mosby, 1996; 1904-51.
3. Pereira G, Barbosa N. Controversies in neonatal nutrition. Pediatr Clin North Am 33:65, 1986.
4. American Academy of Pediatrics (AAP) Committee on Nutrition. Nutritional needs of preterm infants. In: Kleinman RE, ed. Pediatric Nutrition Handbook. 4th edition. Elk Grove Village, Ill.: AAP, 1998; 55-87.
5. Anderson TL, Muttart CR, Bieber MA, et al. A controlled trial of glucose versus glucose and amino acids in premature infants. J Pediatr 94:947, 1979.
6. Zlotkin SH, Bryan MH, Anderson GH. Intravenous nitrogen and energy intakes required to duplicate in utero nitrogen accretion in prematurely born human infants. J Pediatr 99:115, 1981.

7. Heird WC. Parenteral feeding. In: Effective care of the newborn infant. Sinclair JC, Bracken MB, eds. Oxford: Oxford University Press, 1992.
8. Chessex P, Belanger S, Bruno P, et al. Influence of energy substrates on respiratory gas exchange during conventional mechanical ventilation of preterm infants. J Pediatr 126:619, 1995.
9. Rubecz I, Mestyan J, Barga P, et al. Energy metabolism, substrate utilization, and nitrogen balance in parenterally fed postoperative neonates and infants. J Pediatr 98:42, 1981.
10. Pierro A, Carnielli V, Filler R, et al. Characteristics of protein sparing effect of total parenteral nutrition in the surgical infant. J Pediatr Surg 23:538, 1988.
11. VanAerde JE, Sauer PJ, Pencharz PB, et al. Metabolic consequences of increasing energy intake by adding lipid to parenteral nutrition in full-term infants. Am J Clin Nutr 59:659, 1994.
12. Pineault M, Chessex P, Bisailion S, et al. Total parenteral nutrition in the newborn: Impact of the quality of infused energy on nitrogen metabolism. Am J Clin Nutr 47:298,1988.
13. Bresson J, Bader B, Rocchiccioli F, et al. Protein-metabolism kinetics and energy substrate utilization in infants fed parenteral solutions with different glucose-fat ratois. Am J Clin Nutr 54:370, 1991.
14. Salas-Saluado J, Molina J, Figueras J, et al. Effect of the quality of infused energy on substrate utilization in the newborn receiving total parenteral nutrition. Pediatr Res 33:112, 1993.
15. Nose O, Tipton JR, Ament ME, et al. Effect of the energy source on changes in energy expenditure, respiratory quotient, and nitrogen balance during total parenteral nutrition in children. Pediatr Res 21:538, 1987.
16. Bresson JL, Narcy P, Putet G, et al. Energy substrate utilization in infants receiving total parenteral nutrition with different glucose to fat ratios. Pediatr Res 25:645, 1989.
17. Heird WC, Gomez MR. Parenteral nutrition in low-birth-weight infants. Annu Rev Nutr 16:471, 1996.
18. Thureen PJ, Hay WW. Intravenous nutrition and postnatal growth of the micropremie. Clin Perinatol 27(1):197, 2000
19. Hay WW. Lucas A, Heird WC, et al. Workshop summary: Nutrition of the extremely low birth weight infant. Pediatrics 104:1360, 1999.
20. Leitch CA, Denne SC. Energy expenditure in the extremely low-birth weight infant. Clin Perinatol 27(1):181, 2000.
21. Bauer K, Pasel K, Uhrig C, et al. Comparison of face mask, head hood, and canopy for breath sampling in flow-through indirect calorimetry to measure oxygen consumption and carbon dioxide production of preterm infants < 1500 grams. Pediatr Res 41:139, 1997.
22. Dechert R, Wesley J, Schafer L, et al. Comparison of oxygen consumption, carbon dioxide production, and resting energy expenditure in premature and full-term infants. J Pediatr Surg 20:792, 1985.
23. Schafer L, Wesley J, Tse Y, et al. Effects of necrotizing enterocolitis on calculation of resting energy expenditure in infants with gastroschisis. J Parenter Enter Nutr 10:6S, 1986.
24. Kurzner SI, Garg M, Bautista B, et al. Growth failure in bronchopulmonary dysplasia: Elevated metabolic rates and pulmonary mechanics. J Pediatr 112:73, 1988.

25. Yeh TR, McClenan DA, Ajayi OA, et al. Metabolic rate and energy balance in infants with bronchopulmonary dysplasia. J Pediatr 114:448, 1989.

26. Srinivasan G, Pildes RS, Jaspan JB, et al. Metabolic effects of theophylline in preterm infants. J Pediatr 98:815, 1981.

27. Bauer J, Sontheimer D, Fischer C, et al. Metabolic rate and energy balance in very low birth weight infants during kangaroo holding by their mothers and fathers. J Pediatr 129:608, 1996.

28. Pierro A, Jones MO, Hammond P, et al. A new equation to predict the resting energy expenditure of surgical infants. J Pediatr Surg 29:1103, 1994.

29. Heim T. Energy metabolism: Theoretical and practical aspects. In: Brunser O, Carazza F, Graceym, et al., eds. Clinical nutrition of the young child, vol.1. New York: Raven, 1995; 77-92.

30. McGowen JE. The role of glucose in cerebral function. Seminars in Neonatal Nutrition and Metabolism. 4:2, 1997.

31. Tyrala EE, Chen X, and Boden G. Glucose metabolism in the infant weighing less than 1100 grams. J Pediatr 125:283, 1994.

32. Nutritional products. In: Kastrup EK, ed. Facts and Comparisons. St. Louis: Wolters Kluwer Co., 1998; 1-60k.

33. Cochran EB, Phelps SJ, Helms RA. Parenteral nutrition in pediatric patients. Clin Pharm 7:351, 1988.

34. Groh-Wargo S. Prematurity/low birth weight. In: Lang CE, ed. Nutritional support in critical care. Rockville, MD: Aspen, 1987; 287-313.

35. Lifschitz CH. Carbohydrate needs in preterm and term infants. In: Tsang R, Nichols B, eds. Nutrition during infancy. Philadelphia: Hanley and Belfus, 1988; 122.

36. American Academy of Pediatrics (AAP) Committee on Nutrition. Parenteral nutrition. In: Kleinman RE, ed. Pediatric nutrition handbook. 4th ed. Elk Grove Village, IL: AAP, 1998;285-305.

37. Farrag HM, Cowett RM. Glucose homeostasis in the micropremie. Clin Perinatol 27(1):1, 2000.

38. Lee PC, Werlin SL. Carbohydrates. In: Baker RD, Baker SS, and Davis AM, eds. Pediatric Parenteral Nutrition. New York: Chapman and Hall, 1997.

39. Schneling DJ, Coran AG. Hormonal and metabolic response to operative stress in the neonate. J Parenter Enter Nutr 15:215, 1991.

40. Harkavey KL, Scanlon JW, Chowdry PK et al. Dexamethasone therapy for chronic lung disease in ventilator and oxygen dependent infants; a controlled trial. J Pediatr 115:979, 1989.

41. Warner BW, Bower RH. Complications of therapy. In: Lang CE, ed. Nutritional support in critical care. Rockville, MD: Aspen, 1987; 131.

42. McDonald JTJ, Phillips MJ, Jeejeebhoy KN. Reversal of fatty liver by Intralipid in patients on total parenteral alimentation. Gastroenterology 64:885, 1973.

43. Lane RH, Simmons RA. Hyperglycemia and other consequences of aggressive intravenous glucose administration. Semin Neonat Nutr Metab, 4:3, 1997.

44. Vaucher YE, Walson PD, Morrow III G. Continuous insulin infusion in hyperglycemic, very low birth weight infants. J Pediatr Gastroenterol Nutr 1:211, 1982.

45. Binder ND, Raschko PK, Benda GI, et al. Insulin infusion with parenteral nutrition in extremely low birth weight infants with hyperglycemia. J Pediatr 114:273, 1989.
46. Collins JW, Hoppe M, Brown K, et al. A controlled trial of insulin infusion and parenteral nutrition in extremely low birth weight infants with glucose intolerance. J Pediatr 118:921, 1991.
47. Poindexter BB, Karn CA, Denne SC. Exogenous insulin reduces proteolysis and protein synthesis in extremely low birth weight infants. J Pediatr 132:948, 1998.
48. Ostertag SG, Jovanovic L, Lewis B, et al. Insulin pump therapy in the very low birth weight infant. Pediatrics 78:625, 1986.
49. Simeon PS, Geffner ME, Levin SR, et al. Continuous insulin infusions in neonates: Pharmacologic availability of insulin in intravenous solutions. J Pediatr 124:818, 1994.
50. Micheli JL, Schutz Y, Junod S, et al. Early postnatal intravenous amino acid administration to extremely-low-birth-weight preterm infants. Semin Neonat Nutr Metab. 2:1, 1994.
51. Motil KJ. Protein needs for term and preterm infants. In: Tsang RC, Nichols BL, eds. Nutrition during infancy. Philadelphia: Hanley and Belfus, 1988; 100-21.
52. Auld PA, Bhangananda P, Mehta S. The influence of an early caloric intake with IV glucose on catabolism of premature infants. Pediatrics 37:592, 1966.
53. Heird WC, Kashyap S. Protein and amino acid requirements. In: Fetal and neonatal physiology. Polin RA, Fox WW, eds. Philedelphia: Saunders, 1992; 450.
54. Hanning RM, Zlotkin SH. Amino acid and protein needs of the neonate: Effects of excess and deficiency. Semin Perinatol 13:131, 1989.
55. Holt LE, Snyderman SE. Protein and amino acid requirements of infants and children. Nutr Abst Rev 35:1, 1965.
56. Lacey JM, Crouch JB, Benfell K, et al. The effects of glutamine supplemented parenteral nutrition in premature infants. J Parenter Enter Nutr 20:74, 1996.
57. Snyderman, SE. The protein and amino acid requirements of the premature infant. In: Jonxis JHP, Visser HKA, Troelstra JA, eds. Metabolic processes in the fetus and newborn infant. Baltimore: Williams and Wilkins, 1971; 128-41.
58. Fomon SJ. Protein. In: Fomon SJ, ed. Infant nutrition. 2d ed. Philadelphia: Saunders, 1974; 118.
59. Levenson SM, Smith-Hopkins B, Waldron M, et al. Early history of parenteral nutrition. Fed Proc 43:1391, 1984.
60. Ghadimi H. Newly devised amino acid solutions for intravenous administration. In: Ghadimi H, ed. Total parenteral nutrition: Premises and promises. New York: John Wiley and Sons, 1975; 393.
61. Pohlandt TF. Cystine: A semi-essential amino acid in the newborn infant. Acta Paediatr Scand 63:801, 1974.
62. Zlotkin SH, Bryan MH, Anderson GH. Cysteine supplementation to cysteine-free intravenous feeding regimens in newborn infants. Am J Clin Nutr 34:914, 1981.
63. Narkewicz MR, Caldwell S, Jones G. Cysteine supplementation and reduction of total parenteral nutrition-induced hepatic lipid accumulation in the weanling rat. J Pediatr Gastroenterol Nutr 21:18, 1995.

64. Pollack PF, Rivera A, Rassin DK, et al. Cysteine supplementation increases glutathione, but not polyamine, concentrations of the small intestine and colon of parenterally fed newborn rabbits. J Pediatr Gastroenterol Nutr 22:364, 1996.

65. Zlotkin SH, Anderson GH. Sulfur balances in intravenously fed infants: Effects of cysteine supplementation. Am J Clin Nutr 36:862, 1982.

66. Helms RA, Storm MC, Christensen ML, et al. Cysteine supplementation results in normalization of plasma taurine concentrations in children receiving home parenteral nutrition. J Pediatr 134:358, 1999.

67. Zlotkin SH. Nutrient interactions with total parenteral nutrition: Effect of histidine and cysteine intake on urinary zinc excretion. J Pediatr 114:859, 1989.

68. Laine L, Shulman RJ, Pitre D, et al. Cysteine usage increases the need for acetate in neonates who receive total parenteral nutrition. Am J Clin Nutr 54:565, 1991.

69. Geggel HS, Ament ME, Heckenlively JR, et al. Nutritional requirements for taurine in patients receiving long-term parenteral nutrition. N Engl J Med 312:142, 1985.

70. Rassin DK, Malloy MH. Taurine requirement with parenteral nutrition (ltr). N Engl J Med 313:120, 1985.

71. Vandewoude MFJ, DeLeeuw IH. Taurine requirement with parenteral nutrition (ltr). N Engl J Med 313:121, 1985.

72. Vinton NE, Stewart AL, Ament ME, et al. Taurine concentrations in plasma, blood cells, and urine of children undergoing long-term total parenteral nutrition. Pediatr Res 21:399, 1987.

73. Zelikovic I, Chesney RW, Friedman AL, et al. Taurine depletion in very low birth weight infants receiving prolonged total parenteral nutrition: Role of renal immaturity. J Pediatr 116:301, 1990.

74. Heird WC, Dell RB, Helms RA, et al. Amino acid mixture designed to maintain normal plasma amino acid patterns in infants and children requiring parenteral nutrition. Pediatrics 80:401, 1987.

75. Uauy RO, Greene H, Heird W. Conditionally essential nutrients: cyteine, taurine, tyrosine, arginine, glutamine, choline, inositol, and nucleotides. In: Nutritional needs of the preterm Infant. Tsang R, Lucas A, Uauy R, Zlotkin S, eds. Baltimore: Williams and Wilkins, 1993; 267.

76. Abumrad N, Morse EL, Lochslt, et al. Possible sources of glutamine for parenteral nutrition: Impact on glutamine metabolism. Am J Physiol 257:E228, 1989.

77. Furst P, Albers S, Stehle P. Glutamine-containing dipeptides in parenteral nutrition. J Parenter Enter Nutr 14:118s, 1990.

78. Zlotkin SH, Stallings VA, Pencharz PB. Total parenteral nutrition in children. Pediatr Clin North Am 32:381, 1985.

79. Fitzgerald KA, MacKay MW. Calcium and phosphate solubility in neonatal parenteral nutrient solutions containing TrophAmine. Am J Hosp Pharm 43:88, 1986.

80. Fitzgerald KA, MacKay MW. Calcium and phosphate solubility in neonatal parenteral nutrient solutions containing Aminosyn PF. Am J Hosp Pharm 44:1396, 1987.

81. Eggert LD, Rusho WJ, MacKay MW, et al. Calcium and phosphate compatibility in parenteral nutrition solutions for neonates. Am J Hosp Pharm 39:49, 1982.

82. Dunham B, Marcuard S, Khazanie PG, et al. The solubility of calcium and phosphorus in neonatal total parenteral nutrition solutions. J Parenter Enter Nutr 15:608, 1991.

83. Helms RA, Christensen ML, Mauer EC, et al. Comparison of a pediatric versus standard amino acid formulation in preterm neonates requiring parenteral nutrition. J Pediatr 110:466, 1987.

84. Heird WC, Hay W, Helms RA, et al. Pediatric parenteral amino acid mixture in low birth weight infants. Pediatrics 81:41, 1988.

85. Battista MA, Price PT, Kalhan SC. Effect of parenteral amino acids on leucine and urea kinetics in preterm infants. J Pediatr 128:130,1996.

86. Beck R. Use of a pediatric parenteral amino acid mixture in a population of extremely low birth weight neonates: Frequency and spectrum of direct bilirubinemia. Am J Perinatol 7:84, 1990.

87. Helms RA, Johnson MR, Christensen ML, et al. Altered caloric and protein requirement in neonates receiving a pediatric amino acid formulation. Pediatr Res 21:429A, 1987.

88. Raiha NC. Amino acids in premature infants (ltr). Pediatrics 82:680, 1988.

89. Heird WC. Amino acids in premature infants (rep to ltr). Pediatrics 82:680, 1988.

90. Helms RA, Johnson MR, Christensen ML, et al. Evaluation of two pediatric amino acid formulations. J Parenter Enter Nutr 12:422, 1988.

91. Forchelli ML, Gura KM, Sandler R, et al. Aminosyn PF or TrophAmine: Which provides more protection from cholestasis associated with total parenteral nutrition? J Pediatr Gastroenterol Nutr 21:374, 1995.

92. Heird WC, Kashyap S, Gomez MR. Protein intake and energy requirements of the infant. Semin Perinatol 15:438, 1991.

93. Denne S, Karn CA, Ahlrichs JA, et al. Proteolysis and phenylalanine hydroxylation in response to parenteral nutrition in extremely premature and normal newborns. J Clin Invest 97:746, 1996.

94. Rivera A, Bell EF, Bier DM. Effect of intravenous amino acids on protein metabolism of preterm infants during the first three days of life. Pediatr Res 33:106, 1993.

95. Denne SC. Intravenous amino acid nutrition that begins at birth: Effects on protein synthesis and oxidation in the ELBW infant. Semin Neonat Nutr Metab. 5:1, 1998.

96. Schanler RJ, Shulman RJ, Prestridge LL. Parenteral nutrient needs of very low birth weight infants. J Pediatr 125:961, 1994.

97. VanGoudoever JB, Colen T, Wattimena JLD, et al. Immediate commencement of amino acid supplementation in preterm infants: Effect on serum amino acid concentrations and protein kinetics on the first day of life. J Pediatr 127:458, 1995.

98. Thureen P, Sauer P. Modulators of protein metabolism: Catabolic effects. Semin Neonat Nutr Metab. 5:5, 1998.

99. Shulman RJ, DeStefano-Laine L, Pettitt R, et al. Protein deficiency in premature infants receiving parenteral nutrition. Am J Clin Nutr 44:610, 1986.

100. Wahlig TM, Georgieff MK. The effects of illness on neonatal metabolism and nutritional management. Clin Perinatol 22:77, 1995.

101. Heird WC, Kashyap S, Gomez MR. Parenteral alimentation of the neonate. Semin Perinatol 15:493, 1991.

102. Fletcher AB. Nutrition. In: Avery GB, Fletcher MA, MacDonald MG, eds. Neonatology: pathophysiology and management of the newborn. Philadelphia: Lippincott, 1994; 330.

103. Vileisis RA, Inwood RJ, Hunt CE. Prospective controlled study of parenteral nutrition-associated cholestatic jaundice: Effect of protein intake. J Pediatr 96:893, 1980.

104. Kerner JA. Metabolic complications. In: Kerner JA, ed. Manual of pediatric parenteral nutrition. New York: John Wiley and Sons, 1983; 199-215.

105. Gremse DA, Balistreri WE Neonatal cholestasis. In: Lebenthal E, ed. Textbook of gastroenterology and nutrition in infancy. 2d ed. New York: Raven Press, 1989; 909.

106. Hamosh M. Fat needs for term and preterm infants. In: Tsang RC, Nichols BL, eds. Nutrition during infancy. Philadelphia: Hanley and Belfus, 1988; 133-59.

107. Innis SM. Benefits of early IV lipids for nutrition of ELBW/LBW infants. Semin in Neonat Nutr Metab 3:1, 1995.

108. Friedman Z, Danon A, Stahlman MT, et al. Rapid onset of essential fatty acid deficiency in the newborn. Pediatrics 58:640, 1976.

109. Young SL. Pediatric parenteral nutrition. In: DiPiro JT, Talbert RL, Hayes PE, et al., eds. Pharmacotherapy-A pathophysiologic approach. New York: Elsevier, 1989.

110. Knight P, Heer D, Abdenour G. CaxP and Ca/P in the parenteral feeding of preterm infants. J Parenter Enter Nutr 7:110, 1983.

111. Abbott Laboratories. Personal communication, Feb 1999.

112. Holman RT, Johnson SB, Hatch TF. A case of human linolenic acid deficiency involving neurological abnormalities. Am J Clin Nutr 35:617, 1982.

113. Byrne, WJ. Intralipid or Liposyn-comparable products? (edit). J Pediatr Gastroenterol Nutr 1:78, 1982.

114. Cooke RD, Burckhart GJ. Hypertriglyceridemia during the intravenous infusion of a safflower-oil-based fat emulsion. J Pediatr 103:959, 1983.

115. Cooke RJ, Zee P, Yeh Y-Y. Safflower oil emulsion administration during parenteral nutrition in the preterm infant. 1. Effect on essential fatty acid status. J Pediatr Gastroenterol Nutr 4:799, 1985.

116. Cooke RJ, Buis M, Zee P, et al. Safflower oil emulsion administration during parenteral nutrition in the preterm infant. 2. Effect on triglyceride and free fatty acids. J Pediatr Gastroenterol Nutr 4:804, 1985.

117. Nizar L, et al. The risk of hypertriglyceridaemia increases with the duration of intravenous fat administration. Clin Res 38:191A, 1990.

118. Grill B, et al. Prospective comparison of two intravenous lipid emulsions in premature infants: Effects on plasma fatty acids. J Parenter Enter Nutr 14:115, 1990.

119. Malkani A, et al. Evaluation of a new fat emulsion (Liposyn II) in neonates. Clin Res 38:190A, 1990.

120. Bryan H, Shennan A, Griffin E, et al. Intralipid-its rational use in parenteral nutrition of the newborn. Pediatrics 58:787, 1976.

121. Kerner JA, Sunshine P. Parenteral alimentation. Semin Perinatol 3:417, 1979.

122. Levy JS, Winters RW, Heird WC. Total parenteral nutrition in pediatric patients. Pediatr Rev 2:99, 1980.

123. American Academy of Pediatrics Committee on Nutrition: Use of intravenous fat emulsions in pediatric patients. Pediatrics 68:738, 1981.
124. Stahl GR, Spear ML, Hamosh M. Intravenous administration of lipid emulsions to premature infants. Clin Perinatol 13:133, 1986.
125. Farrell PM, Gutcher GR, Palta M, et al. Essential fatty acid deficiency in premature infants. Am J Clin Nutr 48:220, 1988.
126. American Academy of Pediatrics Committee on Nutrition. Fat and fatty acids. In: Kleinman RE, ed. Pediatric nutrition handbook. Elk Grove Village,Ill.: American Academy of Pediatrics, 1998; 213-220.
127. Uauy R, Treen M, Hoffman DR. Essential fatty acid metabolism and requirements during development. Semin Perinatol 13:118, 1989.
128. Gustafson A, Kjellmer I, Olegard R, et al. Nutrition in low-birth-weight infants. I. Intravenous injection of fat emulsion. Acta Paediatr Scand 61:149, 1972.
129. Kao LC, Cheng MH, Warburton D. Triglycerides, free fatty acids, free fatty acids/albumin molar ratio, and cholesterol levels in serum of neonates receiving long-term lipid infusions: Controlled trial of continuous and intermittent regimens. J Pediatr 104:429, 1984.
130. Berkow SE, Spear ML, Gutman A, et al. Lipid clearing in premature infants. Response to increasing doses of Intralipid (IL): II. Free fatty acids (FFA), triglycerides (TG) and cholesterol (CHOL). Pediatr Res 18:135A, 1984.
131. Brans YW, Andrew DS, Carrillo DW, et al. Tolerance of fat emulsions in very low-birth weight neonates. Am J Dis Child 142:145, 1988.
132. Bedrick AD. Metabolic tolerance of parenteral lipid in neonates-Better late than never (edit). Am J Dis Child 142:135, 1988.
133. Marchildon MB. Parenteral 20% safflower oil emulsion safety and effectiveness as a caloric source in newborn infants. J Parenter Enter Nutr 6:25, 1982.
134. Kaminski MU, Abrahamian V, Chrysomilides SA, et al. Comparative study of clearance of 10% and 20% fat emulsion. J Parenter Enter Nutr 7:126, 1983.
135. Haumont D, Richelle M, Deckelbaum RJ, et al. Effect of liposomal content of lipid emulsions on plasma lipid concentrations in low birth weight infants receiving parenteral nutrition. J Pediatr 121:759, 1992.
136. Haumont D, Deckelbaum RJ, Richelle M, et al. Plasma lipid and plasma lipoprotein concentrations in low birthweight infants given parenteral nutrition with twenty or ten percent lipid emulsion. J Pediatr 115:787, 1989.
137. Gohlke BC, Fahnenstich H, Kowalewski S. Serum lipids during parenteral nutrition with a 10% lipid emulsion with reduced phospholipid emulsifier content in premature infants. J Pediatr Endocrinol Metab. 10:505, 1997.
138. Zaidan H, Dhanireddy R, Hamosh M, et al. Effect of continuous herparin administration on Intralipid clearing in very low-birthweight infants. J Pediatr 101:599, 1982.
139. Hathaway WE. Safety of heparin use in the premature infant (edit). J Pediatr 131:337, 1992.
140. Alpan G, Eyal F, Springer C, et al. Heparinization of alimentation solutions administered through peripheral veins in premature infants: A controlled study. Pediatrics 74:375, 1984.

141. Chang GY, Lueder FL, DiMichele PM, et al. Heparin and the risk of intraventricular hemorrhage in premature infants. J Pediatr 131:362, 1997.

142. Schreiner RL, Glick MR, Nordschow CD, et al. An evaluation of methods to monitor infants receiving intranvenous lipids. J Pediatr 94:197, 1979.

143. Coyer W, Groh-Wargo SL, Bates GD. Light scattering index (LSI) norms for the neonatal ICU. Pediatr Res 14:595, 1980.

144. Dahlstrom KA, Goulet OJ, Roberts RL, et al. Lipid tolerance in children receiving long-term parenteral nutrition: A biochemical and immunologic study. J Pediatr 113:985, 1988.

145. Zlotkin SH. Identification of fat overload during total parenteral nutrition. J Pediatr 115:498, 1990.

146. Sentipal-Walerius J, Dollberg S, Mimouni F, et al. Effect of pulsed dexamethasone therapy on tolerance of intravenously administered lipids in extremely low birth weight infants. J Pediatr 134:229, 1999.

147. Pereira GR, Fox WW, Stanley CA, et al. Decreased oxygenation and hyperlipemia during intravenous fat infusion in premature infants. Pediatrics 66:26, 1980.

148. Friedman Z, Marks KH, Maisels MJ, et al. Effect of parenteral fat emulsion on the pulmonary and reticuloendothelial systems in the newborn infant. Pediatrics 61:694, 1978.

149. Hertel J, Tygstrup I, Anderson GE. Intravascular fat accumulation after Intralipid infusion in the very-low birthweight infant. J Pediatr 100:975, 1982.

150. Leven MI, Wigglesworth JS, Desai R. Pulmonary fat accumulation after Intralipid infusion in the preterm infant. Lancet 2:815, 1980.

151. Dahms B, Halpin T. Pulmonary arterial lipid deposit in newborn infant receiving intravenous lipid infusion. J Pediatr 97:800, 1980.

152. Anderson GE, Hertel J, Tygstrup I. Pulmonary fat accumulation in preterm infants (ltr). Lancet 3:441, 1981.

153. Schroder H, Paust H, Schmidt R. Pulmonary fat embolism after Intralipid therapy-a post-mortem artifact? Acta Paediatr Scand 73:461, 1984.

154. Adamkin DH, Gelke KN, Wilkerson SA. Influence of intravenous fat therapy on tracheal effluent phospholipids and oxygenation in severe respiratory distress syndrome. J Pediatr 106:122, 1985.

155. Brans YW, Dutton EB, Andrew DS, et al. Fat emulsion tolerance in very low birth weight neonates: Effect on diffusion of oxygen in the lungs and on blood pH. Pediatrics 78:79, 1986.

156. Hammerman C, Aramburo MJ. Decreased lipid intake reduces morbidity in sick premature neonates. J Pediatr 113:1083, 1988.

157. Frank L, Sosenko IR, Bancalari E, et al. Early lipid intake and bronchopulmonary dysplasia. J Pediatr 115:658, 1989.

158. Gilbertson N, Kovar IZ, Cox DJ, et al. Introduction of intravenous lipid administration on the first day of life in the very low birth weight neonate. J Pediatr 119:615, 1991.

159. Alwaidh MH, Bowden L, Shaw B, Ryan SW. Randomized trial of effect of delayed intravenous lipid administration on chronic lung disease in preterm neonates. J Pediatr Gastroenterol Nutr 22:303, 1996.

160. Sosenko IRS, Rodriguez-Pierce M, Bancalari E. Effect of early initiation of intravenous lipid administration on the incidence and severity of chronic lung disease in premature infants. J Pediatr 123:975, 1993.

161. Fox GF, Wilson DC, Ohlsson A. Effect of early vs. late introduction of intravenous lipid to preterm infants on death and chronic lung disease (CLD)—results of meta-analyses. Pediatr Res 43(4):214A, 1998.

162. Sosenko IR. Intravenous lipids and the management of chronic lung injury: Helpful or harmful. Semina Neonat Nutr Metab 3:3, 1995.

163. Cohen IT, Meunier KM, Hirsh MP. Effects of lipid emulsion on pulmonary function in infants. In: Kinney JM, Borum PR, eds. Perspectives in clinical nutrition. Baltimore: Urban and Schwarzenberg, 1989; 415.

164. Park W, Paust H, Brosicke H, et al. Impaired fat utilization in parenterally fed low-birth weight infants suffering from sepsis. J Parenter Enter Nutr 10:627, 1986.

165. Powell DA, Aungst J, Snedden S, et al. Broviac catheter-related Malassezia furfur sepsis in five infants receiving intravenous fat emulsions. J Pediatr 105:987, 1984.

166. Powell DA, Durell DE, Marcon MJ. Growth of Malassezia furfur in parenteral fat emulsions (Itr). J Infect Dis 153:640, 1986.

167. Dankner WM, Spector SA. Malassezia furfur sepsis in neonate (Itr). J Pediatr 107:643, 1985.

168. Powell DA, Brady MT. Malassezia furfur sepsis in neonates (reply to Itr). J Pediatr 107:644, 1985.

169. Freeman J, Goldmann DA, Smith NE, et al. Association of intravenous lipid emulsion and coagulase-negative staphylococcal bacteremia in neonatal intensive care units. N Engl J Med 323:301, 1990.

170. Avila-Figueroa C, Goldmann DA, Richardson DK, et al. Intravenous lipid emulsions are the major determinant of coagulase-negative staphylococcal bacteremia in very low birth weight newborns. Pediatr Infect Dis J 17:10, 1998.

171. Walterspiel JN. Lipid emulsions and bacteremia in the NICU (Itr). N Engl J Med 324:267, 1991.

172. Perez JL, Linares J, Pallares R, et al. Lipid emulsions and bacteremia in the NICU (Itr). N Engl J Med 324:267, 1991.

173. Freeman J, Goldmann DA, Smith NE, et al. Lipid emulsions and bacteremia in the NICU (reply to Itr). N Engl J Med 342:268, 1991.

174. Andrew G, Chan G, Schiff D. Lipid metabolism in the neonate. II. The effect of Intralipid on bilirubin binding in vitro and in vivo. J Pediatr 88:279, 1976.

175. Burckart GJ, Whitington PF, Helms RA. The effect of two intravenous fat emulsions and their components on bilirubin binding to albumin. Am J Clin Nutr 36:521, 1982.

176. Spear ML, Stahl GE, Paul MH, et al. The effect of 15 hour fat infusions of varying dosage on bilirubin binding to albumin. J Parenter Enter Nutr 9:144, 1985.

177. Brans YW, Ritter DA, Kenny JD, et al. Influence of intravenous fat emulsion on serum bilirubin in very low birthweight neonates. Arch Dis Child 62:156, 1987.

178. Spear ML, Stahl GE, Hamosh M, et al. Effect of heparin dose and infusion rate on lipid clearance and bilirubin binding in premature infants receiving intravenous fat emulsions. J Pediatr 112:94, 1988.

179. Ennever JF, Dresing TJ, Stahl GE, et al. Intralipid: Food for phototherapy? Pediatr Res 23:483A, 1988.

180. Neuzil J, Darlow BA, Inder TE, et al. Oxidation of parenteral lipid emulsion by ambient and phototherapy lights: Potential toxicity of routine parenteral feeding. J Pediatr 126:785, 1995.
181. Spear ML, Spear M, Cohen AR, et al. Effect of fat infusions on platelet concentration in premature infants. J Parenter Enter Nutr 14:165, 1990.
182. Borum PR. Carnitine. Annu Rev Nutr 3:233, 1983.
183. Schmidt-Sommerfeld E, Penn D, Wolf H. Carnitine blood concentrations and fat utilization in parenterally alimented premature newborn infants. J Pediatr 100:260, 1982.
184. Helms RA, Whitington PF, Mauer EC, et al. Enhanced lipid utilization in infants receiving oral L-carnitine during long term parenteral nutrition. J Pediatr 109:984, 1986.
185. Bonner CM, DeBrie KL, Hug G, et al. Effects of parenteral L-carnitine supplementation on fat metabolism and nutrition in premature neonates. J Pediatr 126:287, 1995.
186. Shortland GJ, Walter JH, Stroud C, et al. Randomised controlled trial of L-carnitine as a nutritional supplement in preterm infants. Arch Dis Child Fetal Neonatal Ed 78:F18J, 1998.
187. Yeh Y-Y, Cooke RF, Zee P. Impairment of lipid emulsion metabolism associated with carnitine insufficiency in premature infants. J Pediatr Gastroenterol Nutr 4:795, 1985.
188. Schmidt-Sommerfeld E, Penn D, et al. Carnitine deficiency in premature infants receiving total parenteral nutrition. Effect of L-carnitine supplementation. J Pediatr 102:931, 1983.
189. Penn D, Schmidt-Sommerfeld E, Pascu F. Decreased tissue carnitine concentrations in newborn infants receiving total parenteral nutrition. J Pediatr 98:976, 1981.
190. Schiff D, Chan G, Seccombe D, et al. Plasma carnitine levels during intravenous feeding of the neonate. J Pediatr 95:1043, 1979.
191. Moukarzel AA, Dahlstrom KA, Buchman AL, et al. Carnitine status of children receiving long-term total parenteral nutrition: A longitudinal prospective study. J Pediatr 120:759, 1992.
192. Zamora S, Benador N, Lacourt G, et al. Renal handling of carnitine in ill preterm and term neonates. J Pediatr 127:975, 1995.
193. Winter SC, Szabo-Aczel S, Curry DJR, et al. Plasma carnitine deficiency: Clinical observations in 51 pediatric patients. Am J Dis Child 141:660, 1987.
194. Tao RC, Yoshimura NN. Carnitine metabolism and its application in parenteral nutrition. J Parenter Enter Nutr 4:469, 1980.
195. Innis, SM. Fat. In: Tsang RC, Lucas A, Uauy R, Zlotkin S, eds. Nutritional Needs of the Preterm Infant: Scientific Basis and Practical Guidelines. Baltimore: Williams and Wilkins, 1993; 65-87.
196. Lima LAM. Neonatal parenteral nutrition with medium-chain triglycerides: Rationale for research. J Parenter Enter Nutr 13:312, 1989.
197. Rubin M, Harell D, Naor N, et al. Lipid infusion with different triglyceride cores (long-chain vs medium-chain/long-chain triglycerides): Effect on plasma lipids and bilirubin binding in premature infants. J Parenter Enter Nutr 15:642, 1991.
198. Lima LAM, Murphy JF, Stansbie D, et al. Neonatal parenteral nutrition with a fat emulsion containing medium chain triglycerides. Acta Paediatr Scand 77:332, 1988.

199. Rubin M, Moser A, Naor N, et al. Effect of three intravenously administered fat emulsions containing different concentrations of fatty acids on the plasma fatty acid composition of premature infants. J Pediatr 125:596, 1994.
200. Ghadimi H. Newly devised amino acid solutions for intravenous administration. In: Ghadimi H, ed. Total parenteral nutrition: Premises and promises. New York: Wiley-Liss (div. Wiley and Sons), 1975; 406-07.
201. Snyderman SE. Recommendations for parenteral amino acid requirements. In: Winters RW, Hasselmeyer EG, eds. Intravenous nutrition in the high risk infant. New York: Wiley and Sons, 1975; 422.
202. Neu J, DeMarco V, Weiss M. Glutamine supplementation in low-birth-weight infants: Mechanisms of action. JPEN 23:S49, 1999.
203. Kalhan SC, Iben S. Protein metabolism of the extremely low-birth-weight infant. Clin Perinatol 27(1):23, 2000.
204. Putet G. Lipid metabolism of the micropremie. Clin Perinatol 27(1):57, 2000.
205. Goulet O, de Potter S, Antebi H, et al. Long-term efficacy and safety of a new olive oil–based intravenous fat emulsion in pediatric patients: a double-blind randomized study. Am J Clin Nutr 70:338, 1999.
206. Koletzko B, Gobel Y, Engelsberger I, et al. Parenteral feeding of preterm infants on fat emulsion with soybean and olive oils: Effects on plasma phospholipid fatty acids. Clin Nutr 17(suppl 1):25, 1998.

Nutritional Care for High-Risk Newborns (Rev. 3d. Ed.)
S. Groh-Wargo, M. Thompson, J. Cox, editors
© 2000, Precept Press, Inc., Chicago

11

PARENTERAL NUTRITION: VITAMINS, MINERALS, AND TRACE ELEMENTS

Susan K. Krug, MS, RD, LD

Recommendations for parenteral multivitamins were first prepared in 1975 by the American Medical Association's Nutrition Advisory Group (AMA-NAG).[1] Suggested vitamin intakes were based on the recommended dietary allowances (RDAs), with modifications for differences in utilization and rates of excretion due to route of administration and clinical conditions commonly associated with parenteral nutrition (PN). A separate formulation for infants and children through 10 years of age was proposed.

Shortly thereafter, an expert panel of the AMA's Department of Foods and Nutrition published guidelines on essential trace element preparations for parenteral use.[2] These guidelines recommended trace elements to be included in PN solutions, safe levels for administration based on estimated requirements and contaminants within parenteral solutions, and concentrations for single and multiple trace element formulations.

In the mid-1980s, a subcommittee of the Committee on Clinical Practice Issues of the American Society for Clinical Nutrition (ASCN) was formed to review existing data on the use of parenteral vitamin and mineral supplementation for pediatric patients. The subcommittee report suggested revisions for both sets of AMA guidelines and made recommendations for calcium, phosphorus, and magnesium.[3]

An international panel of infant nutrition experts developed recommended ranges of nutrient intakes for preterm infants in the early 1990s. The "consensus recommendations" included target nutrient ranges for both parenteral and enteral feeding of preterm infants at varying weights and levels of physiologic stability.[4] The parenteral recommendations were consistent with those of ASCN for most nutrients.

Vitamins

The ASCN subcommittee findings support continued use of 1975 AMA-NAG pediatric multivitamin guidelines in term infants and children up to age 11. These guidelines are recommended for both short-term and long-term total parenteral nutrition (TPN). The ASCN subcommittee suggests that patients receiving oral supplements may need adjustments in the parenteral multivitamin dose; however, no specific guidelines are provided.[3]

The 1975 AMA-NAG pediatric multivitamin guidelines, however, do not maintain all serum vitamin levels within acceptable ranges among preterm infants. Therefore, the ASCN subcommittee recommends the development of a multivitamin formulation specifically for high-risk preterm infants. The ASCN subcommittee report includes suggested preterm vitamin dosages based on available research data. In addition, the subcommittee suggests that preterm parenteral multivitamin mixtures (1) include separate water-soluble and lipid-soluble vitamin components, (2) provide lipid-soluble vitamins without the addition of potentially toxic emulifiers, and (3) be sufficiently tested to determine the optimal method of delivery and to ensure nutrient stability under conditions commonly present in intensive care nurseries.[3] The AMA-NAG guidelines for parenteral multivitamins for term infants and children, ASCN suggested dosages for preterm infants, and the recent "consensus recommendations" for stable, growing preterm infants are listed in Table 11.1.

Until a preterm parenteral multivitamin is developed and approved for commercial use, currently available parenteral multivitamins must continue to be used. Both pediatric and adult parenteral multivitamin preparations are given in Table 11.2. The 1988 ASCN subcommittee report suggests giving 40% of the AMA-NAG pediatric multivitamin formulation per kilogram of body weight, with a maximum dose of 100%.[3] Using this guideline, infants weighing 2,500 g receive 100% of the AMA-NAG pediatric multivitamin formulation. The manufacturer of M.V.I.-Pediatric (Astra Pharmaceuticals, Westboro, Mass) currently recommends 100% of the standard dose for infants and children > 3 kg; 65% of the dose for infants 1-3 kg; and 30% of the dose for infants < 1 kg. Table 11.3 compares the calculated vitamin intake per kg for these two sets of recommendations at selected infant weights.

Prolonged, nationwide shortages of parenteral multivitamins have recently occurred in the United States. These shortages have been associated with the development of life-threatening lactic aci-

Table 11.1.   Suggested Daily Intakes of Parenteral Vitamins
              for Infants and Children

Vitamin	Term infants and children dose per day (AMA-NAG)[†]	Preterm infants dose/kg body wt (maximum not to exceed term infant dose)* (ASCN)[3]	Consensus recommendations for stable, growing preterm infants dose/kg body wt[4]
Lipid-soluble			
A (µg)[†]	700	500	700-1,500
w/ lung disease			1,500-2,800
E (mg)[†]	7	2.8	3.5
K (µg)	200[‡]	80[‡]	8-10
D (µg)[†]	10	4	1-4
(IU)	400	160	40-160
Water-soluble			
Ascorbic acid (mg)	80	25	15-25
Thiamin (mg)	1.2	0.35	0.20-0.35
Riboflavin (mg)	1.4	0.15	0.15-0.20
Pyridoxine (mg)	1.0	0.18	0.15-0.20
Niacin (mg)	17	6.8	4.0-6.8
Pantothenate (mg)	5.0	2.0	1-2
Biotin (µg)	20	6.0	5-8
Folate (µg)	140	56	56
Vitamin B_{12} (µg)	1.0	0.3	0.3

*   ASCN best estimate for new preterm parenteral multivitamin formulation.
†   700 µg RE = 2,300 international units (IU); 7 mg alpha tocopherol = 7 IU; 10 µg vitamin D = 400 IU.
‡   This dosage of vitamin K reportedly results in higher blood levels than in control patients and is probably more than needed. However, until more measurements have been conducted using different dosages, ASCN recommends 200 µg/day for term infants and children and 80 µg/kg/day for preterm infants.

dosis secondary to thiamin deficiency in patients who received more than seven days of total parenteral nutrition without multivitamin supplementation.[5] Deficiencies of other B vitamins, folate, vitamin D, vitamin A, and biotin have also been reported. In response to these events, The American Society for Parenteral and Enteral Nutrition (ASPEN) developed guidelines for using available supplies of parenteral multivitamins during periods of shortage, and the U.S. Food and Drug Administration (FDA) permitted the importation of the parenteral multivitamins Multi-12 (Sabex, Boucherville, Quebec) from Canada and Cernavit (Baxter-Clintec, Deerfield, Ill.) from France to help meet the demand for parenteral multivitamins.[6]

When parenteral multivitamin shortages occur, the following guidelines are suggested for infants.[6]

1. Reserve MVI-Pediatric (Astra Pharmaceuticals, Westboro, Mass.) for neonates of < 36 weeks' gestation and infants weighing < 1,500 g.

2. Do not use adult parenteral multivitamins in neonates of < 36 weeks' gestation or infants weighing < 1,500 g. These multivitamins contain the additives propylene glycol, polysorbate 80, and/or polysorbate 20, which may be toxic in young infants.

3. Cernevit (Baxter-Clintec) can be used in neonates/infants and children < 11 years old. The recommended dose is 0.8ml/kg/day up to a maximum of 2.5 ml/day, with additional supplementation of vitamin K at a dose of 80 µg/day for infants < 2,500 g and 200 µg daily for infants and children > 2,500 g. Cernevit does not contain propylene glycol, polysorbate 80, or polysorbate 20. The additives present in Cernevit are not believed to be toxic. Cernevit does increase the glycine content of the parenteral solution.

4. The adult parenteral multivitamins MVI-12 (Astra) and Multi-12 (Sabex) may be used in infants of > 36 weeks gestation and weighing > 1,500 g. The recommended dose is 2 ml/kg body weight to a maximum dose of 5 ml/day. Vitamin K should be supplemented at a dose of 80 µg/day for infants < 2,500 g and 200 µg/day for infants > 2,500 g.

5. MVC (American Pharmaceutical Partners, Santa Monica, Calif.) may be used in infants of > 36 weeks' gestation and weighing > 1500 g. The recommended dose is 0.5 ml/kg body weight to a maximum dose of 1 ml/day. MVC does not contain folic acid, vitamin B_{12}, or biotin. Therefore, a daily supplement of 140 µg folic acid and a monthly injection of 100 µg vitamin B_{12} are recommended. Because no parenteral biotin supplement is available, infants receiving this regimen are at risk of developing biotin deficiency. Vitamin K supplementation is also recommended at a dose of 80 µg/day for infants < 2,500 g and 200 µg daily for those > 2,500 g.

6. All patients > 1,500 g who are able to absorb 50% of nutrients enterally should receive vitamins orally or by gastric tube. Parenteral thiamin should be continued for patients receiving enteral multivitamin supplementation due to the high carbohydrate load provided by parenteral nutrition, which increases the risk of thiamin deficiency. All parenteral nutrition patients receiving enteral multivitamin supplementation should be

observed for evidence of vitamin deficiencies due to poor absorption.

7. Regimens containing MVI-12, Multi-12, Cernevit, and MVC may be further conserved by reducing the daily dose or giving vitamins three times per week. When using this strategy, patients should be carefully observed for evidence of vitamin deficiencies.

8. When multivitamin preparations are not available, individual vitamin preparations (oral and injectable) can be obtained. Recommended intakes include 50 mg I.V. thiamin at least three times a week, 0.4-1.0 mg I.V. folate/day, 100 mg I.V. ascorbic acid/day, 5-10 mg I.V. pyridoxine/day, 40-50 mg I.V. niacin/day, and 100 μg vitamin B_{12} by intramuscular or subcutaneous injection monthly. In home care settings, if the above regimen is not reasonable, the minimum acceptable supplementation provides thiamin and folate three times a week and monthly vitamin B_{12} by injection.

Water-Soluble Vitamins

Intakes of parenteral water-soluble vitamins on a daily basis equal to or greater than the AMA-NAG pediatric multivitamin formulation have been shown to prevent deficiency in term infants and children for periods of three months or more.[7,8] In addition, elevated serum values for several of these vitamins have been reported among pediatric patients with intakes greater than the AMA-NAG pediatric multivitamin guidelines.[7]

Interestingly, infants and children of varying ages and sizes have similar values for biochemical indexes of water-soluble vitamin status when given the AMA-NAG pediatric multivitamin formulation.[8] Because requirements among these children are expected to differ, such findings suggest an efficient elimination of excess water-soluble vitamins. Therefore, continued use of the AMA-NAG pediatric guidelines for water-soluble vitamins appears to be safe and adequate for term infants and children.[3]

Guidelines for using the AMA-NAG pediatric multivitamin formulation in preterm infants have varied from the initial recommendation of 10% of the dose per kilogram of body weight per day to 65% of the total dose per day.[1,3] Intakes of 40-65% of the total dose have been shown to prevent deficiency for all water-soluble vitamins measured.[8,9] However, elevated blood levels for ascorbate, vitamin B_{12}, folate, niacin, and pantothenate in preterm infants receiving 65% of the total dose indicated an excessive intake.[8] The ASCN recommendation for 40% of the AMA-NAG pediatric multivitamin formulation per kilogram of body weight, with a maximum dose of 100%, is also associated with elevated blood levels for pyridoxine and riboflavin.[10-12] Although no clinical symptoms of toxicity have been

Table 11.2. Parenteral Multivitamins—Content per Standard Dose*

	Product* (distributor)[†]			
Vitamin	MVI-Pediatric (Astra)[1]	MVC** (APP)[2]	MVI-12** (Astra)[1] Multi-12** (Sabex)[4]	Cernevit (Baxter)[3]
Lipid-soluble				
A (µg)	700	600	500	530
(IU)	2300	2000	1650	1750
E (mg)	7	1	5	5.6
K (µg)	200	0	0	0
D (µg)	10	5	2.5	2.8
(IU)	400	200	100	110
Water-soluble				
Ascorbic acid (mg)	80	100	50	62.5
Thiamin (mg)	1.2	10	1.5	1.76
Riboflavin (mg)	1.4	2	1.8	2.07
Pyridoxine (mg)	1	3	2	2.27
Niacin (mg)	17	20	20	23
Pantothenate (mg)	5	5	7.5	8.63
Biotin (µg)	20	0	30	34.5
Folate (µg)	140	0	200	207
Vitamin B_{12} (µg)	1	0	2.5	3
Standard unit dose volume (ml)	5	1	5	2.5

* Content data from http://www.clinnutr.org "IV Multivitamin Shortage—Update no. 24" June 10, 1998.

† [1]Astra=Astra Pharmaceuticals, Westboro, Mass.; [2]APP=American Pharmaceutical Partners, Santa Monica, Calif.; [3]Baxter=Baxter-Clintec, Deerfield, Ill. (Imports Cernevit from France. FDA approved as a replacement for MVI-Pediatric during parenteral multivitamin shortage, 1996-1998); [4]Sabex=Sabex, Boucherville, Quebec, Canada (Use in U.S. approved by FDA during parenteral multivitamin shortage, 1996-1998).

** These parenteral multivitamins contain additives such as polysorbate 80, polysorbate 20, propylene glycol, and mannitol. Specific information is given in package inserts. These products meet the 1975 AMA-NAG guidelines for adult parenteral vitamins. Product information indicates that safety and effectiveness in children below the age of 11 years has not been established; however, they have been used in infants and children during periods when supplies of MVI-Pediatric are limited.

identified, preterm infants receiving the 40% of the formulation per kilogram have shown blood pyridoxine values rising to > 10 times cord blood and maternal levels.[11] Blood riboflavin levels dramatical-

Table 11.3. Calculated Vitamin Intake/kg for ASCN and Manufacturer's Recommendations at Selected Preterm Infant Weights Using Current Pediatric Multivitamin Formulation

Weights	ASCN recommended dose* 40% dose/kg body wt (maximum not to exceed term infant dose)	Product guidelines				
		30% dose for infants < 1 kg			65% dose for infants 1-3 kg	
	≤ 2500 g	500 g	950 g	1000 g	2000 g	3000 g
Lipid-soluble						
A (µg)	280	420	221	455	228	152
(IU)	933	1,380	726	1,495	748	498
E (mg)	2.8	4.2	2.2	4.5	2.2	1.5
K (µg)	80	120	63	130	65	43
D (µg)	4	6	3.2	6.5	3.2	2.2
(IU)	160	240	126	260	130	87
Water-soluble						
Ascorbic acid (mg)	32	48	25	52	26	17
Thiamin (mg)	0.48	0.72	0.34	0.78	0.39	0.26
Riboflavin (mg)	0.56	0.84	0.44	0.91	0.46	0.30
Pyridoxine (mg)	0.4	0.6	0.32	0.65	0.33	0.22
Niacin (mg)	6.8	10.2	5.4	11.1	5.6	3.7
Pantothenate (mg)	2.0	3.0	1.4	3.3	1.6	1.1
Biotin (µg)	8.0	12.0	6.3	13.0	6.5	4.3
Folate (µg)	56	84	44	91	46	30
Vitamin B$_{12}$ (µg)	0.4	0.6	0.32	0.65	0.33	0.22

* The 1988 ASCN subcommittee report[3] suggested that until a preterm parenteral multivitamin is available, pediatric formulations meeting the 1975 AMA-NAG pediatric guidelines should be used at 40% of the standard dose per kg. The maximum dose should not exceed 100% of the term infant dose. Infants weighing > 2,500 g receive 100% of the standard dose.

ly increase 20- to 400-fold during the first one to two weeks of PN therapy. During the second to third week, urinary excretion of riboflavin usually increases and is associated with a decrease in blood riboflavin levels.[10] Elevated blood and urine riboflavin levels have raised concerns about the potential for renal toxicity secondary to riboflavin precipitation or cellular damage associated with photoexcitation and photosensitization.[10] These data indicate that current preterm guidelines provide excessive intakes of some water-soluble vitamins and support the development of a preterm parenteral multivitamin formulation that contains more appropriate amounts of water-soluble vitamins.[3,11,13]

Vitamin A

Daily parenteral multivitamin supplementation containing from 700 µg (2,300 IU) to 1,500 µg (5,000 IU) vitamin A maintains normal serum retinol levels in most term infants and children for periods of three months or more.[14-16] Intakes of 250 µg (833 IU) vitamin A per day are inadequate to replete pediatric patients with initial serum retinols below 15 µg/dl.[16] Occasionally, higher intakes may fail to increase serum retinol values in depleted patients.[14,15] Overall, the 700 µg (2,300 IU) vitamin A provided in the AMA-NAG pediatric formulation meets the needs of most term infants and children and continues to be the recommended daily intake.[3]

Preterm infants are born with lower liver stores of vitamin A and have lower serum retinol values than term infants.[17-19] When preterm infants were given 455 µg (1,515 IU) of vitamin A as retinol in amino acid-glucose solutions for periods up to one month, serum retinol values remained low.[14,20] Those with birth weights of < 1,000 g often had a decline in serum retinol.[20] Values of < 10 µg/dl were reported for many parenterally fed preterm infants; such levels are associated with deficiency in older infants and children. Advancement to enteral feedings that provided 200-300 µg (667-1,000 IU) of vitamin A/day was associated with an increase in serum retinol. These data suggest that significant losses of retinol occur during administration of parenteral nutrition.[20]

Administration losses of retinol are reduced when parenteral multivitamins are added to the lipid emulsion rather than the amino acid-glucose solution. The infusion of vitamin-supplemented lipid emulsions providing 280 µg (933 IU) retinol/kg resulted in a progressive increase in serum retinol among preterm infants weighing < 1,500 g at birth.[10] The use of retinyl palmitate instead of retinol in amino acid-glucose solutions also lowered losses during administration. However, increased levels of serum vitamin A occurred primarily as retinyl palmitate, with retinol increasing only slightly.[12]

Another reported approach to optimize vitamin A status has been to give preterm infants up to 5 ml/day intravenous fat emulsion (10% or 20%) supplemented with retinyl palmitate (Aquasol A parenteral) at a standard concentration of 80,000 retinol equivalents (RE) per liter (1 RE = 1 µg retinol) in addition to their standard parenteral multivitamin supplementation. Infants receiving this supplemental regimen achieved intakes 300-400 RE/day higher than infants given standard parenteral multivitamin supplementation alone.[21] These infants maintained or increased their retinol and retinol-binding protein values while receiving parenteral nutrition as their primary nutrient source. Plasma levels collected after several hours off lipid infusion did not suggest an accumulation of retinyl palmitate.

The ASCN guideline to use 40% of the AMA-NAG pediatric multivitamin formulation for preterm infants provides 280 µg (933 IU) of vitamin A/kg/day. This intake may be less than optimal. Future formulations containing up to 500 µg (1,667 IU)/kg may be more appropriate and merit evaluation.[3]

Currently, doses of up to 900 µg (3,000 IU) vitamin A every other day are being evaluated for the prevention of bronchopulmonary dysplasia in high-risk infants. To optimize the delivery of vitamin A to the infant, administration is via intramuscular injection rather than as a component of parenteral nutrition.[22,23]

Vitamin E

Term infants and children who received parenteral nutrition supplemented with 7 mg of vitamin E daily have maintained blood tocopherol levels within a reference range of 0.5 to 1.5 mg/dl for periods up to five months.[14] However, 45% of parenterally fed infants and children supplemented with 2.5 mg vitamin E had blood tocopherol values of < 0.5 mg/dl.[15] These findings support continued use of the AMA-NAG guideline for supplementation with 7 mg of vitamin E/day.

Preterm infants are born with low body stores of vitamin E, and blood tocopherol values on the first day of life are usually < 0.5 mg/dl.[24] The American Academy of Pediatrics (AAP) Committee on the Fetus and Newborn reviewed vitamin E supplementation issues and recommended that blood levels be maintained between 1 and 2 mg/dl.[25] Parenteral supplementation using 65% of the AMA-NAG pediatric multivitamin formulation (4.6 mg vitamin E) in preterm infants may increase blood tocopherol to levels > 3-5 mg/dl.[26-28] However, 30% of the formulation (2.1 mg vitamin E) does not maintain adequate blood levels.[26] The ASCN recommendation to use 40% of the AMA-NAG pediatric multivitamin formulation per kilogram provides 2.8 mg/kg/day. This intake has been shown to maintain acceptable blood tocopherol values whether given in amino acid-glucose solutions or lipid emulsions.[10,12] Amorde-Spalding et al. reported findings for 110 preterm infants with birth weights of ≤ 1000 grams who received 50% of a vial of M.V.I.-Pediatric (3.5 mg vitamin E) per day beginning on the first day of life.[29] Ninety-eight percent of these infants achieved plasma alpha-tocopherol levels between 0.5 mg/dl and 3.0 mg/dl by seven days of life, with 58% having levels within the AAP guidelines. However, additional information concerning vitamin E status beyond seven days is needed to verify the safety of this vitamin E dose.

E-Ferol, an I.V. vitamin E product no longer available, was marketed for use in preterm and low-birth-weight infants as a preventive for retrolental fibroplasia (retinopathy of prematurity). Shortly after its introduction, a clinical syndrome consisting of ascites, hepatomegaly, direct hyperbilirubinemia, thrombocytopenia, and renal failure was identified among infants exposed to E-Ferol at doses of 25-100 mg/day. Toxicological studies have suggested that the emulsifiers, polysorbates 80 and 20, may have been the primary cause for the syndrome. However, vitamin toxicity was not ruled out.[30]

Vitamin K

Long-term PN and frequent use of wide-spectrum antibiotics often impairs endogenous vitamin K production by intestinal flora. Prior to the development of pediatric parenteral multivitamin preparations equivalent to the AMA-NAG guidelines, infants and children received weekly intramuscular injections of 0.5-1 mg vitamin K. With this regimen, evidence of vitamin K deficiency as determined by reduced coagulant activity occurred among preterm infants, but not term infants, between five and seven days following injection.[31] Current pediatric parenteral multivitamins containing vitamin K alleviate the need for these routine injections. Intakes between 70 and 130 µg/day for preterm infants and 200 µg/day for term infants and children are not associated with abnormal clotting times or apparent complications.[3] Current guidelines suggest a dose of 80 µg vitamin K (phylloquinone)/kg/day for preterm infants and 200 µg/day for term infants and children.

Vitamin D

A primary function of vitamin D is to increase intestinal absorption of calcium (Ca) and phosphorus (P); however, it also acts on the kidney and bone to maintain Ca-P homeostasis and may be involved in normal cell differentiation in the bone marrow. Hence, maintenance of vitamin D sufficiency is essential even for patients receiving their total Ca and P intake parenterally.[3] Serum 25-hydroxyvitamin D (25-OHD) is the index that most accurately reflects vitamin D status. Among term infants and children receiving short-term PN supplemented with 400 IU vitamin D, mean values for 25-OHD remained within the normal reference range. Levels of 25-OHD increased over the first three months of supplementation with 400 IU vitamin D in six home parenteral nutrition patients who had normal baseline values. Peak 25-OHD values were not excessive; in two patients monitored beyond three months, a decline toward baseline occurred.[14] This information suggests that supplementation with 400 IU vitamin D is sufficient to maintain normal vitamin D status in most term infants and children with minimal risk for toxicity.

In preterm infants, parenteral vitamin D intakes of 160 IU/kg resulted in progressive increases in serum 25-OHD.[14] Mean baseline values were below the reference range of 15-31 ng/ml and after four weeks equaled 20.2 ± 4.2 ng/ml. Term and preterm infants have been found to maintain normal serum 25-OHD levels with parenteral supplementation as low as 25 IU of vitamin D/dl (about 30-40 IU/kg).[32,33] Of interest, serum 1,25-dihydroxyvitamin D values of parenterally fed preterm infants were elevated when given standard Ca and P intakes (20 mg/dl Ca and 15.5 mg/dl P).[33] Lower 1,25-OH$_2$D values occurred when the content of Ca and P was increased (60 mg/dl Ca and 46.5 mg/dl P). Elevated 1,25-OH$_2$D values suggest that inadequate mineral intake rather than vitamin D deficiency is the primary factor limiting bone mineralization in PN-fed preterm infants. The ASCN guideline to use 40% per kg of the AMA-NAG pediatric multivitamin formulation up to a maximum of 100% provides 160 IU vitamin D/kg. This intake has not been shown to be toxic, and provides a margin of safety in the prevention of vitamin D deficiency.[3]

Vitamin-like Substances

Carnitine. Carnitine is a cofactor required for the transport of carboxylic acids activated with coenzyme A across cellular and subcellular membranes.[34] Neonates, especially preterm infants who receive prolonged TPN, rapidly deplete their limited carnitine reserves and have inadequate rates of biosynthesis to meet their metabolic needs.[35,36] Following a lipid challenge, carnitine-depleted infants have lower levels of beta-hydroxybutarate and acetoacetate and higher levels of triglycerides and free fatty acids than control infants. These findings suggest impaired fatty acid oxidation. Carnitine supplementation has been shown to normalize serum carnitine levels, improve indices of fatty acid metabolism, and improve nitrogen balance.[37,38] Carnitine is now available for general use in I.V. supplementation (Carnitor, Sigma-Tau, Gaithersberg, MD). The dose recommendation made by the manufacturer is between 20 and 50 mg/kg/day. This level of supplementation may be higher than necessary; lower intakes providing 2-10 mg/kg/day have improved carnitine status without the development of adverse events.[34,39] In any case, blood levels should be closely monitored.[39] This nutrient merits consideration in infants who receive TPN for more than four weeks.[34-36]

Inositol. Inositol is a component of membrane phospholipids. In addition, compounds containing inositol are important in signal transduction. Serum inositol levels in newborns are much higher than maternal levels. Human milk, particularly colostrum, is a rich source of inositol. A recent paper reported that inositol supplementation of PN fluids during the first week of life improved survival and reduced bronchopulmonary dysplasia and retrolental fibroplasia (retinopathy of prematurity) among preterm infants with respiratory distress syndrome.[41] The level of supplementation in this study equaled the inositol content of human milk. Additional research supporting these findings is needed before routine supplementation can be recommended.

Major Minerals

Recommendations of the ASCN Subcommittee on Pediatric Parenteral Nutrient Requirements for Ca, P, and magnesium (Mg) are listed in Table 11.4.[3] Mineral guidelines are presented as concentrations per liter rather than daily intakes in order to avoid precipitation of Ca-P salts.[42,43] For infants, these recommendations assume an average fluid intake of 120-150 ml/kg/day with 25 g amino acid/L of a pediatric amino acid solution. Calculated daily mineral intakes for infants given PN within the ASCN guidelines equal 75-90 mg Ca/kg, 48-67.5 mg P/kg, and 6-10.5 mg Mg/kg. The ASCN subcommittee suggests central venous infusion as the preferred route for administration of these concentrations of Ca and P. However, solutions containing 600 mg Ca/L and 465 mg P/L have been given to preterm infants by peripheral venous infusion without complications.[33]

Calcium and Phosphorus

Severe bone demineralization and rickets have been commonly associated with long-term PN in both term and preterm infants.[44] Until recently, PN solutions have provided Ca and P at levels well below reported mineral retention rates for enterally fed infants.[45,46] Reports of low serum phosphorus, increased serum alkaline phosphatase, normal serum 25-OHD, elevated serum 1,25-OH$_2$D, and hypercalciuria in conjunction with tubular phosphorus reabsorption rates of > 90% among PN-fed infants indicated the presence of Ca-P deficiency.[32,33,47,48] By increasing the Ca and P content of PN solutions to levels similar to the ASCN recommendations, serum chemistries and urinary mineral excretion have been normalized, bone mineral content increased, and the incidence of radiographic rickets reduced.[32,33,47-49] Ca and P retention has been reported to approach 85-90% among preterm infants given "high-mineral" parenteral feedings containing 50-80 mg Ca/kg and 35-60 mg P/kg.[50-52] The initiation of parenteral feedings at 70% of the ASCN guidelines, with incremental advances of 10% daily, has been suggested. Daily monitoring of serum Ca and P during the period of advancement is suggested to

Table 11.4. Recommended Intravenous Intakes of Calcium, Phosphorus, and Magnesium

	Preterm infants*	Term infants	Children > 1 yr[†]
	mg/L		
Ca	500-600	500-600	200-400
P	400-450	400-450	150-300
Mg	50-70	50-70	20-40

Reprinted with permission from Greene HL, Hambidge KM, Schanler R, et al.[3]

* To prevent Ca-P precipitation, intakes are described per liter, to prevent administration of high concentrations of Ca and P, which may result if intakes are expressed per kilogram body weight and there is fluid restriction. These recommendations also assume an average fluid intake of about 120-150 ml/kg/day with 25 g amino acid/L of a pediatric amino acid solution. These dosage levels for preterm infants should be given only in central venous infusions.

† Requirements are less with advancing age; few data are available.

detect any tolerance problems such as hyper-hypocalcemia or hyper-hypophosphatemia.[53]

A wide range of Ca:P ratios have been used in PN solutions. Studies using ratios of 1.3:1 to 1.7:1 by weight (1:1 to 1.3:1 by molar ratio) have reported high mineral retention and minimal problems with tolerance.[32,33,48,50,51,54] The use of Ca:P ratios of < 1:1 by weight (0.8:1 by molar ratio) and alternate day infusions of Ca and P are not recommended due to reports of mineral wasting and alterations in Ca and P homeostasis.[29,55-57]

Magnesium

The magnesium content of parenteral nutrition should maintain normal serum magnesium levels. Solutions containing 4.4 mg/dl Mg produced hypomagnesemia in about 25% of infants studied,[58] and transient hypermagnesemia and retention in excess of intrauterine accretion rates have occurred with concentrations of 9.6 mg/dl.[32,50] The ASCN guidelines for infants of 5-7 mg/dl are intermediate to these intakes. Routine monitoring of serum magnesium during the course of PN allows for individualization of the magnesium intake.

Trace Elements

Recommendations of the ASCN Subcommittee on Pediatric Parenteral Nutrient Requirements for trace elements are listed in Table 11.5.[3] These recommendations expand those previously proposed by the AMA.[2] Table 11.6 lists trace element combinations currently available for use with pediatric patients as well as selected adult preparations that contain molybdenum and/or iodine.

Zinc

When PN is supplemental to enteral nutrition or of short duration, zinc is the only trace element that requires supplementation. The ASCN recommendations for parenteral zinc supplementation are calculated from factorial estimates of requirements for growth and endogenous losses. Gestational maturity, postnatal age, and weight are factors considered in these recommendations. Published balance studies and assessments of zinc status among PN-fed infants and children consistently support the ASCN revisions for parenteral zinc recommendations for infants and children.[20,50,59-61]

Some infants and children, however, may require higher intakes of zinc due to increased urinary or G.I. zinc excretion.[62,63] Infants with high-volume stool output or G.I. fluid losses from fistulas/stomas are easily identified as needing additional zinc. Urinary zinc excretion increases with high-output renal failure.[63] In addition, urinary zinc has been shown to increase with the addition of cysteine or histidine to PN solutions.[62] Losses relating to these two amino acids, which can be substantial, should be considered when cysteine supplementation or high histidine amino acid solutions are used.[62]

Copper

The ASCN recommendation for copper supplementation is 20 µg/kg/day for infants and children of all ages who receive prolonged PN (e.g., more than four weeks).[3] Liver stores of copper have been estimated to be sufficient to prevent deficiency for up to two months in preterm infants and four to six months in term infants. Although the current copper recommendations should be adequate to prevent deficiency among preterm infants,[59-64] intakes of 63 µg/kg/day have been estimated for duplication of fetal accretion rates.[50,60] Interestingly, preterm infants given up to five weeks of PN without copper supplementation achieved higher serum copper and ceruloplasmin levels than enterally fed preterm infants.[65] Explanations proposed for this finding include (1) the occurrence of copper depletion among enterally fed infants and (2) the presence of hepatotoxicity or decreased enterohepatic circulation among the parenterally fed infants (bile is the primary route for copper excretion).[65] For most term infants and children on long-term PN therapy, intakes of 20 µg/kg/day maintain normal copper status.[20,60,61]

Copper supplementation is not recommended for infants or children with limited copper excretion due to cholestasis or other conditions that reduce bile excretion. Conversely, infants and children with increased biliary losses due to jejunostomies or external biliary

Table 11.5.   Recommended Intravenous Intakes of Trace Elements*

| Element | Infants | | Children |
	Preterm[†]	Term	
	µg/kg/d		µg/kg/d (max µg/d)
Zinc	400	250 < 3 mo 100 > 3 mo	50 (5,000)
Copper[‡]	20	20	20 (300)
Selenium[§]	2.0	2.0	2.0 (30)
Chromium[§]	0.20	0.20	0.20 (5.0)
Manganese[‡]	1.0	1.0	1.0 (50)
Molybdenum[§]	0.25	0.25	0.25 (5.0)
Iodide	1.0	1.0	1.0 (70)

Iron (see text)

Fluoride (see text)

Reprinted with permission from Greene HL, Hambidge KM, Schanler R, et al.[3]

* When TPN is only supplemental or limited to < 4 weeks, only zinc need be added. Thereafter, addition of the remaining elements is advisable.
† Available concentrations of Mo and Mn are such that dilution of the manufacturer's product may be necessary. Neotrace (American Pharmaceutical Partners, Santa Monica, CA) contains a higher ratio of Mn to Zn than suggested in this table (i.e., Zn = 1.5 mg and Mn = 25 µg/ml).
‡ Omit in patients with obstructive jaundice.
§ Omit in patients with renal dysfunction.

drainage may need an additional 10-15 µg/kg/day of copper supplementation.[3,66]

Selenium

The ASCN recommendation for selenium supplementation, 2 µg/kg/day, is based on estimated intakes of breast-fed infants and is adjusted for absorption.[3] Supplementation is suggested for patients receiving long-term PN (e.g., more than four weeks). It should be lowered or discontinued in patients with renal dysfunction.[3] Selenium deficiency has been well documented among patients receiving more than four weeks of TPN.[67,68] Indicators of selenium depletion, including decreased serum selenium and glutathione per-

Table 11.6. Parenteral Trace Element Combinations*
Content per Milliliter

Product	Zn (mg)	Cu (mg)	Mn (µg)	Cr (µg)	Se (µg)	I (µg)	Mo (µg)
Products for pediatric patients							
PTE-5[1]	1	0.1	25	1	15		
PedTE-Pak-4[2]	1	0.1	25	1			
PTE-4[1]	1	0.1	25	1			
Multiple Trace Element Pediatric[3]	0.5	0.1	30	1			
Pedtrace-4[1]	0.5	0.1	25	0.85			
Neotrace-4[1]	1.5	0.1	25	0.85			
Multiple Trace Element Neonatal[3]	1.5	0.1	36	0.85			
Selected products for adult patients							
MTE-7[†1]	1	0.4	100	4	20	25	25
MTE-6[†1]	1	0.4	100	4	20	25	

Individual trace element solutions available from a number of sources in the following concentrations per milliliter

	Zn	Cu	Mn	Cr	Se	I	Mo
Zinc	1 or 5						
Copper		0.4 or 2.0					
Manganese			100				
Chromium				4 or 20			
Selenium					40		
Iodine						100	
Molybdenum							25

* Content data from Drug facts and comparisons. St. Louis: Facts and Comparisons (div. J.P. Lippincott).
† Currently the only parenteral trace element combinations that contain Mo and/or I are designed for adult use.

1. American Pharmaceutical Partners, Santa Monica, CA.
2. Solo Pak, Elk Grove Village, Ill.
3. American Regent, Shirley, N.Y.

oxidase activity, were present in infants within four weeks of unsupplemented PN.[64,69] In preterm infants, the use of selenium supplemented parenteral nutrition at a mean intake of 1.34 µg/kg/day failed to prevent a decline in serum selenium.[70] However, preterm infants receiving 2.04 µg/kg/day from supplemented parenteral nutrition plus enteral feedings maintained their plasma selenium levels and had higher urinary selenium excretion compared with preterm infants receiving unsupplemented parenteral nutrition plus standard enteral feedings.[71] These data support using a dose closer to the ASCN recommendations. Additional studies are needed to clarify the optimal dose and time for initiation of supplementation.

Chromium

For parenteral chromium intake, the AMA and ASCN both recommend 0.2 µg/kg/day for infants and children of all ages.[1,3] Supplementation is recommended for patients receiving more than four weeks of TPN therapy, but should be discontinued when renal function is impaired.[3] In a study reporting serum chromium and glomerular filtration rates (GFR) in 15 children receiving long-term chromium-supplemented PN, chromium intakes were about 0.15 µg/kg/day.[72] Serum chromium concentrations of the parenterally fed children were about 20 times greater than normal controls. GFR was inversely correlated with chromium intake, serum chromium concentration, and PN duration. Supplemental chromium was discontinued in all patients, and intakes secondary to PN solution contaminants and water were about 0.05 µg/kg/day. After one year, serum values declined but still remained higher than controls. GFR did not change with discontinuation of the chromium supplementation, and its relationship to chromium is not known. These data suggest that the current chromium recommendation of 0.2 µg/kg/day may be too high and that a lower intake such as 0.05 µg/kg/day should be further evaluated.

Manganese

The ASCN recommendation for supplemental manganese is 1 µg/kg/day for patients receiving more than four weeks of TPN. The use of PN solutions containing manganese supplementation of 5 µg/L have resulted in normal serum manganese levels among PN patients free of cholestasis.[73,74] Elevated serum manganese values occur in pediatric patients with cholestasis receiving manganese-supplemented parenteral nutrition. Values decrease when supplemental manganese is reduced or liver function improves.[73] Current guidelines suggest discontinuation of manganese supplementation in patients with cholestasis. Among these patients, the manganese provided as a contaminant in PN solutions appears adequate to meet their needs. Monitoring their serum manganese enables the clinician to determine whether additional modifications are needed. Several case reports of adults and one child on long-term parenteral nutrition have associated elevated levels of blood manganese with manganese deposition in the brain, along with neurologic symptoms that included memory loss, weakness, difficulty walking, slowed response time, and seizures.[75-77]

Molybdenum

Supplemental molybdenum is recommended only for patients receiving TPN for more than four weeks. The ASCN recommendation of 0.25 µg/kg/day is calculated from the estimated intake of 0.3 µg/kg from human milk (assuming 80% absorption). Urine is the primary route of excretion; therefore, supplementation should be withheld in patients with impaired renal function.[3] Investigations continue in the molybdenum requirements for infants.[99]

Iodide

Iodide supplementation is recommended only for patients receiving TPN for more than four weeks. The recommended intake of 1 µg/kg/day is adequate to prevent deficiency and yet avoid toxicity. Because iodide is also absorbed through the skin, contact with iodide-containing disinfectants, detergents, or other environmental sources can affect an individual's iodide status.[3]

Iron

Iron dextran and ferrous citrate have been successfully used to supplement parenteral solutions.[78-81] Because allergic reactions to iron dextran have occurred, patients should be given an initial test dose before routine supplementation is started. Major concerns with iron supplementation relate to problems of iron overload, increased risk for septicemia among malnourished patients with low transferrin levels, and altered requirements for antioxidants such as vitamin E.[3,81] Iron supplementation should be considered among long-term total parenteral nutrition patients who are not receiving frequent blood transfusions.[78] For term infants born with normal iron stores, supplementation may be delayed until 3 months, when body reserves become depleted. A dose of 100 µg/kg should be sufficient. This dose is based on current enteral recommendations of 1 mg/kg, assuming 10% absorption.

Preterm infants are born with reduced body stores of iron and often have increased iron losses due to phlebotomy required for medical care. Current guidelines recommend that parenteral iron supplementation for preterm infants be considered by 2 months of age or 2,000 g body weight. The suggested daily dose is 200 µg/kg.[3,82] This level of intake may promote a positive iron balance in some infants, but will not provide sufficient iron to match fetal accretion rates even if started within the first week of life.[83,84] The use of erythropoetin therapy for preventing anemia of prematurity also demands the initiation of iron supplementation before 2 months of age.[85] Additional research is needed to determine optimal guidelines for parenteral iron supplementation in preterm infants.

Fluoride

Fluoride is beneficial in reducing dental caries; supplementation may be advantageous for infants and children on very long courses of total TPN (e.g., more than three months). No routine recommendations for supplementation have been made and no commercial parenteral supplement is currently available. Since fluoride (Fl) is readily absorbed, parenteral dosages are anticipated to be similar to enteral recommendations.[3] The ASCN subcommittee indicated that a daily dose of 500 µg Fl/day would be reasonable; however, a lower dose of 250 µg/day would meet the AAP Committee on Nutrition guidelines for children 6 months to 3 years.[86] Until a PN solution is available, fluoride supplementation must be limited to infants and children who can tolerate small volumes of an enteral fluoride supplement.

Aluminum

Aluminum is a common contaminant of PN additives. Currently, the highest levels of contamination are associated with calcium and phosphate salts.[87,88] Parenteral administration of aluminum allows increased deposition of aluminum in body tissues because the usual G.I. barrier is bypassed. Aluminum contamination of parenterally administered casein hydrolysates was associated with reduced bone formation and osteomalacia in patients receiving long-term PN.[89,90] The replacement of protein hydrolysates with crystalline amino acids has reduced the incidence of metabolic bone disease in older children and adults.[91] However, aluminum contamination of PN solutions, including albumin and heparin, remains a concern with infants receiving long-term PN.[92-94] In view of these continued concerns, the U.S. Food and Drug Administration has developed a rule for manufacturers concerning the aluminum content in large- and small-volume parenterals in PN.[95-97] For more information on this detailed rule, see reference 97.

Other Trace Elements

Numerous other trace elements may be beneficial in human nutrition. Although serum values for some of these trace elements may be low,[98] there have been no reports of clinical deficiency for any trace element that is not included in the ASCN guideline for trace element supplementation.

References

1. American Medical Association Department of Foods and Nutrition. Multivitamin preparations for parenteral use, a statement by the Nutrition Advisory Group, 1975. J Parenter Enter Nutr 3:258, 1979.
2. American Medical Association Department of Foods and Nutrition. Guidelines for essential trace element preparations for parenteral use, a statement by an expert panel. JAMA 241:2051, 1979.
3. Greene HL, Hambidge KM, Schanler R, et al. Guidelines for the use of vitamins, trace elements, calcium, magnesium, and phosphorus in infants and children receiving total parenteral nutrition: Report of the Subcommittee on Pediatric Parenteral Nutrient Requirements from the Committee on Clinical Practice Issues of The American Society for Clinical Nutrition. Am J Clin Nutr 48:1324, 1988.
4. Tsang RC, Lucas A, Uauy R, et al. Nutrition Needs of the Preterm Infant: Scientific Basis and Practical Guidelines. Baltimore: Williams & Wilkins, 1993; 288.
5. Centers for Disease Control and Prevention. Lactic acidosis traced to thiamine deficiency related to nationwide shortage of multivitamins for total parenteral nutrition—United States, 1997. MMWR 46:523, 1997.
6. http://www.clinnutri.org/m.v.i.htm. IV multivitamin shortage—update #35. Nov 3, 1998.
7. Marinier E, Gorski AM, De Courcy GP, et al. Blood levels of water-soluble vitamins in pediatric patients on total parenteral nutrition using a multiple vitamin preparation. J Parenter Enter Nutr 13:176, 1989.
8. Moore MC, Greene HL, Phillips B, et al. Evaluation of a pediatric multiple vitamin preparation for total parenteral nutrition in infants and children. I. Blood levels of water-soluble vitamins. Pediatrics 77:530, 1986.
9. Levy R, Herzberg GR, Andrews WL, et al. Thiamine, riboflavin, folate, and vitamin B_{12} status of low birth weight infants receiving parenteral and enteral nutrition. J Parenter Enter Nutr 16:241, 1992.
10. Baeckert PA, Greene HL, Fritz I, et al. Vitamin concentrations in very low birth weight infants given vitamins intravenously in a lipid emulsion: Measurement of vitamins A, D, and E and riboflavin. J Pediatr 113:1057, 1988.
11. Greene HL, Baeckert PA, Murrell J, et al. Blood pyridoxine levels in preterm infants receiving TPN. Pediatr Res 25:(4):113A, 1990.
12. Greene HL, Smith R, Pollack P, et al. Intravenous vitamins for very-low-birth-weight infants. J Am Coll Nutr 10:281, 1991.
13. Greene HL, Smidt LJ. Water-soluble vitamins: C, B_1, B_2, B_6, niacin, pantothenic acid, and biotin. In: Tsang RC, Lucas A, Uauy R, et al, eds. Nutritional Needs of the Preterm Infant: Scientific Basis and Practical Guidelines. Baltimore: Williams & Wilkins, 1993; 121.

14. Greene HL, Moore MEC, Phillips B, et al. Evaluation of a pediatric multiple vitamin preparation for total parenteral nutrition. II. Blood levels of vitamins A, D, E. Pediatrics 77:539, 1986.

15. Hack SL, Merritt RJ, Morgan RM, et al. Serum vitamin A and E concentrations in pediatric total parenteral nutrition patients. J Parenter Enter Nutr 14:189, 1990.

16. Ricour C, Navarro J, Duhamel JF. Trace elements and vitamin requirements in infants on total parenteral nutrition (TPN). Acta Chir Scand [suppl] 498:67, 1980.

17. Brandt RB, Mueller DG, Schroeder JR, et al. Serum vitamin A in premature and term neonates. J Pediatr 92:101, 1978.

18. Shenai JP, Chytil F, Jhaveri A, et al. Plasma vitamin A and retinol binding protein in premature and term neonates. J Pediatr 99:302, 1981.

19. Zachman RD. Retinol (vitamin A) and the neonate: Special problems of the human premature infant. Am J Clin Nutr 50:413, 1989.

20. Greene HL, Phillips BL, Franck L, et al. Persistently low blood retinol levels during and after parenteral feeding of very low birth weight infants: Examination of losses into intravenous administration sets and a method of prevention by addition to lipid emulsion. Pediatrics 79:894, 1987.

21. Werkman SH, Peeples JM, Cooke, RJ, et al. Effect of vitamin A supplementation of intravenous lipids on early vitamin A intake and status of premature infants. Am J Clin Nutr 59:586, 1994.

22. Robbins ST, Fletcher AB. Early vs delayed vitamin A supplementation in very-low-birth-weight infants. J Parenter Enter Nutr 17:220, 1993.

23. Kennedy KA, Stoll BJ, Ehrenkranz RA, et al. Vitamin A to prevent bronchopulmonary dysplasia in very-low-birth-weight infants: has the dose been too low? Early Hum Develop 49:19, 1997.

24. Gutcher GR, Raynor WJ, Farrell PM. An evaluation of vitamin E status in premature infants. Am J Clin Nutr 40:1078, 1984.

25. Poland RL. Vitamin E: What should we do? (Ltr). Pediatrics 77:787, 1986.

26. Phillips B, Franck LS, Greene HL. Vitamin E levels in premature infants during and after intravenous multivitamin supplementation. Pediatrics 80:680, 1987.

27. DeVito V, Reynolds JW, Benda GI, et al. Serum vitamin E levels in very low birth weight infants receiving vitamin E in parenteral nutrition solutions. J Parenter Enter Nutr 10:63, 1986.

28. MacDonald MG, Fletcher AB, Johnson EL, et al. The potential toxicity to neonate of multivitamin preparations used in parenteral nutrition. J Parenter Enter Nutr 11:169, 1987.

29. Amorde-Spalding K, D'Harlingue AE, Phillips BL, et al. Tocopherol levels in infants ≤ 1000 grams receiving MVI Pediatric. Pediatrics 90:992, 1992.

30. Arrowsmith JB, Faich GA, Tomita DK, et al. Morbidity and mortality among low birth weight infants exposed to an intravenous vitamin E product, E-Ferol. Pediatrics 83:244, 1989.

31. Goldschmidt B, Bors S, Szabo A. Vitamin K-dependent clotting factors during long-term total parenteral nutrition in full-term and preterm infants. J Pediatr 112:108, 1988.

32. Koo WWK, Tsang RC, Steichen JJ, et al. Vitamin D requirement in infants receiving parenteral nutrition. J Parenter Enter Nutr 11:172, 1987.

33. Koo WWK, Tsang RC, Succop P, et al. Minimal vitamin D and high calcium and phosphorus needs of preterm infants receiving parenteral nutrition. J Pediatr Gastroenterol Nutr 8:225, 1989.

34. Borum, PR. Carnitine in neonatal nutrition. J Child Neurol 10 (suppl):2S26, 1995.

35. Schmidt-Sommerfeld E, Penn D. Carnitine and total parenteral nutrition of the neonate. Biol Neonate 58 (suppl 1):81, 1990.

36. Bonner CM, DeBrie KL, Hug G, et al. Effects of parenteral L-carnitine supplementation on fat metabolism and nutrition in premature neonates. J Pediatr 126:287, 1995.

37. Christensen ML, Helms RA, Mauer EC, et al. Plasma carnitine concentration and lipid metabolism in infants receiving parenteral nutrition. J Pediatr 115:794, 1989.

38. Helms RA, Mauer EC, Hay WW. Effect of intravenous L-carnitine on growth parameters and fat metabolism during parenteral nutrition in neonates. J Parenter Enter Nutr 14:448, 1990.

39. Sulkers EJ, Lafeber HN, Degenhart HJ, et al. Effects of high carnitine supplementation on substrate utilization in low-birth-weight infants receiving total parenteral nutrition. Am J Clin Nutr 52:889, 1990.

40. Innis SM. Fat. In: Tsang RC, Lucas A, Uauy R, et al, eds. Nutritional Needs of the Preterm Infant: Scientific Basis and Practical Guidelines. Baltimore: Williams & Wilkins, 1993.

41. Hallman M, Bry K, Hoppu K, et al. Inositol supplementation in premature infants with respiratory distress syndrome. New Engl J Med 326:1233, 1992.

42. Lenz GJ, Mikrut BA. Calcium and phosphate solubility in neonatal parenteral nutrient solutions containing Aminosyn-PF or TrophAmine. Am J Hosp Pharm 45:2367, 1988.

43. Dunham B, Marcuard S, Khazanie PG, et al. The solubility of calcium and phosphorus in neonatal total parenteral nutrition solutions. J Parenter Enter Nutr 15:608, 1991.

44. Koo WW. Parenteral nutrition-related bone disease. J Parenter Enter Nutr 16:386, 1992.

45. Fomon SJ, Owen GM, Jensen RL, et al. Calcium and phosphorus balance studies with normal full term infants fed pooled human milk or various formulas. Am J Clin Nutr 12:346, 1963.

46. Schanler RJ, Abrams SA, Garza C. Bioavailability of calcium and phosphorus in human milk fortifiers and formula for very low birth weight infants. J Pediatr 113:95, 1988.

47. MacMahon P, Blair ME, Treweeke P, et al. Association of mineral composition of neonatal intravenous feeding solutions and metabolic bone disease of prematurity. Arch Dis Child 64:489, 1989.

48. Koo WWK, Tsang RC, Steichen JJ, et al. Parenteral nutrition for infants: Effect of high versus low calcium and phosphorus content. J Pediatr Gastroenterol Nutr 6:96, 1987.

49. Prestridge LL, Schanler RJ, Schulman RJ, et al. Effect of parenteral calcium and phosphorus therapy on mineral retention and bone mineral content in very low birth weight infants. J Pediatr 122:761, 1993.

50. Schanler RJ, Shulman RJ, Prestridge LL. Parenteral nutrient needs of very low birth weight infants. J Pediatr 125:961, 1994.

51. Pelegano JF, Rowe JC, Carey DE, et al. Simultaneous infusion of calcium and phosphorus in parenteral nutrition for premature infants: Use of physiologic calcium/phosphorus ratio. J Pediatr 114:115, 1989.

52. Chessex P, Pineault M, Brisson G, et al. Role of the source of phosphate salt in improving the mineral balance of parenterally fed low birth weight infants. J Pediatr 116:765, 1990.
53. Koo WWK, Tsang RC. Mineral requirements of low-birth weight infants. J Am Coll Nutr 10:474, 1991.
54. Pelegano JF, Rowe JC, Carey DE, et al. Effect of calcium/phosphorus ratio on mineral retention in parenterally fed premature infants. J Pediatr Gastroenterol Nutr 12:351, 1991.
55. Vileisis RA. Effect of phosphorus intake in total parenteral nutrition infusates in premature neonates. J Pediatr 110:586, 1987.
56. Kimura S, Nose O, Deino Y, et al. Effect of alternate and simultaneous administrations of calcium and phosphorus on calcium metabolism in children receiving total parenteral nutrition. J Parenter Enter Nutr 10:513, 1986.
57. Hoehn GJ, Carey DE, Rowe JC, et al. Alternate day infusion of calcium and phosphate in very low birth weight infants: Wasting of the infused mineral. J Pediatr Gastroenterol Nutr 6:752, 1987.
58. Koo WWK, Fong T, Gupta JM. Parenteral nutrition in infants. Aust Paediatr J 16:169, 1980.
59. Lockitch G, Godolphin W, Pendray MF, et al. Serum zinc, copper, retinol-binding protein, prealbumin, and ceruloplasmin concentrations in infants receiving intravenous zinc and copper supplementation. J Pediatr 102:304, 1983.
60. Zlotkin SH, Buchanan BE. Meeting zinc and copper intake requirements in the parenterally fed preterm and full-term infant. J Pediatr 103:441, 1983.
61. Shulman RJ. Zinc and copper balance studies in infants receiving total parenteral nutrition. Am J Clin Nutr 49:879, 1989.
62. Zlotkin SH. Nutrient interactions with total parenteral nutrition: Effect of histidine and cysteine intake on urinary zinc excretion. J Pediatr 114:859, 1989.
63. Reifen RM, Zlotkin SH. Microminerals. In: Tsang RC, Lucas A, Uauy R, et al, eds. Nutritional Needs of the Preterm Infant: Scientific Basis and Practical Guidelines. Baltimore: Williams & Wilkins, 1993; 195.
64. Huston RK, Shearer TR, Jelen BJ, et al. Relationship of antioxidant enzymes to trace metals in premature infants. J Parenter Enter Nutr 11:163, 1987.
65. Tyrala EE, Manser JI, Brodsky NL, et al. Distribution of copper in the serum of the parenterally fed premature infant. J Pediatr 106:295, 1985.
66. Shike M, Roulet M, Kurian R, et al. Copper metabolism and requirements in total parenteral nutrition. Gastroenterology 81:290, 1981.
67. Kien CL, Ganther HE. Manifestations of chronic selenium deficiency in a child receiving total parenteral nutrition. Am J Clin Nutr 37:319, 1983.
68. Cohen HJ, Chovaniec ME, Mistretta D, et al. Selenium repletion and glutathione peroxidase—differential effects on plasma and red blood cell enzyme activity. Am J Clin Nutr 41:735, 1985.
69. Van Caillie-Bertrand M, Degenhart HJ, Fernandes J. Selenium status of infants on nutritional support. Acta Paediatr Scand 73:816, 1984.
70. Huston RK, Jelen BJ, Vidgoff J. Selenium supplementation in low-birthweight premature infants: Relationship to trace metals and antioxidant enzymes. J Parenter Enter Nutr 15:556, 1991.

71. Daniels L, Gibson R, Simmer K. Randomised clinical trial of parenteral selenium supplementation in preterm infants. Arch Dis Child 74:F158, 1996.
72. Moukarzel AA, Song MK, Buchman AL, et al. Excessive chromium intake in children receiving total parenteral nutrition. Lancet 339:385, 1992.
73. Hambidge KM, Sokol RJ, Fidanza SJ, et al. Plasma manganese concentrations in infants and children receiving parenteral nutrition. J Parenter Enter Nutr 13:168, 1989.
74. Zlotkin SH, Buchanan BE. Manganese intakes in intravenously fed infants: Dosages and toxicity studies. Biol Trace Elem Res 9:271, 1986.
75. Ono J, Harada K, Kodaka R, et al. Manganese deposition in the brain during long-term total parenteral nutrition. J Parenter Enter Nutr 19:310, 1995.
76. Ejima A, Imamura T, Nakamura S, et al. Manganese intoxication during total parenteral nutrition. Lancet 339:426, 1992.
77. Reynolds AP, Kiely E, Meadows N. Manganese in long term paediatric parenteral nutrition. Arch Dis Child 1:527, 1994.
78. Shaw JCL. Iron absorption by the premature infant. The effect of transfusion and iron supplements on the serum ferritin levels. Acta Paediatr Scand Suppl 299:83, 1982.
79. Wan KK, Tsallas G. Dilute iron dextran formulation for addition to parenteral nutrient solutions. Am J Hosp Pharm 37:206, 1980.
80. Sayers MH, Johnson KD, Schumann LA, et al. Supplementation of total parenteral nutrition solutions with ferrous citrate. J Parenter Enter Nutr 7:117, 1983.
81. Burns DL, Mascioli EA, Bistrian BR. Parenteral iron dextran therapy: a review. Nutrition 11:163, 1995.
82. Ehrenkranz RA. Iron requirements of preterm infants. Nutrition 10:77, 1994.
83. Friel JK, Andrews WL, Hall MS, et al. Intravenous iron administration to very-low birth-weight newborns receiving total and partial parenteral nutrition. J Parenter Enter Nutr 19:114, 1995.
84. Friel JK, Penney S, Reid DW, et al. Zinc, copper, manganese and iron balances in parenterally fed very-low-birth-weight preterm infants receiving trace element supplement. J Parenter Enter Nutr 12:382, 1988.
85. Meyer MP, Haworth C, Meyer JH, et al. A comparison of oral and intravenous iron supplementation in preterm infants receiving recombinant erythropoietin. J Pediatr 129:258, 1996.
86. New fluoride schedule adopted. American Dental Association News. 25:12, 1994.
87. Koo WWK, Kaplan LA, Horn JA, et al. Aluminum in parenteral nutrition solutions—sources and possible alternatives. J Parenter Enter Nutr 10:591, 1986.
88. Klein, GL. The aluminum content of parenteral solutions: Current status. Nutr Reviews 49:74, 1991.
89. Klein GL, Targoff CM, Ament ME, et al. Bone disease associated with total parenteral nutrition. Lancet 2:1040, 1980.
90. Klein GL, Alfrey AC, Miller NL, et al. Aluminum loading during total parenteral nutrition. Am J Clin Nutr 35:1425, 1982.

91. Vargas JH, Klein GL, Ament ME, et al. Metabolic bone disease of total parenteral nutrition: Course after changing from casein to amino acids in parenteral solutions with reduced aluminum content. Am J Clin Nutr 48:1070, 1988.

92. Sedman AB, Klein GL, Merritt RJ, et al. Evidence of aluminum loading in infants receiving intravenous therapy. N Engl J Med 312:1337, 1985.

93. Koo WWK, Kaplan LA, Krug-Wispe SK, et al. Response of preterm infants to aluminum in parenteral nutrition. J Parenter Enter Nutr 13:516, 1989.

94. Bishop NJ, Morley R, Day JP, et al. Aluminum neurotoxicity in preterm infants receiving intravenous feeding solutions. N Engl J Med. 336:1557, 1997.

95. Rabinow BE, Ericson S, Shelborne T. Aluminum in parenteral products: Analysis, reduction, and implications for pediatric TPN. J Parenter Sci Technol 43:132, 1989.

96. American Academy of Pediatrics Committee on Nutrition. Aluminum toxicity in infants and children. Pediatrics 97:413, 1996.

97. Klein GL, Leichtner AM, Heyman MB, et al. Aluminum in large and small volume parenterals used in total parenteral nutrition: Response to the Food and Drug Administration notice of proposed rule by the North American Society for Pediatric Gastroenterology and Nutrition. J Pediatr Gastroenterol Nutr 27:457, 1998.

98. Dahlstrom KA, Ament ME, Medhin MG, et al. Serum trace elements in children receiving long-term parenteral nutrition. J Pediatr 109:625, 1986.

99. Friel JK, MacDonald AC, Mercer CN, et al. Molybdenum requirements in low-birth-weight infants receiving parenteral and enteral nutrition. J Parenter Enter Nutr 23:155, 1999.

Nutritional Care for High-Risk Newborns (Rev. 3d. Ed.)
S. Groh-Wargo, M. Thompson, J. Cox, editors
© 2000, Precept Press, Inc., Chicago

12

PARENTERAL NUTRITION: PHARMACEUTICAL CONSIDERATIONS

Marnie I. Levin, Pharm D,
and Kay S. Kyllonen, BS (Pharm), PharmD

PHARMACEUTICAL CONSIDERATIONS PLAY AN important role in the effectiveness of neonatal parenteral nutrition (PN) therapy. Stability and compatibility issues of the solution components can be quite challenging to resolve. Contamination of PN solutions can impose negative patient care outcomes. New technologies are now available to alleviate the tedious preparation of neonatal PN solutions. It is important for practitioners to be knowledgeable in pharmaceutical factors that are involved in neonatal PN therapy. This chapter reviews guidelines for the preparation of neonatal PN solutions as well as pharmaceutical complications.

Dextrose

Dextrose is the most widely used provider of carbohydrate calories in PN. However, dextrose solutions are locally irritating and can shorten the life span of I.V. lines. Infiltration into soft tissues can cause necrosis. Dextrose solutions infused peripherally should be limited to a maximum concentration of 12.5% (631 mOsm/L) to minimize irritation and maximize the life span of venous access.[1-3] Higher concentrations of dextrose may be used in central lines. These solutions can and should be filtered through a 0.22µ filter.

Contributions to the previous version of this chapter by Vernada Hawkins, BS PharmD, are gratefully acknowledged.

Glucose intolerance is common among preterm neonates. This complication is often managed by reducing the amount of glucose provided. If hyperglycemia persists, coadministration of regular insulin by continuous infusion may be beneficial. Because the amount of insulin required can be significantly different from the initial dose, it should be infused separately until the dose is constant.[4] The daily amount of insulin (adjusted for the volume of PN solution needed as below) can then be added directly to the PN solution.[1,4-7] For example:

0.1 units/kg/hour x 1.2 kg x 24 hours = 2.88 units/day
2.88 units/day in 120 ml/day = 0.024 units/ml = 24 units/L

Insulin has been shown to adsorb to glass, polyvinyl chloride tubing, and filters.[8-11] Factors affecting the degree of adsorption include differences in I.V. infusion and administration sets, specific time intervals during an infusion, and various container materials. Specifically, a buretrol with minidrip set, which is often utilized in pediatrics, was associated with significantly more adsorption than other studied infusion sets.[12,13] The addition of albumin to the insulin solution has been suggested to prevent this complication.[13] One study that evaluated the addition of albumin did not find the percentage of decreased insulin adsorption to be clinically significant.[14] A recent survey of neonatal intensive care units did not report routine use of albumin addition for continuous insulin infusions.[15] If the use of albumin is desired, suggested recommendations are to add albumin in a concentration of 0.3 g per 100 ml (0.3%).[16] Careful evaluation of albumin addition should be considered, as insulin infusion has been successful without the concomitant use of albumin,[17] and albumin is an expensive addition.[9] Flushing the administration set with the insulin solution prior to infusion will saturate the binding sites in the tubing and allow a consistent infusion of insulin from the beginning of therapy.[10,18,19]

Amino Acids

Crystalline amino acid solutions are mixtures of essential and nonessential amino acids. Two types of amino acid solutions are routinely used in newborns: (1) standard mixtures, which are based on adult requirements, and (2) pediatric formulations to meet the different needs of infants and young children. (Differences in these two preparations lie in the amounts of amino acids provided; they are delineated in Chapter 10.) The osmolality of these solutions is about 100 mOsm/L for each 1% (10 g/1,000 ml) increase in amino acid content.[1] They can be infused either centrally or peripherally. Amino acid solutions should be protected from light until used.[1,20] Once an amino acid/dextrose/electrolyte solution is compounded, it can be refrigerated for up to 30 days if no multivitamins have been added. Multivitamins should be added immediately prior to administration. Because vitamins A and D and riboflavin degrade, the solution is considered stable for only 24 hours after the addition of multivitamins.[1]

Cysteine

Cysteine supplementation is a controversial issue in neonatal PN therapy (see Chapter 10). Cysteine is thought by many to be an essential amino acid for premature neonates.[21-24] It also acidifies the PN solution and allows the safe addition of more calcium and phosphorus without precipitation.[1] However, the addition of cysteine to neonatal PN is not universal among neonatal nurseries. Since cysteine is unstable in solution with amino acid mixtures and other PN components for extended periods, it must be added separately at the time of compounding.[23,24] The usual dose is 40 mg of cysteine per gram of amino acid.[25,26]

Intravenous Fat Emulsions

Intravenous fat emulsion (IFE) is used in newborns to provide calories and to prevent essential fatty acid deficiency. In infants, each dose of IFE should optimally be infused over 24 hours. It has been suggested that the use of IFE is maximized by continuous versus intermittent administration. Other complications of IFE use such as impaired leukocyte function, negative reticuloendothelial system effects, and hyperlipidemia have been associated with more rapid infusions of IFE.[27-30] The continuous administration of IFE over 24 hours is recommended by the American Academy of Pediatrics.[2,31,32] If this is not feasible, infusions should take place over as long a period as possible.

Both the 10% and 20% IFEs can be used centrally or peripherally, since the osmolality is 268 mOsm/L.[1] The infusion of IFE in the same I.V.. line as the PN solution may protect against phlebitis and I.V. line loss.[33-35] This protection most probably results either from mitigation of the hyperosmolarity of the PN solution or from the physical "coating" of the vein.[27,36,37] Because IFE infusions can cause cracking of ordinary plastic stopcocks, only nylon stopcocks should be used.

Three-in-one Solutions

Infusing IFEs mixed in the same container as the dextrose/amino acid solution is known as a total nutrient admixture (TNA), or three-in-one. The presence of IFE in the TNA obscures the visual inspec-

Table 12.1.   Factors Associated with Solubility of Calcium and Phosphorus in Parenteral Nutrition Solutions

Factors associated with increased solubility	Factors associated with decreased solubility
• Lower concentration of calcium and phosphorus • Calcium gluconate as choice of calcium salt • Higher concentrations of dextrose and amino acids, and addition of cysteine • Cooler temperatures • Very acidic pH • Addition of phosphorus before calcium during compounding • Intravenous fat emulsion delivered by I.V. piggyback	• Higher concentration of calcium and phosphorus • Calcium chloride as choice of calcium salt • Lower concentrations of dextrose and amino acids, and absence of cysteine • Warmer temperatures* • Less acidic pH • Addition of phosphorus after calcium during compounding • Intravenous fat emulsion delivered as part of total nutrient admixture†

* Most commonly the result of lengthy amounts of i.v. tubing running through the isolette.
† Addition of intravenous fat emulsion to amino acid/dextrose mixture results in a more basic pH

tion and detection of physical incompatibilities in the solution. The most common problem is the precipitation of calcium and phosphorus. The presence of such precipitates in TNA solutions has resulted in adverse patient outcomes.[38,39] The maximum amount of calcium and phosphate generally considered acceptable to infuse in a TNA solution is 8.3 mEq/L and 10 mmol/L, respectively.[1] Many neonatal PN solutions contain comparatively increased amounts of calcium and phosphorus to meet the increased requirements of small infants. The higher concentration of these components contributes to the increased risk of precipitation, which would be masked by the milky consistency of IFE. IFE solutions can also cause incompatibilities in the solutions due to inherent phosphorus content and an elevated pH (pH = 8).[1]

TNA solutions require different filtering from that used for standard PN solutions. Standard PN solutions are filtered with a 0.22 micron filter. The 0.22 micron filter removes all contaminating microorganisms and debris particulates. The larger particle size of IFE precludes the use of 0.22 micron filters with TNA solutions. IFE and TNA solutions can be filtered if the pore size of the filter in > 1.2 microns. Using a 1.2 micron filter removes some larger organisms (i.e., candida), certain drug-drug precipitates (i.e., Ca-PO4 salts), some debris particulates, and air.[27] When TNA solutions are used, good clinical practice should include aseptic technique for compounding, use of 1.2 micron filters, and limited hang time to prevent microbial growth.

The risk of disrupting or cracking of the emulsion also complicates the use of TNA solutions.[40] Destabilizing effects on the IFE include higher concentrations of calcium and a lower solution pH.[27] The use of specialized amino acid formulations and cysteine in neonatal PN solutions can significantly decrease the PN solution pH.[1] The lower pH from the PN solution can cause the IFE to degrade and crack the emulsion. The phenomenon looks like salad oil on top of milk. If this is observed, the infusion must be stopped. If the emulsion cracks in a TNA, then both the PN and IFE are wasted, rather than just the relatively inexpensive IFE.[1] Currently, TNA solutions are used more often in adult than in neonatal units.

Calcium and Phosphorus

One of the most challenging issues in PN involves the addition of calcium and phosphorus to the solutions. Compatibilities can be a problem and should be considered in every PN order. Some practitioners will order these ions in milligrams (mg), rather than milliequivalents (mEq) or millimoles (mmol). It is easier for a pharmacist to measure in mEq and mmol. To convert:

224.2 mg calcium gluconate = 1 mEq or 20 mg of elemental calcium

96 mg phosphate (PO_4, HPO_4 and H_2PO_4 can be present) =
1 mmol or 2 mEq of phosphate[5,41]

The solubility of calcium and phosphorus limits the amounts of these ions that can be put into a solution; thus, it is nearly impossible to provide enough to mimic intrauterine accretion.[42] Solubility depends on multiple factors. Sources of alterations in these factors include compounding methods, physicochemical interactions, and external factors. These factors can be summarized as follows:[1,43,44]

- Concentration of calcium and phosphorus
- Salt form of calcium
- Concentration and composition of amino acid solutions
- Concentration of dextrose
- Temperature of solution
- pH of solution
- Order of mixing
- Presence of other additives

Table 12.1 lists specific factors associated with both increased and decreased calcium and phosphorus solubility. Many studies have focused on devising formulas and graphs to predict the maximum soluble concentration of these ions. *The Handbook of Injectable Drugs*[1] is a good resource to predict solubility, as well as original reference articles from journals such as the *American Journal of Health-System Pharmacy*, *Journal of Parenteral and Enteral Nutrition*, and others.[25,45] Appropriate pharmaceutical procedure, including use of available resources, consistent compounding technique, and careful consideration of the factors listed in Table 12.1 will prevent most calcium and phosphorus precipitates. Adverse patient outcomes have been reported from unrecognized precipitates.[38,39] In addition, solutions that include calcium and phosphorus should be filtered with micropore filters. Last, extravasations of calcium- and dextrose-containing solutions can cause soft tissue necrosis, resulting in loss of function or the need for cosmetic surgery.[46] It is very important to ensure the patency of the I.V. line several times daily while infusing these solutions.

Multiple Vitamins and Trace Elements

The pediatric multiple vitamin injection (PMVI) is hyperosmolar and requires dilution prior to administration.[1] Unlike adult preparations, PMVI contains vitamin K. If additional vitamin K is required, it can be safely added to the PN solution, filtered, and infused over 24 hours. In the event of parenteral vitamin shortage, a pediatric multiple vitamin injection should be reserved for use in neonates and premature infants. Adult multivitamin injections should not be substituted, as they may contain propylene glycol or other compounds and preservatives not recommended for infants.[47,90]

The trace elements (TE) for PN infusion in infants generally include zinc (Zn), copper (Cu), manganese (Mn), and chromium (Cr), and, in long-term patients, selenium (Se). Dosage is dependent on weight. Many institutions use a neonatal formula multiple TE solution containing Zn, Cu, Mn, and Cr. More can be added using the individual preparations of these minerals. Trace elements may also be present in variable amounts as contaminants in component parenteral products.[91] If a patient develops cholestasis, Cu and Mn should not be given, because these are excreted in bile. Selenium is recommended for patients on exclusive PN for more than four weeks.[48-51] Iodide intake can be adequate from topical absorption of iodine-containing preparations.[48]

Iron supplementation should be considered if blood transfusions have not been given.[48] Parenteral iron is not for prophylactic use, but it is used in response to depleted iron stores or for infants treated with erythropoietin.[52,53] Further, caution is recommended for infants < 4 months old.[26,92] The dose can be calculated from the formulas below:

Children < 14 kg:

Wt (kg) X [12 (g/dl) - Hgb observed (g/dl)] X 4.5 =
total milligram dosage of iron

Children > 14 kg:

Wt (kg) X [14.8 (g/dl) - Hgb observed (g/dl)] X 4.5 =
total milligram dosage of iron[5]

The maximum daily dose is weight-dependent: for those weighing < 5 kg, the maximum dose is 25 mg; for those weighing 5-10 kg, 50 mg; and for those weighing 10-50 kg, 100 mg. In 1992, iron dextran injection (InFeD®) returned to the market in the United States. In a recent compatibility study, InFeD®, was found to be incompatible with neonatal PN solutions containing < 2% amino acids as a final concentration.[53] Higher concentrations of amino acids decreased the likelihood of precipitation in this study. Although some individual practitioners are currently administering InFeD® in PN solutions, routine use of this practice has not been clearly established.[54] Because of these compatibility concerns, separate infusions of the dextrose-amino acid solution and InFeD® may be favored. Alternately, the product can be given intramuscularly or by slow I.V. administration.

Administration and Preparation Concerns

Compatibilities

In general, medications should not be added to PN solutions because medication compatibilities are difficult to determine. Furthermore, the bioavailability of medications added to PN solutions is unknown; study results usually refer to physical or visual incompatibility (precipitation) rather than chemical incompatibility (drug inactivation without precipitation). General recommendations for compatibility of medications with PN solutions are complicated by wide variations among individual solution components. The use of different amino acid formulations, dextrose and electrolyte concentrations, and other additives can significantly alter the pH of any single solution and impact on its compatibility with medications.[55] If a patient has only one venous access, the PN line should be flushed with a compatible solution before and after the medication is administered. Medication/PN (both additive and Y-site) compatibility questions can be researched in texts by Trissel[1] and King[56] as well as in original reference articles from journals such as the *American*

Journal of Health-System Pharmacy or the *Journal of Parenteral and Enteral Nutrition.*

Filtering

The use of a micropore (0.22 μ) filter may reduce the incidence of phlebitis.[57] The micropore filter can remove particulate debris, impurities, and bacterial contamination from medications, fluids, and administration equipment.[58,59] It cannot remove pyrogens and should not be used with amphotericin or IFEs. PN mixtures should have a micropore in-line filter so that particulate matter that may have formed after admixture is not infused. I.V. lines should be inspected often to detect precipitate in an infusing solution.

Occlusion Clearance

Occlusion of I.V. catheters is not a common occurrence. Clearance with uro- kinase, a thrombolytic enzyme, can be performed when it does happen.[1,60] The procedure is safe for neonates, provided the medication is aspirated out of the line rather than pushed into the patient. For catheter clearance, a volume of urokinase of 5,000 U/ml equal to the volume of catheter should be gently infused into the catheter. After at least 5 minutes, the catheter should be gently aspirated. If unsuccessful, gentle aspirations should be repeated every 5 minutes for 30 minutes. If still unsuccessful, the solution should be left in the catheter for 30-60 minutes (a second injection may be required). Once patency is restored, blood should be aspirated. With a separate syringe, the catheter should then be irrigated with normal saline. Urokinase should be reconstituted immediately prior to use and any unused portion discarded. The product for catheter clearance is stable for 24 hours at room temperature. The urokinase may be filtered. [1,60]

Catheter occlusions may also result from calcium and phosphorus precipitation rather than thrombotic products.[61,62] Sterile dilute (0.1 N) hydrochloric acid may be beneficial in these situations.[63,64] Urokinase is used first, as above, then withdrawn and 0.2-0.5 ml of 0.1 N HCI is instilled. Aspiration is attempted after 20 minutes, and if unsuccessful the process is attempted twice more at 20-minute intervals. Occlusions from IFE have also been reported. The use of ethanol may be useful in clearing occlusions from IFE and alcohol soluble medications.[65,66] Catheters that remain occluded should be replaced.[67]

Osmolality

Osmolality is determined by the behavior of a molecule in solution. If a mole of a certain molecule completely ionizes into 2 ions ($NaCl = Na + Cl$), it exerts twice the osmotic pressure of a molecule that does not ionize (dextrose). Therefore, one mole of NaCl (58 g) in 1 L of water yields a 2-osmolar solution, while one mole of dextrose (180 g) in 1 L of water will yield a 1-osmolar solution.[68] Examples of isotonic solutions are dextrose 5%, normal or 0.9% saline, and dextrose 5% with 0.2% NaCl. It is generally recommended that the osmolality be maintained between 600 and 1,000 mOsm/L in peripheral lines.[2,57,69] *The Handbook on Injectable Drugs*[1] can be used to determine the osmolality of many solutions and additives.

The osmolality of a PN solution can be calculated from the sum of the osmolalities of the components. An example follows (for further information, see Appendix F):

	per liter
Dextrose 12.5% (50.5 mOsm/l1%)[1]	631 mOsm
Amino acid 20g/L (9 mOsm/g)[1]	180 mOsm
Potassium phosphate 25 mEq/L (7.36 mOsm/4.4 mEq)[1]	42 mOsm
Sodium chloride 40 mEq/L (5 mOsm/2.5 mEq)[1]	80 mOsm
Calcium gluconate 15 mEq/L (0.7 mOsm/0.46 mEq)[1]	23 mOsm
	956 mOsm

Contaminants

Infections occurring during PN therapy are a major complication for neonatal patients. These infections may be either cannula- or infusate-related or unrelated to the PN solution. A variety of microorganisms, including *S. aureus*, *S. epidermidis*, candida species, and malassezia furfur have been associated with the use of protein/dextrose solutions and lipid emulsions.[70-73] Other reported organisms associated with contamination of PN solutions include *E. cloacae*, Serratia species, and Acinetobacter.[74-76] Although it is rare that extrinsically contaminated infusates cause sepsis, established procedures for aseptic preparations of these solutions play a major role in eliminating contamination. In-line filters should also be used for PN solutions to reduce the risk of infection from contaminated infusate. Standards of the Joint Commission on Accreditation of Healthcare Organizations (JCAHO) and quality assurance programs should be followed to ensure that the compounded PN product is devoid of microbial contaminants.

Aluminum from components such as calcium and phosphate salts is another significant contaminant of PN solutions (see Table 12.2).[77,78,93] Other sources of potential aluminum contamination include the addition of albumin and/or heparin to PN solutions. Aluminum was first reported to accumulate in the bones of premature infants receiving PN therapy in the 1980s.[77,79] Further evidence of aluminum accumulation in neonates has been documented by both aluminum serum levels and excretion rates in infants maintained on PN therapy.[80] Additionally, the role of aluminum in the neurodevel-

Table 12.2.   Levels of Aluminum in Commonly Administered Intravenous Solutions[77,78]

Solution	µg/L*	mmol/L*
Potassium phosphate (3 mmol/L)	16,598 ± 1,801	615 ± 67
Sodium phosphate (3 mmol/L)	5,977	221
Calcium gluconate (10%)	5,056 ± 335	187 ± 12
Calcium gluceptate	3,645	135
Heparin (1,000 units/ml)	684 ± 761	25 ± 28
Heparin (5,000 units/ml)	359	13
Heparin (10,000 units/ml)	468	17
Human serum albumin (25%)	1,822 ± 2,503	67 ± 93
Intralipid (Baxter-Clintec, Deerfield, Ill.)	195	7
Trace metal solutions	972	36
Multivitamin infusate	891	33
Dextrose (5%)	72 ± 1	2.7
Sodium chloride (4,000 mmol/L)	6 ± 4	0.2 ± 0.15
Potassium chloride (3,000 mmol/L)	6	0.2

Adapted with permission. All rights reserved. Nutrition Reviews 49(3):75. ©1991 by the International Life Sciences Institute, Washington D.C.[78]

Additional Information adapted from Sedman AB, Klein GL, Merritt RJ, et al.[77]

To convert aluminum values from µg per liter to millimoles per liter, divide by 27. Plus-minus values are means ± S.D.

*   Levels may differ depending on manufacturer.

opmental outcome of preterm infants has been debated.[81,82] Premature infants cannot efficiently excrete aluminum via the kidney due to immature renal development and decreased glomerular filtration rate. Thus, they are at increased risk for systemic aluminum toxicity, which includes fracturing osteomalacia, osteopenia, encephalopathy, and microcytic hypochromic anemia.[79] The true extent of the clinical significance of these toxicities is uncertain.

The Food and Drug Administration (FDA) has established an upper limit of 25 µg/L of aluminum content for large-volume parenterals.[83] The FDA's notice of intent also requires that manufacturers of PN additives such as calcium or potassium phosphate injection measure and state the aluminum content on the package label. The American Society for Clinical Nutrition (ASCN) and American

Society for Parenteral and Enteral Nutrition (ASPEN) Working Group on Standards for Aluminum Content of Parenteral Nutrition Solutions further encouraged the FDA to mandate both safe and toxic limits of cumulative aluminum intake in an effort to reduce overall aluminum exposure and toxicity. Possible measures to prevent aluminum contamination of PN solutions for neonates are currently being investigated.[84,85] A recent position paper suggests an upper limit of 5 µg/kg per day of aluminum for preterm infants.[85] Limitation of aluminum content in neonatal PN solutions will be possible once manufactureres comply with FDA new labeling regulations.[86] Until this time, practitioners must continue to use currently marketed calcium and phosphorus salts even though aluminum may be present.

Contamination of pediatric PN solutions with trace elements has been reported.[87,91] Zinc, copper, manganese, chromium, selenium, boron, titanium, barium, vanadium, arsenic, and strontium have been found as contaminants in solutions commonly used in pediatric PN soultions including amino acids, sodium and potassium chloride, and calcium gluconate. The clinical significance of these contaminants is unknown at this time. Further studies of common PN contaminants are needed before changes in the current recommendations can occur.

Peroxidation

Light exposure, especially from phototherapy, induces generation of peroxides in parenteral nutrition solutions.[94] Toxic products resulting from this process may partially explain the chronic lung disease[2] and the alterations in hepatobiliary function associated with TPN.[95] Both intravenous lipids and dextrose/amino acid solutions containing multivitamins, and to some degree, trace elements, are particularly susceptible to peroxidation.[96-98] Protecting solutions from exposure to light by covering solutions bags, covering IV tubing with aluminum foil, or using orange or yellow IV tubing can reduce generation of free radicals and the resultant exposure to peroxidation products.[99,100]

Standardized PN Solutions

Standardized PN solutions for neonates have several advantages, including improved accuracy, efficiency, and cost-effectiveness.[88,89] Standard PN solutions should be formulated to offer the physician a reasonable variety of concentrations of amino acids and dextrose to prescribe for peripheral and central administration. Adequate amounts of electrolytes and minerals should be supplied to the patients by the standard PN solutions when administered at maintenance fluid rates. Standardized PN solutions will not meet the needs of every neonate, however, and may be detrimental in some cases.

Therefore, the option for prescribing nonstandard PN solution should remain. For an example of a standardized neonatal PN order form, see Chapter 8.

A standard PN solution order form for neonates should be used to further promote convenience, accuracy, and cost-effectiveness. Procedures that may be useful when preparing the form include reviewing examples from other hospitals as well as incorporation of guidelines and deadlines for order writing. Multidisciplinary involvement, inservice education, and a pilot study of the TPN form prior to implementation can minimize problems with its use. A follow-up survey or other quality assurance monitor with all involved staff should be conducted periodically to document and assess the impact of the standard solutions and form on the quality of patient care.

The use of automated devices such as the Automix and Micromix compounders (Baxter International, Deerfield, Ill.) by many hospital pharmacies has greatly simplified the preparation of neonatal PN solutions. However, volume limitations do exist for these computerized compounders. Thus, pharmacy personnel should be cautioned that manual addition of amino acids, dextrose, and/or additives may be necessary for neonates who require small volumes of these components. Some hospital pharmacies are using diluted concentrations of PN additives to assure safe and accurate compounding of neonatal PN solutions.

In summary, parenteral nutrition (PN) therapy is widely used in neonates. Appropriate preparation, administration and utilization of these solutions requires a multidisciplinary approach.Understanding the pharmaceutical issues of stability, compatibility, and other potential complications can increase the safety of the use of this therapy in these smallest of patients.

References

1. Trissel LA, ed. Handbook on injectable drugs. 10th ed. Bethesda: American Society of Hospital Pharmacists, 1998.
2. American Academy of Pediatrics. Pediatric Nutrition Handbook. 4th ed. Elk Grove Village, Ill.: AAP, 1998; 285-305.
3. American Academy of Pediatrics, Committee on Nutrition. Commentary on parenteral nutrition. Pediatrics 71:547, 1983.
4. Sajbel TA, Dutro MP, Radway PR. Use of separate insulin infusions with total parenteral nutrition. J Parenter Enter Nutr 11:97, 1987.
5. Benitz WE, Tatro DS. Pediatric drug handbook. 2d ed. Chicago: Year Book Medical Publishers, 1988.
6. Binder ND, Raschko PK, Benda GI, et al. Insulin infusion with parenteral nutrition in extremely low birth weight infants with hyperglycemia. J Pediatr 114:273, 1989.

7. Collins JW, Hopper M, Brown K, et al. A controlled trial of insulin infusion and parenteral nutrition in extremely low birth weight infants with glucose intolerance. J Pediatr 118:921, 1991.

8. Tate JT, Cowan GSM. Insulin kinetics in hyperalimentation solution and routine intravenous therapy. Am Surg 43:811, 1977.

9. Weber SS, Wood WA, Jackson EA. Availability of insulin from parenteral nutrition solutions. Am J Hosp Pharm 34:353, 1977.

10. Peterson L, Caldwell J, Hoffman J. Insulin adsorbance to polyvinyl chloride surfaces with implications for constant-infusion therapy. Diabetes 25:72, 1976.

11. Goldberg NJ, Levin SR. Insulin adsorption to an in-line membrane filter (Itr). N Engl J Med 298:1480, 1978.

12. Whalan FJ, LeCain WK, Latiolais CJ. Availability of insulin from continuous low-dose insulin infusions. Am J Hosp Pharm 36:330, 1979.

13. Seres DS. Insulin adsorption to parenteral infusion systems: Case report and review of the literature. Nutr Clin Prac 5(3):111, 1990.

14. Weber SS, Wood WA, Jackson EA. Availability of insulin from parenteral nutrient solutions. Am J Hosp Pharm 34:353, 1977.

15. Simeon PS, Gottesman MM. Neonatal continuous insulin infusion: A survey of ten level III nurseries in Los Angeles county. Neonatal Network 9(7):19, 1991.

16. Young TE, Mangum OB. Neofax®: A manual of drugs used in neonatal care. 9th ed. Raleigh, N.C.: Acorn Publishing, 1996, 188-189.

17. Niemiec PW, Vanderveen TW. Compatibility considerations in parenteral nutrient solutions. Am J Hosp Pharm 41:893, 1984.

18. Simeon PS, Geffner ME, Levin SR, Lindsey AM. Continuous insulin infusions in neonates: Pharmacologic availability of insulin in intravenous solutions. J Pediatr 124:818, 1994.

19. Simeon PS. The premature infant with hyperglycemia: Use of continuous insulin infusion. J Perinat Neonatal Nurs 6(1):52, 1992.

20. Teasley-Strausberg KM. Cerra FB, Lehmann S, Shronts EP, eds. Nutrition support handbook: A Compendium of products with guidelines. Cincinnati: Harvey Whitney Books, 1992.

21. Zlotkin SH, Bryan MH, Anderson GH. Cysteine supplementation to cysteine free intravenous feeding regimens in newborn infants. Am J Clin Nutr 3:239, 1984.

22. Malloy MH, Rassin DK, Richardson CJ. Total parenteral nutrition in sick preterm infants: Effects of cysteine supplementation with nitrogen intakes of 240 and 400 mg/kg/day. J Pediatr Gastroenterol Nutr 3:239, 1984.

23. Marian, M. Pediatric nutrition support. Nutr Clin Prac 8:199, 1993.

24. Mitton SG. Amino acids and lipid in total parenteral nutrition for the newborn. J Pediatr Gastroenterol Nutr 18:25, 1994.

25. Lenz GT, Mikrut BA. Calcium and phosphate solubility in neonatal parenteral nutrient solutions containing Aminosyn-PF or TrophAmine. Am J Hosp Pharm 45:2367, 1988.

26. Taketomo CK, Hodding JH, Kraus D, eds. Pediatric dosage handbook, 1999-2000. 6th ed. Hudson, Ohio: Lexi-Comp Inc, 1999.

27. Driscoll DF. Clinical issues regarding the use of total nutrient admixtures. DICP An Pharmacother 24:296, 1990.

28. MacFie J, Courtney DF, Brennan TG. Continuous versus intermittent infusion of fat emulsions during total parenteral nutrition: Clinical trial. Nutrition 7(2):99, 1991.

29. Wong AF, Bolinger AM, Edwards RC. Pediatric Nutrition. In: Applied therapeutics: The clinical use of drugs. Young LL, Koda-Kimble MA, eds. 6th ed. Vancouver: Applied Therapeutics, 1995;99.1-99.21.

30. Heird WC. Amino acid and energy needs of pediatric patients receiving parenteral nutrition. Pediatr Clin North Amer 42(4):765, 1995.

31. American Academy of Pediatrics Committee on Nutrition. Use of intravenous fat emulsions in pediatric patients. Pediatrics 68:738, 1981.

32. American Academy of Pediatrics Committee on Nutrition. Nutritional needs of low-birth-weight infants. Pediatrics 75:976, 1985.

33. Phelps SJ, Kamper CA, Helms RA. Comparison of the survival rates of peripheral venous lines in infants receiving peripheral dextrose/amino acid solutions with and without fat emulsion. Abstr #20, J Parenter Enter Nutr 10:6S, 1986.

34. Daly JM, Masser E, Hansen L, et al. Peripheral vein infusions of dextrose/amino acids solutions + 20% fat emulsions. J Parenter Enter Nutr 9:296, 1985.

35. Fujiwara T, Kawarasaki H, Fankelsrud EW. Reduction of post-infusion venous endothelial injury with Intralipid. Surg Gynecol Obstet 158:57, 1984.

36. Pineault M, Chessex P, Piedboeuf B, et al. Beneficial effect of co-infusing a lipid emulsion on venous patency. J Parenter Enter Nutr 13:637, 1989.

37. Matsusue S, Nishimura S, Koizumi S, et al. Preventive effect of simultaneously infused lipid emulsion against thrombophlebitis during postoperative peripheral parenteral nutrition. Surg Today 25:667, 1995.

38. American Society for Parenteral and Enteral Nutrition: Clinical alert. Jan 15-18, 1995.

39. Food and Drug Administration . Safety alert: Hazards of precipitation associated with parenteral nutrition . Am J Hosp Pharm 51:1427, 1994.

40. Mirtallo JM. Should the use of total nutrient admixtures be limited? Am J Hosp Pharm 15:2831, 1994.

41. Baumgartner TG. Phosphate. In: Clinical guide to parenteral micronutrition. Baumgartner TG, ed. 2nd ed. Gainesville, Fla.: Fujisawa, 1991; 79.

42. Gutcher G, Cutz E. Complications of parenteral nutrition. Semin Perinatol 10:196, 1986.

43. Knowles JB, Cusson G, Smith M, et al. Pulmonary deposition of calcium phosphate crystals as a complication of home total parenteral nutrition. J Parenter Enter Nutr 13:209, 1989.

44. Driscoll DF, Newton BW, Bistrian BR. Precipitation of calcium phosphate from parenteral nutrient fluids. Am J Hosp Pharm 51:2834, 1994.

45. Hoie EB, Narducci WA. Laser particle analysis of calcium phosphate precipitate in neonatal TPN admixtures. J Ped Pharm Prac 1:163, 1996.

46. Yosowitz P, Ekland DA, Shaw RC, et al. Peripheral intravenous infiltration necrosis. Ann Surg 182:553, 1975.

47. American Society for Parenteral and Enteral Nutrition: Multivitamin shortage—update no.22, Dec 12, 1997.

48. Greene HL, Hambidge KM, Schanler R, et al. Guidelines for the use of vitamins, trace elements, calcium, magnesium, and phosphorus in infants and children receiving total parenteral nutrition: Report of the Subcommittee on Pediatric Parenteral Nutrient Requirements from the Committee on Clinical Practice Issues of the American Society for Clinical Nutrition. Am J Clin Nutr 48:1324, 1988.

49. Van Caillie-Bertrand M, Degenhart HJ, Fernandes J. Selenium status of infants on nutritional support. Acta Paediatr Scand 73:816, 1984.

50. Kien CL, Ganther HE. Manifestations of chronic selenium deficiency in a child receiving total parenteral nutrition. Am J Clin Nutr 37:319, 1983.

51. Lane HW, Lotspeich CA, Moore CE, et al. The effect of selenium supplementation on selenium status of patients receiving chronic total parenteral nutrition. J Parenter Enter Nutr 11:177, 1987.

52. Friel JK, Andrews WL, Hall MS, et al. Intravenous iron administration to very low birth weight newborns receiving total and partial parenteral nutrition. J Parenter Enter Nutr 19:114, 1995.

53. Mayhew SL, Quick MW. Compatibility of iron dextran with neonatal parenteral nutrient solutions. Am J Health-Syst Pharm 54:570, 1997.

54. Kumpf VJ. Parenteral iron supplementation. Nutr Clin Prac 11(4):139, 1996.

55. Veltri M, Lee CKK. Compatibility of neonatal parenteral nutrient solutions with selected intravenous drugs. Am J Health-Syst Pharm 53:2611, 1996.

56. King JC. Guide to parenteral admixtures. St. Louis: Pacemarq, 1990.

57. Bayer-Berger M, Chiolero A, Freeman J, et al. Incidence of phlebitis in peripheral parenteral nutrition: Effect of the different nutrient solutions. Clin Nutr 8:181, 1989.

58. Bivens BA, Rapp RP, DeLuca PP, et al. Final inline filtration: A means of decreasing the incidence of infusion phlebitis. Surgery 85:388, 1979.

59. Falchuk KH, Peterson L, McNeil BJ. Microparticulate-induced phlebitis. n Engl J Med 312:78, 1985.

60. Abbott Laboratories, Abbokinase Open-cath product information. North Chicago, Il.; Mar 1991.

61. Stennett DJ, Gerwick WH, Egging PK, et al. Precipitate analysis from an indwelling total parenteral nutrition catheter. J Parenter Enter Nutr 12:88, 1988.

62. Robinson LA, Wright BT. Central venous catheter occlusion caused by body-heat mediated calcium phosphate precipitation. Am J Hosp Pharm 39:120, 1982.

63. Hashimoto EG, Morgan D, Kennedy M, et al. Blocked TPN catheter: Clots aren't the only culprit. Abstract 85, J Parenter Enter Nutr 10:17S, 1986.

64. Breaux CW, Duke D, Georgeson KE, et al. Calcium phosphate crystal occlusion of central venous catheters used for TPN in infants and children: Prevention and treatment. J Pediatr Surg 22:829, 1987.

65. Werlin SL, Lausten T, Jessen S, et al. Treatment of central venous catheter occlusions with ethanol and hydrochloric acid. J Parenter Enter Nutr 19:416, 1995.

66. Erdman SH, McElwee CL, Kramer JM, et al. Central line occlusion with three-in-one nutrition admixtures administered at home. J Parenter Enter Nutr 18:177, 1994.

67. Duffy LF, Kerzner B, Gebus V, et al. Treatment of central venous catheter occlusions with hydrochloric acid. J Pediatr 114:1002, 1989.

68. Reich I, Schnaare R, Sugita EI. Tonicity, osmoticity, osmolality, and osmolarity. In: Remington's pharmaceutical sciences. Gennero AR, Chase GD, Gibson MR, eds. 19th ed. Easton,Pa.: Mack Printing, 1995; 613-27.

69. Gazitua R, Wilson K, Bistrian BR. Factors determining peripheral vein tolerance to amino acid infusions. Arch Surg 114:897, 1979.

70. Williams W. Infection control during parenteral nutrition therapy. J Parenter Enter Nutr 9:735, 1985.

71. Powell DA, Aungst J, Snedden S, et al. Broviac catheter related malassezia furfur sepsis in five infants receiving intravenous fat emulsion. J Pediatr 105:987, 1984.

72. D'Angio R, Quercia RA, Treiber NK, et al. The growth of microorganisms in total parenteral nutrition admixture. J Parenter Enter Nutr 11:394, 1987.

73. Ebbert ML, Farraj M, Hwang LT. The incidence and clinical significance of intravenous fat emulsion contamination during infusion. J Parenter Enter Nutr 11:42, 1987.

74. Dugleux G, Le Coutour X, Hecquard C, Oblin I. Septicemia caused by contaminated parenteral nutrition pouches: the refrigerator as an unusual cause. J Parenter Enter Nutr 15:474, 1991.

75. Ng PC, Herrington RA, Beane CA, et al. An outbreak of acinetobacter septicaemia in a neonatal intensive care unit. J Hosp Infect 14:363, 1989.

76. Frean JA, Arntzen L, Rosekilly I, Isaacson M. Investigation of contaminated parenteral nutrition fluids associated with an outbreak of Serratia odorifera septicaemia. J Hosp Infect 27:263, 1994.

77. Sedman AB, Klein GL, Merritt RJ, et al. Evidence of aluminum loading in infants receiving intravenous therapy. N Engl J Med 312:1337, 1985.

78. Klein GL. The aluminum content of parenteral solutions: current status. Nutr Rev 49(3):74, 1991.

79. Koo WWK, Kaplan LA, Krug-Wispe SK, et al. The response of preterm infants to aluminum in parenteral nutrition. J Parenter Enter Nutr 13:516, 1989.

80. Moreno A, Dominguez C, Ballabriga A. Aluminum in the neonate related to parenteral nutrition. Acta Paediatr 83:25, 1994.

81. Bishop NJ, Morley R, Day JP, Lucas A. Aluminum neurotoxicity in preterm infants receiving intravenous-feeding solutions. N Engl J Med 336:1557, 1997.

82. Driscoll WR, Cummings JJ, Zorn W. Aluminum toxicity in preterm infants. N Engl J Med 337:1090, 1997.

83. Klein GL, Alfrey AC, Shike M, et al. Parenteral drug products containing aluminum as an ingredient or a contaminant: Response to Food and Drug Administration notice of intent and request for information. J Parenter Enter Nutr 15:194, 1991.

84. Klein GL. Aluminum in parenteral solutions revisited—again. Am J Clin Nutr 61:449, 1995.

85. Klein GL, Leichtner AM, Heyman MB, et al. Aluminum in large and small volume parenterals used in total parenteral nutrition: Response to the Food and Drug Administration notice of proposed rule by the North American Society for Pediatric Gastroenterology and Nutrition. J Pediatr Gastroenterol Nutr 27:457, 1998.

86. Mouser JF, Wu AH, Herson VC. Aluminum contamination of neonatal parenteral nutrient solutions and additives. Am J Health-Syst Pharm 55:1071, 1998.

87. Hak EB, Storm MC, Helms RA. Chromium and zinc contamination of parenteral nutrient solution components commonly used in infants and children. Am J Health-Syst Pharm 55:150, 1998.

88. Hartwig SC, Gardner DK. Use of standardized total parenteral nutrient solutions for premature neonates. Am J Hosp Pharm 46:993, 1989.

89. Mitchell KA, Jones EA, Meguid MM, Curtas S. Standardized TPN order form reduces staff time and potential for error. Nutrition 6(6):457, 1990.

90. Shulman RJ, Phillips SM, Maciejewski S. An update on a global shortage of intravenous multivitamins. JPGN 28:361, 1999.

91. Pluhator-Murton MM, Fedorak RN, Audette RJ, et al. Trace element contamination of total parenteral nutrition. 1. Contribution of component solutions. JPEN 23:222, 1999.

92. Young TE, Mangum OB. NeoFax®: A Manual of Drugs Used in Neonatal Care, ed 12. Raleigh, North Carolina: Acorn Publishing, USA, 1999, p. 205.

93. Davis AM, et al. Aluminum: A problem trace element in nutrition support. Nutr Clin Prac 14:227, 1999.

94. Putet G. Lipid metabolism of the micropremie. Clin Perinatol 27 (1):57, 2000.

95. Bhatia J, Moslen MT, Haque AK, et al. Total parenteral nutrition—associated alterations in hepatobiliary function and histology in rats: Is light exposure a clue? Pediatr Res 33:487, 1993.

96. Helbock HJ, Motchnik PA, Ames BN. Toxic hydroperoxides in intravenous lipid emulsions used in preterm infants. Pediatrics 91:83, 1993.

97. Lavoie JC, Belanger S, Spalinger M, et al. Admixture of a multivitamin preparation to parenteral nutrition: The major contributor to in vitro generation of peroxides. Pediatrics 99:6, 1997.

98. Steger PJK, Muhlebach SF. Lipid peroxidation of intravenous lipid emulsions and all-in-one admixtures in total parenteral nutrition bags: The influence of trace elements. JPEN 24:37, 2000.

99. Neuzil J, Darlow BA, Inder TE, et al. Oxidation of parenteral lipid emulsion by ambient and phototherapy lights: Potential toxicity of routine parenteral feeding. J Pediatr 126:785, 1995.

100. Laborie S. Lavoie JC, Pineault M, Chessex P. Protecting solutions of parenteral nutrition from peroxidation. JPEN 23:104, 1999.

Nutritional Care for High-Risk Newborns (Rev. 3d. Ed.)
S. Groh-Wargo, M. Thompson, J. Cox, editors
© 2000, Precept Press, Inc., Chicago

13

PARENTERAL NUTRITION: NURSING CARE FOR THE INFANT RECEIVING PARENTERAL NUTRITION

*Rebecca L. Hoagland, BSN, RNC, CNSN, and
Bonnie Foster Gahn, RNC, MA, MSN*

THE INFANT RECEIVING PARENTERAL NUTRITION (PN) is comprehensively managed by a multidisciplinary health care team. The nurse, or nurse case manager, along with the physician, coordinates services provided by this team. The bedside nurse has the most thorough and constant interaction with the infant. Nursing services must offer consistency and provide an overall plan of care that is both developmentally and physiologically focused.

It is the aim of this chapter to provide an overview of nursing care designed to meet the multiple needs of parenterally nourished high-risk neonates and their families. Topics covered include descriptions of complications of vascular access devices (VADs), infusion pumps, individualized care, and home parenteral nutrition.

Vascular Access Devices

Parenteral nutrition is provided to infants through various VADs. These devices are a lifeline for many neonates, but are also associated with risks. Each device has advantages and disadvantages (see Table 13.1). Nurses play an important role in catheter selection, maintenance, and identification of complications.

Table 13.1. Advantages and Disadvantages of Central and Peripheral Lines

Central	Peripheral
Advantages	
Can administer glucose concentrations > 12.5%	Low risk of sepsis
Decreased risk of phlebitis or extravasation	No surgical insertion
	Lower cost
	Lower risk of mechanical injury (e.g., hemothorax, hydrothorax, pneumothorax)
	Lower risk of air embolism
	Lower risk of venous obstruction
Disadvantages	
Greater risk of bacterial colonization and sepsis	Limited glucose concentration to ≤ 12.5%
Surgical insertion	Requires adequate peripheral I.V. access
May require general anesthesia	Higher risk of phlebitis or extravasation
Risk of vessel wall thrombosis	
Increased cost	
Greater risk of mechanical injury (e.g., hemothorax, hydrothorax, pneumothorax)	
Higher risk of air embolism	
Greater risk of venous obstruction	

Peripheral Intravenous Lines

The traditional peripheral I.V. catheter and the newer midline peripheral catheters have several advantages and minimal risks. Midline peripheral I.V.s may be considered whenever I.V. therapy will be required for an intermediate duration of 1 to 4 weeks. These small-bore catheters may be inserted by a procedure-trained nurse typically into one of the antecubital vessels with the tip of the catheter in the peripheral circulation. Midline and peripheral I.V. catheters are available in various materials. Many soften and expand in the vein to extend the dwell time of the catheter[1,2] and are less irritating to the vascular surface than traditional Teflon plastic I.V. catheters. However, because the catheter tip is below the axilla in a peripheral vessel, it is not suited for the delivery of hyperosmolar solutions. The maximum dwell time should be limited to 2 to 4 weeks[3] to minimize the risk of phlebitis. Phlebitis is a commonly reported complication of infusion therapy which may lead to thrombus formation or infection.[2-6]

The greatest advantage of a peripheral device is a low septicemia rate due to the distance of the catheter from central circulation. Other advantages include minimal mechanical complications and lower cost of insertion by nursing staff members trained in insertion and care of such catheters instead of insertion by surgical staff members.

Central Venous Catheters (CVC)

A CVC is a device whose tip is located in the central circulation. CVCs are usually indicated when I.V. therapy is needed for a longer duration or peripheral I.V. therapy is unavailable. A peripherally inserted central catheter (PICC) is a small gauge silastic or polyurethane catheter inserted into a peripheral vein and threaded into the central circulation.

PICC placement must be confirmed by X-ray examination before use. The use of PICCs is increasing with the proficiency of procedure-trained nurses to insert them. PICCs have advantages of both peripheral and central catheters. However, mechanical complications such as kinking, dislodgement, and occlusion may affect the longevity of the catheter and overall cost[7]. The distance of the catheter exit site from central circulation can decrease the risk of sepsis, and the position in the superior vena cava allows the use of hyperosmolar solutions.[6,8]

Percutaneous. Percutaneous central venous catheters (PCVCs) are inserted directly into the central venous circulation. Insertion sites may vary with the size of the infant and the availability of accessible veins, including the internal and external jugular, subclavian, and femoral veins.[2] These catheters have a high risk of septicemia associated with them, but allow central venous access immediately. They are available with single, double, and triple lumens. Each lumen is a separate catheter into the central circulation, making it possible to infuse several different solutions simultaneously and medications that may be incompatible. The use of multiple lumens may also increase the risk of infection.[9,10]

Tunneled Silastic Catheters. Tunneled Silastic catheters (e.g., Broviac Catheters, Davol Inc., Cranston, R.I.) are the devices of choice when anticipating long-term I.V. therapy. They are widely used in the neonatal population. These vascular catheters are inserted in the operating room or in a designated area in the neonatal intensive care unit (NICU), using either general or local anesthesia. The subclavian or saphenous veins are used most often. In the extremely premature neonate, the femoral vein is used when the saphenous vein is too small. The tip of the catheter is placed in the vena cava or right atrium. A subcutaneous tunnel is created to provide a distance between the exit site at the skin surface and the bloodstream. A Dacron cuff on the catheter allows ingrowth of tissue inside the tunnel to act as a barrier against infection ascending from the exit site. The cuff also anchors the catheter once tissue ingrowth is complete (three to six weeks), allowing the sutures to be removed. Occasionally, immunosuppressed patients who have poor healing capabilities may not have ingrowth of the Dacron cuff and therefore should not have sutures removed from the exit site.[9]

Complications

Various complications associated with the use of VADs can compromise the infant's clinical status (see Table 13.2).

Mechanical Complications

Mechanical complications can be related to catheter insertion or use. Pneumothorax, hydrothorax, and hemothorax can be associated with any catheter threaded into the thoracic area.[6,8,11] Respiratory distress or circulatory collapse may be clinical indicators of these conditions which should alert the nurse. A chest X-ray will confirm these complications.

A commonly reported complication seen with peripheral catheters is phlebitis due to infiltration.[4] Phlebitis is characterized by swelling, redness, pain, and tenderness over the vein; it is treated with heat and elevation. In severe cases of infiltration, extravasation and tissue necrosis have been reported.[12]

To minimize the complications of infiltration, peripheral I.V. sites should be assessed hourly and rotated at the first sign of injury. Additionally, dextrose solutions in peripheral I.V.s should not exceed 12.5% concentration. Prolonged exposure to hyperosmolar solutions increases the risk of vessel wall injury and thrombosis.[12]

Venous thrombosis can occur secondary to vessel wall injury associated with catheter placement or administration of hyperosmolar solutions. The nurse should observe for distended veins or swelling in the catheter extremity. Silastic catheters are less thrombogenic than polyurethane,[2,11] but they are more likely to rupture with excessive infusion pressure.[13] Rupture in the subcutaneous tunnel usually results in swelling in the area, hypoglycemia, and leakage around the catheter exit site. Assessing the site drainage with a reagent strip for blood glucose will result in an abnormally high

Table 13.2. Catheter-Related Complications of Parenteral Nutrition

Mechanical complications

Catheter insertion
  Pneumothorax
  Hemothorax
  Hydromediastinum
  Subclavian artery injury
  Subclavian hematoma
  Subclavian vein laceration
  Arteriovenous fistula
  Air embolism
  Catheter embolism
  Catheter malposition
  Thoracic duct laceration
  Cardiac perforation and tamponade
  Brachial plexus injury
  Horner's syndrome
  Phrenic nerve paralysis
  Carotid artery injury

Catheter Use
  Venous thrombosis
    Superior vena cava syndrome
    Pulmonary embolus
  Catheter dislodgement
  Perforation and/or infusion leaks (pericardial, pleural, mediastinal)

Infectious Complications

Catheter
  Contamination and infection at catheter site
  Catheter "seeding" from distant site infection
Parenteral nutrition solution
  Contamination in mixing/handling/administration of solutions

reading if dextrose-containing solutions are leaking. A fluoroscopic contrast study may confirm catheter leakage. Externally ruptured catheters may be detected by wet bed linens or CVC dressings. Ruptured catheters should be clamped upon discovery and repaired by procedure-trained nurses immediately. The patient may need additional I.V. access during this time.

Catheter occlusion is a complication of peripheral and central venous catheters. Peripheral catheters are usually removed and replaced when occluded. However, salvaging an occluded CVC may be more cost-effective and safer than placing a new device. At the first sign of resistance during catheter flushing, impending occlusion should be suspected. Before using any pharmacologic agent to restore catheter patency, the catheter should be inspected for kinking under the dressing or malposition. Injecting contrast under fluoroscopy will rule out an internally kinked catheter or malpositioned tip.

Catheter clotting may be due to a fibrin sheath formation or thrombus at the catheter tip. This is commonly associated with frequent blood withdrawals from the catheter. Catheter occlusion may also be caused by waxy lipid deposits (from I.V. fat emulsions) or by calcium-phosphate or other mineral precipitates. The catheter-clearing agent should be selected according to the type of occlusion and the use of the catheter.[14-17] Published algorithms are available to assist the health care team in selecting the appropriate pharmacologic agent for management of occluded catheters[17]. All catheter-clearing agents should be administered slowly (by a physician or procedure-trained nurse) in an amount equal to the catheter volume. No smaller than a 5 ml syringe should be used in order to prevent excessive pressure that may dislodge the clot or rupture the catheter.[18] Using a three-way stopcock to create negative pressure within the catheter will reduce the risk of catheter rupture when dealing with a complete occlusion[13].

Sepsis

The most prevalent, costly, and life-threatening complication of indwelling vascular devices is sepsis. The pathogens seen most often are coagulase-negative staphylococci (CNS), candida, enterococci, and staphylococcus aureus. CNS, the most frequent pathogen, is associated with the skin flora of patients and contamination of the hands of healthcare workers. The increase in catheter-related infections may also be attributed to the increased survival rates of low birth weight infants and the increased use of vascular access devices and intravenous fat emulsions (IFEs)[19]. Thus, infants receiving central PN are at risk for CVC-related infection, with those weighing <1,000 g having the greatest risk[20].

Several studies over the last decade have documented sepsis as a significant problem in neonates with percutaneous central venous catheters. Catheter-related sepsis has been reported to be anywhere from 19 to 31 percent. A range of contributing variables exist in these studies, including: patient characteristics, catheter insertion techniques, and maintenance procedures[21]. Manipulation of the central venous catheter has been identified as an important factor in the development of CVC-related infection[22,23].

It is often necessary to interrupt the sterile closed catheter system to administer I.V. medication, change I.V. tubing, or draw blood specimens. When interrupting the line, strict sterile technique according to individual unit protocols must be followed. Contamination may also be due to colonization at the catheter exit site or seeding of the catheter tip from another infection site within the body or from the G.I. tract.

Dextrose solutions and IFEs contribute to the risk of catheter contamination by providing substrate for bacterial and fungal growth. Malassezia furfur has been reported in neonates receiving IFEs through CVCs.[24] When this lipophilic yeast is isolated, both the CVC and the IFE are discontinued and an antifungal agent is administered.

Astute nursing assessment for CVC sepsis is essential. Early identification will facilitate prompt treatment. Symptoms of sepsis include apnea and bradycardia, temperature instability, lethargy, feeding intolerance, mottling, cyanosis, and irritability. Laboratory data may reflect an increase or decrease in white blood cell (WBC) count, decrease in platelets, increase in band count, and hyperglycemia.

Infusion Pumps

Many safe and user-friendly infusion pumps are currently in use in hospitals. Pumps and their specific tubing for neonatal patients require some unique features to minimize the risk of error. Pumps should be accompanied by the manufacturer's statement that they are appropriate for use with infants and are able to deliver small volumes. It should be possible to set flow rates as low as any infusion may require. The pump should be volumetric and have a documented accuracy of ± 2% to assure precise and controlled delivery. The pump should also protect against the inadvertent delivery of a bolus. If the tubing is removed from the pump, the solution should not flow by gravity. The occlusion pressure setting should be low so that infiltration and impending catheter occlusion can be detected promptly. If an occlusion occurs, the system should be able to relieve pressure so that a bolus is not delivered when the occlusion is removed. An air-in-line alarm is important to prevent air embolism.

Nursing Guidelines

Each institution should have established policies, procedures, or protocols to direct staff in care of the infant with a VAD and PN. These protocols may differ from institution to institution, but they should be strictly enforced. Most hospitals have a mandatory competency-based educational program for care of VADs to maintain quality of care.

Peripheral catheters are generally inserted by procedure-trained nurses using aseptic technique. The site if cleansed with an antimicrobial solution before insertion. When the catheter is in place, a sterile transparent dressing typically is applied. The site should be evaluated hourly for cannula-related complications. At the first sign of infiltration or phlebitis, the catheter should be removed and a new one inserted in a different location. The Intravenous Nursing Standards of Practice recommends removing peripheral catheters every 48 to 72 hours, even if there are no signs of complications[3]. Since vascular access is limited in small babies, however, this recommendation is not routinely practiced in most NICUs.

Umbilical vessels are used for the infusion of parenteral nutrition in some NICUs. This practice is controversial due to the many possible complications including sepsis, tip malposition, liver abscess, portal vein thrombosis, and perforation into the peritoneal cavity[25,26]. Whenever umbilical vessels are used, the catheter should be stabilized to prevent it from becoming dislodged. If the umbilical catheter is not stabilized properly, it may slip out. The catheter should never be advanced secondary to the risk of infection.

According to the Centers for Disease Control (CDC) guidelines, PN solutions and IFE administration sets should be changed every 24 hours to reduce the risk of bacterial growth[3,19]. However, these recommendations for tubing changes are not specific to pediatric patients. Between changes, a closed system should be maintained as much as possible. Stopcocks should never be used on CVCs. All entries into the system for I.V. medication administration should be made through injection ports that have been appropriately disinfected.

Proper handling and maintenance of central lines are essential aspects of nursing care. In 1996, the CDC stated that strict adherence to handwashing and aseptic technique remains the cornerstone to prevention of catheter-related infection[19].

The specifics of CVC site care may vary from institution to institution. However, an antiseptic skin preparation and a sterile dressing are essential and universal in the hospital setting. The advantage of transparent dressings versus gauze and tape remains controversial but both are widely accepted[27]. Transparent dressings have been associated with increased colonization at the catheter site, however, this colonization is not reported to lead to increased site infections[28].

If the catheter dressing is in the groin or adjacent to a stoma, a transparent dressing may be preferable, or used in addition to the gauze and tape. This protects the dressing from stool, urine, or secretions. These dressings may be changed more frequently to reduce the risk of bacterial colonization at the catheter exit site and to allow examination of the site for complications. All CVC dressings should be changed whenever soiled, wet, or no longer occlusive.

Individualized Infant Care

The delivery of PN to the high-risk infant is considered an aspect of routine care for many infants in the NICU. However, there is increasing concern regarding the environmental iatrogenic effects of routine neonatal intensive care. A study by Als demonstrated a dramatic improvement in the outcome of very low birth weight preterm infants when behavioral observations were used to modify the environment and care-giving techniques.[29] The challenge to the neonatal nurse is to optimize the infant's developmental outcome while providing the necessary interventions. The nurse can do this only through a comprehensive understanding of the premature infant's phases of development and associated cues of infant behavior. The nurse should incorporate theories of development into the assessment of each infant's response to care-giving techniques, including I.V. insertion. Without compromising medical management of the infant, nurses should assume a developmental approach to care. Developmental considerations related to PN include:

1. *Type of catheter*. The type of catheter used is dependent on weight and gestational age of the infant. It has been demonstrated that highly intrusive interventions (such as needle sticks) significantly increase heart and respiratory rates and decrease oxygen saturation, thus resulting in an increase in energy expenditure in these infants[30]. PICCs are recommended for infants weighing < 1,200 g and/or < 30 weeks' gestation. Placing these lines within the first few days of hospitalization spares infants the stress of repeated venipunctures and infiltration.[31] Thus, they may demonstrate behavioral organization and steady weight gain at an earlier age than infants stressed by repeated venipunctures.
2. *I.V. insertion techniques*. Infants should be swaddled or contained as much as possible during painful procedures. Swaddling the infants' extremities assists them in behavioral and autonomic regulation.[32] The use of topical anesthesia for line insertion in infants should also be considered. It has been demonstrated that topical lidocaine and prilocaine cream application minimized the autonomic system response without evidence of toxicity during PCVC insertion[33].
3. *I.V. maintenance and positioning*. Peripheral and central lines should be taped and/or dressed with a product conducive to integrity of the premature skin. Infants should be positioned so that I.V. insertion sites are protected without requiring extremity restraints.[34]
4. *Nonnutritive sucking (NNS)*. NNS increases transcutaneous arterial oxygen levels and decreases heart rate for preterm infants.[35] Therefore, NNS should be used for infants who are autonomically

stable and can benefit from a comfort intervention. This is particularly true for infants receiving PN without any oral feedings.[35]

5. *Parent involvement*. Parent participation should be encouraged throughout the infant's hospitalization. Behavioral and developmental assessment information provides parents with anticipatory guidance as they respond to their infant and gain confidence in their ability to provide care.

Home Parenteral Nutrition

Home parenteral nutrition (HPN) for infants is coming into wider use, in part because it enables the family to regain a more normal, nurturing life-style. If prolonged PN is indicated, technologies exist to enable its safe and efficient delivery in the home. HPN decreases hospital stay, cost of care, and complications associated with prolonged hospitalization[36,37].

In planning discharge, there are many issues for the nursing staff to consider. Among them are the following:

1. *The family must be ready*. The family must want to take their child home with this therapy and be responsible for the care. The parents or designated care-givers must demonstrate competency in the skills needed for safely administering HPN and anticipating complications. Skills may be taught through a training program designed by the hospital's nutrition support service or the home care agency.

2. *The infant must be ready*. The infant must be medically and nutritionally stable on the HPN regimen before discharge. Accurate physical assessment should be expected of the infant's care-givers, since laboratory assessment of nutritional status will not be readily available.

3. *Financial support must be identified*. Financial coverage must be established. Although it is not as costly as continued hospitalization, HPN is still a costly program.[37]

4. *Responsibility for follow-up must be assigned*. A case manager in coordination with a home care agency should be responsible for the training, coordination of discharge, and follow-up of these infants and families, as well as for providing necessary supplies and solutions at home.[38] The hospital may have a nutrition support service to meet these needs. In most institutions, a case manager will assume responsibility for facilitating discharge. Additionally, a nutrition support team or a physician familiar with outpatient parenteral nutrition is necessary for follow up care of the patient.

Home care agencies should be selected according to strict criteria assuring the best possible care for the infant. Service companies must be licensed and Medicare-Medicaid approved, certified by the Joint Commission on Accreditation of Healthcare Organizations, and should employ experienced pediatric nurses. A collaborative relationship between the hospital and home care agency should be fostered to facilitate frequent communications related to the family's progress. Although licensed, these agencies may not have pharmacists or nutritionists familiar with neonatal PN on their staffs. A nursing visit should be scheduled at least three times the first week the infant is home to reinforce teaching that the family received. The home care nurse should always be available to the family when problems arise. The nutrition support team should also be available to the agency nurse so that consistent and safe home care is assured. Some nutrition support services also provide for scheduled patient follow-up visits with the physician at least every two to four weeks in order to promote the transition to enteral feedings.

References

1. Wheeler C, Frey AM. Intravenous therapy in children. In: Terry J, Baranowski L, Lonsway RA, et al, eds. Intravenous Therapy, Clinical Principles and Practice. Intravenous Nurses Society. Philadelphia: W.B. Saunders, 1995.
2. Baranowski L. Central venous access devices, current technologies, uses, and management strategies. J Intraven Nurs 16:167, 1993.
3. Intravenous Nurses Society. Revised intravenous nursing standards of practice. J Intrav Nurs 21:1S, 1998.
4. Carey BE. Major complications of central lines in neonates. Neonatal Network 7:17, 1989.
5. Ryder MA. Device selection: a critical strategy in the reduction of catheter-related complications. Nutrition 12:143, 1996.
6. Duck S. Neonatal intravenous therapy. J Intraven Nurs 20:121, 1997.
7. Hinson EK, Blough L. Skilled IV therapy clinicians' product evaluation of open-ended versus closed-ended valve PICC lines. J Intrav Nurs 19:195, 1996.
8. Ryder MA. Peripherally inserted central venous catheters. Nurs Clin North Am 28:936, 1993.
9. Hoagland R, Stewart B. Central venous catheter related sepsis: A closer look. Heartbeat 2:1 Children's Hospital, Columbus, Ohio, 1991.
10. Clark-Christoff N, Walters VA, Sparks W, et al. Use of triple lumen subclavian catheters for administration of total parenteral nutrition. J Parent Ent Nutr 16:403, 1992.
11. Viall CD. Your complete guide to central venous catheters. Nursing 90, 1:34, 1990.
12. Cochran EB, Phelps SJ. Parenteral nutrition in pediatric patients. Clin Pharm 7:19, 1988.
13. Bonstell R, Brown B. Declotting peripherally inserted central catheters with a new technique using urokinase. J Vasc Acc Devices 2:10, 1992.

14. Cunliffe MT, Polomano RC. How to clear clots with urokinase. Nursing '86 16:40, 1986.
15. Pennington CR, Pithie AD. Ethanol lock in the management of catheter occlusion. J Parenter Enter Nutr, 11:507, 1987.
16. Kupensky DT. Use of hydrochloric acid to restore patency in an occluded implantable port. J Intrav Nurs 18:198, 1995.
17. Holcombe BJ, Forloines-Lynn S, Garmhausen LW. Restoring patency of long-term central venous access devices. J Intraven Nurs 15:36, 1992.
18. Catheter Technology Corp., Salt Lake City. Unpublished data, 1989.
19. Centers for Disease Control and Prevention. Guidelines for prevention of intravascular device-related infections. Amer J Infect Control 24:262, 1996.
20. Gaynes RD, Martone WJ, Culver DH, et al. Comparison of rates of nosocomial infections in neonatal intensive care units in the United States. Am J Med 91(3B):192S, 1991.
21. Trotter CW. A national survey of percutaneous central venous catheter practices in neonates. Neonatal Network 17:31, 1998.
22. Maki D. Infections due to infusion therapy. In: Bennett J, Bractiman P, ed. Hospital Infections, 2nd Ed. Boston: Little Brown & Co. 1986; 561-80.
23. Lucas JW, Berger AM, Fitzgerald A, et al. Nosocomial infections in patients with central catheters. J Intrav Nurs 15:44, 1992.
24. Carey BE. Malassezia furfur infection in the NICU. Neonatal Network 9:19, 1991.
25. Athersen HB, Hebra A, Chessman KH, et al. Central lines in parenteral nutrition. In: Baker RD, Baker SS, Davis AM, ed. Pediatric Parenteral Nutrition. New York: Chapman & Hall, 1997; 254-272.
26. Green C, Yohannan MD. Umbilical arterial and venous catheters: placement, use, and complications. Neonatal Network 17:23, 1998.
27. Lau CE. Transparent and gauze dressings and their effect on infection rates of central venous catheters: a review of past and current literature. J Intraven Nurs 19:240, 1996.
28. Taylor D, Myers ST, Monarch K, et al. Use of occlusive dressings on central venous catheter sites in hospitalized children. J Pediatr Nurses 11:169, 1996.
29. Als H, Lawhorn G, Brown E, et al. Individualized behavioral and environmental care for the very low birth weight infant at high risk for BPD: Neonatal intensive care and developmental outcome. Pediatrics 78:1123, 1986.
30. Zahr LK, Balin S. Responses of premature infants to routine nursing interventions and noise in the NICU. Nurs Res 44:179, 1995.
31. Storroff M, Teague WG. Intravenous access in infants and children. Pediatr Clin North Am 45:1373, 1998.
32. Short MA, Brooks-Brunn JA, Reeves DS, et al. The effects of swaddling versus standard positioning on neuromuscular development in VLBW infants. Neonatal Network 15(4):25, 1996.
33. Garcia O, et al. Topical anesthesia for line insertion in VLBW infants. J Perinatol 17:477, 1997.
34. Kuller JM, Lund CH. Assessment and management of integumentary dysfunction. In: Kenner C, Lott JW, Flandermeyer AA, ed. Comprehensive Neonatal Nursing. Philadelphia: WB Saunders Co., 1998; 648-681.

35. Lawhon G. Providing developmentally supportive care in the NICU: an evolving challenge. J Perinat Neonat Nurs 10:48, 1997.
36. Misra S, Ament ME, Reyen L. Home parenteral nutrition. In: Baker RD, Baker SS, Davis AM, ed. Pediatric Parenteral Nutrition. New York: Chapman & Hall, 1997; 354.
37. Prabashni R, Malone M. Cost and outcome analysis of home parenteral and enteral nutrition. J Parent Ent Nutr 22:302, 1998.
38. Forsyth TJ, Maney LA, Ramirez A, et al. Nursing case management in the NICU: enhanced coordination for discharge planning. Neonatal Network 17:23, 1998.

Bibliography

Als H, Gilkerson L. The role of relationship-based developmentally supportive newborn intensive care in strengthening outcome of preterm infants. Semin Perinatol 21:178, 1997.

Baker RD, Baker SS, Davis AM, ed. Pediatric Parenteral Nutrition. New York: Chapman and Hall, 1997.

Bender JH. Parenteral nutrition for the pediatric patient. Home Healthcare Nurse, 3:32, 1985.

Fay MJ. The positive effects of positioning. Neonatal Network 6:23, 1988.

Feaster SJ. Evaluating new intravenous catheters in the NICU. Neonatal Network 10:3, 1991.

MacDonald M, Clou M. Preventing complications from lines and tubes. Semin Perinatol 10:224, 1986.

Moore MC. Total parenteral nutrition for infants. Neonatal Network 6:33, 1987.

Murphy LM, Lipman TO. Central venous catheter care in parenteral nutrition, a review. J Parenter Enter Nutr, 11:190, 1987.

Reid S, Frey AM. Techniques for administration of IV medications/parenteral nutrition via central lines in the NICU: A pilot study. Neonatal Network, 11:6, 1992.

Sterk MB. Understanding parenteral nutrition: A basis for neonatal nursing care. J Obstet Gynecol Neonatal Nurs 12(3) suppl:45, 1983.

Trotter C, Carey BE. Tearing and embolization of Pcvcs. Neonatal Network. 17:67, 1998.

SECTION III

ENTERAL NUTRITION

Nutritional Care for High-Risk Newborns (Rev. 3d. Ed.)
S. Groh-Wargo, M. Thompson, J. Cox, editors
© 2000, Precept Press, Inc., Chicago

14

GASTROINTESTINAL DEVELOPMENT

Sharon Groh-Wargo, MS, RD, LD

BIRTH AND THE ABRUPT interruption of the placental flow of nutrients from mother to fetus normally requires the newborn infant's G.I. tract to adapt to extrauterine life. Months of gestation usually prepare this relatively untested, untried system to perform its functions of assimilation and movement of food and digestion and absorption of nutrients. When premature birth intervenes, the normal sequence of events is altered. The challenge of feeding smaller and sicker infants requires understanding of G.I. development. Because the components of the G.I. system do not evolve concurrently, all aspects of the activities and their sequence must be studied to understand their interaction and analyze the impact on feeding.

During fetal life, the alimentary canal evolves as a digestive/absorptive organ with a massive surface area, the pancreas differentiates into an organ with both endocrine and exocrine functions, and the liver prepares to function as the metabolic factory of the body.[1] As proposed by Lebenthal and Lee, this development is governed by four interacting determinants:[2,3]

- *Genetic endowment*—The programmed nucleotide sequence of DNA that controls the progression and expression of the organism's development.
- *Biological clock*—The predetermined temporal sequence of events that is genetically controlled and species-specific.
- *Regulatory mechanisms*—The hormonal, neurological, and endocrinological influences that affect the expression of the genetic endowment.

• *Environmental influences*—Factors such as quality or quantity of food that can change the potential for development inherent in the genetic endowment.

With these general concepts in mind, the purpose of this chapter is to briefly outline normal human G.I. development. The goal is to be able to plan reasonable feeding regimens for high-risk newborns.

Anatomic Development

Specialized features of the G.I. tract become discernible in the second to third trimester (see Table 14.1). By 14 weeks, the pancreas has differentiated into its two cell types, the stomach and liver have formed their distinctive tissue separations, and the crypts and villi unique to the small intestine are present. In the human, anatomic differentiation of the fetal gut at 20 weeks' gestation closely resembles that of the newborn infant.

Data on stomach capacity are limited. Data from animal studies suggest a rapid increase (within hours) in stomach and intestinal mass following the initiation of enteral nutrition.[5] Scammon and Doyle reviewed 14,571 individual feeding records in 323 newborns with birth weights of > 2,000 g.[6] Gestational age of the subjects was not specified. Physiologic capacity was determined by weighing before and after feeding. All infants were breast-fed. Their data reveal a rapid gain in capacity during the first four days of life resulting in a physiologic capacity that approximates 15-30 ml/kg. The term human fetus swallows as much as 750 ml/day.[7] Others have estimated that the volume of fluid swallowed at one time by the fetus may be as large as 100-200 ml—roughtly equivalent to 3-5 % of body weight.[8]

Of practical significance are data on elongation of the small and large bowel. At four weeks' gestation, the intestine is a simple tube. By the fifth week, it begins elongating faster than the trunk, so that by 40 weeks the intestine is 1,000 times longer than it was at 5 weeks.[4] Average newborn infants have crown-heel lengths of 45.5-53.5 cm. The length of their small intestine is reported to be 200-300 cm.[10,11] Small bowel lengths have a fairly predictable relationship of four to five times the crown-heel length.[10,11] Congenital anomalies such as omphalocele can vary this ratio. A small bowel of 253 cm would be divided roughly into 5.0 cm of duodenum and 248 cm of jejunum and ileum.[6] The newborn colon averages 45 cm, which is about one-sixth the length of the small intestine.[12]

Table 14.1.   Temporal Sequence of Anatomic Development
              of the G.I. Tract in the Human Fetus

Esophagus	
Superficial glands develop	20 wk
Squamous cells appear	28 wk

Stomach	
Gastric glands form	14 wk
Pylorus and fundus defined	14 wk

Pancreas	
Differentiation of endo- and exocrine tissue	14 wk

Liver	
Lobules form	11 wk

Small intestine	
Crypt-villi develop	14 wk
Lymph nodes appear	14 wk

Colon	
Diameter increases	20 wk
Villi disappear	20 wk

Adapted from Lebenthal E, Lee PC, Heitlinger, LA[4] with permission of Mosby Year Book (1983).

Motor Development

Intestinal motor activity moves the intraluminal contents from one specialized region of the gut to the next. The term *motility*, used to embrace all aspects of motor development, includes the G.I. functions of sucking, swallowing, gastric emptying, and intestinal transit. Figure 14.1 shows schematically the temporal sequence in the development of several of these activities.[13]

Sucking and Swallowing

In general, swallowing activity develops earlier than sucking behavior. Gryboski defined three developmental stages of suck-swallow coordination:[14]

1. *The mouthing stage*: characterized by mouthing movements alone, with no accompanying sucking or swallowing
2. *The immature suck and swallow pattern*: characterized by short bursts of four to seven sucks at a rate of 1-1.5 per second; swallows do not occur during sucking bursts but rather during resting periods between bursts of sucking
3. *The mature suck and swallow pattern*: characterized by prolonged bursts of at least 30 sucks at a rate of two per second, and by swallowing without interruption of respiratory rhythm; associated with propulsive peristaltic waves in the esophagus

The mature pattern is attained within days by full-term infants. Preterm infants generally display a nutritive suck by about 34 weeks, although it may exhibit the immature pattern.[15] Nipple feeding prior to 30 weeks could cause apnea or aspiration as airway-protective mechanisms may not be intact.[16] The mature suck and swallow pattern is rarely seen before 34 weeks' gestation. The maturation of the suck and swallow reflex is also related to postnatal age. For example, an infant born at 28 weeks' gestation may be able to suck four weeks after birth; however, an infant born at 32 weeks would generally not be able to effectively suck during the first few days of life.[17]

Non-nutritive sucking is the sucking behavior exhibited by infants when a pacifier is offered. It is characterized by series of shorter bursts and pauses when compared with nutritive sucking. The physiologic function of non-nutritive sucking is not well understood. Its role in promoting growth and gastrointestinal maturation is controversial.[18] Some evidence supports non-nutritive sucking's soothing effect and its role as a stress reducer.[19,20] (See Chapter 18.)

Gastric Emptying

Passage of food from mouth to stomach requires a functional lower esophageal sphincter. Premature infants, especially those less than 33 weeks gestation, often experience a higher rate of regurgitation after feeding than term infants because of decreased lower esophageal sphincter pressure.[21]

Gastric emptying begins at midgestation, but is thought to remain relatively immature even at term. This may be due to the newborn's thin stomach muscular layer, which results in weak mixing action of the organ.[22] The preterm infant may have an additional handicap, inasmuch as an infant of 27-28 weeks' gestation can generate only 20-

Figure 14.1. Ontogeny of Motor Function[13]

MMC = Migrating motor complex.
Reprinted with permission from Premji, SS. Ontogeny of the gastrointestinal system and its impact on feeding the preterm infant. Santa Rosa, CA: Neonatal Network, 17(2):17-24, 1998.

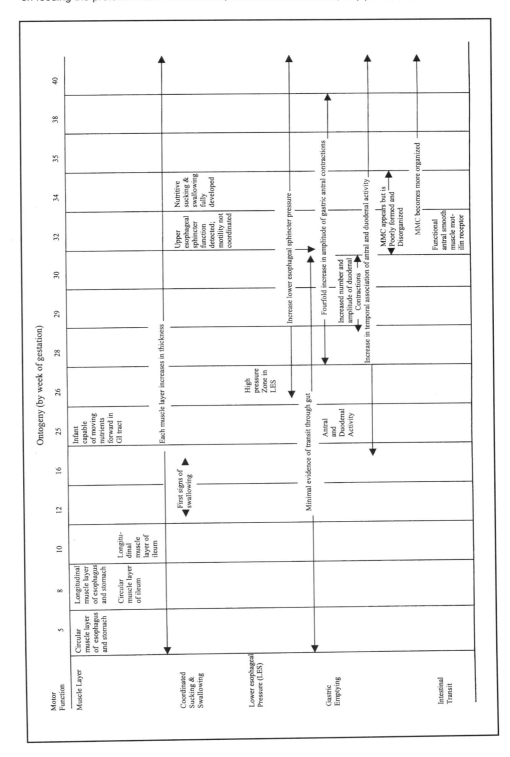

25% of the pressure in the gastric antrum that a term infant can.[23] Despite this and although it is widely believed that gastric emptying is delayed in the premature neonate, studies comparing term and preterm infants are conflicting.[24-28] Factors such as gestational and postnatal age and the type and volume of feeding can affect results and need to be considered when studies are compared. The following conclusions about gastric emptying can be stated with some assurance:

- Gastric emptying is significantly delayed in the first 12 hours of life for both term and preterm infants.[26]
- After the first few days of life, preterm infants of ≥ 32 weeks' gestation and term infants have similar gastric emptying times when all factors, such as age and volume and content of feeding, are held constant.[25,27]
- In infants of < 32 weeks' gestation the time in minutes for half-antral clearance (i.e., the time required for the volume of liquid in the stomach to fall by half, a measure of gastric emptying) decreases with increasing postnatal age.[29]
- Independent of gestational age, size and surface area may affect gastric emptying, such that larger infants have faster emptying rates than smaller infants.[28]
- A 20-30 ml/kg oral feeding has a gastric emptying half-time of about 45-60 minutes.[28,30]
- Most infants have a biphasic pattern of gastric emptying, with an initial rapid phase lasting about 20 minutes.[28-30]
- Body position does not affect gastric emptying in infants, at least not after the first few days of life.[27,31]
- The pattern of gastric emptying appears to be affected by the composition of the feeding, so that
  —medium-chain triglycerides empty faster than long-chain triglycerides
  —glucose polymers empty faster than lactose or glucose
  —caloric density is directly related to stomach emptying (i.e., the higher the caloric density, the longer the emptying time)[32,33]
  —human milk empties faster than formula[29,34]
- Electrolyte abnormalities, endocrinopathies, and central nervous system disorders are likely to disturb gastric emptying.[16]

Intestinal Transit

During fasting, a cyclic pattern of contractions progresses from the antrum of the stomach to the ileum. This activity is called the migrating motor complex (MMC)[16] (see Figure 14.1). It consists of four distinct phases and is interrupted by feeding. A progression from disorganized intestinal contractile activity to organized MMC patterns is observed among infants of increasing gestational age.[35] The term newborn displays a nearly adult-like MMC pattern.

Although the MMC pattern appears to be a marker of increasing neuronal maturation, it is not necessary for normal peristalsis.[16] The development of low-compliance, continuous-perfusion manometry has improved the study of intestinal motility in infants[36] and can predict feeding readiness in preterm infants, but the technology is not yet available clinically.[16,37]

Intestinal motility development between 29 and 31 weeks is impressive.[38] Contractile activity becomes increasingly coordinated and capable of generating greater pressure. Associated with gaining the ability to suck, a more mature motor pattern emerges at about 34-35 weeks.[35] Intestinal motility development may be inducible by maternal and neonatal corticosteroid therapy and early, hypocaloric feeding.[35,38-40]

Gastric and transpyloric feeding appear to be equal in stimulating intestinal motility.[36] Trophic feedings shorten intestinal transit times.[36,41] Volumes as low as 4 ml/kg are effective.[36] Slow infusion (over 2 hours) feedings may enhance both duodenal motor responses as well as gastric emptying in preterm infants more than rapid bolus (over 15 minutes) feedings.[37] Dilute formula (6.6 cal/oz) may not be as effective as more concentrated feedings (13.2-21.0 cal/oz) in stimulating intestinal motility.[36] Human milk has been shown to have positive effects on intestinal motility.[3]

Infants with feeding intolerance have significantly longer gastric emptying time[29] and abnormal intestinal motor activity.[42] Immaturity of neural regulation is thought to be the primary cause of this delay in G.I. development[35] and appears to be transient as most infants become tolerant of feedings with two to four weeks.[42] Calorically dense formulas (24 cal/oz) may inhibit the G.I. response in infants with feeding intolerance.[43] A change to 20 cal/oz formula with progression to 24 cal/oz feedings may be beneficial for those infants.

Small intestine transit time decreases with increasing gestational age. It takes nine hours for contrast material introduced into the oral cavity to enter the colon in premature infants of 32 weeks' gestational age, but only 4.5 to 7.0 hours are required in full-term infants.[17] Reasons for the prolonged transit time in the preterm baby include (1) immature muscular layer of the intestine, (2) uncoordinated peristaltic waves, (3) increase in the number of antiperistaltic waves, and (4) decreased secretion of several G.I. hormones.[22] The slower transit time of preterm infants could actually facilitate greater absorption of nutrients secondary to longer exposure to digestive mechanisms.

Colonic motility is poorly developed until close to term.[16] This is based on the observation that preterm infants frequently have delayed passage of their first stool. Nearly all normal full-term infants pass their first meconium stool within 48 hours of birth, while many preterm infants may not pass a stool until more than one week after birth.[16] Total G.I. transit time (mouth to anus) for full-term newborns approximates 13.4 ± 4.4 hours.[44]

Many questions remain about G.I. motor development in the fetus and newborn and the significance of various factors in its progression. In addition, a variety of disease entities and disorders are associated with disturbances in gastric emptying and intestinal motility.[45]

Functional Development

The appearance of enzymes and the sequential development of digestive capability are important factors involved in the choice of enteral feeding. Unlike anatomic development, which is nearly mature by 20 weeks' gestation, intestinal absorptive processes are only partially available at 26 weeks. Figure 14.2 summarizes major milestones in digestion.[46] Figure 14.3 illustrates nutrient-specific sites of absorption.[47-49]

Carbohydrate

Although sucrase-isomaltase and lactase both appear at about 10 weeks of gestation, their functional development follows different timelines. Sucrase-isomaltase reaches about 70% of term newborn levels at 28-34 weeks of gestation. At this same gestational age, however, lactase has attained only about 30% of that found at term.[50-52] Studies have demonstrated that although preterm infants malabsorb significant lactose in the small bowel, it is fairly efficiently salvaged by colonic flora when it reaches the large bowel.[53,54] This is accomplished by bacterial fermentation of unabsorbed carbohydrate to short-chain fatty acids that are reabsorbed into circulation. Interruption of the normal pattern of intestinal flow eliminates this compensatory mechanism. This could occur, for example, when an ileostomy is performed following bowel resection. Additionally, administration of broad-spectrum antibiotics may alter the colonic flora and interfere with this retrieval system.[55]

There is no agreement on whether or not the ingestion of lactose enhances lactase activity.[53,56,57] There is evidence of accelerated intestinal maturation in the preterm newborn with time. During the first few weeks, whether enterally or parenterally fed, preterm infants show a rapid rise in lactase actitvity.[58-60] Preterm infants given early trophic feedings have increased lactase activity by 10 days of age, especially if fed human milk.[61] Small-for-gestational-age (SGA) term infants with birthweights < 1500 g may have decreased capacity to absorb lactose compared with their appropriately grown counterparts.[53] Preliminary experimental data have shown that administration of dexamethasone and epidermal growth factor may also induce an increase in lactase levels.[62,63]

Despite low levels of alpha amylases in newborns and virtually no alpha amylase activity in premature infants of 32-34 weeks' gesta-

Figure 14.2. Origin and activity level of digestive enzymes in the newborn.[46]

Activity level in the newborn is indicated by: bold print = high activity; regular print = adequate activity; italics = low or trace level activity. ? = level of activity and/or function in the newborn infant unknown. While pepsin expression is evident in the mucosa and gastric content of newborn infants, the high postprandial pH of the stomach (5.0-6.0) precludes a meaningful contribution of this enzyme to protein digestion.

Adapted with permission from
Hamosh M. Digestion in the newborn.
Philadelphia: Saunders, 1996.

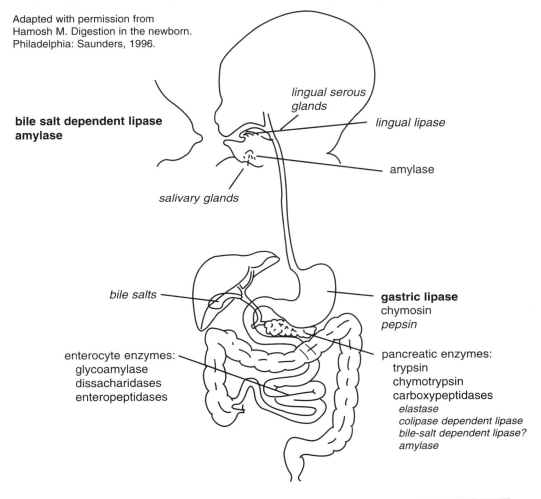

tion, most infants tolerate moderate amounts of starch.[64] This is most likely due to moderate activity of glucoamylase, an enzyme capable of hydrolyzing starch and glucose polymers. Studies suggest that premature infants can hydrolyze and absorb glucose polymers to an extent similar to that of lactose.[65]

Although the mechanisms for active transport of monosaccharides develop fairly early in intrauterine life, they remain relatively deficient in the term newborn as compared to the adult. This imma-

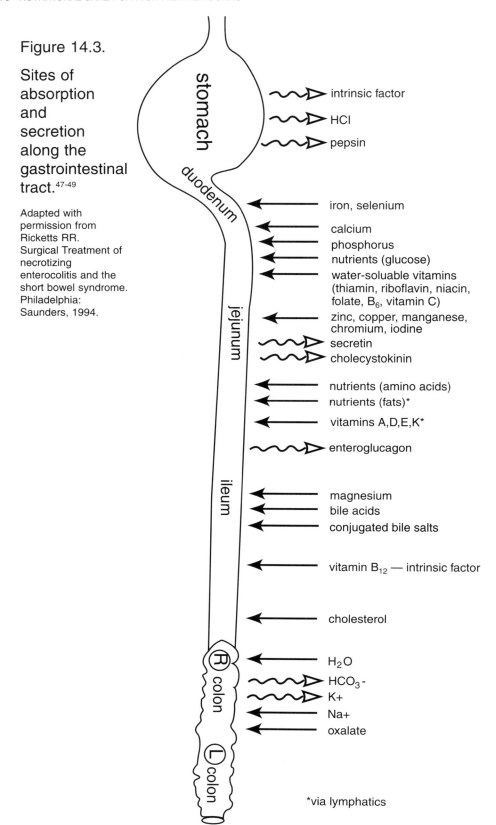

Figure 14.3.

Sites of absorption and secretion along the gastrointestinal tract.[47-49]

Adapted with permission from Ricketts RR. Surgical Treatment of necrotizing enterocolitis and the short bowel syndrome. Philadelphia: Saunders, 1994.

stomach

duodenum

jejunum

ileum

R colon

L colon

intrinsic factor

HCl

pepsin

iron, selenium

calcium

phosphorus

nutrients (glucose)

water-soluable vitamins (thiamin, riboflavin, niacin, folate, B_6, vitamin C)

zinc, copper, manganese, chromium, iodine

secretin

cholecystokinin

nutrients (amino acids)

nutrients (fats)*

vitamins A,D,E,K*

enteroglucagon

magnesium

bile acids

conjugated bile salts

vitamin B_{12} — intrinsic factor

cholesterol

H_2O

HCO_3-

K+

Na+

oxalate

*via lymphatics

turity does not appear to be the rate-limiting step in carbohydrate absorption. The availability and function of the various carbohydrases are more important in determining what is retained.[4,53]

Protein

Proteolysis usually begins in the stomach. This process is limited in infants due to low levels of pepsin and hydrochloric acid.[53,66] Little intragastric digestion of protein is noted in very young infants.[67] As a result, smaller peptides, the products of pepsin hydrolysis of protein, are scarce. It is peptides that stimulate gastrin and cholecystokinin (CCK) release. Consequently, these important G.I. hormones may be less available in the newborn period.[68]

Most protein digestion takes place in the small bowel. Both enterokinase and trypsin are important activators of pancreatic proteases. Although enterokinase activity is low, trypsin concentration and activity are adequate in the infant after about 24-28 weeks' gestation.[51,69,70] Concentrations of trypsinogen, chymotrypsinogen, and procarboxypeptidase are also adequate, so that intraluminal digestion of protein in newborn infants is assumed to be relatively efficient.[4]

The lack of CCK is one factor that limits the output of pancreatic proteases. Enteral feeding may stimulate CCK secretion almost immediately in SGA infants and, after 3-4 days, in other infants.[71] Function of the G.I. tract is modulated by the autonomic nervous system, especially the vagus nerve. Breast-feeding, and possibly pleasant sensory contact during other types of feeding, may enhance the release of CCK.[71] Clinically, the ability to digest protein appears adequate unless the protein load is increased. This situation can occur for the premature infant whose protein requirement may exceed the intestinal capacity.[17]

Brush border enteropeptidases are present by the second trimester, but little is known about the postnatal changes in these enzymes following birth.[53] Activity is higher in term than in preterm infants, and near adult levels at term.[4,53]

Active transport of amino acids into circulation is well developed in newborns. Various studies have shown that about 85% of food nitrogen is absorbed independent of age, type of diet, or maturity.[53] There is also some degree of macromolecular absorption in young infants. Whole proteins and/or peptides of various sizes may pass through the so-called 'leaky' gut, increasing, for example, the likelihood of allergic reactions. This characteristic of the newborn gut, more pronounced in the premature and SGA infant than in the mature infant, decreases progressively with age.[4,53,72-75] Early trophic feedings, antenatal glucocorticoids, and human milk may decrease intestinal permeability in preterm infants.[76]

Lipid

Lingual lipase, an enzyme secreted from lingual serous glands, and gastric lipase, an enzyme secreted from glands within the gastric mucosa, initiate fat digestion in the stomach of the newborn.[77-79] They appear before 26 weeks of gestation and have high activity levels at birth.[80,81] Although present in the adult, they are functionally more important to the infant who has low levels of pancreatic lipase and colipase. Apparently stimulated by sucking, these lipases are active at gastric pH and do not require bile salts.[82] Continuous, or near-continuous, infusion of intravenous fat emulsion (IFE) may be more effective in maintaining postnatal levels of preduodenal lipases than IFE given over shorter periods of time.[81] Medium-chain triglycerides released by the action of lingual and gastric lipases in the stomach are absorbed directly through the gastric mucosa of the infant.[83,84]

Intraluminal fat digestion is restricted in all neonates, especially those born prematurely, by:

- Diminished enterohepatic circulation
- Depressed secretory response to stimuli
- Bile acid concentrations below the critical micellar concentration
- Decreased levels of pancreatic lipase
- An immature lymphatic system[17,85-88]

Human milk lipase (also called bile salt-dependent lipase) enhances fat digestion and the hydrolysis of retinol esters in the intestine of breast-fed infants.[53,77] It is present in the milk of mothers of both term and preterm infants.[77] This lipase is stable at gastric pH, functional in the duodenum, and, at least in part, accounts for the superior absorption of the fat from human milk. It is also stable in expressed human milk that is refrigerated or frozen.[78] Both human milk lipase and pancreatic lipase activity are enhanced by lingual lipase.[82]

Table 14.2 summarizes digestive enzyme function in preterm and term newborns.

Vitamins, Minerals, Water, and Electrolytes

The ability of newborns to absorb vitamins is not completely understood. Folic acid is absorbed in the proximal jejunum. It is apparently absorbed more slowly than in adults,[89,90] although the ability to accumulate folate against a concentration gradient-and to incorporate the vitamin into red blood cells-is present from at least 20 weeks' gestation.[91] The relative inefficiency of fat absorption in infants-especially preterm infants-may adversely affect the absorption of fat-soluble vitamins.[72] The relatively low gastric secretion of

Table 14.2. Summary of Digestive Enzyme Function[†] in Preterm (PT) and Term (FT) Newborns[4,46,53,123,124]

Protein:

- Hydrochloric Acid (HCl) (stomach; stomach): secretion PT < FT < adult
- Chymosin (stomach; stomach): AKA rennin; primary gastric protease in newborns
- Pepsin (stomach; stomach): secretion PT < FT < adult; activity limited in newborns secondary to low HCl output
- Trypsin, Chymotrypsin and Carboxypeptidases (pancreas; intestine): present by 5 months gestation; increase rapidly following birth for both PT and FT newborns resulting in adequate proteolytic function in early infancy
- Elastase (pancreas; intestine): low activity throughout infancy
- Enteropeptidase (intestine; intestine): key activator of proteolysis; present by 5-6 months gestation; activity PT < FT < 1 year old infant

Carbohydrate:

- Salivary Amylase (salivary glands; stomach?/intestine): detectable by 4 months gestation; moderate activity in FT newborns but functional significance unclear
- Pancreatic Amylase (pancreas; intestine): virtually absent until approximately 6 months of age
- Lactase (intestine; intestine): low levels until close to term; functional significance controversial in PT; activity FT > adult
- Sucrase-Isomaltase (intestine; intestine): significant levels of this disaccharidase appear earlier in gestation than lactase; FT functioning is equivalent to adult
- Glucoamylase (intestine; intestine): significant levels along entire length of small intestine make this enzyme important for both starch and glucose polymer digestion; activity PT < FT

Fat:

- Lingual Lipase (lingual serous glands; stomach): present and functional in both PT and FT newborns
- Gastric Lipase (stomach; stomach): structurally very similar to lingual lipase; present early in gestation; contributes significantly to fat digestion, especially fat from human milk, in both PT and FT newborns and facilitates action of milk BSDL and pancreatic colipase
- Colipase Dependent Lipase (pancreas; intestine): little contribution to fat digestion in newborns
- Pancreatic Lipase (pancreas; intestine): major digestive lipase in adults but contribution limited in newborns; PT < FT and SGA < AGA; fat digestion improves rapidly during infancy
- Bile Salt Dependent Lipase (BSDL) (pancreas; intestine): structurally similar to milk BSDL but contribution to digestion unknown in human newborns
- Bile Salts (liver; intestine): levels PT < FT < adults

Human Milk Enzymes:

- Bile Salt Dependent Lipase (mammary gland; intestine): AKA human milk lipase and bile salt stimulated lipase; significant contribution to fat digestion in both PT and FT newborns
- Amylase (mammary gland; stomach?/intestine): equally present in milk of women who deliver prematurely and at term; stable during storage; structurally identical to salivary amylase but, unlike this isoenzyme, milk amylase makes a significant contribution to starch digestion in both PT and FT newborns

† Factor/Enzyme (origin; site of action): function/activity

intrinsic factor may affect vitamin B_{12} absorption in both premature and term newborns.[72]

Calcium is absorbed throughout most of the small intestine.[92] The efficiency of calcium absorption is lower in preterm than in more mature infants.[92,93] Vitamin D, and to some degree increasing gestational and postnatal age, improves calcium absorption.[94,95] The literature is controversial regarding the effects of lactose and fat on calcium absorption.[94,96-98] Recent evidence would suggest that calcium absorption is higher when the fat source is medium-chain triglycerides.[99] Iron is absorbed in the duodenum and the upper segment of the jejunum.[90] The capacity to absorb iron is well developed at birth in both term and preterm infants.[90] Zinc absorption, although sufficient in term newborns, is less efficient in premature infants.[72]

The primary function of the colon is to conserve water and electrolytes. This role becomes even more important in the newborn because reserves are smaller and diarrhea is more frequent than in the adult. Based on animal studies, the newborn colon is probably less efficient in performing this primary function.[72] The fetal and newborn colon, as distinct from the adult colon, almost resembles the small intestine in that it may (1) contain villi or dissaccharidases, (2) actively transport glucose, (3) tolerate high concentrations of bile acids, and (4) conserve nutrients, particularly carbohydrate.[100]

Enhancement of G.I. Function

Several factors regulate intrauterine and newborn G.I. development:

- Amniotic fluid. The hormonal and nutritive components of amniotic fluid appear to enhance intestinal growth.[101]
- Nongastrointestinal hormones. The glucocorticoid hormone cortisone and thyroxine promote maturation of enzyme concentrations.[102,103]
- Gastrointestinal hormones. Preliminary work has suggested a role for insulin, insulin-like growth factors, growth hormone, gastrin, cholecystokinin, enteroglucagon, and epidermal growth factor in G.I. maturation.[72,102,103]
- Polyamines and prostaglandins. Further work is need to elucidate the role of these two factors.[72,103]
- Drugs. Antenatal steroids, specifically dexamethasone, may speed maturation of the infant G.I. tract.[38,76,104-106]
- Nucleotides. Preliminary studies in animals suggest that formula supplementation with dietary nucleotides, present in generous quantities in human milk, may promote gut growth and maturation.[107] More study is needed to clarify the role of nucleotide supplementation in humans.[103,108]
- Glutamine. A primary fuel for the enterocyte, glutamine is absent in parenteral nutrition solutions and may be present in insuffi-

cient quantities in commercial infant formulas. Preliminary studies in infants suggest supplementation with glutamine may improve G.I. integrity resulting in improved feeding tolerance and a lower incidence of sepsis.[103,125]

• Enteral feeding. The introduction of food into the newborn gut is a key environmental trigger that causes a cascade of developmental changes.[103,109] Provision of an I.V. regimen does not support the structural or hormonal alterations in the G.I. tract that an isocaloric enteral intake supports.[110,111] Preterm infants appear to benefit from even very small enteral feedings.[39,41,112-115] Human milk, with its unique hormonal, enzymatic, and nutritive composition, stimulates G.I. development in a special way.[46,61,76,116-119]

Liver and Endocrine Pancreas

Hepatic excretory and metabolic functions are immature in the newborn. Low levels of bile secretion and diminished enterohepatic circulation have already been mentioned. Gall bladder contractibility is probably decreased.[120] The immaturity of hepatic metabolic function is best reflected in bilirubin physiology. There is decreased activity of UDP-glucuronyl transferase, the rate-limiting enzyme in the secretion of bilirubin.[121] Maturation of this enzyme seems to occur postnatally regardless of gestational age.[22,121] There is generalized hepatic biochemical immaturity in the premature infant. The pathways involved are mostly in amino acid and nitrogen metabolism, specifically methionine-cystine, phenylalanine-tyrosine and ammonia-urea.[1] Newborns, especially preterm newborns, exhibit a decreased capacity to metabolize and detoxify drugs.[122] This inefficiency is probably related to the low levels of activity of the hepatic cytochrome P450 monooxygenase system.[22] Insulin and glucagon, important hormones in intermediary metabolism, are detectable very early in fetal life-by the eighth to tenth week of development.[1] Premature infants, when compared to their full-term counterparts, however, are equipped with less than fully functional metabolic machinery. They are more likely, therefore, to experience intolerance when forced to metabolize full exogenous dietary loads.

To summarize this chapter, the human G.I. tract follows a dynamic course of development during fetal and newborn life governed by genetics, the biological clock, intrinsic regulatory mechanisms, and environmental influences. Although anatomically complete by about 22 weeks of gestation, the gut has many motor and functional deficiencies until close to term.[126] These immaturities have major implications for feeding premature infants.

References

1. Neu J. Functional development of the fetal gastrointestinal tract. Semin Perinatol 13:224, 1989.
2. Lebenthal E, Lee PC. Interactions of determinants in the ontogeny of the gastrointestinal tract: A unified concept. Pediatr Res 17:19, 1983.
3. Lebenthal E. Gastrointestinal maturation and motility patterns as indicators for feeding the premature infant. Pediatrics 95:207, 1995.
4. Lebenthal E, Lee PC, Heitlinger LA. Impact of development of the gastrointestinal tract on infant feeding. J Pediatr 102:1, 1983.
5. Berseth CL, Lichtengerger LM, Morris FH. Comparison of the gastrointestinal growth-promoting effects of rat colostrum and mature milk in newborn rats in vivo. Am J Clin Nutr 37:52, 1983.
6. Scammon RE, Doyle LO. Observations on the capacity of the stomach in the first ten days of postnatal life. Am J Dis Child 20:516, 1920.
7. Pritchard J. Fetal swallowing and amniotic fluid volume. Obstet Gynecol 28:606, 1966.
8. Brace RA. Fluid distribution in the fetus and neonate. In: Polin RA, Fox WW, eds. Fetal and neonatal physiology. 2d ed. Philadelphia: Saunders, 1998; 1703-13.
9. Arey LB. Developmental anatomy. Philadelphia: Saunders, 1974; 245-262.
10. Reiquam CW, Allen RP, Akers DR. Normal and abnormal small bowel lengths. Am J Dis Child 109:447, 1965.
11. Siebert J. Small-intestine length in infants and children. Am J Dis Child 134:593, 1980.
12. Benson CD. Resection and primary anastomosis of the jejunum and ileum in the newborn. Ann Surg 142:478, 1955.
13. Premji SS. Ontogeny of the gastrointestinal system and its impact on feeding the preterm infant. Neonatal Network 17(2):17, 1998.
14. Gryboski J. Suck and swallow in the premature infant. Pediatrics 43:96, 1969.
15. Herbst JJ. Development of suck and swallow. In: Lebenthal E, ed. Human gastrointestinal development. New York: Raven Press, 1989; 229-39.
16. Dumont RC and Rudolph CD. Development of gastrointestinal motility in the infant and child. Gastroenterol Clin North Am 23(4):655, 1994.
17. Lebenthal E, Leung YK. Developmental changes of the gastrointestinal tract in the newborn. In: Stern L, ed. Feeding the sick infant. New York: Raven Press, 1987; 1-24.
18. Lau C and Schanler RJ. Oral motor function in the neonate. Clin Perinatol 23(2):161, 1996.
19. DiPietro JA, Cusson RM, Caughy MO, et al. Behavioral and physiologic effects of nonnutritive sucking during gavage feeding in preterm infants. Pediatr Res 36:207, 1994.
20. Field T. Sucking for stress reduction and growth and development during infancy. Pediatric Basics 64:13, 1993.
21. Omari TI, Rudolph CD. Gastrointestinal motility. In: Polin RA, Fox WW, eds. Fetal and neonatal physiology, 2d ed. Philadelphia: Saunders, 1998; 1373-83.

22. Balistreri WF. Anatomic and biochemical ontogeny of the gastrointestinal tract and liver. In: Tsang RC, Nichols BL, eds. Nutrition during infancy. Philadelphia: Hanley and Belfus, 1988; 33-57.
23. Bisset WM, Watt JB, Rivers JPA, et al. The ontogeny of fasting small intestinal motor activity in the human infant. Gut 29:483, 1988.
24. Cavell B. Gastric emptying in infants. Acta Paediatr Scand 60:370, 1971.
25. Signer E, Fridrich R. Gastric emptying in newborns and young infants. Acta Paeadiatr Scand 64:525, 1975.
26. Gupta M, Brans YW. Gastric retention in neonates. Pediatrics 62:26, 1978.
27. Blumenthal I, Ebel A, Pildes RS. Effect of posture on the pattern of stomach emptying in the newborn. Pediatrics 63:532, 1979.
28. Cavell B. Gastric emptying in preterm infants. Acta Paediatr Scand 68:725, 1979.
29. Carlos MA, Babyn PS, Marcon MA, Moore AM. Changes in gastric emptying in early postnatal life. J Pediatr 130:931, 1997.
30. Pildes RS, Blumenthal I, Abel A. Stomach emptying in the newborn. Pediatrics 66:482, 1980.
31. Yu VYH. Effect of body position on gastric emptying in the neonate. Arch Dis Child 50:500, 1975.
32. Siegel M, Lebenthal E, Krantz B. Effect of caloric density on gastric emptying in premature infants. J Pediatr 104:118, 1984.
33. Siegel M, Krantz B, Lebenthal E. Effect of fat and carbohydrate composition on the gastric emptying of isocaloric feedings in premature infants. Gastroenterology 89:785, 1985.
34. Ewer AK, Durbin GM, Morgan MEI, Booth IW. Gastric emptying in preterm infants. Arch Dis Child 71:F24, 1994.
35. Berseth CL. Gut motility and the pathogenesis of necrotizing enterocolitis. Clinics Perinatol 21(2):263, 1994.
36. Koenig WJ, Amarnath RP, Hench V, Berseth CL. Manometrics for preterm and term infants: A new tool for old questions. Pediatrics 95:203, 1995.
37. deVille K, Knapp E, Al-Tawil Y, Berseth CL. Slow infusion feedings enhance duodenal motor responses and gastric emptying in preterm infants. Am J Clin Nutr 68:103, 1998.
38. Morriss FH, Moore M, Weisbrodt NW, et al. Ontogenic development of gastrointestinal motility. IV. Duodenal contractions in preterm infants. Pediatrics 78:1106, 1986.
39. Berseth CL. Effect of early feeding on maturation of the preterm infant's small intestine. J Pediatr 120:947, 1992.
40. Berseth CL and Nordyke C. Enteral nutrients promote postnatal maturation of intestinal motor activity in preterm infants. Am J Physiol 264:G1046, 1993.
41. Schanler RJ, Shulman RJ, Lau C, et al. Feeding strategies for premature infants: randomized trial of gastrointestinal priming and tube-feeding method. Pediatrics 103:434, 1999.
42. Berseth CL and Nordyke CK. Manometry can predict feeding readiness in preterm infants. Gastroenterology 103:1523, 1992.
43. Jadcherla SR and Berseth CL. Acute and chronic intestinal motor acctivity responses to two infant formulas. Pediatrics 96:331, 1995.
44. Morriss FH. Neonatal gastrointestinal motility and enteral feeding. Semin Perinatol 15:478, 1991.

45. Siegel M, Lebenthal E. Development of gastrointestinal motility and gastric emptying during the fetal and newborn periods. In: Lebenthal E, ed. Human gastrointestinal development. New York: Raven Press, 1989; 277-98.

46. Hamosh M. Digestion in the newborn. Clin Perinatology 23(2):191, 1996.

47. Ricketts RR. Surgical treatment of necrotizing enterocolitis and the short bowel syndrome. Clin Perinatol 21(2):365, 1994.

48. Ernst JA, Neal PR. Minerals and trace elements. In: Polin RA, Fox WW, eds. Fetal and neonatal physiology. 2d ed. Philadelphia: Saunders, 1998; 332-43.

49. Moran JR and Greene HL. Vitamin requirements. In: Polin RA, Fox WW, Eds. Fetal and Neonatal Physiology. 2d ed. Philadelphia: Saunders, 1998; 344-53.

50. Dahlqvist A, Lindberg T. Development of the intestinal disaccharidase and alkaline phosphatase activities in the human fetus. Clin Sci 30:517, 1966.

51. Antonowicz I, Lebenthal E. Developmental pattern of small intestinal enterokinase and disaccharidase activities in the human fetus. Gastroenterology 72:1299, 1977.

52. Antonowicz I, Milunsky A, Lebenthal E, et al. Disaccharidase and lysosomal enzyme activities in amniotic fluid, intestinal mucosa and meconium. Biol Neonate 32:280, 1977.

53. Koldovsky O. Digestive-Absorptive functions in fetuses, infants, and children. In: Walker WA, Watkins JB, eds. Nutrition in pediatrics. London: BC Decker, 1997; 233-47.

54. Kien CL, Liechty EA, Myerberg DZ, et al. Dietary carbohydrate assimilation in the premature infant: Evidence for a nutritionally significant bacterial ecosystem in the colon. Am J Clin Nutr 46:456, 1987.

55. Bhatia J, Prihoda AR, Richardson CJ. Parenteral antibiotics and carbohydrate intolerance in term neonates. Am J Dis Child 140:111, 1986.

56. Kien CL, McClead RE, Cordero L. Effects of lactose intake on lactose digestion and colonic fermentation in preterm infants. 133:401, 1998.

57. Montgomery RK, Buller HA, Rings EHHM, et al. Lactose intolerance and the genetic regulation of intestinal lactase-phlorizin hydrolase. FASEB J 5:2824, 1991.

58. Raul F, Lacroix B, Aprahamian M. Longitudinal distribution of brush border hydrolases and morphological maturation in the intestine of the preterm infant. Early Human Dev 13:225, 1986.

59. Auricchio S, Rubino A, Murset G. Intestinal glycosidase activities in the human embryo, fetus and newborn. Pediatrics 35:944, 1965.

60. Mayne A, Hughes CA, Sule D, et al. Development of intestinal disaccharidases in preterm infants. Lancet 2:622, 1983.

61. Shulman RJ, Schanler RJ, Lau C, et al. Early feeding, feeding tolerance, and lactase activity in preterm infants. J Pediatr 133:645, 1998.

62. Auricchio S, and Sebastio G. Development of disaccharidases. In: Lebenthal E, ed. Human gastrointestinal development. New York: Raven Press, 1989; 451-70.

63. Menard D, Pothier P, Arsenault N, et al. Epidermal growth factor binding and biologic effects in human fetal small intestine (abstr). Gastroenterology 92:1531, 1987.

64. Zoppi G, Andreotti G, Pajno-Ferrara F, et al. Exocrine pancreas function in premature and full term neonates. Pediatr Res 6:880, 1972.

65. Cicco R, Holzman IR, Brown DR, et al. Glucose polymer tolerance in premature infants. Pediatrics 67:498, 1981.
66. Kelly EJ, Brownlee KG. When is the fetus first capable of gastric acid, intrinsic factor and gastrin secretion? Biol Neonate 63:153, 1993.
67. Harries JT, Fraser AJ. The acidity of the gastric contents of premature babies during the first 14 days of life. Biol Neonate 12:186, 1966.
68. Defize J. Development of pepsinogens. In: Lebenthal E, ed. Human gastrointestinal development. New York: Raven Press, 1989; 299-324.
69. Borgstrom B, Lindquist B, Lundh G. Enzyme concentration and absorption of protein and glucose in duodenum of premature infants. Am J Dis Child 99:338, 1960.
70. Boehm G, Bierbach U, DelSanto A, et al. Activities of trypsin and lipase in duodenal aspirates of healthy preterm infants: effects of gestational and postnatal age. Biol Neonate 67:248, 1995.
71. Tornhage C-J, Serenius F, Uvnas-Moberg K, Lindberg T. Plasma somatostatin and cholecystokinin levels in response to feeding in preterm infants. J Pediatr Gastroenterol Nutr 27:199, 1998.
72. Lebenthal E, Leung YK. Feeding the premature and compromised infant: Gastrointestinal considerations. Pediatr Clin North Am 35:215, 1988.
73. Committee on Nutrition, American Academy of Pediatrics. Use of whole cow's milk in infancy. Pediatrics 89:1105, 1992.
74. Kuitunen OOM, Savilahti E, Sarnesto A. Human α-lactalbumin and bovine β-lactoglobulin absorption in premature infants. Pediatr Res 35:344, 1994.
75. D'Netto M, Knox I, Herson V, et al. Allergic gastroenteropathy in preterm infants. J Pediatr Gastroenterol Nutr 25:472, 1997.
76. Shulman RJ, Schanler RJ, Lau C, et al. Early feeding, antenatal glucocorticoids, and human milk decrease intestinal permeability in preterm infants. Pediatr Res 44:519, 1998.
77. Hamosh M. Lingual and breast milk lipases. Adv Pediatr 29:33, 1982.
78. DeNigris SJ, Hamosh M, Kasbekar DK, et al. Secretion of human gastric lipase from dispersed gastric glands. Biochim Biophys Acta 836:67, 1985.
79. Menard D, Monfils S, Tremblay RE. Ontogeny of human gastric lipase and pepsin activities. Gastroenterology 108:1650, 1995.
80. Hamosh M, Scanlon JW, Ganot D, et al. Fat digestion in the newborn: Characterization of the lipase in gastric aspirates of premature and term infants. J Clin Invest 67:838, 1981.
81. Lee P-C, Borysewicz R, Struve M, et al. Development of lipolytic activity in gastric aspirates from premature infants. J Pediatr Gastroenterol Nutr 17:291, 1993.
82. Hamosh M, Hamosh P. Lingual and gastric lipases during development. In: Lebenthal E, ed. Human gastrointestinal development. New York: Raven Press, 1989; 251-76.
83. Hamosh M, Bitman J, Mehta NR, et al. Medium chain fatty acids are absorbed directly from the stomach of premature infants. Pediatr Res 21:429A, 1987.
84. Iverson SJ, Kirk CL, Hamosh M. Fat digestion in the newborn: In vitro studies greatly underestimate the high extent of intragastric digestion of fat. Pediatr Res 27:107A, 1990.
85. Watkins JB. Lipid digestion and absorption. Pediatrics 75 (suppl):151, 1985.

86. Katz L, Hamilton JR. Fat absorption in infants of birth weight less than 1300 gm. J Pediatr 85:608, 1974.

87. Lebenthal E, Lee PC. Development of functional response in human exocrine pancreas. Pediatrics 66:556, 1980.

88. Watkins JB. Mechanism of fat absorption and the development of gastrointestinal function. Pediatr Clin North Am 22:721, 1975.

89. Shojania AM, Hornady G. Folate metabolism in newborns and during early infancy. I. Absorption of pteroylglutamic (folic) acid in newborns. Pediatr Res 4:412, 1970.

90. Oski FA. Development of the small intestine's capacity to absorb iron and folic acid. In: Lebenthal E, ed. Human gastrointestinal development. New York: Raven Press, 1989; 487-490.

91. Ek J. Plasma and red cell folate values in newborn infants and their mothers in relation to gestational age. J Pediatr 96:288, 1980.

92. Toverud SU. Calcium absorption and vitamin D function in the small intestine during development. In: Lebenthal E, ed. Human gastrointestinal development. New York: Raven Press, 1989; 471-86.

93. Lyon AJ, McIntosh N. Calcium and phosphorus balance in extremely low birth weight infants in the first six weeks of life. Arch Dis Child 59:1145, 1984.

94. Koo, WWK, Tsang RC. Calcium, magnesium, phosphorus, and Vitamin D. In: Tsang RC, Lucas A, Uauy R, Zlotkin S, eds. Nutritional needs of the preterm infant: Scientific basis and practical guidelines. Baltimore: Williams and Wilkins, 1993; 135-55.

95. Senterre J, Salle B. Calcium and phosphorus economy of the preterm infant and its interaction with vitamin D and its metabolites. Acta Paediatr Scand (suppl) 296:85, 1982.

96. Ziegler EE, Fomon SJ. Lactose enhances mineral absorption in infancy. J Pediatr Gastroenterol Nutr 2:288, 1983.

97. Allen LH. Calcium bioavailability and absorption: A review. Am J Clin Nutr 35:783, 1982.

98. Wirth FH, Numerof B, Pleban P, et al. Effect of lactose on mineral absorption in preterm infants. J Pediatr 117:283, 1990.

99. Sulkers EJ, Lafeber HN, Degenhart HJ, et al. Comparison of two preterm formulas with and without addition of medium-chain triglycerides (MCT'S). II. Effects on mineral balance. J Pediatr Gastroenterol Nutr 15:42, 1992.

100. Potter GD. Development of colonic function. In: Lebenthal E, ed. Human gastrointestinal development. New York: Raven Press, 1989; 545-58.

101. Klein RM. Cell proliferative regulation in developing small intestine. In: Lebenthal E, ed. Human gastrointestinal development. New York: Raven Press, 1989; 367-92.

102. Lebenthal E. Concepts in gastrointestinal development. In: Lebenthal E, ed. Human gastrointestinal development. New York: Raven Press, 1989, 3-18.

103. Carver JD, Barness LA. Trophic factors for the gastrointestinal tract. Clin Perinatol 23(2):265, 1996.

104. Pang KY, Newman AP, Udall JN, et al. Development of gastrointestinal mucosal barrier. VII. In utero maturation of microvillus surface by cortisone. Am J Physiol 249:85, 1984 (suppl).

105. Neu J, Ozaki CK, Angelides KJ. Glucocorticoid-mediated alteration of fluidity of brush border membrane in rat small intestine. Pediatr Res 20:79, 1986.

106. Bauer CR, Morrison JC, Poole WK, et al. A decreased incidence of necrotizing enterocolitis after prenatal glucocorticoid therapy. Pediatrics 73:682, 1984.

107. Uauy R, Stringel G, Thomas R, et al. Effect of dietary nucleosides on growth and maturation of the developing gut in the rat. J Pediatr Gastroenterol Nutr 10:497, 1990.

108. Quan R, Barness L, Uauy R. Do infants need nucleotide supplemented formula for optimal nutrition? J Pediatr Gastroenterol Nutr 11:429, 1990.

109. Johnson LR. Effects of enteral feeding on GI growth and function. In: Enteral feeding: Scientific basis and clinical applications. Report of the 94th Ross Clinical Conference on Pediatric Research, Columbus, Ohio, 1988.

110. Johnson LR, Copeland EM, Dudrick SJ, et al. Structural and hormonal alterations in the GI tract of parenterally fed rats. Gastroenterology 68:1177, 1975.

111. Lucas A, Bloom SR, Aynsley-Green A. Metabolic and endocrine consequences of depriving preterm infants of enteral nutrition. Acta Paediatr Scand 72:245, 1983.

112. Lucas A, Bloom SR, Aynsley-Green A. Gut hormones and "minimal enteral feeding." Acta Paediatr Scand 75:719, 1986.

113. Slagle TA, Gross SJ. Effect of early low-volume enteral substrate on subsequent feeding tolerance in very low birth weight infants. J Pediatr 113:526, 1988.

114. Dunn L, Hulman S, Weiner T, et al. Beneficial effects of early hypocaloric enteral feeding on neonatal gastrointestinal function: Preliminary report of a randomized trial. J Pediatr 112:622, 1988.

115. Meetze WH, Valentine C, McGuigan JE, et al. Gastrointestinal priming prior to full enteral nutrition in very low birth weight infants. J Pediatr Gastroenterol Nutr 15:163, 1992.

116. Sheard NF, Walker WA. The role of breast milk in the development of the gastrointestinal tract. Nutr Rev 46:1, 1988.

117. Zumkeller W. Relationship between insulin-like growth factor I and II and IGF-binding proteins in milk and the gastrointestinal tract: Growth and development of the gut. J Pediatr Gastroenterol Nutr 15:357, 1992.

118. Perin NM, Clandinin MT, Tromson ABR. Importance of milk and diet on the ontogeny and adaptation of the intestine. J Pediatr Gastroenterol Nutr 24:419, 1997.

119. Catassi C, Bonucci A, Coppa V, et al. Intestinal permeability changes during the first month: Effect of natural versus artificial feeding. J Pediatr Gastroenterol Nutr 21:383, 1995.

120. Denehy CM, Ryan JR. Development of gallbladder contractibility in the guinea pig. Pediatr Res 20:214, 1986.

121. Kawade N, Onishi S. The prenatal and postnatal development of UDP-glucuronyltransferase activity toward bilirubin and the effect of premature birth on this activity in the human liver. Biochem J 196:257, 1983.

122. Soyka LF, Redmond GP, eds. Drug metabolism in the immature human. New York: Raven Press, 1981.

123. Manson WG, Coward WA, Harding M, Weaver LT. Development of fat digestion in infancy. Arch Dis Child Fetal Neonatal Ed 80:F183, 1999.
124. Christian M, Edwards C, Weaver LT. Starch digestion in infancy. J Pediatr Gastroenterol Nutr 29:116, 1999.
125. Neu J, DeMarco V, Weiss M. Glutamine supplementation in low-birth-weight infants: mechanisms of action. JPEN 23:S49, 1999.
126. Lebenthal A, Lebenthal E. The ontogeny of the small intestinal epithelium. JPEN 23:S3, 1999.

Nutritional Care for High-Risk Newborns (Rev. 3d. Ed.)
S. Groh-Wargo, M. Thompson, J. Cox, editors
© 2000, Precept Press, Inc., Chicago

15

RECOMMENDED ENTERAL NUTRIENT INTAKES

Sharon Groh-Wargo, MS, RD, LD

The most widely accepted nutrient recommendations for term, healthy infants are the Recommended Dietary Allowances (RDA) from the Food and Nutrition Board of the National Research Council[1] (see Appendix G). These levels are set using the bioavailability and nutrient content of human milk and the growth and estimated intakes of the breast-fed infant as the model. The RDA's may be too generous for some infants; they are intended to meet the highest requirements observed within an infant group.

Dietary Reference Intakes (DRIs) are being issued by the Food and Nutrition Board and are intended to eventually expand and replace the RDAs.[2] The DRIs are being issued in seven separate nutrient groups and include recommendations for adequate intakes (AI), estimated average requirements (EAR), recommended dietary allowances (RDA), and/or tolerable upper intake levels (UL). The AI is provided instead of an RDA when sufficient scientific evidence is not available to calculate an EAR.[2] AIs for infants 0-6 months are based on the mean nutrient intakes supplied by human milk. Appendix G summarizes DRIs for infants that are available at this time.[3,4,204]

Appropriate nutrient intakes are difficult to determine for preterm infants. Incomplete stores, high accretion rates, suboptimal digestion and absorption, and related diseases of prematurity affect the need for many nutrients. In addition, the ideal growth rate remains unclear. The healthy, breast-fed infant is a clearly appropriate model for term babies, but there is no such model for the preterm infant. Several professional organizations and groups of experts have issued nutrient recommendations for preterm and low-birth-weight (LBW) infants.[5-8] These can be compared when expressed as units per 100 kcal of energy (see Appendix G). A summary of recommended daily enteral nutrient intakes for stable, low-birth-weight infants in units per kg per day can be found in Table 15.1. Energy requirements are increased following major surgery (20-30% increase) and when fever is present (12% increase for each degree above 37° C).[9] Several conditions such as extreme low birth weight, intrauterine growth retardation, and neonatal diseases can affect specific nutrient requirements[10-12] (Tables 15.2 and 15.3).

Because the enteral intake of infants is predominantly human milk or infant formula, the content of infant formula is closely related to nutrient recommendations for infants. Several proposed standards exist for formulas.[8,13-16]

There is mounting evidence that nutrition in early life may have a profound effect on long-term health and development.[17] Undernutrition during a period of rapid cell division could have a permanent effect on the physiology and metabolism of those cells.[18] The critical period of growth for the central and enteric nervous system is from 25-26 weeks' gestation through 18 months postterm.[17] It has been suggested, for example, that deficiencies of specific nutrients such as iron and long chain polyunsaturated fatty acids (LC-PUFAs) may have negative effects on neurocognition[19] and visual development,[20] respectively. In addition, preterm infants fed human milk with its unique nutritional, hormonal, and immunological components, may have significantly higher intelligence quotient (IQ) scores in early childhood than similar children who received formula.[21] These so-called "programming" effects may continue to affect health into adulthood.[18,22,23] These data underscore the importance of nutrition for small, sick newborns.

This chapter presents guidelines for nutrient intakes for enterally fed newborns, with discussions of some of the more controversial issues. Emphasis is on the stable, growing preterm infant. Suggested intakes for the preterm infant in transition from parenteral to enteral nutrition exist but are not discussed in this chapter.[5] Recommended parenteral nutrient intakes are found in Chapters 9, 10, and 11.

Fluid

For the critically ill newborn, initial fluids are generally managed intravenously. Some guidelines for enteral fluids, however, do exist. Fluid management is especially important in infants due to (1) large body surface area, (2) high percentage of body water and its high rate of turnover, (3) limited renal capacity for handling solute load, and (4) susceptibility to dehydration due to inability to express thirst.[1]

The RDA fluid recommendation for infants of 1.5 ml/kcal of energy expenditure corresponds to the water-to-energy ratio in human milk.[1] Fluid needs of preterm infants are more variable.[205] Although preterm infants are more susceptible to dehydration, they are also more likely to suffer complications of overhydration, such as patent ductus arteriosus and bronchopulmonary dysplasia.[24,25]

Enteral fluid requirements for preterm infants are given as both ml/100 kcal in a range of 100-167 ml/100 kcal,[5,26] and as ml/kg in a range of 120-200 ml/kg[7,24] (see Appendix G). The intake of water should maintain serum sodium within the normal range, produce urine with a specific gravity of 1.010-1.016 g/ml and a flow of 2-6 ml/kg/hour, and maintain urine osmolality around 200-400 mOsm/kg water.[25-27]

Energy

The energy requirement of infants is determined by three variables: energy expended, energy stored, and energy lost. The energy expenditure component consists of the basal metabolic rate, an activity factor, the cost of thermoregulation or "cold stress," the energy cost of tissue synthesis, and the thermic effect of food or "specific dynamic action." Energy storage includes both fat and lean body mass accretion. Energy losses, often due to incomplete digestion and absorption, are generally greater in the infant, especially the preterm infant, than in the adult. Using these factors, estimates of the energy requirement of premature infants are available (Table 15.4).[6,28] The total energy cost of growth is estimated to be between 3.0-4.5 kcal/g weight gain.[29,30] About 70 kcal/kg, on top of the maintenance energy requirement of approximately 50 kcal/kg, should support a daily weight gain of 15 g/kg.[30,31]

Many studies of energy balance in preterm infants have been reported.[31-46] Intakes ranging from 92-183 kcal/kg/day support growth ranging from 14-29 g/kg/day. Although these various recommendations are difficult to compare because of variations in feeding composition, postnatal age, degree of prematurity, etc., excessive energy intake (> 165 kcal/kg/day) appears to promote excessive fat accumulation, while inadequate intake (< 110 kcal/kg/day) is associated with growth retardation.[8] Average energy intakes of 105-130 kcal/kg/day are recommended based on an assessment of all factors.[5-8,12,30] Specific groups of infants, such as those small for gestational age (SGA) or of extremely low birth weight, or those diagnosed with BPD, may have increased energy needs.[6,11,37,45,47,48,206] After protein and essential fatty acid needs are met, the remaining energy requirement is usually divided between fat and carbohydrate. An intake with approximately 40-50% of total calories from carbohydrate and 40-50% from fat results in an appropriate distribution of energy.[30]

Table 15.1. Recommended Daily Enteral Nutrient Intakes for Stable, Preterm, Low-Birth-Weight Infants[5,30]

Nutrient	Recommended intake
Fluid (ml/kg)[5]	150-200
Energy (kcal/kg)[5,30]	105-130
Protein (g/kg)[5,30]	3.0-4.0
Carbohydrate (% of total energy)[30]	40-50
Fat (% of total energy)[5]	40-55
Linoleic and linolenic acids (% of total energy)[30]	3.0
Minerals (mg/kg)[5]	
Calcium	120-230
Phosphorus	60-140
Magnesium	7.9-15.0
Electrolytes (mEq/kg)[5,30]	
Sodium	2.0-3.0
Potassium	2.0-3.0
Magnesium	2.0-3.0
Trace elements (µg/kg)[5]	
Zinc	1000
Copper	120-150
Selenium	1.3-3.0
Chromium	0.1-0.5
Molybdenum	0.3
Manganese	0.75-7.5
Iodine	30-60
Vitamins (fat soluble)[5]	
Vitamin A (IU/kg)	700-1500
Vitamin D (IU/d)	400
Vitamin E (IU/kg)	6.0-12.0
Vitamin K (µg/kg)	8.0-10.0
Vitamins (water soluble)[5]	
Vitamin C (mg/kg)	18-24
Thiamin (µg/kg)	180-240
Riboflavin (µg/kg)	250-360
Niacin (mg/kg)	3.6-4.8
Pyridoxine (µg/kg)	150-210
B_{12} (µg/kg)	0.3
Folic Acid (µg/kg)	25-50
Pantothenic acid (mg/kg)	1.2-1.7
Biotin (µg/kg)	3.6-6.0

Table 15.2.   Special Nutritional Conditions in Extremely Low Birth Weight Infants[11]

1. Low energy reserves (both carbohydrate and fat)
2. Higher metabolic rate (intrinsically, due to a higher body content of more metabolically active organs: brain, heart, liver)
3. Higher protein turnover rate (especially when growing)
4. Higher glucose needs for energy and brain metabolism
5. Higher lipid needs to match the in-utero rate of fat deposition and the unique requirements of essential fatty acids for brain, neural and vascular development
6. Excessive evaporative rates and occasionaly very high urinary water and solute losses
7. Low rates of gastrointestinal peristalsis
8. Limited production of gut digestive enzymes and growth factors
9. High incidence of stressful events (hypoxemia, respiratory distress, sepsis)
10. Abnormal neurological outcome if not fed adequately

Reprinted with permission from Hay WW. Nutritional requirements of extremely low birth-weight infants. Stockholm, Sweden: Scandinavian University Press, 1994.

Protein

Many factors affect the protein requirements of infants. They include (1) gestational age and chronological age, (2) clinical condition, (3) quality of protein consumed, (4) energy intake, and (5) availability of nutrients such as sodium and phosphorus.[49,50]

Common clinical conditions experienced by the preterm infant, such as surgery, sepsis, and BPD, increase protein turnover rates and urinary nitrogen excretion.[10,51,52,207] Steroid therapy has known catabolic effects.[53] Further studies are needed to define differences in protein metabolism in appropriate-for-gestational-age (AGA) versus SGA, LBW infants.[54]

Protein quality alters the amount of protein required. The most recognizable example of this is the lower rates of weight gain and nitrogen retention observed in infants fed early soy protein formulas, which were not fortified with methionine.[55] Glutamine may improve gut integrity and decrease sepsis but data to date do not support routine supplementation of LBW infant diets.[208,209] Human milk protein (60-80% whey and 20-40% casein) and modified bovine milk (60% whey and 40% casein) are the common proteins fed to preterm infants. The minimum mean amount of protein apparently required to support fetal nitrogen accretion of individual amino acids in LBW infants is estimated to be less for human milk (2.6-2.8 g/kg/day) than

Table 15.3. The Effects of Neonatal Diseases on Specific Nutrient Requirements[10]

Nutrient	RDS	BPD	Cyanotic HD	CHF	Sepsis	IUGR
Free H$_2$0	⇓	⇓	⇔	⇓	⇔	⇑
Energy	⇑	⇑⇑	⇑	⇑⇑	⇑	⇑
Fat	⇔	⇑	⇑	⇑	⇔	⇑
CHO	⇑	⇓	⇑	⇑	⇑	⇑
Protein	⇔	⇑	⇑	⇑	⇑⇑	⇑
Calcium	⇔	⇑*†	⇑*‡	⇑*†‡	⇔	⇑
Iron	⇔	⇑*	⇑	⇔	⇓	⇑
Vitamin A	⇑*	⇑*	⇔	⇔	⇔	⇔
Vitamin E	⇔	⇑	⇔	⇔	⇔	⇔

RDS = respiratory distress syndrome
HD = heart disease
IUGR = intrauterine growth retardation
* in < 1,500 g infant
‡ especially postoperatively

BPD = bronchopulmonary disease
CHF = congestive heart failure
CHO = carbohydrate
† especially if on calciuric diuretic (furosemide)

Reprinted with permission from Wahlig TM, Georgieff MK. Clinics in Perinatology, 1995.

for modified bovine milk (3.0 g/kg/day).[56,57] The superior protein quality of human milk is the most likely explanation for this difference.

It is difficult to consider protein and energy needs separately, as they are uniquely symbiotic in the following ways:

- Protein synthesis for maintenance and growth is energy-expensive.
- If energy intake is inadequate, protein synthesis will be depressed and amino acid oxidation may be increased.
- Protein retention becomes more a function of protein intake if energy intake is adequate.
- Higher energy intake alone does not guarantee improved weight gain.
- Excessive energy intake, especially without adequate protein, can produce increased body fat.
- Excessive protein intake, especially without adequate energy, can be potentially harmful to the preterm infant due to renal and metabolic immaturity.[53,58-60]

Clinical studies using a variety of techniques have shown that intakes of 3.5-4.0 g protein/kg/day are well tolerated.[49,58,61] Weight gain and nitrogen accretion are maximized when protein intake is accompanied by energy intakes of at least 130 kcal/kg.[49,61] To preserve the

Table 15.4.   Estimates of Energy Requirement (kcal/kg/day) for the Preterm Infant[6,28]

| | AAP* | ESPGAN† | |
		Average	Range
Energy expenditure			
Resting metabolic rate	50	2.5	45-60
Activity	15	7.5	5-10
Cold stress	10	7.5	5-10
Synthesis/thermic effect of food	8	17.5	10-25
Energy stored	25	25.0	20-30
Energy excreted	12	20.0	10-30
Estimated energy requirement	120	130	95-165

*American Academy of Pediatrics
†European Society of Pediatric Gastroenterology and Nutrition

appropriate protein/energy ratio recommendations for both kcal/g of protein and g protein/100 kcal are available. With few exceptions, the data support provision of 33-43 kcal/g of protein and 2.5-3.3 g protein/100 kcal.[5-8,30,59,60,62] Infants weighting < 1000 g are more likely than larger infants to benefit from intakes in the lower end of the kcal/g of protein range, and in the upper end of the g protein/100 kcal range.[5,7]

The recommended protein intake for preterm infants is 2.5-4.0 g/kg/day.[5,11,30,58,63] This relatively wide range reflects the variety of research methods used to study protein requirements, as well as the heterogeneous nature of the population. Specific advisable intakes based on body weight are available.[58]

| Body weight (g) | Protein intake (g/kg/day) | |
	Low	High
700-1,000	2.6	3.9
1,000-1,500	3.1	4.1
1,500-2,000	3.0	3.9
2,000-2,500	3.0	3.7

Intakes of < 2.5 g/kg/day are associated with poor outcomes.[56,64-66] Excessive intakes (> 6g/kg/day) are poorly tolerated[64,67] (Table 15.5).

Carbohydrate

Specific requirements for carbohydrate are not well defined.[5,210] Emphasis is on providing energy from both carbohydrate and fat. Carbohydrate may be more effective than fat in sparing protein.[69,70,211] Based on parenteral nutrition studies and on the energy breakdown in human milk, a diet providing approximately 40-50% of the calories as carbohydrate is usually recommended.[30,71] As little as 35% of energy as carbohydrate may be acceptable, especially in infants with chronic lung disease.[7,10]

For the preterm infant, the type of carbohydrate is also important. Glucose alone delivers an excessive osmotic load. Glucose polymers are well tolerated and minimize the osmotic load.[6] Low intestinal lactase levels may limit the amount of lactose preterm infants can tolerate.[72] Early trophic feedings may enhance enzyme activity.[73] Studies suggest that these infants have bacteria in the colon that are able to salvage the malabsorbed carbohydrate and convert it to usable short-chain fatty acids.[74] The galactose liberated from lactose digestion appears to have a special role in maintaining blood glucose between feedings, for the reason that it more directly and effectively produces glycogen.[75-77] Lactose also appears to enhance the absorption of calcium and other minerals, although this is controversial.[78,79] These issues related to carbohydrate intake remain under study.

Fat

Recommendations for fat intake are based on human milk composition, energy needs, and requirements for the essential fatty acids linoleic acid (LA) and linolenic acid (LNA). Overall, fat provides about half of total energy, and 5-7 g/kg/day.[30] Both LA, an ω-6 fatty acid, and LNA, an ω-3 fatty acid, are precursors to long-chain polyunsaturated fatty acids (LC-PUFAs). Through desaturation and elongation, LA and LNA become arachidonic acid (AA) and docosahexanoic (DHA), respectively. These LC-PUFAs produce eicosanoids. Eicosanoids include prostaglandins, prostacyclins, thromboxanes and leukotrienes. They are metabolically active in a variety of biological functions, such as regulation of blood pressure and modulation of platelet function and immunological status.[80,212] The metabolic pathways of the series-3 and the series-6 fatty acids are competitive.[81]

Attention in the perinatal literature has focused on DHA and AA because of their presence in human milk and because they are found in concentrated amounts in neural and retinal tissue.[82-85] Multiple clinical trials of both term and preterm infants fed human milk, com-

Table 15.5. Consequences for Preterm Infants of Deviations in Protein Intake

Excessive intake[64,67,68]	Inadequate intake[56,64]
Abnormal metabolic measures	
Aminoacidemia	Decreased nitrogen retention
Metabolic acidosis	Low serum albumin and transthyretin
Elevated BUN	
Hyperammonemia	
Poor clinical responses	
Lethargy	Slow growth
Diarrhea	
Increased mortality	
Edema	
Strabismus	
Poor developmental outcome	
Lower I.Q. scores	Lower scores on the Bayley Psychomotor Developmental Index and Neonatal Behavior Assessment Scale

mercially available infant formulas, and infant formulas supplemented with various sources of LC-PUFAs have been conducted. Results of these ongoing studies related to neurocognition, visual acuity, and growth are inconclusive and controversial.[86-112]

Neither the American Academy of Pediatrics (AAP) nor the Canadian Pediatric Society have specific recommendations for LC-PUFAs. An analysis of current data do not support specific recommendations at this time.[213,214] European recommendations are more detailed.[113] At present, commercial infant formulas in the United States and Canada do not contain derivatives of LA or LNA. Fatty acid recommendations from several sources are summarized in Table 15.6.[5,7,30,80,113] While human milk is assumed to be the best model on which to base the fat composition of the infant diet, further studies are needed to identify the optimal balance in artificial feedings.[112,114]

A dietary supply of the antioxidant alpha-tocopheral is required to prevent auto-oxidation of unsaturated lipids in food and tissues.[113] The vitamin E requirement increases with the amount of supplemental iron and the concentration of PUFAs in the diet.[30] Prematurity is presumed to be an additional risk for deficiency due to poor vitamin stores and impaired digestion of fat. Infants require approximately 0.6-0.7 IU (mg)/ 100 kcal.[30,115] A ratio of $\geq$ 0.9 mg vitamin E/g PUFA[115] or 1 mg vitamin E/g linoleic acid[30] is recommended.

Table 15.6. Fatty Acid Recommendations for Preterm Infants[5,7,30,80,113]

Fat	40-55% of total energy[5,7,113]
	4.5-6.0 g/100 kcal[30]
	5-7 g/kg/d[30]
Linoleic* plus Linolenic* acids	3%[30] to 4-12%[80] of total energy
	0.6-1.5 g/kg/day[80]
ω-6 Fatty Acids	
Linoleic acid	0.5-0.7 g/kg/day[80]
	4-5% of total energy[5,7,113]
	12% of total energy (maximum)[80]
Arachidonic acid*	40-60 mg/kg/d[80]
Total ω-6 (C20 and C22)	1% of total energy[113]
ω-3 Fatty Acids	
Linolenic Acid	0.5-1.0 % of total energy[5,7,113]
Docosahexaenoic Acid*	35-75 mg/kg/day[80]
Total ω-3 (C20 and C22)	0.25-0.50% of total energy[5,113]
	70-150 mg/kg/day[80]
Ratios	
ω-6 to ω-3	5:1 to 15:1[5,80,113]
DHA to AA*	1:1 to 1:2[5,80]

* Linoleic acid (C18:2ω-6); linolenic acid (C18:3ω-3); arachidonic (AA) acid (C20:4ω-6); docosahexaenoic (DHA) acid (C22:6ω-3).

The amount of fat required is influenced by the type of fat consumed. It is usually reported that medium-chain triglycerides (MCT) are more efficiently absorbed and utilized than long-chain triglycerides by the preterm infant.[116-120] Presumably this is because MCTs are not dependent on duodenal intraluminal bile salt levels, which are low in the premature infant.[6] MCTs are also absorbed in the stomach of the newborn.[120] This superior performance of MCTs appears to be particularly true in preterm infants of < 34 weeks postconceptual age[120] and may have beneficial effects on mineral absorption.[121,122] The concentration of MCTs in human milk is between 10% (full-term) and 15% (preterm).[123] ESPGAN has recommended that formulas for preterm infants contain no more than 40% of total energy as MCT.[113]

Calcium, Phosphorus, Magnesium, and Vitamin D

Calcium (Ca), phosphorus (P), and magnesium (Mg) are primary components of skeletal tissue making up 99%, 80-85%, and 60-65%, respectively, of bone mass.[124] They are also important constituents of extracellular fluid, intracellular structures, cell membranes, muscles and soft tissues.[124] Vitamin D's principle physiologic function is to maintain serum calcium and phosphorus in a range that supports cellular processes, neuromuscular function, and bone ossification.[125] This is accomplished by enhancing absorption of calcium and phosphorus in the small intestine and mobilizing stores from bone.[125] The goal of nutritional management for VLBW infants is to achieve intrauterine mineral accretion and minimize the risk of osteopenia and fractures.[126,127]

Preterm infants require higher intakes of Ca, P and Mg per unit of body weight than do term infants. Recommendations are usually based on the expected gains in body minerals had the infant remained in utero until term.[128,129] The intrauterine accretion rates of Ca, P and Mg have been measured by a variety of techniques including carcass chemical analysis, factorial calculation, and direct measurement of bone mass using dual energy x-ray absorptiometry.[215] More than 75% of intrauterine bone mineralization occurs in the third trimester[130] and between 25-36 weeks gestation averages for Ca 118mg/kg/d,[129,131-134] for P 70 mg/kg/d,[129,131,132] and for Mg 3.1 mg/kg/d.[129,131,132] Retention of minerals fed to infants varies considerably, but averages 56-64% for Ca, 69-71% for P, and 41-59% for Mg.[127,131] Retention is primarily determined by intestinal absorption. Absorption may be facilitated by:

- Increasing the mineral content of the enteral feeding[127]
- Supplementing with vitamin D (enhances Ca absorption only)[135]
- Providing carbohydrate as lactose, although this is controversial[78,79]
- Providing fat as medium-chain triglycerides[131]
- Maintaining a calcium-to-phosphorus ratio of 1.8-2:1[127]

Chronic diuretic therapy, especially furosemide, and treatment with theophylline and caffeine can increase urinary calcium loss.[127,136-139] Steroid therapy for prevention and treatment of chronic lung disease theoretically impairs mineral retention.[140]

Published recommendations for Ca, P, and Mg intake in preterm infants are available.[5-8] Recommended intake ranges for Ca are 120-230 mg/kg/day; P, 60-140 mg/kg/day; and Mg, 7.9-15.0 mg/kg/day.[5] Special attention should be given to the balance of minerals and energy when the caloric density of formulas is manipulated. Suggested ratios (in mg/100 kcal) are Ca, 100-192; P, 50-117; Mg, 6.6-12.5.[5]

Preterm infants appear to have the ability to absorb vitamin D, perform 25-hydroxylation in the liver, and produce active 1,25 hydroxyvitamin D in the kidney.[131] Although intakes of vitamin D as low as 160 IU/day appear to maintain normal vitamin D status, bone mineralization, and growth if the diet is high in Ca and P,[141] most recommendations for LBW infants are 400-800 IU/day.[5,7,30,216]

Iron

Iron requirements of preterm infants during the first year of life are determined by birth weight, initial hemoglobin concentration, rate of growth, and magnitude of iron losses during this period.[142] Preterm infants start out with a lower absolute amount of storage iron than term infants, because neonatal iron stores are roughly proportional to body weight.[30,143] A pregnant woman must be extremely iron deficient to significantly affect fetal iron stores; however, maternal hypertension or diabetes can result in reduced placental transfer of iron.[143] SGA infants have lower iron stores than their AGA counterparts.[10] The bulk of fetal iron, about 75%, is present as hemoglobin: 1 g hemoglobin contains 3.4 mg of iron.[144] If no supplemental iron is given, the weight at which iron depletion will occur can be approximated using the following formula:[142]

percent of birth weight at which iron depletion will be present = cord blood hemoglobin (g/dl) x 11.5

For example, a 1 kg infant with a cord blood hemoglobin concentration of 17 g/dl will become iron depleted at a weight of 1,955 g:

percent of birth weight = 17 x 11.5 = 195.5% of birthweight

As illustrated by the above example, doubling of birth weight is the approximate time of iron depletion. The initial hemoglobin concentration directly affects this sequence.

Postnatal iron needs are greater in the preterm than the full-term infant.[1,30] Frequent blood sampling is also a factor in determining iron requirements. About 1 mg iron is lost with each 1-2 ml of blood.[145,146] Removal of 4 ml of red blood cells, without replacement, accelerates by about 100 g the weight at which iron depletion will occur.[146] Infections may also increase iron requirements.[144]

Postnatal iron metabolism is divided into three stages for the preterm infant: [142,144]

- Decreased erythropoiesis. This stage begins after birth. The hemoglobin falls, with lower nadirs associated with lower birth weights. This so-called "physiologic anemia of prematurity" cannot be prevented by administration of iron.

- Renewed erythropoiesis. This stage begins at 1-3 months of age. The hemoglobin rises as active red cell production resumes. Iron supplementation is required at this time.
- Exhausted iron stores. This stage is observed if iron supplementation is inadequate or absent. Anemia, with a fall in hemoglobin concentration, follows. This is the so-called "late anemia of prematurity."

These stages occur for full-term infants, but iron supplementation is not required until four to six months because of their greater reserves at birth.

Preterm infants are at risk for developing hemolytic anemia. This can occur if the supply of the antioxidant vitamin E is deficient; if an adequate quantity of suitable substrate, such as polyunsaturated fatty acids (PUFA), is present; and if excessive iron (a powerful oxidant) is provided.[147,148] Vitamin E-deficient preterm infants given 8 mg/kg ferrous sulfate per day develop hemolytic anemia.[147] It is characterized by red cell morphological alterations, thrombocytosis, edema, and a plasma tocopherol level of < 0.5 mg/dl.[146] Contemporary formulas now have a suitable E/PUFA ratio for preterm infants. This ratio is expressed as IUS of vitamin E per gram of linoleic acid. If vitamin E intake is within recommended levels, the E/linoleic acid ratio is 1, and iron supplementation is appropriate and delayed until after 2-3 weeks of age, the risk of hemolytic anemia virtually disappears.6,149,150

The recommended intake of iron for preterm infants is 2-4 mg/kg/day by 2 months of age or when the birth weight has doubled, whichever comes first.[5,7,8,30] It can be safely started at 2-3 weeks.[30] The maximum intake recommended is 15 mg/day.[30] If the initial hemoglobin is < 17 mg/dl, or if substantial blood loss has occurred without replacement, an iron supplement of 1-2 mg/kg/day can be considered earlier than 2 months.[142,144] The use of recombinant erythropoietin to prevent or treat anemia of prematurity increases the need for supplemental iron.[30]

Specific daily iron doses are suggested based on both gestational age and birthweight, and on treatment with recombinant erythropoietin as follows:[1,7,30,143,217,218]

Newborn category:	Daily iron dose (mg/kg)
Term, AGA	1
Term, SGA	3
Preterm, AGA, LBW	2
Preterm, AGA, VLBW	3
Preterm, AGA, ELBW	4
Erythropoietin Therapy	6

Premature infants may absorb iron more efficiently than full-term infants.[142,143] Nearly 50% of the iron in human milk is absorbed.[143] The time to give exogenous iron to infants fed human milk is unclear. In general, no distinction is made between human-milk-fed and formula-fed preterm infants regarding the time or dose of supplemental iron. Iron-fortified formula provides about 2 mg/kg/day when fed at 120 kcal/kg/day. If additional iron is required, or when human milk is fed, ferrous sulfate drops may be given (see Appendix L). Iron drops are better absorbed when given before or between feedings than with feedings.[145] There may be a small but significant improvement in iron absorption when iron is given as a supplement as opposed to iron-fortified formula.[151] Intestinal intolerance is rarely a problem with iron in either form.[145]

Sodium, Potassium, and Chloride

Preterm infants need more sodium (Na) per unit of body weight than full-term infants. This is due to immature renal Na conservation mechanisms that result in increased urinary Na losses.[152] An inverse correlation exists between urinary Na excretion and gestational age, so that the most immature infants are at the greatest risk for renal Na wasting. This physiological imbalance in the renal system usually improves after about 3 weeks postnatal age.[153,154] Monitoring of serum Na is imperative. Intake is adjusted to avoid both hypo- and hypernatremia, although the amount of Na excreted may not always be directly related to the Na intake.[152] Preterm infants need more Na during the first few weeks of life than older preterm infants.[153] During this time, infants < 32 weeks' gestation may require 5-6 mEq/kg/day Na; more mature preterm infants may require about 3-5 mEq/kg/d.[153] Na requirements vary, especially in relation to water intake.[5]

Human milk provides inadequate Na for the rapidly growing VLBW infant.[6,8] Infants fed human milk, and others whose serum Na drops below 130-132 mEq/L, need Na supplementation. This is usually provided as sodium chloride in a dose of 2-3 mEq/kg/day.[8,152] Late hyponatremia (after 3 weeks of age) is more likely to be due to inappropriate antidiuretic hormone secretion than to negative Na balance.[152] Urine osmolality is determined to evaluate this possibility.

Infants require more potassium per unit of body weight than adults to support their increasing lean body mass.[1] Although specific recommendations exist for preterm infants,[5,6] they are not greatly different from those for full-term infants.[1] Chloride needs parallel those for sodium.[5,6]

In summary, stable and growing preterm infants require approximately 2-3 mEq/kg/d of Na.[5,30,153] Equal amounts of both potassium and chloride are also needed.[5,30,153] Commercial infant formulas designed for preterm infants and fortified human milk provide close to these levels when fed in amounts to meet energy needs.

Trace Elements

Nine trace elements are currently considered to be of practical importance in human nutrition.[1] These are iron, zinc, copper, iodine, selenium, chromium, molybdenum, manganese, and fluoride. (Iron is discussed earlier in this chapter.) Accretion of all trace elements occurs during the third trimester of pregnancy placing the preterm infant at risk for deficiency.[155,206] Limited data exist to support intake recommendations for preterm infants for iodine, selenium, chromium, molybdenum, and manganese.[155-157,206,217] (Fluoride is discussed later in this chapter under supplementation.) Overt clinical deficiency of both zinc and copper has been described in enterally-fed premature infants.[158,159] Somewhat more data exist to support intake recommendations for these two trace elements.

The classical sign of zinc deficiency is an erythematous skin rash involving the perioral, perineal, and facial areas and the extremities.[144,159] Although there are significant limitations to the assay, a plasma zinc of < 50 µg/dl is highly suggestive of zinc deficiency.[144] In addition, alkaline phosphatase activity is usually below normal.[155] Zinc's central role in immunity and in growth and development is becoming increasingly apparent.[160] Many factors influence the zinc requirement of enterally fed premature infants. They include:

- Intrauterine accretion. Fetal accretion of zinc is about 850 µg/kg/day during the third trimester.[155]
- Growth. Growth is the major determinant of the zinc requirement.[144]
- Absorption. Net absorption of zinc is about 20-25% from formula; about 60% from preterm human milk; and about 36% from fortified preterm human milk.[144,159,161] Despite the superior absorption from human milk, the absolute amount of zinc in human milk may be inadequate for the rapidly growing preterm infant.[30,156,162] Bioavailability of zinc varies in casein-predominant and soy formulas.[163,219,220]
- Losses. The major excretion route is gastrointestinal.[155,156] Total urinary, fecal, and dermal losses are estimated at 115-125 µg/kg/day.[144]
- Drug/nutrient interactions. High dietary intakes of zinc, such as those prescribed for zinc deficiency, have a significant negative interaction on copper absorption and utilization.[144,155,164] Dexamethasone may impair zinc absorption.[165]

Rapidly growing preterm infants are at risk for zinc deficiency. Conditions that increase zinc losses, especially large stool or ostomy output, may magnify this risk. Boys are at greater risk than girls.[217] Intake of zinc is generally sufficient in the stable preterm infant if premature formula or fortified human milk is fed.[30,156,166] Recommendations range from 600 µg/kg/d[30] to 700-1500 µg/kg/d.[8,166,217]

The premature infant is at risk for copper deficiency because of limited hepatic copper stores.[144,167] Rapid growth in VLBW infants increases the risk.[168,217] Symptoms of copper deficiency include osteoporosis, neutropenia, and a hypochromic anemia that is unresponsive to iron therapy.[144,155,156] Diagnosis is usually confirmed with plasma copper concentration, although erythrocyte copper, zinc-superoxide dismutase may be a more appropriate indicator of copper status in VLBW infants.[144,168] Factors that affect the copper requirement of the enterally-fed premature infant include:

- Intrauterine accretion. 75% of newborn stores are accreted in the third trimester and average about 50-60 µg/kg/day during this time period. Two-thirds of all copper accreted during gestation is stored in the liver.[144,156]
- Absorption. Net absorption of copper from the diet is about 10-30% and varies by source similarly to zinc.[144,159,161,163]
- Losses. The major excretion route of copper is bile.[144]
- Drug/nutrient interactions. High levels of either dietary zinc or iron decrease copper absorption.[144,155,164,167] Dexamethasone may impair copper aborption.[165]

Intake of copper is generally sufficient in the preterm infant if premature formula or fortified human milk is fed.[30,155,156] Recommendations range from 108-156 µg/kg/d.[8,30,217]

Water-Soluble Vitamins

Nine water-soluble vitamins are considered essential in human nutrition: vitamin C, thiamine (B_1), riboflavin (B_2), niacin, pyridoxine (B_6), B_{12}, folic acid, pantothenic acid, and biotin.[1] Although water-soluble vitamins are not stored in the body, they may accumulate in the fetus because of favorable transplacental mechanisms.[169] Little information is available on specific requirements for preterm infants.[30,170,221] Fortified human milk and commercial infant formulas fed to meet energy needs of preterm infants approximate their estimated vitamin requirements.[221] The preterm infant is at risk of deficiency because intake and absorption may be limited, requirements are high, and, with the exception of vitamin B_{12}, water-soluble vitamins are not conserved to any appreciable extent following birth.[169-171] Continued intake at frequent intervals is required to avoid deficiency; dietary excesses are thought to be largely excreted in urine (vitamin C, thiamin, riboflavin, niacin, pyridoxine, folic acid, pantothenic acid and biotin) and bile (B_{12}).[170,171] Renal regulatory capacity may be limited in preterm infants, so that excessive intakes may result in supraphysiologic serum levels of some water-soluble vitamins (ex., riboflavin and pyridoxine).[170-173]

Factors related to specific water-soluble vitamin requirements are listed in Table 15.7. These can be used in conjunction with the estimated requirements for preterm infants given in Table 15.1 and Appendix G. Thorough reviews of the biochemistry, metabolism, assessment of vitamin status, deficiency, and toxicity of these vitamins are available.[169,171,221] The effects of specific drugs on vitamin status are reviewed in Appendix E.

Vitamins A, E, and K

Vitamin A's biological roles include preservation of vision, growth and differentiation of epithelial tissues, and support of the immune response.[170,176] Preterm infants have virtually no hepatic reserves of vitamin A at birth.[30,170] Placental transfer of retinol-binding protein, the chief carrier protein for circulating retinol, is relatively poor until the third trimester of pregnancy.[171] Vitamin A requires pancreatic enzymes and bile acids for absorption; consequently, pancreatic insufficiency and cholestatic conditions impede its availability.[171] Because vitamin A is stored when intake exceeds needs, toxicity is a concern. Olson has suggested 750-1,000 IU/100 kcal as a maximum safe dose.[177] Oral intakes of > 4,300 IU/kg/day of vitamin A over several weeks increases the risk of toxicity in preterm infants.[170] Vitamin A requirements are reported as either µg retinol or IU vitamin A (1 µg retinol = 3.33 IU vitamin A).[170] Current recommendations for stable, growing preterm infants range from 700-1,500 IU/kg/day.[5,7,221] The smallest infants may benefit from the highest doses.[7] Intakes of < 400 IU/kg/day in VLBW infants results in laboratory evidence of vitamin A deficiency.[178] Several studies suggest that oral intakes from 1,500-4,000 IU/day[179-182] or periodic intramuscular injections averaging approximately 2,000 IU/day[183,222,223] improve vitamin A status, and/or prevent or minimize chronic lung disease. The evidence regarding lung disease is very conflicting.[221,224] These generous amounts of vitamin A are not used in most clinical situations.[7,30,170]

Vitamin E's most important biological function is as an antioxidant. All infants are born with low body stores of vitamin E; plasma and tissue levels rise after birth with feeding.[184,185] This rise occurs more slowly after preterm birth because of less efficient tocopherol absorption.[186-188] Both bile acids and pancreatic enzymes are required for absorption. Poor stores, relative malabsorption, potentially inad-

Table 15.7.   Factors Related to Water-Soluble Vitamin Requirements in Preterm Infants

Vitamin C	Protein intakes of > 4 g/kg/d or consumption of casein-predominant formula may increase requirement[8,30,170,221]
	Hyperoxic environments may increase the need for vitamin C as a functional antioxidant[169,170,221]
	Storage adversely affects concentration in human milk[1,30,221]
	Supplementation may be necessary to meet requirement[8,169,170]
Thiamin	Requirement is related to the carbohydrate content of the diet[169,170]
	No evidence preterm infants fed human milk need supplementation[80,30,169]
	Intake from formulas designed for preterm infants appears to be adequate[173]
Riboflavin	Phototherapy may increase requirement[30,170,174,221]
	Exposure to light destroys riboflavin in milk[169,170]
	Requirement appears to be related more to tissue growth and nitrogen balance than to caloric intake[169]
	Intake from human milk may not be adequate for preterm infants[8,169,170]
	Formulas designed for preterm infants may have excessive amounts[172,173]
Niacin	Requirement is directly related to energy expenditure[169]
	Although there are no specific studies, intake from fortified human milk and preterm infant formula appears to be adequate for preterm infants[8,30,170]
Pyridoxine	Requirement is directly related to protein intake[169,170]
	Destruction by light of the vitamin present in human milk may reduce its availability[169]
	LBW infants fed human milk may need supplement in order to achieve an intake of at least 15 µg/g protein and/or 35µg/100 kcal[8,175]
	Formulas designed for preterm infants may have excessive amounts[30,172]
Folic acid	Requirement is substantially higher for preterm and LBW infants than for full-term, appropriately grown infants[1,5,30,221]
	High folic acid intake may mask vitamin B_{12} deficiency, resulting in irreversible neurological damage[142]
	Nutritional value of folate is higher in human milk than in formula based on cow's milk, but the total concentration in human milk may not be adequate for preterm infants[8,142,170]
Vitamin B_{12}	Intake from fortified human milk and formulas designed for preterm infants appears to be adequate for preterm infants[8,30,170,173]
	Stores are lower in preterm than in term infants[221]
Biotin and pantothenic acid	Endogenous synthesis from intestinal microorganisms is present but not well understood[170,171]
	Although there are no specific studies, intake from fortified human milk and preterm infant formula appears to be adequate for preterm infants[8,30,170,221]

equate intake, greatly increased requirements for rapid growth, and oxidative stresses of the neonatal intensive care environment all place the VLBW infant at increased risk of developing deficiency when compared with the adult.[170,171] Significant nutrient interactions occur among vitamin E, fat, and iron (see previous sections on fat and iron). Vitamin E toxicity can occur at plasma concentrations close to those considered therapeutic.[189] Aggressive vitamin E supplementation in preterm infants is associated with increased risk of necrotizing enterocolitis and infection, especially in infants whose serum vitamin E levels exceed 3.5 mg/dl.[190,191]

Recommendations for vitamin E intake for preterm infants vary. Consensus recommendations suggest 6-12 IU/kg/day with a maximum of 25 IU/kg/day for formula-fed preterm infants.[5] A supplement of 3.5 IU/kg/day is recommended for preterm infants fed human milk by some,[5] but not others.[8,186,192] Pharmacologic doses of tocopherol have been recommended in the past to prevent or minimize oxygen toxicity and associated conditions such as bronchopulmonary dysplasia, retinopathy of prematurity, and intraventricular hemorrhage.[221] Evidence is conflicting and needs further study.[225-227] At present, pharmacologic doses of vitamin E are not given in most clinical situations.[221] Additional recommendations for vitamin E suggest a diet that provides 0.7 IU/100 kcal and 1.0 IU/g linoleic acid,[7,30,193] and maintains plasma vitamin E concentrations of 10-30mg/L.[7]

Vitamin K is essential for normal blood clotting.[170] Transport of vitamin K across the placenta appears to be poor, based on the increased incidence of hemorrhagic disease in preterm infants due to vitamin K deficiency.[171] Maternal anticonvulsant therapy during pregnancy may precipitate bleeding in the newborn due to poorly understood mechanisms.[194] Vitamin K produced by colonic bacteria may be an important source in infancy.[171] Antibiotic treatment, bowel resection, or other therapies that disrupt normal gut flora may interfere with vitamin K production and result in symptomatic deficiency.[195,196]

The AAP Committee on Nutrition recommends that all newborn infants receive either an intramuscular injection of 0.5 to 1.0 mg of vitamin K or an oral dose of 1.0 to 2.0 mg of vitamin K on the day of delivery for routine prophylaxis of hemorrhagic disease of the newborn.[197] Specifically, the AAP recommends that preterm infants > 1 kg receive a one-time IM dose of 1 mg, and those infants < 1 kg receive a one-time IM dose of 0.3 mg/kg.[30] Deficiency of vitamin K can occur more rapidly than other fat-soluble vitamins because of vitamin K's relatively short half-life.[171] Absorption of dietary vitamin K from the small intestine requires both bile acids and pancreatic enzymes.[170,171] Despite one initial report, no relationship between IM vitamin K and childhood cancer has been substantiated.[194,198] There are no data to support claims that vitamin K deficiency is a cause of intraventricular hemorrhage in the preterm infant.[194,221] Maintenance dietary recommendations for preterm infants are 7-9 µg/kg/day[30] to

Table 15.8   Vitamin and Mineral Supplementation Guidelines for Hospitalized Newborns*

Nutrition	Suggested Supplement
Full-term, formula-fed	Provide iron fortified formula no later than 4 mo
Full-term, breast-fed	Consider vitamin D supplement of 400 IU/d Provide another dietary source of iron no later than 6 mo
Preterm, formula-fed	Consider supplement of vitamins A, D, and/or E (preterm infant formula) Consider multivitamin supplement (formula not designed for preterm infant) Provide another dietary source of iron no later than 2 mo
Preterm, human milk–fed	Fortify human milk provided to VLBW infants (see Chapter 16) Consider supplement of vitamins A, D and/or E (fortified human milk) Consider multivitamin supplement (unfortified human milk) Provide another dietary source of iron no later than 2 mo

*   See Appendix L for composition of selected supplements

8-10 µg/kg/day.[5] Human milk has low vitamin K content and preterm infants given human milk are at increased risk for deficiency.[30,170,194] Commercial human milk fortifiers bring the vitamin K intake to within the recommended range.[30,195] Alternately, a daily supplement of 2-3 µg/kg can be given to the preterm infant fed unfortified human milk.[8]

Carnitine

Carnitine is essential for the metabolism of long-chain fatty acids. Newborn infants, especially premature babies, are born with limited tissue reserves of carnitine.[199] Biosynthesis of carnitine is not fully developed in the newborn, and lack of dietary carnitine results in significantly lower plasma carnitine concentrations.[200] Human milk is a rich source of carnitine, containing about 10 µmol (1.6 mg)/dl at 2 weeks and about 6 µmol (1.0 mg)/dl at 4 months.[201] Similar amounts are present in commercial formulas either inherent in the cow's milk base for standard formulas[113] or fortified in soy, protein hydrolysate, and preterm formulas. Tentative recommendations are set at ≥ 7.5 µmol/100 kcal,[113] or 2.9 mg/kg/day.[5] These amounts are approximated by human milk or most commercial infant formulas in the United States. If deficiency is confirmed, the usual oral dose of supplemental carnitine is 100 mg/kg/day given in two to three divided doses.[202] The manufacturers of Carnitor (Levocarnitine) Oral Solution (Sigma-Tau Pharmaceuticals, Gaithersburg, MD) recommend an initial dose of 50 mg/kg/day followed by monitoring of the therapeutic response. Oral carnitine supplements are suspended in hyperosmolar syrup and may cause G.I. upset.

Supplementation

General guidelines for vitamin and mineral supplementation are reviewed in Table 15.8. Some preterm newborns may require supplementation if the daily volume consumed is inadequate to meet daily micronutrient requirements. This is more likely to occur when unfortified human milk or a formula not designed for preterm infants is fed. A useful exercise for NICU nutrition staff is to calculate the volume at which all recommended vitamin and mineral levels are satisfied using the typical products fed in the intensive care unit.[12] A supplement may be indicated for the infant whose intake falls below this number. Micronutrients of particular concern are the fat-soluble vitamins A, D and E; the water-soluble vitamins C, B_6 and folic acid; the minerals calcium, phosphorus, and iron; the trace element zinc; and sodium. Fluoride supplementation is no longer recommended for infants 0-6 months.[203] There are no specific fluoride recommendations for preterm newborns.

Low birth weight, preterm delivery, and medical complications increase the nutritional risk of newborns. Consideration of dietary intake adequacy is a vital part of the nutrition assessment. Appropriate reference values, such as those reviewed in this chapter, provide the context for evaluating the diets of high-risk newborns. Individualized nutrition care plans based on these values, as well as anthropometric, biochemical, and clinical data can improve outcome in these special patients.

References

1. National Research Council, Food and Nutrition Board. Recommended Dietary Allowances. 10th ed. Washington, D.C.: National Academy of Sciences, 1989.
2. Yates AA, Schlicker SA, Suitor CW. Dietary Reference Intakes: The new basis for recommendations for calcium and related nutrients, B vitamins and choline. JADA 98:699, 1998.

3. Institute of Medicine, Food and Nutrition Board. Dietary reference intakes for calcium, phosphorus, magnesium, vitamin D and fluoride. Washington, D.C.: National Academy Press, 1997.

4. Institute of Medicine, Food and Nutrition Board. Dietary reference intakes for thiamin, riboflavin, niacin, vitamin B-6, folate, vitamin B-12, pantothenic acid, biotin, and choline. Washington, D.C.: National Academy Press, 1998.

5. Tsang RC, Uauy R, Lucas A, Zlotkin S, eds. Nutritional needs of the preterm infant: Scientific basis and practical guidelines. Baltimore: Williams and Wilkins, 1993; 288-95.

6. American Academy of Pediatrics Committee on Nutrition. Nutritional needs of low-birth-weight infants. Pediatrics 75:976, 1985.

7. Nutrition Committee, Canadian Paediatric Society. Nutrient needs and feeding of premature infants. Can Med Assoc J 152(11):1765, 1995

8. ESPGAN Committee on Nutrition of Preterm Infants. Nutrition and feeding of pre-term infants. Acta Paediatr Scand (suppl) 336:1, 1987.

9. Kerner JA. Parenteral nutrition. In: Walker WA, ed. Pediatric gastrointestinal disease, vol. 2. Philadelphia: Decker, 1991; 228-58.

10. Wahlig TM and Georgieff MK. The effects of illness on neonatal metabolism and nutritional management. Clin Perinatol 22(1):77, 1995.

11. Hay WW. Nutritional requirements of extremely low birthweight infants. Acta Paediatr (suppl) 402:94, 1994.

12. Pereira GR. Nutritional care of the extremely premature infant. Clin Perinatol 22(1):61, 1995.

13. American Academy of Pediatrics Committee on Nutrition. Commentary on breast-feeding and infant formulas, including proposed standards for formulas. Pediatrics 57:278, 1976.

14. Food and Drug Administration Rules and Regulations: Nutrient requirements for infant formulas. Fed Register 50:45106, 1985.

15. Fomon SJ, Ziegler EE, eds. Upper limits of nutrients in infant formulas. J Nutr 119(12S):1763-1873, 1989.

16. LSRO Assessment of nutrient requirements for infant formulas. J Nutr 128:2059S, 1998.

17. Milla PJ. Influence of nutrition on psychomotor development. JPGN 25:S9, 1997.

18. Lucas A. Programming by early nutrition in man. In: Bock GE, Whelan J, eds. The childhood environment and adult disease. Chicester: Wiley, 1991; 38-55.

19. Lozoff B, Jimeney E, Wolf AB. Long term developmental outcome of infants with iron deficiency. N Engl J Med 325:687, 1991.

20. Carlson SE, Werkman SH, Rhodes PG, Tolley EA. Visual acuity development in healthy preterm infants: effects of marine oil supplementation. Am J Clin Nutr 58:35, 1993.

21. Lucas A, Morley R, Cole TJ, et al. Breastmilk and subsequent intelligence quotient in children born preterm. Lancet 339:261, 1992.

22. Lucas A. Role of nutrition programming in determining adult morbidity. Arch Dis Child 71:288, 1994.

23. Barker DJP, Gluckman PD, Godfrey KM, et al. Fetal nutrition and cardiovascular disease in adult life. Lancet 341:938, 1993.

24. Micheli J-L, Pfister R, Junod S, et al. Water, energy and early postnatal growth in preterm infants. Acta Paediatr (suppl) 405:35, 1994.

25. Hay WW. Nutritional needs of the extremely low-birthweight infant. Semin Perinatol 15:482, 1991.

26. Liechty EA. Water requirements. In: Polin RA, Fox WW, eds. Fetal and neonatal physiology. 2d ed. Philadelphia: Saunders, 1998; 305-07.
27. Holliday MA. Requirements for sodium chloride and potassium and their interrelation with water requirement. In: Tsang RC, Nichols BL, eds. Nutrition during infancy. Philadephia: Hanley and Belfus, 1988; 160-174.
28. Committee on Nutrition of the Preterm Infant, European Society of Paediatric Gastroenterology and Nutrition. Nutrition and feeding of preterm infants. Oxford, England: Blackwell Scientific Publications, 1987.
29. Denne SC. Energy requirements. In: Polin RA, Fox WW, eds. Fetal and neonatal physiology. 2d ed. Philadelphia: Saunders, 1998; 307-14.
30. American Academy of Pediatrics Committee on Nutrition. Nutritional needs of preterm infants. Pediatric nutrition handbook. 4th ed. Elk Grove Village, Ill.: AAP, 1998; 55-87.
31. Towers HM, Schulze KF, Ramakrishnan R, Kashyap S. Energy expended by low birth weight infants in the deposition of protein and fat. Pediatr Res 41:584, 1997.
32. Brooke OG. Energy balance and metabolic rate in preterm infants fed with standard and high energy formulas. Br J Nutr 44:13, 1980.
33. Reichman B, Chessex P, Putet G, et al. Diet, fat accretion, and growth in preterm infants. N Engl J Med 305:1495, 1981.
34. Reichman B, Chessex P, Verellen G, et al. Dietary composition and macronutrient storage in preterm infants. Pediatrics 72:322, 1983.
35. Whyte RK, Haslam R, Vlainic C, et al. Energy balance and nitrogen balance in growing low birth weight infants fed human milk or formula. Pediatr Res 17:891, 1983.
36. Putet G, Senterre J, Rigo J, et al. Nutrient balance, energy utilization, and composition of weight gain in very-low-birth weight infants fed pooled human milk or a preterm formula. J Pediatr 105:79, 1984.
37. Chessex P, Reichman B, Verellen G, et al. Metabolic consequences of intrauterine growth retardation in very low birth weight infants. Pediatr Res 18:709, 1984.
38. Sauer PJJ, Dane HJ, Visser HKA. Longitudinal studies on metabolic rate, heat loss and energy cost of growth in low birth weight infants. Pediatr Res 18:254, 1984.
39. Whyte RK, Campbell D, Stanhope R, et al. Energy balance in low birth-weight infants fed formula of high or low medium-chain triglyceride content. J Pediatr 108:964, 1986.
40. Freymond D, Schutz Y, Decombaz J, et al. Energy balance, physical activity, and thermogenic effect of feeding in pre-term infants. Pediatr Res 20:638, 1986.
41. Roberts SB, Lucas A. Energetic efficiency and nutrient accretion in preterm infants fed extremes of dietary intake. Hum Nutr Clin Nutr 41C:105, 1987.
42. Putet G, Rigo J, Salle B, Senterre J. Supplementation of pooled milk with casein hydrolsate energy and nitrogen balance and weight gain composition in very low birth weight infants. Pediatr Res 21:458, 1987.
43. Catzeflis C, Schutz Y, Micheli, JL, et al. Whole body protein synthesis and energy expenditure in very low birth weight infants. Pediatr Res 19:679, 1985.

44. Reichman BL, Chessex P, Putet G, et al. Partition of energy metabolism and energy cost of growth in very low birth weight infants. Pediatrics 69:446, 1982.

45. Cauderay M, Schutz Y, Micheli J-L, et al. Energy-nitrogen balances and protein turnover in small and appropriate for gestational age low birthweight infants. Eur J Clin Nutr 42:125, 1988.

46. Roberts SB, Young VR. Energy costs of fat and protein deposition in the human infant. Am J Clin Nutr 48:951, 1988.

47. Wilson DC, McClure G. Energy requirements in sick preterm babies. Acta Paediatr Supp 405:60, 1994.

48. Picaud J-C, Putet G, Rigo J, et al. Metabolic and energy balance in small- and appropriate-for-gestational-age, very low-birth-weight infants. Acta Paediatr Supp 405:54, 1994.

49. Kashyap S, Forsyth M, Zucker C, et al. Effects of varying protein and energy intakes on growth and metabolic response in low birth weight infants. J Pediatr 108:955, 1986.

50. Raiha NCR, Heinonen K, Rassin DK, et al. Milk protein quality in low birth weight infants. I. Metabolic response and effects on growth. Pediatrics 57:659, 1976.

51. Duffy B, Pencharz P. The effects of surgery on the nitrogen metabolism of parenterally fed human neonates. Pediatr Res 20:32, 1986.

52. Boehm G, Handrick W, Spencker FB, et al. Effects of bacterial sepsis on protein metabolism in infants during the first week. Biomed Biochim Acta 45:813, 1986.

53. VanGoudolver JB, Wattemena JD, Cornielle VP, et al. Effect of dexamethasone on protein metabolism in infants with bronchopulmonary dysplasia. J Pediatr 124:112, 1994.

54. Bronstein MN. Energy requirements and protein energy balance in preterm and term infants. In: Hay WW, ed. Neonatal nutrition and metabolism. St. Louis: Mosby Year Book, 1991; 42-70.

55. Fomon SJ, Ziegler EE, Filer LJ, et al. Methionine fortification of a soy protein formula fed to infants. Am J Clin Nutr 32:2460, 1979.

56. Kashyap S, Schulze KF, Forsyth M, et al. Growth, nutrient retention and metabolic response of low-birthweight infants fed supplemented and unsupplemented preterm human milk. Am J Clin Nutr 52:254, 1990.

57. Heird WC, Kashyap S, Gomez MR. Protein intake and energy requirements of the infant. Semin Perinatol 15:438, 1991.

58. Denne SC. Protein requirements. In: Polin RA, Fox WW, eds. Fetal and neonatal physiology. 2d ed. Philadelphia: Saunders, 1998; 315-25.

59. Kashyap S. Schulze KF, Ramakrishnan F, et al. Evaluation of a mathematical model for predicting the relationship between protein and energy intakes of low-birth-weight infants and the rate and composition of weight gain. Pediatr Res 35:704, 1994.

60. Bell EF. Diet and body composition of preterm infants. Acta Paediatr Suppl 405:25, 1994.

61. Kashyap S, Schulze KF, Forsyth M, et al. Growth, nutrient retention and metabolic response in low birth weight infants fed varying intakes of protein and energy. J Pediatr 113:713, 1988.

62. Fairey AK, Butte NF, Mehta N, et al. Nutrient accretion in preterm infants fed formula with different protein:energy ratios. JPGN 25:37, 1997.

63. Ziegler EE. Protein requirements of preterm infants. In: Fomon SJ, Heird WC, eds. Energy and protein needs during infancy. New York: Academic Press, 1986; 69-85.

64. Rassin DKD. Nutritional requirements for the fetus and the neonate. In: Ogra PL, ed. Neonatal infections: Nutritional and immunologic interactions. New York: Grune and Stratton, 1984; 205-27.

65. Lucas A, Morley R, Cole TJ, et al. Early diet in preterm babies and developmental status at 18 months. Lancet 335:1477, 1990.

66. Bhatia J, Rassin DK, Cerreto MC, et al. Effect of protein/energy ratio on growth and behavior of premature infants: Preliminary findings. J Pediatr 119:103, 1991.

67. Goldman AHI, Liebman DB, Freudenthal R, et al. Effects of early dietary protein intake on low-birthweight infants: Evaluation at 3 years of age. J Pediatr 78:126, 1971.

68. Polberger SKT, Axelsson IE, Raiha NCR. Amino acid concentrations in plasma and urine in very low birth weight infants fed protein-unenriched or human milk protein-enriched human milk. Pediatrics 86:909, 1990.

69. Munro HN. General aspects of the regulation of protein metabolism by diet and by hormones. VI. Influence of dietary carbohydrate and fat on protein metabolism. In: Munro HN, ed. Mammalian protein metabolism. San Diego: Academic Press, 1964; 412-47.

70. Long JM, Wilmore DW, Mason AD, et al. Effect of carbohydrate and fat intake on nitrogen excretion during total intravenous feeding. Ann Surg 185:417, 1977.

71. Denne SC. Carbohydrate requirements. In: Polin RA, Fox WW, eds. Fetal and neonatal physiology. 2d ed. Philadelphia: Saunders, 1998; 325-27.

72. MacLean WC, Fink BB. Lactose malabsorption by premature infants: Magnitude and clinical significance. J Pediatr 97:383, 1980.

73. Shulman RJ, Schanler RJ, Lau C, et al. Early feeding, feeding tolerance, and lactase activity in preterm infants. J Pediatr 133:645, 1998.

74. Kien CL, Kepner J, Grotjohn KA, et al. Efficient assimilation of lactose carbon in premature infants. JPGN 15:253, 1992.

75. Sparks JW, Lynch A, Ginsmann WH. Regulation of rat liver glycogen synthesis and activities of glycogen cycle enzymes by glucose and galactose. Metabolism 25:47, 1976.

76. Spedale SB, Battaglia FC, Sparks JW. Hepatic carbohydrate utilization after milk feeding in the newborn lamb. Pediatr Res 27:117A, (abstr), 1990.

77. Kaempf JW, Li H-Q, Groothuis JR, et al. Galactose, glucose, and lactate concentrations in the portal venous and arterial circulations of newborn lambs after nursing. Pediatr Res 23:598, 1988.

78. Ziegler EE, Fomon SJ. Lactose enhances mineral absorption in infancy. J Pediatr Gastroenterol Nutr 2:288, 1983.

79. Wirth FH, Numerof B, Pleban P, et al. Effect of lactose on mineral absorption in preterm infants. J Pediatr 117:283, 1990.

80. Uauy-Dagach R, Mena P. Nutritional role of omega-3 fatty acids during the perinatal period. Clin Perinatol 22(1):157, 1995.

81. Uauy R, Hoffman DR. Essential fatty acid requirements for normal eye and brain development. Semin Perinatol 15:449, 1991.

82. Kolezko B, Thiel I, Abiodun PO. The fatty acid composition of human milk in Europe and Africa. J Pediatr 120:S62, 1992.

83. Neuringer M, Connor WE, Lin DS, et al. Biochemical and functional effects of prenatal and postnatal ω3 fatty acid deficiency on retina and brain in rhesis monkeys. Proc Natl Acad Sci USA 83:4021, 1986.

84. Martinez M. Tissue levels of polyunsaturated fatty acids during early human development. J Pediatr 120:S129, 1992.

85. Farquharson J, Cockburn F, Patrick WA, et al. Infant cerebral cortex phospholipid fatty-acid composition and diet. Lancet 340:810, 1992.

86. Carlson SE, Cooke RJ, Rhodes PG, et al. Effect of vegetable and marine oils in preterm infant formulas on blood arachidonic and docosa-hexaenoic acids. J Pediatr 120:S159, 1992.

87. Birch EE, Birch DG, Hoffman DR, Uauy R. Dietary essential fatty acid supply and visual acuity development. Invest Ophthalmol Vis Sci 33:3242, 1992.

88. Agostoni C, Trojan S, Beller R. Neurodevelopmental quotient of healthy term infants at 4 months and feeding practice: The role of long-chain polyunsaturated fatty acids. Pediatr Res 38:262, 1995.

89. Agostoni C, Trojan S, Bellu R, et al. Developmental quotient (DQ) and fatty acid (FA) status in 24-months old children fed different diets in infancy. JPGN 22:412, 1996.

90. Auestad N, Montalto MB, Hall RT, et al. Visual acuity, erythrocyte fatty acid composition, and growth in term infants fed formulas with long chain polyunsaturated fatty acids for one year. Pediatr Res 41:1, 1997.

91. Carlson SE, Cooke RJ, Werkman SH, Tolley EA. First year growth of preterm infants fed standard compared to marine oil n-3 supplement-ed formula. Lipids 27:901, 1992.

92. Carlson SE, Werkman SH, Rhodes PG, Tolley EA. Visual-acuity devel-opment in healthy preterm infants: effect of marine-oil supplementa-tion. Am J Clin Nutr 58:35, 1993.

93. Carlson SE, Werkman SH, Peeples JM, et al. Arachidonic acid status correlates with first year growth in preterm infants. Proc Natl Acad Sci USA 90:1073, 1993.

94. Carlson SE, Werkman SH, Peeples JM, Wilson WM. Growth and devel-opment of premature infants in relation to ω3 and ω6 fatty acid status. Work Rev Nutr Diet 75:63, 1994.

95. Carlson SE, Ford AJ, Werkman SH. Visual acuity and fatty acid status of term infants fed human milk and formulas with and without docosa-hexaenoate and arachidonate from egg yolk lecithin. Pediatr Res 39:882, 1996.

96. Carlson SE, Werkman SH, Tolley EA. Effect of long-chain n-3 fatty acid supplementation on visual acuity and growth of preterm infants with and without bronchopulmonary dysplasia. Am J Clin Nutr 63:687, 1996.

97. Carlson SE, Werkman SH. A randomized trial of visual attention of preterm infants fed docosahexaenoic acid until two months. Lipids 31:85, 1996.

98. Hartmann EE, Neuringer M. Longitudinal behavioral measures of visual acuity in full-term human infants fed different dietary fatty acids. Invest Ophthalmol Vis Sci 36:S869, 1995.

99. Innis SM, Nelson CM, Rioux MF, King DJ. Development of visual acu-ity in relation to plasma and erythrocyte n-6 and n-3 fatty acids in healthy term gestation infants. Am J Clin Nutr 60:347, 1994.

100. Innis SM, Nelson CM, Lwanga D, et al. Feeding formula without arachidonic acid and docosahexaenoic acid has no effect on preferential looking acuity or recognition memory in healthy full-term infants at 9 mo of age. Am J Clin Nutr 64:40, 1996.

101. Jorgensen MH, Hernell O, Lund P, et al. Visual acuity and erythrocyte docosahexaenoic acid status in breast-fed and formula-fed infants during the first four months of life. Lipids 31:99, 1996.

102. Neuringer M, Fitzgerald KM, Weleber RG, et al. Electroretinograms in four-month-old fullterm human infants fed diets differing in long-chain n-3 and n-6 fatty acids. Invest Ophthalmol Vis Sci 36:S48, 1995.

103. Werkman SH, Carlson SE. A randomized trial of visual attention of preterm infants fed docosahexaenoic acid until nine months. Lipids. 31:91, 1996.

104. Hoffman DR, Birth EE, Birch DG, et al. Effects of ω-3 long chain polyunsaturated fatty acid supplementation on retinal and cortical development in premature infants. Am J Clin Nutr 57:807S, 1993.

105. Makrides M, Simmer K, Goggin M, et al. Erythrocyte docosahexaenoic acid correlates with the visual response of healthy, term infants. Pediatr Res 34:425, 1993.

106. Uauy R, Hoffman DR, Birch EE, et al. Role of ω-3 fatty acids in the nutrition of very-low-birthweight infants: Soy and marine oil supplementation of formula. J Pediatr 124:612, 1994.

107. Carlson SE, Montalto MB, Ponder DL, et al. Lower incidence of necrotizing enterocolitis in infants fed a preterm formula with egg phospholipids. Pediatr Res 44:491, 1998.

108. Jorgensen MH, Holmer G, Lund P, et al. Effect of formula supplemented with docosahexaenoic acid and γ-linolenic acid on fatty acid status and visual acuity in term infants. JPGN 26:412, 1998.

109. O'Connor DL, Hall RT, Adamkin D, et al. Growth, tolerance, and morbidity of preterm infants fed exclusively human milk, exclusively preterm infant formula, or a combination of human milk and a preterm infant formula until term corrected age (CA). Pediatr Res 45(4):287A, 1999.

110. O'Connor DL, Hall RT, Adamkin D, et al. Randomized trial of premature infants fed human milk and/or a nutrient enriched formula with and without a source of arachidonic acid (AA) and docosahexaenoic acid (DHA). Pediatr Res 45(4):288A, 1999.

111. Ryan AS, Montalto MB, Groh-Wargo S, et al. Effect of DHA-containing formula on growth of preterm infants to 59 weeks postmenstrual age. Am J Hum Biol 11:457, 1999.

112. Udall JN. Fish oil: For use in infant formula? JPGN 28:244, 1999.

113. ESPGAN Committee on Nutrition: Comment on the content and composition of lipids in infant formulas. Acta Paediatr Scand 80:887, 1991.

114. Innis SM. Human milk and formula fatty acids. J Pediatr 120(4):S56, 1992.

115. ESPGAN Committee on Nutrition. Comment on the vitamin E content in infant formulas, follow-up formulas, and formulas for low birth weight infants. JPGN 26:351, 1998.

116. Roy CC, Ste-Marie M, Chartrand L, et al. Correction of the malabsorption of the preterm infant with a medium-chain triglyceride formula. J Pediatr 86:446, 1975.

117. Huston RK, Reynolds JW, Jensen C, et al. Nutrient and mineral retention and vitamin D absorption in low-birth-weight infants: Effect of medium-chain triglycerides. Pediatrics 72:44, 1983.

118. Hamosh M, Mahta NR, Fink CS, et al. Fat absorption in premature infants: Medium-chain triglycerides and long-chain triglycerides are absorbed from formula at similar rates. J Pediatr Gastroenterol Nutr 13:143, 1991.

119. Sulkers EJ, Goudoever JB, Leunisse C, et al. Comparison of two preterm formulas with or without addition of medium-chain triglycerides (MCTS). I: Effects on nitrogen and fat balance and body composition changes. J Pediatr Gastroenterol Nutr 15:34, 1992.

120. Hamosh M, Bitman J, Liao TH, et al. Gastric lipolysis and fat absorption in preterm infants: Effect of medium-chain triglyceride or long-chain triglyceride-containing formulas. Pediatrics 83:86, 1989.

121. Tantibhedhyangkul P, Hashim SA. Medium-chain triglyceride feeding in premature infants: Effects on calcium and magnesium absorption. Pediatrics 61:537, 1978.

122. Sulkers EJ, Lafeber HN, Degenhart HJ, et al. Comparison of two preterm formulas with or without addition of medium-chain triglycerides (MCTS). II. Effects on mineral balance. J Pediatr Gastroenterol Nutr 15:42, 1992.

123. Leitch CA. Fat metabolism and requirements. In: Polin RA, Fox WW, eds. Fetal and neonatal physiology. 2d ed. Philadelphia: Saunders, 1998; 328-32.

124. Ernst JA, Neal PR. Mineral and trace elements. In: Polin RA, Fox WW, eds. Fetal and neonatal physiology. 2d ed. Philadelphia: Saunders, 1998; 332-43.

125. Holick MF. Vitamin D. In: Shils ME, Olson JA, Shike M, eds. Modern nutrition in health and disease. 8th ed. Philadelphia: Lea & Febiger; 1994, 308-25.

126. Schanler RJ, Rifka M. Calcium, phosphorus and magnesium needs for the low-birth-weight infant. Acta Paediatr (suppl) 405:111, 1994.

127. Koo WWK, Tsang RC. Mineral requirements of low-birth-weight infants. J Am Coll Nutr 10:474, 1991.

128. Widdowson EM, McCance RA. The metabolism of calcium, phosphorus, magnesium and strontium. Pediatr Clin North Am 12:595, 1965.

129. Ziegler EE, O'Donnell AM, Nelson SE, et al. Body composition of the reference fetus. Growth 40:329, 1976.

130. Koo WWK, Steichen JJ. Osteopenia and rickets of prematurity. In: Polin RA, Fox WW, eds. Fetal and neonatal physiology, 2d ed. Philadelphia: Saunders, 1998; 2335-49.

131. Koo WWK, Tsang RC. Calcium, magnesium, phosphorus, and vitamin D. In: Tsang RC, Lucas A, Uauy R, Zlotkin S, eds. Nutritional needs of the preterm infant: Scientific basis and practical guidelines. Baltimore: Williams and Wilkins, 1993; 135-55.

132. Shaw JCL. Parenteral nutrition in the management of sick low birth-weight infants. Pediatr Clin North Am 20:333, 1973.

133. Forbes GB. Calcium accumulation by the human fetus. Pediatrics 57:976, 1976.

134. Koo, WWK, Walters J, Bush AJ, et al. Dual-energy x-ray absorptiometry studies of bone mineral status in newborn infants. J Bone Min Res 11:997, 1996.

135. Senterre J, Salle B. Calcium and phosphorus economy of the preterm infant and its interaction with vitamin D and its metabolites. Acta Paediatr Scand 296(suppl):85, 1982.

136. Ezzedeen F, Adelman RD, Ahlfors CE. Renal calcification in preterm infants: pathophysiology and long-term sequelae. J Pediatr 113:532, 1988.

137. Jacinto JS, Modanlou HD, Crade M, et al. Renal calcification incidence in very low birth weight infants. Pediatrics 81:31, 1988.

138. Vileisis RA. Furosemide effect on mineral status of parenterally nourished premature neonates with chronic lung disease. Pediatrics 85:316, 1990.

139. Zanardo V, Dani C, Trevisanuto D. Methylxanthines increase renal calcium excretion in preterm infants. Biol Neonate 68:169, 1995.

140. Weiler HA, Wang Z, Atkinson SA. Dexamethasone treatment impairs calcium regulation and reduces bone mineralization in infant pigs. Am J Clin Nutr 61:805, 1995.

141. Koo WWK, Krug-Wispe S, Neylan M, et al. Effect of three levels of vitamin D intake in preterm infants receiving high mineral-containing milk. JPGN 21:182, 1995.

142. Ehrenkranz RA. Iron, folic acid, and vitamin B,2. In: Tsang RC, Lucas A, Uauy R, Zlotkin S, eds. Nutritional needs of the preterm infant: Scientific basis and practical guidelines. Baltimore: Williams and Wilkins, 1993; 177-94.

143. Guiang SF, Georgieff MK. Fetal and neonatal iron metabolism. In: Polin RA, Fox WW, eds. Fetal and neonatal physiology. 2d ed. Philadelphia: Saunders, 1998; 401-10.

144. Hambidge KM. Trace minerals. In: Hay WW, ed. Neonatal nutrition and metabolism. St. Louis: Mosby Year Book, 1991; 203-33.

145. Dallman PR. Nutritional anemia of infancy: Iron, folic acid, and B_{12}. In: Tsang RC, Nichols BF, eds. Nutrition during infancy. Philadelphia: Hanley and Belfus, 1988; 216-35.

146. Oski FA. Iron requirements of the premature infant. In: Tsang RC, ed. Vitamin and mineral requirements in preterm infants. New York: Marcel Dekker, 1985; 9-21.

147. Melhorn DK, Gross S. Vitamin E-dependent anemia in the premature infant. I. Effects of large doses of medicinal iron. J Pediatr 79:569, 1971.

148. Williams ML, Shott RJ, O'Neal PL, et al. Role of dietary iron and fat on vitamin E deficiency of infancy. N Engl J Med 292:887, 1975.

149. Gross SJ, Gabriel E. Vitamin E status in preterm infants fed human milk or infant formula. J Pediatr 106:635, 1985.

150. Zipurski A. Vitamin E deficiency anemia in newborn infants. Clin Perinatol 11:393, 1984.

151. McDonald MC, Abrams SA, Schanler RJ. Iron absorption and red blood cell incorporation in premature infants fed an iron-fortified infant formula. Pediatr Res 44:507,1998.

152. Arant BS, Sodium, chloride, and potassium. In: Tsang RC, Lucas A, Uauy R, Zlotkin S, eds. Nutritional needs of the preterm infant: Scientific basis and practical guidelines. Baltimore: Williams and Wilkins, 1993; 157-75.

153. Herin P, Zetterstrom R. Sodium, potassium and chloride needs in low-birth-weight infants. Acta Paediatr Suppl 405:43, 1994.

154. Al-Dahhan J, Haycock GB, Chantler C, et al. Sodium homeostasis in term and preterm neonates. I. Renal aspects. Arch Dis Child 58:335, 1983.
155. Zlotkin SH, Atkinson S, Lockitch G. Trace elements in nutrition for premature infants. Clin Perinatol 22(1):223, 1995.
156. Tyrala EE. Trace element metabolism in the fetus and neonate. In: Polin RA and Fox WW, eds. Fetal and Neonatal Physiology, 2nd Edition. Philadelphia: WB Saunders Co, 1998, pp 410-420.
157. Milner JA. Trace minerals in the nutrition of children. J Pediatr 117:S147, 1990.
158. Ziegler EE. Infants of low birthweight: Special needs and problems. Am J Clin Nutr 41:440, 1985.
159. Ehrenkranz RA. Mineral needs of the very-low-birthweight infant. Semin Perinatol 13:142, 1989.
160. Black RE. Preface: Zinc for child health. Am J Clin Nutr 68(2):409S, 1998.
161. Ehrenkranz RA, Gettner PA, Nelli CM, et al. Zinc and copper nutritional studies in very low birthweight infants: Comparison of stable isotope extrinsic tag and chemical balance methods. Pediatr Res 26:298, 1989.
162. Wauben I, Gibson R, Atkinson S. Premature infants fed mothers' milk to 6 months corrected age demonstrate adequate growth and zinc status in the first year. EarlyHum Develop 54:181, 1999.
163. Lonnerdal B. Trace element absorption in infants as a foundation to setting upper limits for trace elements in infant formulas. J Nutr 119:1839, 1989.
164. O'Dell BL. Mineral interactions relevant to nutrient requirements. J Nutr 119:1832, 1989.
165. Wang Z, Weiler H, Atkinson SA. Long-term dexamethasone therapy ± high dietary zinc alters intestinal zinc uptake in the piglet model. Proc Can Fed Biol Soc 36:144, 1993.
166. Wastney ME, Angelus PA, Barnes RM, Siva Subramanian KN. Zinc absorption, distribution, excretion, and retention by healthy preterm infants. Pediatr Res 45:191, 1999.
167. Lonnerdal B. Copper nutrition during infancy and childhood. Am J Clin Nutr 67(5):1046S, 1998.
168. L'Abbe MR, Friel JK. Copper status of very low birth weight infants during the first 12 months of infancy. Pediatr Res 32:183, 1992.
169. Greene HL, Smidt LJ. Water-soluble vitamins: C, B_1, B_2, B_6, niacin pantothenic acid, and biotin. In: Tsang RC, Lucas A, Uauy R, Zlotkin S, eds. Nutritional needs of the preterm infant: Scientific basis and practical guidelines. Baltimore: Williams and Wilkins, 1993; 121-33.
170. Moran JR, Greene HL. Vitamin requirements. In: Polin RA and Fox WW, eds. Fetal and Neonatal Physiology, 2nd Edition. Philadelphia: WB Saunders Co, 1998, pp 344-353.
171. Riedel BD, Greene HL. Vitamins. In: Hay WW, ed. Neonatal nutrition and metabolism. St. Louis: Mosby Year Book, 1991; 143-70.
172. Porcelli PJ, Adcock EW, DelPaggio D, et al. Plasma and urine riboflavin and pyridoxine concentrations in enterally fed very-low-birth-weight neonates. JPGN 23:141, 1996.
173. Friel JK, Andrews WL, Long DR, et al. Thiamine, riboflavin, folate, and vitamin B12 status of infants with low birth weights receiving enteral nutrition. JPGN 22:289, 1996.

174. Hovi L, Hekali R, Siimes MA. Evidence of riboflavin depletion in breastfed newborns and its further acceleration during treatment of hyperbilirubinemia by phototherapy. Acta Paediatr Scand 68:567, 1979.

175. Kang-Yoon SA, Kirksey A, Giacoia GP, West KD. Vitamin B-6 adequacy in neonatal nutrition: associations with preterm delivery, type of feeding, and vitamin B-6 supplementation. Am J Clin Nutr 62:932, 1995.

176. Greene HL. Vitamin A in preterm infants. In: Polin RA and Fox WW, eds. Fetal and Neonatal Physiology, 2nd Edition. Philadelphia: WB Saunders Co, 1998, pp 420-425.

177. Olson JA. Upper limits of vitamin A in infant formulas, with some comments on vitamin K. J Nutr 119:1820, 1989.

178. Koo WWK, Krug-Wispe S, Succop P, et al. Effect of different vitamin A intakes on very-low-birth-weight infants. Am J Clin Nutr 62:1216, 1995.

179. Shenai JP, Chytil F, Stahlman MT. Vitamin A status of neonates with bronchopulmonary dysplasia. Pediatr Res 19:185, 1985.

180. Shenai JP, Kennedy KA, Chytil F, et al. Clinical trial of vitamin A supplementation in infants susceptible to bronchopulmonary dysplasia. J Pediatr 111:269, 1987.

181. Pearson E, Bose C, Snidow T, et al. Trial of vitamin A supplementation in very low birth weight infants at risk for bronchopulmonary dysplasia. J Pediatr 121:420, 1992.

182. Schwarz KB, Cox JM, Sharma S, et al. Possible antioxidant effect of vitamin A supplementation in premature infants. JPGN 25:408, 1997.

183. Kennedy KA, Stoll BJ, Ehrenkranz RA, et al. Vitamin A to prevent bronchopulmonary dysplasia in very-low-birth-weight infants: has the dose been too low? Early Human Devel 49:19, 1997.

184. Dju MY, Mason KE, Filer LJ Jr. Vitamin E (tocopherol) in human tissues from birth to old age. Am J Clin Nutr 6:50, 1958.

185. Phelps DL. Current perspectives on vitamin E in infant nutrition. Am J Clin Nutr 46:187, 1987.

186. Gross SJ, Gabriel E. Vitamin E status in preterm infants fed human milk or infant formula. J Pediatr 106:635, 1985.

187. Bell EF, Brown EJ, Milner R, et al. Vitamin E absorption in small premature infants. Pediatrics 63:830, 1979.

188. Melhorn DK, Gross S. Vitamin E-dependent anemia in the premature infant: Relationship between gestational age and absorption of vitamin E. J Pediatr 79:581, 1971.

189. Law MR, Wijewardene K, Wald NJ. Is routine vitamin E administration justified in very low-birthweight infants? Develop Med Child Neuro 32:442, 1990.

190. Johnson L, Bowen FW, Abbasi S, et al. Relationship of prolonged pharmacologic serum levels of vitamin E to incidence of sepsis and necrotizing enterocolitis in infants with birth weights 1,500 grams or less. Pediatrics 75:619, 1985.

191. Finer NN, Peters KL, Hayek Z, et al. Vitamin E and necrotizing enterocolitis. Pediatrics 73:387, 1984.

192. Kaempf DE, Linderkamp O. Do healthy premature infants fed breast milk need vitamin E supplementation: α- and γ-tocopherol levels in blood components and buccal mucosal cells. Pediatr Res 44:54, 1998.

193. Johnson L. Vitamin E nutrition in the fetus and newborn. In: Polin FA and Fox WW, eds. Fetal and Neonatal Physiology, 2nd Edition. Philadelphia: WB Saunders Co, 1998, pp 425-442.

194. Greer FR. Vitamin K deficiency and hemorrhage in infancy. Clin Perinatol 22(3):759, 1995.
195. Greer FR. Vitamin K. In: Tsang RC, Lucas A, Uauy R, Zlotkin S, eds. Nutritional Needs of the Preterm Infant. Baltimore: Williams and Wilkins, 1993, pp 111-119.
196. Moran JR, Greene HL. Nutritional biochemistry of fat-soluble vitamins, In: Grand RJ, Sutphen JL, Dietz WH Jr, eds. Pediatric nutrition. Theory and practice. Boston: Butterworths, 1987; 69-85.
197. American Academy of Pediatrics, Committee on Nutrition. Vitamins. Pediatric Nutrition Handbook, 4th Edition. Elk Grove Village, IL: American Academy of Pediatrics, 1998, pp 267-281.
198. Brousson MA, Klein MC. Controversies surrounding the administration of vitamin K to newborns: A review. Can Med Assoc J 154(3):307, 1996.
199. Shenai JP, Borum PR. Tissue carnitine reserves of newborn infants. Pediatr Res 18:679, 1984.
200. Borum PR. Carnitine. Ann Rev Nutr 3:233, 1983.
201. Atkinson SA, Lonnerdal B. Nonprotein nitrogen fractions of human milk. In: Jensen RG, ed. Handbook of milk composition. New York: Academic Press, 1995; 369-387.
202. Zinn AB. Inborn errors of metabolism. In: Fanaroff AA, Martin RJ, eds. Neonatal-perinatal medicine. St. Louis: Mosby Year Book, 1992; 1147.
203. American Academy of Pediatrics, Committee on Nutrition. Fluoride supplementation for children: Interim Policy Recommendations. Pediatrics. 95:777,1995.
204. Institute of Medicine, Food and Nutrition Board. Dietary reference intakes for vitamin C, vitamin E, selenium, and carotenoids. Washington, D.C.: National Academy Press, 2000.
205. Baumgart S, Costarino AT. Water and electrolyte metabolism of the micropremie. Clin Perinatol 27(1):131, 2000.
206. Hay WW, Lucas A, Heird WC, et al. Workshop summary: Nutrition of the extremely low birth weight infant. Pediatrics 104:1360, 1999.
207. Mrozek JD, Georgieff MK, Blazar BR, et al. Effect of sepsis syndrome on neonatal protein and energy metabolism. J Perinatol 2:96, 2000.
208. Neu J, DeMarco V, Weiss M. Glutamine supplementation in low-birth-weight infants: Mechanisms of action. JPEN 23:S49, 1999.
209. Tubman TRJ, Thompson SW. Glutamine supplementation for prevention of morbidity in the preterm infant. (Cochrane Review). In: The Cochrane Library, 2/22/99. Oxford: Update Software.
210. Kalhan SC, Kilic I. Carbohydrate as nutrient in the infant and child: range of acceptable intake. Eur J Clin Nutr 53 (Suppl 1):S94, 1999.
211. Kashyap S, Ohira-Kist K, Abildskov K, et al. Effects of quality of energy on enterally fed low birth weight infants. Pediatr Res 45:284A, 1999.
212. Uauy R, Mena P, Rojas C. Essential fatty acid metabolism in the micropremie. Clin Perinatol 27(1):71, 2000.
213. Gibson RA, Makrides M. n-3 Polyunsaturated fatty acid requirements of term infants. Am J Clin Nutr 71:S251, 2000.
214. Uauy R, Hoffman DR. Essential fat requirements of preterm infants. Am J Clin Nutr 71:S245, 2000.
215. Rigo J, DeCurtis M, Pieltain C, et al. Bone mineral metabolism in the micropremie. Clin Perinatol 27(1):147, 2000.

216. Backstrom MC, Maki R, Kuusela A-L, et al. Randomised controlled trial of vitamin D supplementation on bone density and biochemical indices in preterm infants. Arch Dis Child Fetal Neonatal Ed 80:F161, 1999.
217. Aggett PJ. Trace elements of the micropremie. Clin Perinatol 27(1):119, 2000.
218. Widness JA. Pathophysiology, diagnosis, and prevention of neonatal anemia. NeoRev 1 (4):e61, 2000.
219. Krebs NF, Reidinger CJ, Miller LV, Borschel MW. Zinc homeostasis in healthy infants fed a casein hydrolysate formula. JPGN 30:29, 2000.
220. Atkinson SA. Zinc absorption from infant formulas. JPGN 30:8, 2000.
221. Greer FR. Vitamin metabolism and requirements in the micropremie. Clin Perinatol 27(1):95, 2000.
222. Tyson JE, Wright LL, Oh W, et al. Vitamin A supplementation for extremely-low-birth-weight infants. N Engl J Med 340:1962, 1999.
223. Shenai JP. Vitamin A supplementation in very low birth weight neonates; Rationale and evidence. Pediatrics 104:1369, 1999.
224. Darlow BA, Graham PJ. Vitamin A supplementation for preventing morbidity and mortality in very low birthweight infants. (Cochrane Review). In: The Cochrane Library, 10/21/99. Oxford: Update Software.
225. Raju TNK, Langenberg P, Bhutani V, Quinn GE. Vitamin E prophylaxis to reduce retinopathy of prematurity: A reappraisal of published trials. J Pediatr 131, 844, 1997.
226. Zamora SA, Maret A. Vitamin E for ROP (ltr). J Pediatr 134:249, 1999.
227. Raju TNK, Langenberg P, Bhutani V, Quinn GE. Reply to ltr: Vitamin E for ROP. J Pediatr 134:249, 1999.

Nutritional Care for High-Risk Newborns (Rev. 3d. Ed.)
S. Groh-Wargo, M. Thompson, J. Cox, editors
© 2000, Precept Press, Inc., Chicago

16

HUMAN MILK AND ENTERAL NUTRITION PRODUCTS

Amy L. Sapsford, RD, CSP, LD

This chapter encompasses a review of the nutrient composition of human milk and infant formulas, especially products for premature infants. It includes the rationale for use of formulas with specific components and discusses osmolality, renal solute load, and concentration of formulas. Information on selected nutrients in human milk, many commercial infant formulas, modular additives, and vitamin and mineral supplements, as well as preparation guidelines for a variety of concentrations of formulas using liquid concentrate or powder are presented in Appendixes I, J, K and L.

Human Milk

Human milk is the preferred source of enteral nutrition for all infants, including premature and sick newborns. Policy statements from the American Academy of Pediatrics (AAP) and the American Dietetic Association (ADA) support this recommendation.[1,2] Although the decision to provide breast milk or to breast-feed ultimately lies with the mother, physicians, nurses, dietitians, and other health care providers can provide the education and encouragement that a mother may need to make the decision. Although many pediatricians agree with the AAP's recommendations, these physicians may not have sufficient educational background or experience to provide effective breast-feeding management.[3] Professionals certified in lactation management through organizations such as International Lactation

Table 16.1. Selected Benefits of Use of Human Milk and Breastfeeding[1]

Health of Infant

- Decreased incidence or severity of diarrhea
- Lower risk of infection
- Protective effect against some illnesses/conditions

Health of Mother

- Less bleeding/More rapid uterine involution
- Earlier return to prepregnant weight
- Improved bone remineralization
- Reduces risk of some cancers

Nutritional

- Species-specific composition
- Low renal solute load
- Ease of digestion

Immunologic

- Antimicrobial agents
- Anti-inflammatory agents
- Immunomodulating agents

Developmental

- Enhances Cognitive Development
- Promotes maternal infant attachment

Economic

- Reduces health care costs
- Decreases cost to feed infant

Environmental

- Reduces waste

Table 16.2   Circumstances to Avoid or Temporarily Discontinue Use of Human Milk[1,8-15]

- Infant with galactosemia

- Infant whose mother has active, untreated tuberculosis

- Possibly infant whose mother has cytomegalovirus (CMV)

- Infant in the United States whose mother is infected with human T-Cell Leukemia Virus Type I or Type II (HTLV-I or II)

- Infant whose mother has herpetic lesions on breasts from Herpes Simplex Virus Type I (HSV-I).

- Infant in the United States whose mother is infected with human immunodeficiency virus (HIV).

- Mother's use of the following general classes of medications

Radioactive Compounds	Ethanol
Drugs of Abuse	Gold
Ergot Alkaloids	Antimetabolites
Cancer Chemotherapy Agents	CNS-acting drugs
Lithium	Nicotine
Oral Contraceptives (may decrease milk supply)	

Consultant Association (ILCA) can provide these educational opportunities to physicians so that they can better support mothers.

Most term infants and some preterm infants may be able to nurse soon after delivery to establish lactation. If the infant is not able to nurse, the mother must establish lactation by expressing her milk and storing it until the infant is ready to take it. Strategies used in a successful hospital-based lactation program have been described.[4] (See Chapter 17 for detailed information on supporting a mother who is expressing milk for her sick newborn.) Even though many high-risk newborns, including premature, low-birth-weight (LBW) infants, are not able to nurse, expressed human milk is the preferred initial feeding and is usually well tolerated.[5] Some centers support the use of banked donor milk when the mother is not able to provide it for her newborn. This practice is well recognized around the world.[6] Standards and guidelines for banked donor milk in the United States have been established by the Human Milk Banking Association of North America[6] (see Appendix M). The benefits of breast-feeding or use of human milk are outlined in Table 16.1.

There are few circumstances in which the use of human milk would not be in the best interest of the infant, as summarized in Table 16.2.[1,8-13] Recommendations related to the transmission of infectious agents through human milk have been published.[9,13-15] Special attention must be given to storage and labeling policies in hospitals, particularly in the neonatal intensive care unit (NICU). For example, a mother who is positive for Hepatitis B surface antigen may breast-

Table 16.3. General Comparisons in Variations: Human Milk Composition for Selected Nutrients[21]

Composition of Selected Nutrients	Gestation		During a Feeding		Diurnal		Stage of Lactation		Maternal Diet	
	Preterm	Mature	Fore-milk	Hind-milk	Early a.m.	Late p.m	Colostrum 1-5 days	Mature > 30 days	Mal-nourished	Well nourished
Lactose	Lower	Higher	Higher	Lower	Lower	Higher	Lower	Higher	Same	Same
Protein	Higher	Lower	Lower	Higher	Lower	Higher	Higher	Lower	Same	Same
Fat	Higher	Lower	Lower	Higher	Lower	Higher	Lower	Higher	Same	Same
Enegy	Higher	Lower	Lower	Higher	Lower	Higher	Lower	Higher	Same	Same
Volume	Same	Same			Lower	Higher	Lower	Higher	Lower	Higher
Water Soluble Vitamins	Varies	Varies			Lower	Higher	Lower	Higher	Lower	Higher
Fat Soluble Vitamins	Varies	Varies					Higher	Lower	Lower	Higher
Calcium/ Phosphorus	Same	Same					Same	Same	Same	Same
Iron	Higher	Lower					Higher	Lower	Same	Same
Sodium	Higher	Lower					Higher	Lower	Same	Same
Potassium	Same	Same					Higher	Lower	Same	Same

feed her baby after the baby has received hepatitis B immune glob-ulin and vaccine. Milk that is potentially contaminated with hepatitis B should not be stored in the nursery due to the risk to the other infants.[14] If the other babies are not immunized and a baby is inad-vertently fed the contaminated milk, disease transmission may occur. A unique labeling system has been developed to help prevent feeding a baby another mother's breastmilk.[267] Specific recommen-dations on the transfer of drugs and other chemicals in breast milk have been published.[10-12,16]

The unique composition of human milk is "the gold standard" upon which all other infant formulas are modeled and compared. The com-position of human milk varies with gestation, within a feeding, during the day, throughout lactation and with variations in the maternal diet.[17-28] Table 16.3 summarizes changes in milk composition in a vari-ety of situations.[21] Milk from mothers who deliver prematurely may vary from those who deliver at term.[22-28] Donor milk varies in its com-position of fat, protein, and calories.[26] The fat and energy content of human milk can be estimated using the creamatocrit (see Chapter 17).

The principal carbohydrate in human milk is lactose, which pro-vides about 40% of the total energy content.[29] It is synthesized in the mammary gland.[21] Lactase is required for hydrolysis of lactose to glucose and galactose. Premature infants have low mucosal lactase activity; however, they seem to tolerate lactose well when they are challenged with this disaccharide.[30]

Human milk proteins differ significantly from cow's milk pro-teins in quality and quantity.[31-35] The casein to whey ratio in cow's milk is 18:82. Casein synthesis varies in human milk from colostrum to mature milk. The ratio of whey or lactalbumin protein to casein changes from 90:10 in early milk to 60:40 in mature milk. Later in lac-tation, the whey component decreases further to 50:50.[33] The amino acid content of human milk differs from cow's milk as well. The tau-rine concentration is high in human milk and is nearly absent in bovine milk. The methionine to cysteine ratio in human milk is close to one, which is much lower than most mammalian milks. The pheny-lalanine and tyrosine levels of human milk are low. This is advanta-geous for preterm infants who may have low levels of the enzymes required to metabolize aromatic amino acids.[21]

Many compounds contribute to the protein and nonprotein nitro-gen (NPN) present in human milk.[35,36] The NPN may provide addi-tional benefits for the premature infant, such as stimulation for gut maturation and resistance to infection.[27,37] These NPN components in human milk vary greatly from bovine milk, providing about 25-33% of the total nitrogen in human milk.[27,36] (See Appendix K for nutrient composition of preterm and mature human milk compared to infant formulas and cow milk.)

Human milk contains 3.5-4.5% fat, which provides about 40-50% of the total calories.[38] Triglycerides contribute about 98% of the total fat content of human milk.[38,39] Fat is synthesized in the mammary alveolar cells and is stimulated by emptying the breast and by prolactin secretion.[39] The fatty acid content of human milk and infant formulas has been reviewed.[40] Arachidonic acid (AA) and docosahexaenoic acid (DHA), two important fatty acids that are uniquely present in human milk, are involved in brain and retinal development. AA and DHA may be essential for infants unable to synthesize optimal levels from linoleic and linolenic acid.[41] AA and DHA may be higher in preterm human milk than in term human milk.[42] Human milk contains factors that improve fat absorption, including human milk lipoprotein lipase (LL) and bile salt-stimulated lipase (BSSL), which are complementary to pancreatic lipase.[32,38,43,44] Use of hindmilk, which is higher in fat and calories, may improve weight gain in LBW infants fed human milk.[45] Optimal delivery methods are necessary to ensure maximum energy and nutrient delivery when tube feedings are necessary[4,46,47] (see Chapter 18).

There may be neurodevelopmental advantages to using human milk compared with formula. Breast-fed infants may have advanced cognitive abilities when compared with formula-fed infants.[48-51] Other advantages for the use of human milk in the premature infant include:

- Whey predominant protein[52]
- Ease of digestion and absorption of fat, zinc, and iron[44,53,54]
- Low renal solute load[55]
- Presence of antiinfective factors[56,57]
- Promotion of maternal-infant attachment[58]
- Possible protection against necrotizing enterocolitis (NEC) and late-onset sepsis[59-61]

Although these advantages support the use of human milk in the high-risk newborn, some nutrient needs may not be met in the growing preterm infant. These nutrients include protein, calcium, phosphorus, magnesium, sodium, copper, zinc, and vitamins B_2, B_6, C, D, E, K, and folic acid.[62,63] These nutrient deficiencies can result in clinical manifestations of kwashiorkor,[64-66] osteopenia or rickets,[32,67-69] hyponatremia,[70] and zinc deficiency.[71] Fortifying human milk can minimize these nutrient deficiencies.

Human Milk Fortification

Nutrient fortification of human milk can be accomplished by adding liquid or powdered commercially available fortifiers, premature infant formulas, powdered formulas, modular supplements, or vitamin/mineral supplements. The commercially available fortifiers are Similac Human Milk Fortifier (SHMF) (Ross Products Division of Abbott Laboratories, Columbus, OH),[268] Enfamil Human Milk Fortifier (EHMF) (Mead Johnson Nutritionals, Evansville, IN),[72] and Similac

Natural Care (SNC) Human Milk Fortifier (Ross).[73] A comparison of the commercially available fortifiers is summarized in Table 16.4. The nutrient content and source of macronutrients of the fortifiers and the content of the fortifiers mixed with human milk is summarized in Appendix K. Altering the nutrient composition of human milk with modular supplements or powdered formulas may result in either an unbalanced or inadequate nutrient composition, or high osmolality. An analysis of the nutrient content of the special formulation will reveal any imbalances or inadequacies. Studies on human milk fortification for premature infants have encompassed the effects on development, growth, body composition, nutritional status, and morbidity.[74]

A randomized, controlled trial of fortified human milk studied 275 premature infants < 1,850 g on a multinutrient powdered fortifier (EHMF) versus a control liquid supplement containing only phosphate and vitamins.[75] Preterm formula was used when breast milk was not available. Compared with the control group, developmental scores at 18 months were slightly but not significantly higher in the multinutrient-fortified group, and short-term growth was improved when human milk provided a greater proportion of total intake than preterm formula.[75]

A prospective, randomized, double-blinded multicenter study evaluated growth and serum biochemistries in preterm infants less than or equal to 1600 grams and less than or equal to 33 weeks gestation receiving preterm human milk supplemented with either EHMF or SHMF.[269] Overall growth was better in the SHMF group compared to the EHMF group with the SHMF group reaching 1800 grams one week sooner than the EHMF group. Length and head circumference gains were improved as well showing proportional growth across all parameters.[269]

A study of 108 infants < 1,250 g compared infants fed human milk fortified with EHMF with those exclusively fed preterm formula.[61] Infants fed fortified human milk grew significantly slower than those fed preterm formula. There were no differences in tolerance, and the incidence of NEC and late-onset sepsis were less in the fortified human milk group.

The unique properties of human milk appear to promote improved host defense and G.I. function compared with formula feeding.[61] EHMF versus SNC was fed to healthy preterm infants. Results showed there was no significant difference in growth, but calcium levels were elevated and alkaline phosphatase levels were lower in the EHMF group.[76] The authors speculated that this finding could be related to the variation in vitamin D content in the fortifiers.

A multinutrient powdered fortifier versus a calcium/phosphorus supplement alone was studied in a randomized, controlled trial in preterm infants in Canada.[77] Use of the multinutrient fortifier resulted in improved linear growth but did not offer advantages to bone mineral content when compared with supplementing with calcium and phosphorus alone.[77] Infants fed EHMF with calcium glycerophosphate

Table 16.4 Comparison of Commercially Available Human Milk Fortifiers

	Similac Human Milk Fortifier (SHMF)[#]	Enfamil Human Milk Fortifier (EHMF)*	Similac Natural Care[#]
Macronutrient Composition	Corn syrup solids, whey protein concentrate, fractionated coconut oil (MCT) (balanced composition)	Corn syrup solids, lactose, whey protein concentrate, sodium caseinate, no added fat	Corn syrup solids, lactose, nonfat milk and whey (60:40) MCT oil, soy and coconut oil (balanced formula)
Energy	3.5 kcal/pkt.	3.5 kcal/pkt.	24 kcal/oz.
Calcium/ Phosphorus	Calcium phosphate tribasic, calcium carbonate (No hypercalcemia reported despite higher levels compared to EHMF)	Calcium gluconate and calcium glycerophosphate (Hypercalcemia has been reported in infants < 1000 gm)	Calcium phosphate tribasic, calcium carbonate (Levels greater than Similac Special Care [SSC])
Fat Soluble Vitamins	Adequate levels	Adequate levels Monitor if more than 16-20 packets/day are used	Same levels as SSC
Mixing	1 pkt./25 ml human milk equals 24 kcal/oz	1 pkt./25 ml human milk equals 24 kcal/oz	Add to human milk or alternate with human milk
Maximum caloric density	24 kcal/oz Do not add SHMF in ratio greater than than 1 pkt./25 ml	24 kcal/oz Do not add EHMF in ratio greater than than 1 pkt./25 ml	≈23 kcal/oz mixed 3:1 with human milk 22 kcal/oz mixed 1:1
Milk Supply	No formula supplement necessary	No formula supplement necessary	Extends mother's milk if supply is low
Osmolality (mOsm/kg H_2O)	385	410-440 (varies)	285
Packaging	Unit dose packets	Unit dose packets	4 oz. Bottles

[#] Ross Product Handbook, Ross Products Division, Columbus, OH, March, 1999.
* Mead Johnson Product Handbook, Mead Johnson Nutritionals, Evansville, IN, November, 1999.

Table 16.5 Guidelines for Use of Fortified Human Milk for Premature Infants

- Infants < 34 weeks gestation

- Infants < 1500 grams at birth

- Infants on TPN for greater that 2 weeks

- Infants > 1500 grams at birth with suboptimal growth

- Infants > 1500 grams at birth with limited ability to tolerate increased volume intake

---

(CaGP), the current formulation, achieved intrauterine accretion rates for calcium and phosphorus; however, fat absorption was significantly lower when compared with similar infants fed preterm formula.[78,79] Fat absorption was directly related to weight gain.[79] Total fat, free fatty acids (FFA), and mineral-bound fatty acids (MBFA) were measured in EHMF fortified human milk and preterm formula. There was a rapid decrease in human milk FFA after fortification which was significantly associated with the amount of fortifier added. The authors suggest there is very strong binding of MBFA and increased fat excretion.[79]

When protein versus carbohydrate was added to fortified human milk in a double-blind study, infants in the fortified human milk group with additional protein grew better than those fortified with additional carbohydrate.[80] Protein may be the limiting nutrient even in fortified human milk, and is likely the most important nutrient required for improved short-term growth.[75,80,270,271] Other studies related to growth, body composition, and tolerance support fortification of human milk for preterm infants.[81-88,272]

The effects of nutrient fortification on osmolality, storage conditions, and host defense properties of human milk have been studied. The addition of human milk fortifiers, formula powders, and some modular products increases the osmolality of human milk[89,273] (see Table 16.4). As storage time increases, total bacterial colony counts are significantly greater in fortified versus unfortified human milk. Fortification or storage does not affect IgA.[90,91] These studies support current recommendations of using fortified human milk within 24 hours. Very low birth rate (VLBW) preterm infants fed fortified human milk have a significantly lower incidence of NEC, sepsis and meningitis compared with formula-fed VLBW prematures.[61,92] These findings demonstrate the protective effect of breast milk on the high-risk preterm infant and support the recommendation of providing fortified human milk to hospitalized infants.[5,92]

Fortification of human milk has been reviewed and is widely recognized as a standard of care.[93-95,274-276] Although there are no universally accepted recommendations for use of human milk fortifiers,

Table 16.6   Daily Feeding Plans for Former Preterm Infants* to be Breastfed or Given Human Milk at Discharge: Comparison of Selected Nutrients

	Breastfeeding[+] or Human Milk with No Supplement		Human milk plus Similac Human Milk Fortifier to equal 24 kcal/oz[t‡]		Breastfeeding[+] alternated with Similac NeoSure 22 kcal/oz		Human Milk plus Similac NeoSure Powder to equal 24 kcal/oz[‡]		Recommendations Stable/Growing Preterm Infant[1-2]
Volume ml/kg	150	180	150	180	150	180	150	180	150-200
Energy kcal/kg	102	122	119	142	107	128	121	145	105-130
Protein g/kg	1.6	1.9	3.5	4.1	2.2	2.7	2.1	2.5	3-4
Calcium[#] mg/kg	42	50	207	248	80	96	63	75	120-230
Phosphorus[#] mg/kg	21	26	117	140	45	54	34	41	60-140
Sodium mEq/kg	1.1	1.4	2.5	3	1.3	1.6	1.4	1.7	2-3
Vitamin D IU/D[§]	6	7	179	214	81	98	34	42	150-400
Iron mg/kg[§]	trace	trace	0.7	0.8	1.0	1.2	0.4	0.5	2-4
Zinc µg/kg	178	214	201	241	761	913	412	494	1000

*   Assumes a weight of 2 kg.
+   Breastfeeding volumes are estimated to equal other feedings for comparison.
†   Calculations derived from Product Monograph 62352, Ross Products Division, October, 1999.
‡   When mother chooses not to breastfeed or has weaned but still has stored milk.
#   Infants with hypophosphatemia or osteopenia may require additional supplementation of calcium and phosphorus with some regimens. Infants on SHMF only require 170 ml/kg/day to meet calcium needs.
§   Supplemental vitamin D and iron needed; evaluate need for other vitamin/mineral supplementation.

NEONOVA Nutrition Optimizer (4.2P), Ross Products Division, Columbus, OH
1. Tsang RC, Lucas A, Uauy R, Zlotkin S (eds). Nutritional Needs of the Preterm Infant: Scientific Basis and Practical Guidelines. Baltimore: Williams and Wilkins, 1993, pp 288-289.
2. American Academy of Pediatrics (AAP). Nutritional Needs of Preterm Infants. In Kleinman, RE (ed). Pediatric Nutrition Handbook, 4th ed. Elk Grove Village: AAP, 1998, pp 55-87.

practical guidelines are outlined in Table 16.5. Clinical condition of the infant is considered when evaluating the need for fortification. This includes growth history, fluid tolerance, estimation of energy and protein needs, and the risk of osteopenia from long-term total parenteral nutrition, low intake of calcium/phosphorus, and/or the use of diuretics or steroids. Term infants who may benefit from fortification with either a commercially available fortifier or supplement include infants with cardiac or renal anomalies or those requiring fluid restriction.

Preterm infants are discharged at weights often less than 2000 grams. Reasonable guidelines must be developed to provide adequate nutrients and energy for growth while also supporting breast-feeding success. Commercial fortifiers are not readily available for retail purchase. Although there are no research-based, generally accepted recommendations for breast-feeding the prematurely born infant after hospital discharge, suggestions are given in Table 16.6 and in Chapters 17, 33, and 34. Further research is needed to determine the most appropriate nutrition plan for this population. If other modular supplements or infant formulas are used, a complete nutrient analysis is recommended to avoid inadequate or excessive nutrient intake. When commercial fortifiers are used after discharge, intake should be monitored to avoid excessive consumption of nutrients, especially fat soluble vitamins, as volumes increase beyond 360-400 ml/day. The discharge nutrition plan is given to the parents and all health care professionals who participate in follow-up of the infant after discharge, including the community pediatrician, infant follow-up clinic, and WIC clinic.

Premature Formulas

Premature infants whose mothers have decided not to breast-feed may be given a formula specifically designed for preterm infants. These formulas include Similac Special Care (SSC) (Ross), and Enfamil Premature Formula (EPF) (Mead Johnson).[65,66] SSC and EPF are available in 20 and 24 kcal/oz dilutions and with and without supplemental iron. The AAP recommends the use of iron-fortified infant formulas for all infants.[96] Although SSC and EPF are both "premature formulas," they vary in their nutrient content. Careful comparison of current nutrient composition prior to choosing a formula for premature babies is advised.

The carbohydrate composition of premature formulas is a combination of lactose and glucose polymers. In theory, the preterm infant's ability to use lactose is marginal as a result of lactase activity that develops late in gestation[97,98] (see Chapter 14). Early feeding may increase intestinal lactase activity in premature infants.[99] In practice, lactose intolerance is rarely a problem, as evidenced by the many VLBW babies who tolerate human milk and lactose-containing formulas with little or no difficulty. This may be explained in part by the utilization of undigested lactose in the colon.[97] The presence of lactose may facilitate absorption of calcium and other minerals,[100] although recent studies do no support this claim.[101,102] Glucose polymers may enhance calcium absorption in premature infants.[102] The use of glucose polymers results in low osmolality,[102] and they appear to be well tolerated and well utilitzed.[102-105]

The protein in premature formulas is whey-predominant protein derived from cow's milk. Whey protein contains more cystine and less methionine than casein, which may be more suitable for a preterm infant who has limited enzymes to convert methionine to cystine.[106] Premature infants fed a whey-predominant protein may not have improved growth or nitrogen retention compared with those given casein-predominant protein.[107] There may be differences, however, in both plasma and urinary amino acid concentrations between the two groups. Infants fed whey-predominant protein may have greater cystine intake and retention as well as greater taurine stores. Although the issue is controversial, there does not appear to be a difference in gastric emptying rates in infants fed whey versus casein predominant formulas.[108,109] Use of a whey-predominant formula may decrease the potential for development of lactobezoars in premature infants.[110-113] Overall, the above data support the theoretical advantages of whey-predominant protein for the premature infant.

All premature formulas contain greater amounts of protein than do standard infant formulas. This increased protein provides optimal protein intake of > 3 g/kg/day at an intake of 120 kcal/kg/day. Nitrogen retention is directly related to protein intake; the ratio of protein to energy may affect the composition of deposited tissue.[114-116] Studies suggest that intakes of about 3.5 g/kg/day of protein and 110-130 kcal/kg/day are well tolerated metabolically, support better nitrogen retention, and result in more rapid weight gain than intakes of 2.24 g/kg/day of protein.[116-118] The AAP currently recommends 3.5-4.0 g/kg/day of protein and 2.9-3.3 g protein/100 kcal for infants weighing < 1800 g at birth.[119] Similar recommendations by others are available.[120,121] These recommendations are easily met by premature formulas commercially available in the United States.

Fats provide about 47% of the total calories in premature formulas. The fat consists of a combination of vegetable oils providing both long-chain and medium-chain triglycerides (MCTs). Low concentrations of duodenal bile acids and pancreatic lipase found in both full-term and preterm infants explain the fat malabsorption sometimes observed in the neonatal period.[122,123] Intravenous lipid emulsions may promote the development of lipase activity in gastric aspirates.[124] Fat from human milk or formula (different fat blends) and different fat particle sizes does not appear to affect the level of activity of gastric enzymes.[125] The contribution of gastric lipase to overall fat absorption may be greater in the newborn (a period of pancreatic insufficiency) compared with adults.[125]

About 50% of the fat in premature formulas is in the form of MCTs. The addition of MCT to these formulas does not affect G.I. tolerance, and may enhance calcium absorption, promote nitrogen retention, lipogenesis, and weight gain, and improve fat absorption,[126-129] although the effect on fat absorption is controversial.[130,131] MCTs are absorbed as medium-chain free fatty acids (MCFA) without requiring micelle formation with bile salts.[132] MCTs are absorbed in the newborn's stomach.[133] Most MCFAs enter the mitochondria independent of carnitine. This may be significant in premature infants born with low carnitine tissue reserves and limited capability to synthesize carnitine.[132]

Dietary nonessential fatty acids such as MCTs may interfere with metabolism of DHA, an important long-chain polyunsaturated fatty acid (LC-PUFA).[129] Multiple clinical trials of preterm infants fed human milk, commercial infant formulas, and infant formulas supplemented with various sources of LC-PUFAs have been conducted. Effects on visual acuity and neurocognition are conflicting.[134-139] There is evidence of slower growth in preterm infants[140,141] and in infants with bronchopulmonary dysplasia fed formula supplemented with DHA and AA.[134] A randomized trial of premature infants fed human milk and/or nutrient-enriched formulas with and without AA and DHA showed no significant benefit or disadvantage.[142] Research in this area is ongoing. Commercially available premature formulas in the United States are not supplemented with DHA or AA. Current recommendations do not support the addition of AA or DHA to infant formulas at this time.[143,144]

Recommendations for linoleic acid and linolenic acid and vitamin E to PUFA ratios have been reviewed and are available.[106,118-120,143,144-147] The premature formulas meet or exceed the recommendations (see Chapter 15).

Mineral content of the premature formulas is higher compared with term infant formulas. The calcium (Ca) and phosphorus (P) content is probably one of the most important differences in formula composition. Ca and P, along with magnesium (Mg) and vitamin D, play a vital role in bone mineralization in the preterm infant. Ca needs of up to 200 mg/kg/day and P needs of up to 113 mg/kg/day[148] or higher[120] can be met by SSC or EPF. The Ca to P ratio is 2:1 in both formulas. The Mg content of EPF and SSC is 55 mg/dl and 100 mg/dl, respectively. As VLBW infants achieve intakes of Ca and P to allow retention equivalent to in-utero accretion rates, Mg absorption and retention decreases, suggesting that Mg needs are increased as well.[149] Both EPF and SSC exceed the recommendations for Mg content.[144] Numerous metabolic balance studies using SSC have been conducted and summarized.[150] Infants fed SSC absorb and retain enough calcium to match in-utero accretion.[151] Bone mineralization and growth have not been studied in the new (present) formulation of EPF; however, good mineralization and growth would be expected.[152] Macromineral needs and bone mineralization in preterm infants have been reviewed[153] and are discussed in Chapter 29. The early nutritional environment of the preterm infant may play an important role in determining later skeletal growth and mineralization.[154]

Both SSC and EPF are available iron fortified. Iron was well absorbed in infants fed EPF with added iron.[155] A study using SSC with high iron (15 mg/L) versus low iron (3 mg/L) suggests that preterm infants < 1,800 g benefit from the high-iron formula.[156] An intake of 150 ml/kg/day provides about 2 mg/kg/day of iron. Additional iron may be needed for VLBW infants.[119,157] The electrolyte content of premature formulas is greater than that in standard formulas in order to support growth and to replace dermal, urine, and stool losses.[150]

Levels of vitamin supplementation are higher in the premature formulas than in standard infant formulas. Increased concentration is necessary for the premature infant taking relatively small volumes of formula. Premature infants also have altered vitamin needs compared with term infants. Vitamin supplementation may be necessary in some clinical situations. Guidelines for vitamin supplementation have been established[118-120] (see Chapter 15).

Nutrient-Enriched Follow-up Formulas for Premature Infants

Nutrition management of the premature infant after discharge is an active area of research. Infants once given a premature formula and hospitalized until they reached five pounds are now being discharged at a weight less than half that of a term baby and often on formulas not designed for their needs. Casey et al. followed 985 premature LBW infants until 3 years corrected age.[158] Growth patterns for these infants were lower than published standards for term infants of the same age and sex. There was little catch-up growth by 36 months.[158] Hack and co-workers followed 249 VLBW infants born from 1977 to 1979 for eight years.[159] At 40 weeks, 54% of infants were subnormal in weight; at 8 months 33% were subnormal in weight; and by 8 years, 8% were subnormal in weight.[159] Inappropriate feeding during infancy may contribute to poor growth at 1 year of age.[160]

In a randomized, double-blind trial, a nutrient enriched "postdischarge" formula was compared with standard infant formula in 32 formula-fed infants < 1,850 g at birth.[161] Infants fed the enriched formula up to a postnatal age of 9 months had significant increases in linear growth and weight gain.[161] Premature infants fed a standard versus a nutrient-enriched formula ad libitum voluntarily consumed similar volumes, but those given the nutrient-enriched formula had greater energy, protein, and mineral intake.[162] Lucas evaluated bone mineralization in 31 infants fed either standard or nutrient-enriched formula after discharge and noted a significant increase in bone mineral content for the enriched group at 3 and 9 months corrected age.[163]

Wheeler and Hall, who evaluated use of term versus premature formula or human milk after discharge, found infants < 1,800 g at birth may benefit from continuation of a preterm formula.[164] With only one exception,[165] these and other studies support the use of nutrient-enriched formulas for preterm infants after discharge.[161-164,166,167]

The AAP recommends use of a nutrient-enriched formula to a corrected postnatal age of 9 months.[119]

Similac NeoSure (formerly Similac NeoCare) (Ross) and Enfamil EnfaCare (formerly Enfamil 22) (Mead Johnson) are two nutrient-enriched formulas available for feeding preterm infants after discharge from the hospital. (A nutrient comparison is included in Appendix K.) Both formulas are available ready to feed for hospital use and in powdered form for home use. When prepared according to directions from the manufacturer, both formulas are 22 cal/oz. Scoop sizes are altered to provide the appropriate dilution at the higher calorie level compared to other 20 cal/oz formulas.

The nutrient composition of these two formulas vary, but in general they are similar to the formulation used by Lucas et al.[161] The carbohydrate source is lactose and glucose polymers and the protein is 60:40 whey/casein for EnfaCare and 50:50 for NeoSure. The fat source is a blend of MCT and vegetable oils. Both have higher levels of protein, minerals, and vitamins compared with term infant formulas, but they have lower levels of these nutrients than premature formulas. Studies conducted documenting the efficacy of Similac NeoSure include those on growth,[166,168,169] fat, nitrogen, and mineral retention,[170] and plasma amino acid profiles.[171] Infants fed Similac NeoSure compared with Similac With Iron (both Ross products) had improved weight gain to two months adjusted age and better length gains over the entire study period.[172] Limited clinical studies using EnfaCare were conducted prior to its release; however there is a clinical trial in progress at this writing.[173] The issue of postdischarge feeding of premature infants has been reviewed.[174] Follow-up after discharge by clinicians knowledgeable in nutrition management for premature infants is essential (see Chapters 33 and 34).

Standard Infant Formulas

When breast-feeding is not possible, or breast milk supply is inadequate, an iron-fortified formula is recommended for feeding the term infant. Standard cow's milk-based formulas are the feeding of choice.[175] Enfamil (Mead Johnson) and Improved Similac (Ross) are both available in a hospital feeding system and as powder, concentrated liquid, and ready-to-feed in the retail market. The generic store brands sold at grocery stores and discount department stores is the formula formerly known as SMA (Wyeth Laboratories, Philadelphia, PA).

Cow's milk-based formulas for special circumstances include Enfamil Lacto-Free, Enfamil AR (both Mead Johnson), and Similac Lactose Free and Similac PM 60/40 (both Ross). These formulas are not reviewed in detail; their nutrient composition is outlined in Appendix K. Lactose is the primary carbohydrate source with the exception of the lactose-free formulas. Lactose-free formulas contain glucose polymers but are not indicated for galacotsemia, as they contain trace amounts of lactose.[175] The protein and fat compositions of the formulas vary.

Enfamil and generic store brands have a 60:40 whey/casein ratio. Improved Similac contains 50:50 whey/casein. Previously, Similac was casein-predominant 18:82. The protein source in standard formulas is bovine protein. While whey-predominant formulas may appear "closer to human milk" in the ratio of protein than casein-predominant formulas, bovine whey is a different protein from human milk whey and has an amino acid composition that is quite different from human milk.[176,177] The benefit of using a whey-predominant protein in term infants is not clear.[178,179]

Altering the whey/casein ratio to 60:40 will not achieve the desired blood levels unique to infants fed human milk unless the total N content of the formula is reduced.[178] Likewise, use of whey-predominant formulas for term infants results in no nutritional advantages with respect to growth, estimated body fat, or lean body tissue compared to casein-predominant formula or human milk.[179] Infants on Improved Similac have serum amino acid profiles similar to those of breast-fed infants.[180] Many factors influence serum amino acid patterns, including protein fed, time of blood sampling, age of infant, laboratory procedure and equipment used, and interpretation of results.[181]

Data from eight studies were collected to evaluate stool consistency in infants fed Enfamil, Improved Similac, and human milk. Appropriate combinations and ratios of protein and vegetable oils may modify stool consistency to be similar to that of breast-fed infants.[182]

Standard infant formulas contain a variety of vegetable oils that provide nearly 50% of the total calories. Fat blends are formulated to provide a desired concentration of saturated, monounsaturated, and polyunsaturated fatty acids. Corn oil is a good source of the essential fatty acid (EFA) linoleic acid, while soy oil provides both linoleic and α-linolenic acid.[181] Ratios of these EFAs have been recommended in order to achieve adequate production of AA and DHA.[143,144,183] Biochemistry of fats and fatty acids has been reviewed.[181,184] Palm olein is present in Enfamil and Lacto-free to provide levels of palmitic and oleic acids similar to breast milk. The calcium and fat is less well absorbed from formulas that contain palm olein and soy oil as compared with formulas with soy and coconut oils, presumably because of the formation of insoluble calcium soaps with unabsorbed palmitic acid.[185-187]

The addition of preformed long-chain polyunsaturated fatty acids such as DHA and AA is not recommended at this time.[143] No infant formula currently on the market in the United States contains supplemental DHA and AA. It is an area of intense research. The role of nutrition in the development of normal cognition has been reviewed.[188] A prospective, longitudinal study of healthy term infants resulted in no detectable enhancement in visual acuity from DHA/AA supplemented formula compared with the standard fat blend.[189] Growth was similar in both groups. The authors did not support adding DHA or AA to standard infant formulas.[189] Infants fed formula with no supplemental DHA or AA compared with others fed human milk had no significant differences in visual acuity or cognitive development, suggesting that DHA and AA are not essential for development of these parameters in healthy term infants.[190] Other studies have been done on infants fed formula supplemented with cholesterol.[191-193] There are no recommendations for the addition of cholesterol to infant formula at this time.[143]

Supplementation of infant formula with nucleotides is another area of much research. Nucleotides are precursors of nucleic acid synthesis[194] and are a source of nonprotein nitrogen. The possible benefits of nucleotides include:[195]

- Enhanced immune response
- Greater iron availability
- Modifications in intestinal microflora
- Changes in plasma lipoproteins and other lipids
- Promotion of gut growth and maturation

Nucleotide nitrogen accounts for 0.4-0.6% of the nonprotein nitrogen content of human milk.[196] A new method to determine the nucleotide content of human milk has been developed.[197] Recent data suggest that the traditional method used to measure free nucleotide content of human milk underestimates the total nucleotides available to the infant by $\geq 50\%$. Studies prior to 1995 may not have used high enough levels of supplemental nucleotides to achieve the average total potentially available nucleosides (TPAN) available in human milk.[197-199] A recent 12-month, controlled, randomized and blinded multisite trial was conducted with 370 term infants fed infant formula with or without nucleotides, or human milk plus formula without nucleotides.[200] The formula group with supplemented nucleotides received nucleotides at a level of 72 mg/L and a ratio of individual nucleotides patterned after those available in human milk. In this study, infant formula fortified with nucleotides enhanced the Haemophilus influenzae type b (HIB) and diptheria humoral antibody responses, and human milk enhanced the antibody response to oral polio virus. These findings suggest that nutrition factors play a role in the antibody response of infants to immunization.[200] Nucleotides may also decrease diarrheal disease in infants.[198,199,201] The Life Science Research Office (LSRO) does not recommend the addition of nucleotides at this time, however; they consider the safe upper limit to be 16 mg/100 cal.[143] The Infant Formula Act has no minimum recommendations.[144]

Standard infant formulas are available low-iron and iron-fortified. No significant differences have been reported in the prevalence of fussiness, cramping, regurgitation, colic, and flatus or in stool characteristics (except color) between term infants fed low-iron and iron-fortified formulas.[202] Infants receiving therapeutic doses of iron up to 6 mg/kg/day tolerate it well.[203] The AAP's newest recommendations state that:[96]

- Infants who are not breastfed should receive a formula containing between 4.0-12.0 mg/Liter of iron from birth to 12 months.
- The manufacturing of "low-iron" formulas containing < 4.0 mg/L should be discontinued.
- If low-iron formulas continue to be made, a warning label should notify consumers of potential risks of iron deficiency anemia.
- The "with iron" statement should be removed from the label and iron content should be included in the nutrition information.
- Parents and clinicians should be educated about the role of iron in growth and cognitive development.

All standard infant formulas are supplemented with taurine in concentrations similar to those of human milk. Taurine has many biological roles, and research findings suggest that supplementation in formulas is indicated.[204] The Infant Formula Act has no recommendations for taurine, but the LSRO recommends a maximum of 12 mg/dl.[143,144]

Soy Formulas

Soy protein formulas differ from standard cow's milk-based formulas in carbohydrate and protein content. The fat blends in each soy formula, however, are similar to the standard formula made by the same company, and all soy formulas have added L-carnitine.[181] Soy formulas are lactose-free, with varying carbohydrate sources. Isomil (Ross) contains corn syrup and sucrose, Prosobee (Mead Johnson) contains corn syrup solids, and the generic store brands, formerly Nursoy (Wyeth), contain sucrose. Ross Carbohydrate Free (RCF, Ross) contains no carbohydrate; thus, any carbohydrate can be added that meets the infant's needs.

If an infant cannot tolerate lactose, as in galactosemia or in primary lactase deficiency, a soy formula may be appropriate. A secondary lactase deficiency can occur with acute diarrhea. Other disaccaridases may be affected as well.[181] Formula choice in refeeding infants with acute diarrhea is controversial. Some recommend use of a lactose-free formula for severe or persistent gastroenteritis,[205-207] but infants with mild, acute diarrhea may not require a lactose-free formula.[175,206,208,209] Rationale for use of the sucrose-free formulas has been reviewed,[210] as has carbohydrate intolerance.[211] Isomil DF (Ross) is a soy formula with added dietary fiber. Clinical trials suggest that use of fiber-supplemented soy formula may reduce the duration of symptoms in older infants and children with diarrhea.[212,213]

Soy formulas contain soy protein isolate with L-methionine added to improve protein quality in comparison with casein in cow's milk. The quantity of protein is higher in soy formula than in standard formulas in order to compensate for the lower biological value of soy protein. The increased amount of protein does not excessively increase the renal solute load.[214,215] Although cow's milk protein allergy is relatively uncommon, some clinicians would consider use of a soy formula in patients with a strong family history of allergy, or IgE-associated cow's milk allergy.[216,277] Soy protein can be as allergenic as cow's milk protein, and is not recommended for the routine management of cow's milk protein allergy or for colic.[217-219]

Soy formulas have been shown to promote normal growth in healthy, full-term infants, but several issues should be considered when feeding soy formulas to these infants as well as to high-risk infants.[219] Bone mineral content (BMC) may be decreased in term infants fed soy formula compared with infants fed cow's milk-based formula but is about the same as in infants given human milk.[220,221] If vitamin D is sufficient, however, term infants fed human milk, cow's milk-based formula, or soy formula attain similar levels of serum minerals and BMC.[222] Routine use of a soy formula is undesirable in feeding VLBW infants.[223] Premature infants fed soy formula have significantly lower serum phosphorus levels than milk-fed infants.[223] Premature infants who require soy for extended periods due to feeding intolerance should be monitored for potential adverse effects on bone mineralization.[219,223]

The AAP recommends the use of soy formula for:[219]

- Term infants whose nutritional needs are not met from breast milk or cow's milk formulas. There is no advantage of soy formulas over milk-based formulas for breastfed infants
- Infants with galactosemia
- Infants with hereditary lactase deficiency
- Parents who desire a vegetarian-based diet for their infant
- Infants with documented lactose intolerance
- Infants with documented IgE-mediated allergy to cow's milk protein

Soy formulas are not recommended for:[219]

- Premature infants who weigh < 1,800 g at birth
- Routine use in the prevention of atopic disease in healthy or high-risk infants
- Infants with documented cow's milk protein-induced enteropathy

Elemental and Semi-elemental Formulas

Dietary protein, specifically cow's milk protein and soy protein, are the most commonly implicated dietary proteins causing adverse reactions in infants.[224] Terminology for adverse reactions to ingested food is standardized to include three general categories:[225]

- *Food anaphylaxis*—classic, immediate allergic reaction involving IgE antibody and release of chemical mediators

- *Food hypersensitivity*—immunologic reaction which may or may not involve IgE antibody

- *Food Intolerance*—abnormal physiologic response including idiosyncratic, metabolic, pharmacologic or toxic reactions

Diagnosis for food allergy in infants has been reviewed.[226,227] Three reasons infants are prone to protein-induced intestinal hypersensitivity are: immaturity of the mucosal immune defense system;[228] the large antigenic load resulting from use of formulas with intact protein; and disorders that increase intestinal permeability, such as prematurity or reflux esophagitis.[224,229] If breast milk is not available, most of these infants will respond to use of a casein or whey hydrolysate.[230] Alimentum (Ross), Nutramigen, and Pregestimil (both Mead Johnson) contain enzymatically hydrolyzed casein (casein hydrolysate). The amino acids L-cystine, L-tyrosine, and L-tryptophan are decreased in the manufacturing process. The formulas are then supplemented with these three amino acids to restore the products to appropriate levels. All three formulas are considered to be hypoallergenic based on the molecular weight of the peptides, which is < 1,200 daltons.[231] Good Start (Carnation, Glendale, CA), derived from whey, contains some peptides with a molecular weight > 2,000 daltons.[231] This formula may be more pleasant-tasting and smelling, as it does not contain free amino acids, but is not considered "hypoallergenic." There have been case reports of anaphylaxis in infants fed a whey hydrolysate formula.[232] No evidence supports the use of hydrolysates in the treatment of colic, sleeplessness, and irritability unless these symptoms are due to cow's milk allergy.[231]

An amino-acid–based, elemental formula powder for infants has been developed. Neocate (SHS North America, Gaithersburg, MD) contains 100% free amino acids and may be indicated for infants with multiple food allergies.[233] Although most infants with protein-induced colitis respond to a casein hydrolysate, some infants demonstrate resolution of their symptoms only when changed from a casein hydrolysate to a free amino acid formula.[234]

The fat and carbohydrate composition of the semielemental and elemental formulas varies and affects their indications for use.

Nutramigen is the only one of these formulas with no MCT as part of the fat component. Corn and soy oils used in infant formulas are highly refined and purified and can be used in hypoallergenic formulas without concern for allergic reactions.[181] Alimentum is the only one of these formulas with part of the carbohydrate from a source other than corn syrup solids. (See Appendix K for details concerning sources of macronutrients.)

Infants with chylothorax or chylous ascites may benefit from a formula that contains MCT oil. Portagen (Mead Johnson) contains > 80% of the fat as MCT but has intact cow's milk protein (and therefore is not considered semi-elemental). Infants fed Portagen may be at risk for essential fatty acid deficiency, and supplementation with EFAs may be necessary.[235,236]

Literature has been published on the indications and use of elemental and semi-elemental infant formulas.[224,233,234,237-248] Elemental/semi-elemental products for infants over 1 year of age include EleCare (Ross), Neocate One+ (SHS North America), Vivonex Pediatric (Novartis, Minneapolis, MN), and Peptamen Jr. (Nestle, Deerfield, IL). Nutrient compositions are included in Appendix K.

Increased Caloric Density Formulas

Many infants require formulas greater than the standard 20 kcal/oz for a variety of reasons, including:

- Maintenance of a fluid restriction with or without increased energy needs
- Decreased energy or strength to take all formula by nipple
- Increased energy expenditure
- Malabsorption of carbohydrate or fat
- Earlier transition from gavage feedings to nipple feedings

These infants may benefit from a formula with increased caloric density. Increasing the caloric density increases the osmolality of the formula, but most infants will tolerate gradual, incremental changes. Some formulas are available in ready-to-feed, calorically dense forms, whereas others must be prepared from available concentrates or powders. Creative "recipes" often provide the nutrients needed when ready-to-feed formulas are not available. (See Appendices I and J for examples of these.)

A detailed monograph has been published on preparation and use of concentrated formulas and calorie supplements.[249] Modular supplements, such as glucose polymers and oils, can be added to increase caloric density,[250] but provision of nonprotein calories alone will alter the nutrient ratios of the formula. Concentrating a formula by adding less water to a concentrated liquid or powder usually results in a more balanced solution. Registered dietitians are uniquely qualified to assess the composition of an altered infant formula and monitor an infant's response.[250,251] Practical suggestions to consider when using an increased caloric density formula at discharge are listed below.

- Ensure appropriate measuring devices are available in the home
- Communicate the follow-up plan to the pediatrician, infant follow-up clinic and/or WIC clinic
- Use concentrated liquid in recipes as often as possible to increase the accuracy of the caloric density
- Use formula powders only in carefully selected situations, as they can result in inconsistent caloric density, depending on how the measuring device or scoop is packed
- Choose concentrating formula as the preferred method of increasing caloric density to maintain balance of nutrients and increase ease of mixing
- Choose modular supplements when additional calories or protein are needed, but other nutrient requirements are met; assess nutrient balance
- Analyze the nutrient content of all special formulations and compare to intake recommendations for age (Use of a computer program, such as Neonova Nutrition Optimizer [Ross], is recommended—see Chapter 6).

Osmolality

Osmolality is the measurement of the osmotic concentration of a solution. It represents the dissociation of particles in the solution and is expressed as milliosmoles per kilogram of water (mOsm/kg H_2O). The osmolality of serum is approximately 300 mOsm/kg H_2O. Feedings higher or lower than 300 mOsm/kg H_2O are hyperosmolar or hypoosmolar, respectively. Osmolality is affected most by the carbohydrate and mineral content of the formula; protein and fat contribute to a lesser extent.[181] Fortification increases the osmolality of human milk (see Table 16.4).[273] Hyperosmolar products have been known to cause osmotic diarrhea.[252] The AAP recommends that formulas for infants have concentrations of no greater than 450 mOsm/kg water.[253] Most infants have no difficulty tolerating formulas up to 30 kcal/oz if the caloric density is gradually increased. Medications, including vitamin/mineral supplements, given with formula often alter the osmolality to a much greater extent than the formula composition itself. Use of an I.V. preparation of a medicine, e.g., potassium chloride administered orally with feedings, may cause less of a rise in osmolality than that caused by drugs suspended in syrups. Values for osmolalities of products used in the NICU are available.[250,252,254-258] (Appendixes C, H and K list the osmolality of selected medications and enteral products, respectively; Appendix H describes methods for calculating the osmolality of formula/medication mixtures.)

Renal Solute Load

Renal solute load (RSL) refers to all solutes, either endogenous or dietary, that must be excreted by the kidneys. RSL is derived primarily from the nitrogen and electrolyte content of the diet.[259] *Potential renal solute load* (PRSL) refers to solutes that must be excreted in the urine if none are used for protein synthesis or are lost through other nonrenal routes.[259] PRSL is expressed as mOsm/L or as mOsm/100 kcal. Upper limits of 277 mOsm/L and 30-35 mOsm/100 kcal have been proposed for infant formulas.[143,259-261] Actual renal solute load is calculated by subtracting the portion of RSL used for growth and lost through nonrenal routes from the PRSL.[259] (Calculations for PRSL, estimated actual renal solute load, and urine osmolality are included in Appendix H.)

Knowledge of PRSL is important when (1) fluid intake is low, (2) fluid losses are high, (3) growth is suboptimal, (4) highly concentrated formulas are ingested, and/or (5) renal concentrating ability is limited.[262] If one or several of these conditions occur, the infant may mobilize body water for excretion of solute. This could possibly lead to dehydration. Infants may require additional free water during febrile illness, especially when formulas with increased caloric density are fed.[259]

Preparation of Formula for Hospitalized Infants

Guidelines for preparation of special formulas for health care facilities have been published.[263] Development of the guidelines was accomplished with the cooperation and contribution of many organizations, including the ADA, the AAP, the American Nurses Association, and the Food and Drug Administration. Although the recommendations are not "regulations," they furnish guidelines for providing optimal care for infants with special nutritional needs.[263] Important points are highlighted:[263]

- Aseptic technique is recommended over terminal sterilization, reducing the risk of nutrient loss.
- Commercially prepared sterile water supplied by manufacturers of infant formulas is the preferred 'ingredient water' to reconstitute concentrated liquid or formula powders.

- Municipal, distilled, or other bottled water may be used if it has been brought to a full rolling boil for five minutes.
- Powdered ingredients are weighed using a gram scale.
- Formulas are mixed with a blender or other appropriate device until all lumps disappear.
- Microwave ovens are never used in the formula room or for warming formula in the patient care area.
- Infant formula orders are documented in writing.
- Bottles are labeled with patient's name, medical record number, location, formula name plus additives, caloric density, volume, expiration date and time; labels state "for enteral use only" and "refrigerate until used."
- Refrigerator temperatures are maintained between 35° and 45° F
- Flowing warm water, or warmers that do not permit contact of bottles or hands with standing water, are used to warm formula in bottles.

Summary

Human milk has distinct advantages for all infants, including preterm and high-risk newborns. Human milk's composition is complex and variable. Excellent resources are available.[264,278] Infant formulas are almost constantly changing. Recommendations for composition are published,[143,144] and opportunities for improvements have been outlined.[265] Use of modular products may be indicated and requires careful assessment and follow-up.[250] Despite the best efforts of professional staff, the intake of critically ill infants often falls short of known nutrient needs.[266] Understanding the composition of and indications for the wide variety of enteral products available presents a unique opportunity for improving the nutritional status of the high-risk newborn.

References

1. American Academy of Pediatrics Work Group on Breastfeeding. Breastfeeding and the use of human milk. Pediatrics 100:1035, 1997.
2. American Dietetic Association. Position of the American Dietetic Association: promotion of breast feeding. J Am Diet Assoc 86:1580, 1986.
3. Schanler RJ, O'Connor KG, Lawrence RA. Pediatricians' practices and attitudes regarding breastfeeding promotion. Pediatrics 103(3):E35, 1999.
4. Hurst NM, Myatt A, Schanler RJ. Growth and development of a hospital-based lactation program and mother's own milk bank. J Obstet Gynecol Neonatal Nurs 27:503, 1998.

5. Schanler RJ, Hurst NM, Lau C. The use of human milk and breast-feeding in premature infants. Clin Perinatol 26(2):379, 1999.
6. Arnold LDW. Use of banked donor milk in the United States. Building block for life, Pediatric Nutrition Practice Group, American Dietetic Association, 23(1):1, 1999.
7. Human Milk Banking Association of North America, Inc: Guidelines for the establishment and operation of a donor human milk bank. Arnold LDW, Tully MR, eds. Sandwich, Mass.:HMBANA. 1998.
8. American Academy of Pediatrics Committee on Pediatric AIDS, Human milk, breastfeeding and transmission of human immunodeficiency virus in the United States. Pediatrics. 96:977, 1995.
9. American Academy of Pediatrics Committee on Infectious Diseases. Recommendations for care of children in special circumstances: Human milk. In: 1997 Red book, report of the Committee on Infectious Diseases. 24th ed. Elk Grove Village, Ill.: AAP, 1997; pp. 73-79.
10. American Academy of Pediatrics Committee on Drugs. The transfer of drugs and other chemicals into human milk. Pediatrics 93(1):137, 1994.
11. Bailey B, Ito S. Breast-feeding and maternal drug use. Pediatr Clin North Am 44(1):41, 1997.
12. Howard CR, Lawrence RA. Drugs and breastfeeding. Clin Perinatol 26(2):447, 1999.
13. Lawrence RA, Howard CR. Given the benefits of breastfeeding: Are there any contraindications? Clin Perinatol 26(2):479, 1999.
14. American Academy of Pediatrics, American College of Obstetricians and Gynecologists. Maternal and newborn nutrition. In: Guidelines for perinatal care. 4th ed. Elk Grove Village, Ill.:AAP, 1997.
15. World Health Organization. Consensus statement from the WHO/UNICEF consultation on HIV transmission and breast feeding; April 20–May 1, 1992; Geneva, Switzerland.
16. Briggs GG, Freeman RK, Yaffe JS. In: Drugs in pregnancy and lactation. Baltimore:Williams and Wilkins, 1994.
17. Hytten FE. Clinical and chemical studies in human lactation. II. Variations in major constituents during a feeding. Br Med J 1:176, 1954.
18. Hytten FE. Clinical and chemical studies in human lactation. III. Diurnal variations in major constituents of milk. Br Med J 1:179, 1954.
19. Hytten FE. Clinical and chemical studies in human lactation. IV. Trends in milk composition during course of lactation. Br Med J 1:239, 1954.
20. Macy IG, Mims G, Brown M, et al. Human milk studies. VII. Chemical analysis of milk representative of the entire first and last halves of the nursing period. Am J Dis Child 42:569, 1931.
21. Lawrence, RA, Lawrence RM, eds. Breastfeeding: A guide for the medical profession. 5th ed. St. Louis: Mosby, 1999; 95-158, 451.
22. Anderson GH, Atkinson SA, Bryan MH. Energy and macronutrient content of human milk during early lactation from mothers giving birth prematurely and at term. Am J Clin Nutr 34:258, 1981.
23. Gross SJ, Geller J, Tomarelli RM. Composition of breast milk from mothers of preterm infants. Pediatrics 68:490, 1981.
24. Lemons JA, Moye L, Hall D, et al. Differences in the composition of preterm and term human milk during early lactation. Pediatr Res 16:113, 1982.

25. Sann L, Bienvenu F, Lahet C, et al. Comparison of the composition of breast milk from mothers of term and preterm infants. Acta Paediatr Scand 70:115, 1981.

26. Anderson DM, Williams FH, Merkatz RB, et al. Length of gestation and nutritional composition of human milk. Am J Clin Nutr 37:810, 1983.

27. Kunz C, Rodriquez-Palmero M, Koletzko B, Jensen R. Nutritional and biochemical properties of human milk, Part I: General aspects, proteins and carbohydrates. Clin Perinatol 26(2):307, 1999.

28. Rodriquez-Palmero M, Koletzko B, Kunz C, Jensen R. Nutritional and biochemical properties of human milk, Part II: Lipids, micronutrients, and bioactive factors. Clin Perinatol 26(2):335, 1999.

29. Garza C, Schanler RJ, Butte NF, et al. Special properties of human milk. Clin Perinatol 14:11, 1982.

30. Klish WJ, Udall JN, Rodriguez JT, et al. Intestinal surface area in infants with acquired monosaccharide intolerance. J Pediatr 92:566, 1978.

31. Lonnerdal B, Forsum E. Hambraeus L. A longitudinal study of the protein, nitrogen, and lactose contents of human milk from Swedish well-nourished mothers. Am J Clin Nutr 29:1127, 1976.

32. Steichen JJ., Krug-Wispe SK, Tsang RC. Breastfeeding the low birth weight preterm infant. Clin Perinatol 14:131, 1987.

33. Kunz C, Lönnerdal B. Re-evaluation of whey protein/casein ratio of human milk. Acta Paediatr Scand 81:107, 1992.

34. Lonnerdal B, Forsum E. Casein content of human milk. Am J Clin Nutr 41:113, 1985.

35. Montagne P, Cuilliere ML, Mole C, et al. Immunological and nutritional composition of human milk in relation to prematurity and mothers' parity during the first 2 weeks of lactation. J Pediatr Gastroenterol Nutr 29:75, 1999.

36. Forsum E, Lönnerdal B. Protein evaluation of breast milk and breast milk substitutes with special reference to the nonprotein nitrogen: effect of protein intake on protein and nitrogen composition of breast milk. Am J Clin Nutr 33:1809, 1980.

37. Carlson SE. Human milk nonprotein nitrogen: occurrence and possible function. Adv Pediatr 32:43, 1985.

38. Hamosh M, Bitman J, Wood DL, et al. Lipids in milk and the first steps in their digestion. Pediatrics 75(suppl):146, 1984.

39. Koletzko, B. Importance of dietary lipids. In: Tsang RC, Zlotkin SH, Nichols BL, Hansen JW, eds. Nutrition during infancy 2d ed. Cincinnati: Digital Educational Publishing, 1997; 123-53.

40. Innis SM. Human milk and formula fatty acids. J Pediatr 120:S56, 1992.

41. Wagner CL, Anderson DM, Pittard WB. Special properties of human milk. Clin Pediatr 35(6):283, 1996.

42. Luukkainen P, Salo MK, Nikkari T. Changes in the fatty acid composition of preterm and term human milk from 1 week to 6 months of lactation. J Pediatr Gastroenterol Nutr 18:355, 1994.

43. Schanler RJ. Human milk for preterm infants: Nutritional and immune factors. Semin Perinatol 13:69, 1989.

44. Hamosh M. Fat needs for term and preterm infants. In: Tsang RC, Nichols BL, eds. Nutrition during infancy. Philadelphia: Hanley and Belfus, 1988; 133-59.

45. Valentine CJ, Hurst NM, Schanler RJ. Hindmilk improves weight gain in low-birth-weight infants fed human milk. J Pediatr Gastroenterol Nutr 18:474, 1994.
46. Greer FR, McCormick A, and Joker J. Changes in fat concentration of human milk during delivery by intermittent bolus and continuous mechanical pump infusion. J Pediatr 105:745, 1984.
47. Brennan-Behm M, Carlson GE, Meier P, Engstrom J. Caloric loss from expressed mother's milk during continuous gavage infusion. Neonatal Network 12(2):27, 1994.
48. Bauer G, Ewald LS, Hoffman J, Dubanoski R. Breastfeeding and cognitive development of three-year-old children. Psychol Rep 68(2):1218, 1991.
49. Lucas A, Morley R, Cole TJ. Early diet in preterm babies and later intelligence quotient: a randomised trial. BMJ 317:1481, 1998.
50. Rogan WJ, Gladen BC. Breastfeeding and cognitive development. Early Hum Dev 31(3):181, 1993.
51. Morley R, Lucas A. Influence of early diet on outcome in preterm infants. Acta Paediatrica. 405:123, 1994.
52. Raiha NCR, Heinonen K, Rassin DK, et al. Milk protein quantity and quality in low-birthweight infants. I. Metabolic responses and effects on growth. Pediatrics 57:659, 1976.
53. Hambidge KM, Walravens PA, Casey CE, et al. Plasma zinc concentrations of breast-fed infants. J Pediatr 94:607, 1979.
54. McMillan JA, Landaw SA, Oski FA. Iron sufficiency in breast-fed infants and the availability of iron from human milk. Pediatrics 58:686, 1976.
55. Fomon SJ, Ziegler EE. Renal solute load and potential renal solute load in infancy. J Pediatr 134(1):11, 1999.
56. Pittard WB. Breast milk immunology. A frontier of infant nutrition. Am J Dis Child 133:83, 1979.
57. Slusser W, Powers NG. Breastfeeding update 1: Immunology, nutrition, and advocacy. Pediatr Rev 18(4):111, 1997.
58. Klaus MH, Kennell JH. Care of the parents. In: Klaus MH, Fanaroff AA, eds. Care of the high-risk neonate. Philadelphia: Saunders, 1986; 147-70.
59. Lucas A, Cole TJ. Breastmilk and neonatal necrotizing enterocolitis. Lancet 336:1519, 1990.
60. Kliegman RM, Pittard WM, Fanaroff AA. Necrotizing enterocolitis in neonates fed human milk. J Pediatr 95:450, 1979.
61. Schanler RJ, Shulman RJ, Lau C. Feeding strategies for premature infants: Beneficial outcomes of feeding fortified human milk versus preterm formula. Pediatr 103(6):1150, 1999.
62. Lucas A. Enteral nutrition. In: Tsang RC, Lucas A, Uauy R, Zlotkin S, eds. Nutritional needs of the preterm infant: Scientific basis and practical guidelines. Baltimore:Williams and Wilkins; 1993, 209-223.
63. American Academy of Pediatrics. Nutritional needs of preterm infants. In: Kleinman RE, ed. Pediatric nutrition handbook. 4th ed. Elk Grove Village, Ill.: AAP, 1998, 55 -87.
64. Schanler RJ. Human milk for the very low birthweight infant. Perinatol Neonatol 7:17, 1983.
65. Schanler RJ, Garza C, Nichols BL. Fortified mother's milk for very low birth weight infants: Results of growth and nutrient balance studies. J Pediatr 107:437, 1985.

66. Motil KJ. Protein needs for term and preterm infants. In: Tsang RC, Nichols BL, eds: Nutrition during infancy. Philadelphia: Hanley and Belfus, 1988; 100-21.

67. Fomon SJ, Ziegler EE, Vasquez HD. Human milk and the small premature infant. Am J Dis Child 131:463, 1977.

68. Mendelson RA, Bryan MH, Anderson GH. Trace mineral balances in preterm infants fed their own mother's milk. J Pediatr Gastroenterol Nutr 2:256, 1983.

69. Koo WWK, and Tsang RC: Calcium, Magnesium, Phosphorus, and Vitamin D. In: Tsang RC, Lucas A, Uauy R, Zlotkin S, eds. Nutritional needs of the preterm infant: Scientific basis and practical guidelines. Baltimore:Williams and Wilkins; 1993, 135-155.

70. Engelke SC, Shah BL, Vasan U, Raye JR. Sodium balance in very low-birth-weight infants. J Pediatr 93:837, 1978.

71. Zlotkin SH. Assessment of trace element requirements in newborns and young infants, including the infant born prematurely. In: Chandra RK, ed. Trace elements in nutrition of children-II. New York:Raven Press, 1991.

72. Mead Johnson. Enfamil Family Pediatric Products Handbook. Evansville, Ind.: Mead Johnson Nutritionals, 1999.

73. Pediatric Nutritionals Product Guide. Columbus, Ohio:Ross Products Division, Abbott Laboratories Inc., March, 1999.

74. Schanler RJ. Human milk fortification for premature infants (edit). Am J Clin Nutr 64:249, 1996

75. Lucas A, Fewtrell MS, Morley R, et al. Randomized outcome trial of human milk fortification and developmental outcome in preterm infants. Am J Clin Nutr 64:142, 1996.

76. Sankaran K, Papageorgiou A, Ninan A, et al. A randomized, controlled evaluation of two commercially available human breast milk fortifiers in healthy preterm neonates. J Am Diet Assoc 96:1145, 1996.

77. Wauben IP, Atkinson SA, Grad TL, et al. Moderate nutrient supplementation of mother's milk for preterm infants supports adequate bone mass and short-term growth: a randomized, controlled trial. Am J Clin Nutr 67:465, 1998.

78. Schanler RJ, Abrams SA. Postnatal attainment of intrauterine macromineral accretion rates in low birth weight infants fed fortified human milk. J Pediatr 126:441, 1995.

79. Schanler RJ, Henderson TR, Hamosh M. Fatty acid soaps may be responsible for poor fat absorption in premature infants fed fortified human milk (FHM). Pediatr Res 45(4):290A, 1999.

80. Carlson SJ, Johnson KJ, Cress, GA, et al. Higher protein intake improves growth of VLBW infants fed fortified breast milk. Pediatr Res 45(4):278A, 1999.

81. Wauben IP, Atkinson SA, Shah JK, et al. Growth and body composition of preterm infants: influence of nutrient fortification of mother's milk in hospital and breastfeeding post-hospital discharge. Acta Paediatr 87(7):780, 1998.

82. Warner JT, Linton HR, Dunstan FD, et al. Growth and metabolic responses in preterm infants fed fortified human milk or a preterm formula. Int J Clin Pract 52(4):236, 1998.

83. Kashyap S, Schulze KF, Forsyth M, et al. Growth, nutrient retention, and metabolic response of low-birth-weight infants fed supplemented and unsupplemented preterm human milk. Am J Clin Nutr 52:254, 1990.

84. Chan GM, Mileur L, and Hansen JW. Effects of increased calcium and phosphorus formulas and human milk on bone mineralization in preterm infants. J Pediatr Gastroenterol Nutr 5:444, 1986.

85. Greer F, McCormick A. Improved bone mineralization and growth in premature infants fed fortified own mother's milk. J Pediatr 112:961, 1988.

86. Moyer-Mileur L, Chan GM, McInnes R, et al. Effect on growth and bone mineralization status of preterm infants fed enriched human milk or formulas. Am J Clin Nutr 47:779, 1988.

87. Schanler RJ, Garza C. Improved mineral balance in very low birth-weight infants fed fortified human milk. J Pediatr 112:452, 1988.

88. Ventkataraman PS, Blick KE. Effect of mineral supplementation of human milk on bone mineral content and trace element metabolism. J Pediatr 113:220, 1988.

89. Fenton TR, Delisle SA, Tough SC. Osmolality of breast milk enriched with added formula powders. Pediatr Res 45(4):281A, 1999.

90. Jocson MAL, Mason EO, Schanler RJ. The effects of nutrient fortification and varying storage conditions on host defense properties of human milk. Pediatrics 100:240, 1997.

91. Quan R, Yang C, Rubinstein S, et al. The effect of nutritional additives on anti-infective factors in human milk. Clin Pediatr 33:325, 1994.

92. Hylander MA, Strobina DM, Dhanireddy R. Human milk feedings and infection among very low birth weight infants. Pediatrics 102(3):e38, 1998.

93. Thompson M, McClead RE. Human milk fortifiers. J Pediatr Perinatal Nutr 1:65, 1987.

94. Schanler RJ. Fortified human milk: Nature's way to feed premature infants. J Hum Lact 14(1):5, 1998.

95. Schanler RJ. The role of human milk fortification for premature infants. Clin Perinatol 25(3):645, 1998.

96. American Academy of Pediatrics Committee on Nutrition. Iron fortification of infant formulas. Pediatrics 104(1):119, 1999.

97. MacLean WC, Fink BB. Lactose malabsorption by premature infants: Magnitude and clinical significance. J Pediar 97:383, 1980.

98. Lebenthal E, Lee PC, Heitlinger LA. Impact of development of the gastrointestinal tract on infant feeding. J Pediatr 102:1, 1983.

99. Shulman, RJ, Schanler RJ, Lau C, et al. Early feeding, feeding tolerance, and lactase activity in preterm infants. J Pediatr 133(5):645, 1998.

100. Ziegler EE, Fomon SJ. Lactose enhances mineral absorption in infancy. J Pediatr Gastroenterol Nutr 2:288, 1983.

101. Wirth FH, Numerof B, Pleban P, et al. Effect of lactose on mineral absorption in preterm infants. J Pediatr 117:283, 1990.

102. Stathos TH, Shulman RJ, Schanler RJ, et al. Effect of carbohydrates on calcium absorption in premature infants. Pediatr Res 39(4):666, 1996.

103. Smith L, Darling P, Roy CC. Pitfalls in the design and manufacture of infant formulas. In: Lebenthal E, ed. Textbook of gastroenterology and nutrition in infancy. 2d ed. New York: Raven Press, 1989; 435-48.

104. Cicco R, Holzman IR, Brown DR, et al. Glucose polymers tolerance in premature infants. Pediatrics 67:498, 1981.

105. Williams PR, Andrews A, Penn D, et al. Comparison of glucose tolerance and and insulin responses of term infants fed glucose polymers (GP), glucose (G), and preterm infants fed glucose polymers (abstr). Clin Res 27:800A, 1979.

106. Brady MS, Rickard KA, Ernst JA, et al. Formulas and human milk for premature infants: A review and update. J Am Diet Assoc 81:547, 1982.

107. Kashyap S, Okamoto E, Kanaya S, et al. Protein quality in feeding low birth weight infants: A comparison of whey-predominant versus casein-predominant formulas. Pediatrics 79:748, 1987.

108. Lindberg T, Engberg S, Sjoberg LB, et al. In vitro digestion of proteins in human milk fortifiers and in preterm formulas. J Pediatr Gastroenterol Nutr 27:30, 1998.

109. Thorkelsson T, Mimouni F, Namgung R, et al. Similar gastric emptying rates for casein- and whey-predominant formulas in preterm infants. Pediatr Res 36:329, 1994.

110. Duritz G, Oltorf C. Lactobezoar formation with high-density caloric formula. Pediatrics 63:647, 1979.

111. Erenberg A, Shaw RD, Yousefzadeh D. Lactobezoar in the low-birth-weight infant. Pediatrics 63:642, 1979.

112. Schreiner RL, Brady MS, Franken EA, et al. Increased incidence of lactobezoars in low birth weight infants. Am J Dis Child 133:936, 1979.

113. Schreiner RL, Brady MS, Ernst JA, et al. Lack of lactobezoars in infants given predominantly whey protein formulas. Am J Dis Child 136:437, 1982.

114. Fairey AK, Butte NF, Mehta N, et al. Nutrient accretion in preterm infants fed formula with different protein:energy rations. J Pediatr Gastroenterol Nutr 25(1):37, 1997.

115. Kashyap S, Schulze KF, Ramakrishnan R, et al. Evaluation of a mathematical model for predicting the relationship between protein and energy intakes of low-birth-weight infants and the rate of composition of weight gain. Pediatr Res 35(6):704, 1994.

116. Towers HM, Schulze KF, Ramakrishnan R, et al. Energy expended by low birth weight infants in the deposition of protein and fat. Pediatr Res 41(4):584, 1997.

117. Schulze KF, Stefanski M, Masterson J, et al. Energy expenditure, energy balance, and composition of weight gain in low birthweight infants fed diets of different protein and energy content. J Pediatr 110:753, 1987.

118. American Academy of Pediatrics Committee on Nutrition. Nutritional needs of low-birth-weight infants. Pediatrics 75:976, 1985.

119. American Academy of Pediatrics. Nutritional Needs of Preterm Infants. In: Kleinman RE, ed. Pediatric nutrition handbook. 4th ed. Elk Grove Village, Ill.: AAP, 1998; 55.

120. Tsang RC, Lucas A, Uuay R, et al. Nutritional needs of the preterm infant: Scientific basis and practical guidelines. Baltimore: Williams and Wilkins, 1993.

121. Kashyap S, Heird WC. Protein requirements of low birthweight, very low birthweight, and small for gestational age infants. In: Niels C, Raiha R., eds. Protein metabolism during infancy. New York:Raven Press, 1994; 133.

122. Norman A, Strandik B, Ojame O. Bile acids and pancreatic enzymes during absorption in the newborn. Acta Paediatr Scand 61:571, 1972.

123. Signer E, Murphy GM, Edkins S. The role of bile salts in the fat malabsorption of premature infants. Arch Dis Child 49:174, 1974.

124. Lee PC, Borysewicz R, Struve M, et al. Development of lipolytic activity in gastric aspirates from premature infants. J Pediatr Gastroenterol Nutr 17:291, 1993.

125. Armand M, Hamosh M, Mehta, NR, et al. Effect of human milk or formula on gastric function and fat digestion in the premature infant. Pediatr Res 40(3):429, 1996.

126. Roy CR, Ste-Marie M, Chartrand L, et al. Correction of the malabsorption of the preterm infant with a medium-chain triglyceride formula. J Pediatr 86:446, 1975.

127. Huston RK, Reynolds JW, Jensen C, et al. Nutrient and mineral retention and vitamin D absorption in low birth weight infants: The effect of medium chain triglycerides. Pediatrics 72:44, 1983.

128. Wu PY, Edmond J, Morrow JW, et al. Gastrointestinal tolerance, fat absorption, plasma ketone and urinary dicarboxylic acid levels in low-birth-weight infants fed different amounts of medium-chain triglycerides in formula. J Pediatr Gastroenterol Nutr 17:145, 1993.

129. Carnielli VP, Rossi K, Badon T, et al. Medium-chain triacylglycerols in formulas for preterm infants: effect on plasma lipids, circulating concentrations of medium-chain fatty acids, and essential fatty acids. Am J Clin Nutr 64:152, 1996.

130. Whyte RK, Campbell D, Stanhope R, et al. Energy balance in low birth weight infants fed formula of high or low medium-chain triglyceride content. J Pediatr 108:964, 1986.

131. Hamosh M, Mehta NR, Fink CS, et al. Fat absorption in premature infants: Medium-chain triglycerides and long-chain triglycerides are absorbed from formula at similar rates. J Pediatr Gastroenterol Nutr 13:143, 1991.

132. Penn D, Schmidt-Sommerfeld E. Lipids as an energy source for the fetus and newborn infant. In: Lebenthal E, ed. Textbook of gastroenterology and nutrition in infancy, 2d ed. New York: Raven Press, 1989; 293.

133. Hamosh M, Bitman J, Liao TH, et al. Gastric lipolysis and fat absorption in preterm infants: Effect of medium-chain triglyceride or long-chain triglyceride-containing formulas. Pediatrics 83:86, 1989.

134. Carlson SE, Werkman SH, Tolley EA. Effect of long-chain n-3 fatty acid supplementation on visual acuity and growth of preterm infants with and without bronchopulmonary dysplasia. Am J Clin Nutr 63:687, 1996.

135. Carlson SE, Werkman SH, Peeples JM, Wilson WM. Growth and development of premature infants in relation to ω3 and ω6 fatty acid status. World Rev Nutr Diet 75:63, 1994.

136. Carlson SE. Lipid requirements of very-low-birth-weight infants for optimal growth and development. In Dobbing J, ed. Lipids, learning and the brain: fats in infant formulas, Report of 103rd Ross Conference on Pediatric Research. Columbus, Ohio: Ross Laboratories, 1993; 188-214.

137. Carlson SE, Werkman SH, Rhodes PG, Tolley EA. Visual-acuity development in healthy preterm infants: Effect of marine-oil supplementation. Am J Clin Nutr 58:35, 1993.

138. Carlson SE, Werkman SH. A randomized trial of visual attention of preterm infants fed docosahexaenoic acid until two months. Lipids 31:85, 1996.

139. Werkman SH, Carlson SE. A randomized trial of visual attention of preterm infants fed docosahexaenoic acid until nine months. Lipids 31:91, 1996.

140. Carlson SE, Cooke RJ, Werkman SH, Tolley EA. First year growth of preterm infants fed standard compared to marine oil n-3 supplemented formula. Lipids 27:901, 1992.

141. Carlson SE, Werkman SH, Peeples JM. Arachidonic acid status correlates with first year growth in preterm infants. Proc Natl Acad Sci USA 90:1073, 1993.

142. O'Connor DL, Hall RT, Adamkin, D, et al. Randomized trial of premature infants fed human milk and/or a nutrient enriched formula with and without a source of arachidonic acid (AA) and docosahexanoic acid (DHA). Pediatr Res 45(4):288A, 1999.

143. Life Sciences Research Office. LRSO report: Assessment of nutrient requirements for infant formulas. J Nutr 128:2059S, 1998.

144. U.S. Congress. Infant Formula Act of 1980 (Public Law 96-359). Sept 26, 1980.

145. Slagle TA, Gross SJ. Vitamin E. In: Tsang RC, Nichols BL, eds. Nutrition during infancy. Philadelphia: Hanley and Belfus, 1988; 277.

146. Dallman P. Nutritional anemia of infancy: Iron, folic acid and vitamin B12. In: Tsang RC, Nichols BL, eds. Nutrition during infancy. Philadelphia: Hanley and Belfus, 1988; 216.

147. Aggett P, Bresson JL, Hernell O, et al., ESPGHAN Committee on Nutrition. Comment on the vitamin E content in infant formulas, follow-on formulas, and formulas for low birth weight infants. J Pediatr Gastroenterol Nutr 26:351, 1998.

148. Tsang RC. Vitamin and mineral requirements in preterm infants. New York: Marcel Dekker, 1985; vii.

149. Giles MM, Laing IA, Elton RA, et al. Magnesium metabolism in preterm infants. Effects of calcium, magnesium, and phosphorus, and of postnatal and gestational age. J Pediatr 117:147, 1990.

150. Ross Pediatrics. Meeting the special nutrient needs of low-birth-weight and premature infants in the hospital. Columbus, Ohio: Ross Products Division, Abbott Laboratories, Jan 1998.

151. Steichen JJ, Gratton TL, Tsang RC: Osteopenia of prematurity: The cause and possible treatment. J Pediatr 96:528, 1980

152. Welch NJ, Personal communication. Mead Johnson Nutritionals. May 8, 1997.

153. Koo WWK, Tsang RC. Mineral requirements of low-birthweight infants. J Am Coll Nutr 10:474, 1991.

154. Bishop NJ, Dahlenburg SL, Fewtrell MS, et al. Early diet of preterm infants and bone mineralization at age five years. Acta Paediatr 85:230, 1996.

155. McDonald MC, Abrams SA, Schanler RJ. Iron absorption and red blood cell incorporation in premature infants fed an iron-fortified infant formula. Pediatr Res 44(4):507, 1998.

156. Hall RT, Wheeler RE, Benson J, et al. Feeding iron-fortified premature formula during initial hospitalization to infants less than 1800 grams birth weight. Pediatrics 92(3):409, 1993.

157. Roth P. Anemia in preterm infants. Pediatr in Rev 17(10):370, 1996.

158. Casey PH, Kraemer HC, Bernbaum, J, et al. Growth status and growth rates of a varied sample of low birth weight, preterm infants: A longitudinal cohort from birth to three years. J Pediatr 119:599, 1991.

159. Hack, M, Weissman B, Borawski-Clark, E. Catch-up growth during childhood among very low-birth-weight children. Arch Pediatr Adolesc Med 150:1122, 1996.

160. Ernst JA, Bull MJ, Rickard KA, et al. Growth outcome and feeding practices of the very low-birth-weight infant (less than 1500 grams) within the first year of life. J Pediatr 117(s):S156, 1990.

161. Lucas A, Bishop NJ, King FJ, et al. Randomised trial of nutrition for preterm infants after discharge. Arch Dis Child 67:324, 1992.

162. Lucas A, King F, Bishop NB. Postdischarge formula consumption in infants born preterm. Arch Dis Child 67:691, 1992.

163. Bishop NJ, King FJ, Lucas A. Increased bone mineral content of preterm infants fed with a nutrient enriched formula after discharge from hospital. Arch Dis Child 68:573, 1993.

164. Wheeler RE, and Hall RT. Feeding of premature infant formula after hospital discharge of infants weighing less than 1800 grams at birth. J Perinatol 16:111, 1996.

165. Chan GM, Borschel MW, Jacobs JR. Effects of human milk or formula feeding on the growth, behavior, protein status of preterm infants discharged from the newborn intensive care unit. Am J Clin Nutr 60:710, 1994.

166. Friel JK, Andrews WL, Matthew JD, et al. Improved growth of very low birthweight infants. Nutr Res 13:611, 1993

167. Cooke RJ, Griffin IJ, McCormick K, et al. Feeding preterm infants after hospital discharge: Effect of dietary manipulation on nutrient intake and growth. Pediatr Res 43(3), 355, 1998.

168. Ross Products Division. Ross Clinical Trial AF51, 1996.

169. Ross Products Division. Ross Clinical Trial AH25, 1997.

170. Ross Products Division. Ross Clinical Trial AA93, 1994.

171. Ross Products Division. Ross Clinical Trial AB16, 1994.

172. Blennemann, B. Ross Products Division, Columbus, OH. Personal communication, February, 1997.

173. Engelland, M. Mead Johnson Nutritionals, Evansville, IN. Personal communication, July, 1999.

174. Hay WW, and Lucas A (Co-chair). Posthospital Nutrition in the Preterm Infant. Report of the 106th Ross Conference on Pediatric Research. Columbus, Ohio:Ross Products Division, Abbott Laboratories, 1996.

175. American Academy of Pediatrics. Formula Feeding of Term Infants. In: Kleinman RE, ed. Pediatric nutrition handbook, 4th ed. Elk Grove Village, Ill.: AAP, 1998; 29.

176. Gurr MI. Review of the progress of dairy science: Human and artificial milks for infant feeding. J Dairy Res 48:519, 1981.

177. Lonnerdal B, Forsum E, Hambraeus L. The protein content of human milk. I. A transversal study of Swedish normal material. Nutr Rep Int 13:125, 1976.

178. Janas LM, Picciano MF, Hatch TF. Indices of protein metabolism in term infants fed human milk, whey-predominant formula, or cow's milk formula. Pediatrics 75:775, 1985.

179. Harrison GG, Graver EJ, Vargas M, et al. Growth and adiposity of term infants fed whey-predominant or casein-predominant formulas or human milk. J Pediatr Gastroenterol Nutr 6:739, 1987.

180. Paule C, Wahrenberger D, Jones W, et al. A novel method to evaluate the amino acid response to infant formulas. FASEB J 10:1749, 1996.

181. Hansen, JW, and Boettcher JA. Human milk substitutes. In: Tsang RC, Zlotkin SH, Nichols BL, and Hansen JW., eds. Nutrition during infancy: principles and practice, 2d ed. Cincinnati:Digital Educational Publishing. 1997; 441.

182. Halter R, Masor M, Paule C, et al. Stool consistency of formula-fed and breast-fed infants. FASEB J 10(3):A230, No. 1326, 1996.

183. Gibson RA, Makrides M, Neumann MA, et al. Ratios of linoleic to α-linolenic acid in formulas for term infants. J Pediatr 125:248, 1994.

184. American Academy of Pediatrics Committee on Nutrition. Fats and Fatty Acids. In Kleinman RE, ed. Pediatric nutrition handbook, 4th ed. Elk Grove Village, Ill.: AAP, 1998; 213.

185. Nelson SE, Rogers RR, Frantz JA, Ziegler EE. Palm olein in infant formula: absorption of fat and minerals by normal infants. Am J Clin Nutr 64:291, 1996.

186. Nelson SE, Frantz JA, Ziegler EE. Absorption of fat and calcium by infants fed a milk-based formula containing palm olein. J Am Col Nutr 17(4):327, 1998.

187. Lien EL. The role of fatty acid composition and positional distribution in fat absorption in infants. J Pediatr 125:S62, 1994.

188. Kretchmer N, Beard JL, Carlson S. The role of nutrition in the development of normal cognition. Am J Clin Nutr 63:997S, 1996.

189. Auestad N, Montalto MB, Hall RT, et al. Visual acuity, erythrocyte fatty acid composition, and growth in term infants fed formulas with long chain polyunsaturated fatty acids for one year. Pediatr Res 41(1):1, 1997.

190. Innis SM, Nelson CM, Rioux FM, et al. Visual acuity, cognitive development and nutrition in term infants. Pediatr Res 37:310A, 1995.

191. Van Biervliet JP, Vinaimont N, Bercaemst R, et al. Seum cholesterol, cholesteryl ester, and high-density lipoprotein development in newborn infants: Response to formulas supplemented with cholesterol and γ-linolenic acid. J Pediatr 120:S101, 1992.

192. Hayes KC, Pronczuk A, Wood RA, et al. Modulation of infant formula fat profile alters the low-density lipoprotein/high-density lipoprotein ratio and plasma fatty acid distribution relative to those with breast-feeding. J Pediatr 120:S109, 1992.

193. Clark KJ, Makrides M, Beumann MA, et al. Determination of the optimal ratio of linoleic acid to α-linoleic acid in infant formulas. J Pediatr 120:S151, 1992.

194. Uuay R. Dietary nucleotides and requirements in early life. In: Lebenthal E, ed.: Textbook of gastroenterology and nutrition in infancy. 2d ed. New York: Raven Press, 1989; 265.

195. Quan R, Barness LA, Uuay R. Do infants need nucleotide-supplemented formula for optimal nutrition? (edit). J Pediatr Gastroenterol Nutr 11:429, 1990.

196. Greer FR. Formulas for the healthy term infant. Pediatr in Rev 16(3):107, 1995.

197. Leach JL, Baxter JH, Molitor, BE, et al. Total potentially available nucleosides of human milk by stage of lactation. Am J Clin Nutr 61:1224, 1995.

198. Sanchez-Pozo A, Pita ML, Martinez A, et al. Effects of dietary nucleotides upon lipoprotein pattern of newborn infants. Nutr Res 6:763, 1986.

199. DeLucchi C, Pita ML, Faus MJ, et al. Effects of dietary nucleotides on the fatty acid composition of erythrocyte membrane lipids in term infants. J Pediatr Gastroenterol Nutr 6:568, 1987.
200. Pickering LK, Granoff DM, Erickson JR, et al. Modulation of the immune system by human milk and infant formula containing nucleotides. Pediatrics 101(2):242, 1998.
201. Brunser O, Espinoza J, Araya, M, et al. Effect of dietary nucleotide supplementation on diarrhoeal disease in infants. Acta Paediatr 83:188, 1994.
202. Nelson SE, Ziegler EE, Copeland AM, et al. Lack of adverse reaction to iron-fortified formula. Pediatrics 81:360, 1988.
203. Reeves JD, Yip R. Lack of adverse side effects of oral ferrous sulfate therapy in 1-year old infants. Pediatrics 75:352, 1985.
204. Gaull GE. Taurine in pediatric nutrition: Review and update. Pediatrics 83:433, 1989.
205. Dagan R, Gorodischer R, Moses S, et al. Lactose-free formulas for infantile diarrhea. Lancet 326:207, 1980.
206. Haffejee IE. Cow's milk-based formula, human milk, and soya feeds in acute infantile diarrhea: A therapeutic trial. J Pediatr Gastroenterol Nutr 10:193, 1990.
207. Lifshitz F, Neto UF, Olivo CAG, et al. Refeeding of infants with acute diarrheal disease. J Pediatr 118:599, 1991.
208. Brown KH. Dietary management of acute childhood diarrhea: Optimal timing of feeding and appropriate use of milks and mixed diets. J Pediatr 118:S92, 1991.
209. Donovan GK, Torres-Pinedo R. Chronic diarrhea and soy formulas: Inhibition of diarrhea by lactose. Am J Dis Child 141:1069, 1987.
210. Brady MS, Rickard KA, Fitzgerald JF, et al. Specialized formulas and feedings for infants with malabsorption or formula intolerance. J Am Diet Assoc 86:191, 1986.
211. Lifshitz F. Carbohydrate intolerance in infancy. New York: Marcel Dekker, 1982; 3-255.
212. Brown KH, Perez F, Peerson JM, et al. Effect of dietary fiber (soy polysaccharide) on the severity, duration, and nutritional outcome of acute, watery diarrhea in children. Pediatrics 92:241, 1993.
213. Vanderhoof JA, Murray ND, Paule CL, Ostrom KM. Use of soy fiber in acute diarrhea in infants and toddlers. Clin Pediatr 36(3):135, 1997.
214. Nichols BL. Infant feeding practice. In: Tsang RC, Nichols BL, eds. Nutrition during infancy. Philadelphia: Hanley and Belfus, 1988, 367.
215. Fomon SJ, Thomas LN, Filer LJ, et al. Requirements for protein and essential amino acids in early infancy. Studies with a soy-isolate formula. Acta Paediatr Scand 72:33, 1973.
216. Bahna SL, Heiner DC. Allergies to milk. New York: Grune and Stratton, 1980; 137-140.
217. Eastham EJ, Lichauco T, Grady MI, et al. Antigenicity of infant formulas: Role of immature intestine on protein permeability. J Pediatr 93:561, 1978.
218. Benkov KJ, LeLeiko NS. A rational approach to formulas. Pediatr Ann 16:225, 1987.
219. American Academy of Pediatrics Committee on Nutrition. Soy protein-based formulas: Recommendations for use in infant feeding. Pediatrics 101(1), 1998.

220. Steichen JJ, Tsang RC. Bone mineralization and growth in term infants fed soy-based or cow milk-based formula. J Pediatr 110:687, 1987.
221. Greer FR, Searcy JE, Levin RS, et al. Bone mineral content and serum 25–hydroyvitamin D concentrations in breastfed infants with and without supplemental vitamin D. J Pediatr 98:696, 1981.
222. Hillman LS, Chow W, Salmons SS, et al. Vitamin D metabolism, mineral homeostasis, and bone mineralization in term infants fed human milk, cow milk-based formula, or soy-based formula. J Pediatr 112:864, 1988.
223. Shenai JP, Jhaveri BM, Reynolds JW, et al. Nutritional balance studies in very low-birth-weight infants: Role of soy formula. Pediatrics67:631, 1981.
224. Lake AM. Beyond hydrolysates: Use of L-amino acid formula in resistant dietary protein-induced intestinal disease in infants. J Pediatr 131:658, 1997
225. American Academy of Allergy and Immunology Committee on Adverse Reactions to foods. Washington, D.C.:U.S. Department of Health and Human Services; NIH pub no. 84-2442, 1984.
226. Ferguson A. Definitions and diagnosis of food intolerance and food allergy: consensus and controversy. J Pediatr 121:S7-11, 1992.
227. Lake AM. Food protein-induced colitis and gastroenteropathy in infants and children. In: Metcalfe DD, Sampson HA, Simon RA, eds. Food allergy: adverse reactions to food and food additives. 2d ed. Cambridge: Blackwell Science; 1996; 277-286.
228. Walker WA. Host defense mechanisms in the gastrointestinal tract. Pediatrics 57:901, 1976.
229. D'Netto M, Knox I, Herson V, et al. Allergic gastroenteropathy in preterm infants. J Pediatr Gastrenterol Nutr 25(4):472, 1997.
230. Kleinman RE, Bahna S, Powell GF, Sampson HA. Use of infant formulas in infants with cow milk allergy: A review and recommendations. Pediatr Allergy Immunol 2:146, 1991.
231. American Academy of Pediatrics Committee on Nutrition. Hypoallergenic infant formulas. Pediatrics 83:1068, 1989.
232. Businco L, Cantani A, Longhi A, et al. Anaphylactic reactions to a cow's milk whey protein hydrolysate (Alfa-Re, Nestle) in infants with cow's milk allergy. Ann Allergy 62:333, 1989.
233. Isolauri E, Sutas Y, Makinen-Kiljunen S, et al. Efficacy and safety of hydrolyzed cow milk and amino acid-derived formulas in infants with cow milk allergy. J Pediatr 127:550, 1995.
234. Vanderhoof JA, Murray N, Kaufman SS, et al. Intolerance to protein hydrolysate infant formulas: An under recognized cause of gastrointestinal symptoms in infants. J Pediatr 131:741, 1997.
235. Kaufmann SS, Scrivner KJ, Murray ND, et al. Influence of Portagen and Pregestimil on essential fatty acid status in infantile liver disease. Pediatrics 89:151, 1992.
236. Pettei MJ, Daftary S, Levine J. Essential fatty acid deficiency associated with the use of a medium-chain-triglyceride infant formula in pediatric hepatobiliary disease. Am J Clin Nutr 53:1217, 1991.
237. Lifshitz F. Nutrition for special needs in infancy: Protein hydrolysates. New York: Marcel Dekker, 1985; 1-312.
238. Merritt RJ, Carter M, Haight M, et al. Whey protein hydrolysate formula for infants with gastrointestinal intolerance to cow milk and soy protein in infant formulas. J Pediatr Gastroenterol Nutr 11:78, 1990.

239. Greene HL, McCabe DR, Merenstein GB. Protracted diarrhea and malnutrition in infancy: Changes in intestinal morphology and disaccharidase activities during treatment with total intravenous nutrition or oral elemental diets. J Pediatr 87:695, 1975.

240. Cordle CT, Mahmoud MI, Moore V. Immunogenicity evaluation of protein hydrolysates for hypoallergenic infant formulae. J Pediatr Gastroenterol Nutr 13:270, 1991.

241. Chandra RK, Singh G, Shridhara B. Effect of feeding whey hydrolysate, soy and conventional cow milk formulas on incidence of atopic disease in high risk infants. Ann Allergy 63:102, 1989.

242. Forsyth BWC. Colic and the effect of changing formulas: A double-blind, multiple-crossover study. J Pediatr 115:521, 1989.

243. Vandenplas Y, Malfroot A, Dab I. Short-term prevention of cow's milk protein allergy in infants. Immunol Allergy Pract 11:17, 1989.

244. Erickson J, Auerbach B, Callie A, et al. Stool characteristics of healthy term (T) infants fed different protein hydrolysate formulas (HF). J Parenter Enter Nutr 13:19S, 1989.

245. Sampson HA. Safety of casein hydrolysate formula in children with cow's milk protein sensitivity. Pediatr Res 25:123A, 1989.

246. deBoissieu D, Matarazzo P, DuPont C. Allergy to extensively hydrolyzed cow milk proteins in infants: Identification and treatment with an amino acid-based formula. J Pediatr 131:744, 1997.

247. Hill DJ, Heine RG, Camden DJS, et al. The natural history of intolerance to soy and extensively hydrolyzed formula in infants with multiple food protein intolerance. J Pediatr 135:118, 1999.

248. Kerner JA. Formula allergy and intolerance. Gastroenterol Clin North Am 24(1):1, 1995.

249. Ross Laboratories. Using concentrated formulas and caloric supplements to meet special infant feeding needs (G 477). Columbus, Ohio: Ross Laboratories, 1987.

250. Davis A, Baker S. The use of modular nutrients in pediatrics. J Parenter Enter Nutr 20(3):228, 1996.

251. Schanler RJ. The low-birth-weight infant. In: Walker WA, Watkins JB, eds. Nutrition in pediatrics. Hamilton:Decker, 1997; 405.

252. Zenk L, Huztable R. Osmolality of infant formulas, tube feedings, and total parenteral nutrition solutions. Hosp Formulary 577, Aug 1978.

253. Committee on Nutrition, American Academy of Pediatrics. Commentary on breastfeeding and infant formula, including proposed standards for formulas. Pediatrics 57:278, 1976.

254. Niemiec PW, Vanderveen TW, Morrison JI, et al. Gastrointestinal disorders caused by medication and electrolyte solution osmolality during enteral nutrition. J Parenter Enter Nutr 7:387, 1983.

255. Paxson C, Adcok III E, Morriss E. Osmolalities of infant formulas. Am J Dis Child 131:139, 1977.

256. Ernst JA, Williams JM, Glick MR, et al. Osmolality of substances used in the intensive care nursery. Pediatrics 72:347, 1983.

257. White KC, Harkarvy KL. Hypertonic formula resulting from added oral medications. Am J Dis Child 136:931, 1982.

258. Jew RK, Owen D, Kaufman D, et al. Osmolality of commonly used medications and formulas in the neonatal intensive care unit. Nutr Clin Prac 12:158, 1997.

259. Fomon SJ, Ziegler EE. Renal solute load and potential renal solute load in infancy. J Pediatr 134:11, 1999.

260. Ziegler EE, Ryu J. Renal solute load and diet in growing premature infants. J Pediatr 89:609, 1976
261. Hay WW. Nutritional needs of the extremely low-birth-weight infant. Semin Perinatol 15:482, 1991.
262. Aperia A, Broberger O, Zetterstrom R. Implications of limitation of renal function for the nutrition of low birthweight infants. Acta Paediatr Scand (suppl) 294:48, 1982.
263. American Dietetic Association. Preparation of formula for infants: Guidelines for health care facilities. Chicago: The American Dietetic Association, 1991.
264. Jensen RG, ed. Handbook of milk composition. New York: Academic Press, 1995.
265. Lo CW, Kleinman RE. Infant formula, past and future: opportunities for improvement. Am J Clin Nutr 63:646S, 1996.
266. Carlson SJ, Ziegler EE. Nutrient intakes and growth of very low birth weight infants. J Perinatol 18(4):252, 1998.
267. Sapsford A. Children's Hospital Medical Center, Cincinnati, OH. Expressed Human Breastmilk Labeling and Tracking System. Patent Pending, 2000.
268. Ross Products Division, Product Monograph 62352, Columbus, OH. October, 1999.
269. Barrett Reis B, Hall R, Schanler R, et al. An evaluation of growth and serum biochemistries of preterm infants fed preterm human milk fortified with a new powdered human milk fortifier. Pediatrics, In Press.
270. Kuschel C. Protein supplementation of human milk to promote growth in preterm infants. (Cochrane Review). In: The Cochrane Library, 2/23/99. Oxford: Update Software.
271. Carlson SJ, Johnson KL, Cress GA, et al. Higher protein intake improves growth of VLBW infants fed fortified breast milk. Pediatr Res 46:278A, 1999.
272. Moody GJ, Schanler RJ, Lau C, Shulman RJ. Feeding tolerance in premature infants fed fortified human milk. J Pediatr Gastroenterol Nutr 30:408, 2000.
273. DeCurtis M, Candusso M, Pieltain C, Rigo J. Effect of fortification on the osmolality of human milk. Arch Dis Child Fetal Neonatal Ed 81:F141, 1999.
274. Kuschel C. Multicomponent fortification of human milk for premature infants. (Cochrane Review). In: The Cochrane Library, 8/19/98. Oxford: Update Software.
275. Atkinson SA. Human milk feeding of the micropremie. Clin Perinatol 27(1):235, 2000.
276. Hay WW, Lucas A, Heird WC, et al. Workshop summary: Nutrition of the extremely low birth weight infant. Pediatrics 104:1360, 1999.
277. Zeiger RS, Sampson HA, Bock SA, et al. Soy allergy in infants and children with IgE-associated cow's milk allergy. J Pediatr 134:614, 1999.
278. Atkinson SA, Lemons JA. Eds. Human milk for very-low-birth-weight infants, Report of the 108th Ross Conference on Pediatric Research. Columbus, OH: Ross Products Division, Abbott Laboratories, 1999.

Nutritional Care for High-Risk Newborns (Rev. 3d. Ed.)
S. Groh-Wargo, M. Thompson, J. Cox, editors
© 2000, Precept Press, Inc., Chicago

17

LACTATION ISSUES

Joy G. Kubit, RN, BSN, IBCLC

EVERY WOMAN WHO DELIVERS a sick or preterm infant who is hospitalized should be given the option to provide milk for her baby. Of special importance to the preterm infant are human milk's unique immunological components, easy digestibility, and special properties that may aid maturation of the gut,[1] improve cognitive function,[2] and protect against necrotizing enterocolitis.[3,66] Providing milk for her infant has psychological benefits for the mother as well. Being able to express milk for her baby offers the mother a tangible means of contributing to her infant's care, which may help promote mother-infant attachment and increase the mother's self-esteem.[4,67]

Mothers face major barriers to successful breast-feeding when confronted with long-term separation from their infants. Maintaining a milk supply by mechanical methods, coping with the responsibility of home and family, early return to employment, difficulty establishing breast-feeding with an immature or compromised infant, and conflicting advice from health care professionals often lead to premature discontinuation of lactation.[5,6]

Knowledgeable health care professionals are instrumental in providing information about pumping and techniques to facilitate breast-feeding and in offering support for the lactating mother. Some hospitals have a certified lactation consultant on staff available to counsel the breast-feeding mother during and after the infant's hospitalization. The infant's primary nurse, neonatal nutritionist, and social worker are important sources of support, and contact with other women who have breast-fed a high-risk infant may be helpful. Mothers of preterm infants who receive support from several different sources produce more milk and continue breast-feeding longer than women with little or no support.[7] When continuing to express milk leads to unrelieved stress, the mother may decide to

Table 17.1. Tips to Maintain or Increase Milk Production

Express regularly 6-10 times daily with a double piston-style electric pump[11,12,15,16]

Increase pumping frequency for 2-3 days between 2 and 3 weeks postpartum or when supply decreases

Pump once between midnight and 6 a.m.

Massage breasts prior to or during pumping[17]

Practice relaxation and visual imagery[18]

Have frequent mother-baby contact, especially skin-to-skin holding[19-21]

Place baby's picture and an article of clothing near breast pump

Listen to soft music during pumping sessions

Apply warm, moist packs to breasts prior to pumping

Maintain adequate fluids and nourishment

Use fenugreek tea or tablets (2-3 tablets three times a day)

Combine manual expression with electric breast-pumping

---

stop pumping; the health care provider can affirm and support whatever decision is made.

Physiology of Lactation

During pregnancy, glandular tissue of the breast proliferates rapidly under the influence of estrogen and progesterone. At 16 weeks of pregnancy, the breast is fully able to support lactation.[8] After the delivery of the placenta at birth, blood levels of estrogen and progesterone fall rapidly. Suckling or breast-pumping stimulates nerve endings in the nipple to send impulses to the hypothalamus, which controls the release of prolactin and oxytocin from the anterior and posterior pituitary gland, respectively. Prolactin stimulates alveolar milk production in the breast, and oxytocin stimulates myoepithelial cells surrounding the alveoli to contract, ejecting milk into the ducts. This release of milk into the ducts is called "letdown," or milk ejection reflex (MER). Maternal signs of an effective MER are thirst and/or sleepiness, uterine contractions, "tingling" or "tightening" sensations in the breast, and leaking from the contralateral breast during pumping or breast-feeding.[9] Another factor affecting milk production is the presence of suppressor peptides in human milk that signal the breast to decrease milk production.[10] Poor milk removal from the breasts leads to a buildup of suppressor peptides, which results in decreased milk supply. An understanding of milk production, milk ejection reflex, and role of suppressor peptides in the milk is necessary when assisting the mother in initiating and maintaining lactation.

Breast-Pumping

When a woman delivers a sick or preterm baby, a period of several days, weeks, or months may elapse before the infant may be able to effectively breast-feed. Milk expression should be initiated as soon as possible after delivery. The earlier milk expression is begun, the greater the milk production in the first two weeks postbirth.[11] Recommendations regarding frequency of expression range from five or more expressions per day with a duration of 100 minutes/day[11] to 8 or more expressions per day.[12] Considerations, such as the mother's physical condition, family responsibilities, time management, and physiological principles that support production, need to be addressed. During the weeks or months of pumping, a woman will at times feel discouraged with providing milk for her baby and will need extra support to continue.

Many types of breast pumps are available for breast-feeding mothers. These pumps are reviewed elsewhere.[12,13] Manual and battery-operated pumps may be used successfully for short-term pumping (infant is discharged within a week). However, for the woman who needs to express milk regularly to maintain lactation, a piston-style electric pump has several advantages. This type of pump stimulates increased prolaction levels, expresses milk with higher fat content, increases yield, and is easy to use.[13,14] Medela Inc. (McHenry, Ill.) and Hollister, Inc. (Libertyville, Ill.) contract with pharmacies and individuals nationwide to offer electric pumps on a rental basis (see Appendix M). A computerized listing of local breast pump depots is distributed by both companies and is available in many neonatal intensive care units. Rental fees vary, depending on the length of time that the pump will be rented. Parents should be instructed to contact individual pump depots for specific costs. Some third-party medical insurance programs offer reimbursement for breast pump rental with a medical prescription. Both companies have a charity program to cover rental fees when there is a financial and medical need. Both single and double (both breasts simultaneously) pumping systems are available for use with the electric pump. In studies of mothers of preterm infants, double pumping has been shown to decrease pumping time[15,16] and may increase milk yield and prolactin levels.[16]

Pumping Techniques

In addition to information about breast pumps and frequency and duration of milk expression, every mother needs information from the health care provider about expression techniques that may increase milk yield. (See Table 17.1) When milk production is low and the techniques in Table 17.1 do not stimulate increased output, medications have been used with varying degrees of success. Metoclopramide, given three times a day for one week, has been used to increase milk production.[22] Human growth hormone therapy in women with lactational insufficiency may improve breast milk volumes[23] (see section on discharge planning).

Collection, Storage, and Feeding of Human Milk

Strict hygiene needs to be practiced when expressing milk for a sick or preterm infant. All expressed human milk contains nonpathogenic bacteria. Thorough hand and nail cleansing helps to minimize contamination of human milk during expression and storage. The breast should be wiped with a clean wet cloth from the nipple outward prior to pumping. One researcher showed reduced bacteria levels when the nipple is cleansed with soap and water prior to pumping.[24] A daily shower, clean bra, and frequent change of breast pads help keep the breast area clean. The milk collection unit needs to be washed well with hot, soapy water and rinsed with hot water after every use. Once a day, the mother should clean the unit either in a dishwasher or by sterilizing it by boiling for 15 minutes in a covered pan.

Expressed milk should be stored in a sterile plastic or glass container; neither of these materials interacts with the nutrients in human milk.[25,26] Viable cells, such as leukocytes, may adhere to glass more than to plastic,[27] but after refrigeration for 12 hours, the adherence is equal in both types of containers.[27] Rigid polypropylene plastic containers maintain the stability of all constituents in human milk collections and may be easier and safer to handle than plastic bags or glass bottles.[28]

Written guidelines for parents on the handling of human milk assure safety and quality. Each container should be marked with the name, date, and time of expression, and transported on ice from home to hospital. The small amounts of colostrum collected during the first days of pumping are ideal for the preterm infant's first feedings. Multiple expressions of milk can be layered in the same container if each addition is chilled prior to adding more milk.[74] Mothers are encouraged to collect and store milk in feeding size portions.

Initially, the milk should be given in the order expressed because human milk composition changes as the infant's needs change.[4] Fresh human milk is preferable to frozen milk because the viability of lymphocytes and macrophages is conserved.[28]

Guidelines for storage vary from institution to institution. Freshly expressed human milk can be safely refrigerated for two days, kept for 6 months in a self-defrosting freezer, or for 12 months in a freezer that maintains a constant temperature of 0°F (-20° C).[29,30] Human milk can safely be defrosted in the refrigerator, or more quickly, under running tap water. Some experts recommend defrosting in a small standard laboratory incubator.[31] Microwaving is not recommended because it destroys immunoglobulins in the milk.[32] In addition, because microwaves heat unevenly, hot spots can be present having the potential for scalding. Thawed human milk and fortified human milk should be used within 24 hours of preparation.[33]

There are no research-based recommendations for how frequently expressed human milk should be cultured for the presence of bacteria. Some experts recommend an initial culture the first week, followed by subsequent cultures at intervals from weekly to monthly, depending on the condition of the baby and the results of the first culture. Other experts culture only when giving human milk via continuous feedings or when an infant shows signs of feeding intolerance. Guidelines for acceptable bacteria levels in human milk are: absence of enterobacteria or other potentially pathogenic organisms and presence of modest amounts of nonpathogenic bacteria (usually 10^3 to 10^5 cfu/ml).[34-37] Human milk given via continuous feedings should have levels of nonpathogenic bacteria of $\leq 10^4$ cfu/ml.[38]

The advantages of giving expressed human milk via intermittent bolus feedings rather than continuous feedings to the preterm infant are decreased fat loss and lower risk of bacterial contamination.[39,40] When continuous feedings are used, collection techniques must be strictly followed, and fresh milk rather than frozen milk is recommended. Ideally, the infusion syringe is angled in a semiupright position, the feeding equipment is changed every four hours, and small-lumen tubing attached to a syringe-loaded infusion pump is used to minimize bacterial growth and fat loss.[40]

Fortification of human milk is recommended for infants weighing < 1,500 g at birth.[68] Several commercial products are available (see Chapter 16). Significant changes in rate of infant growth have been documented with the use of hindmilk to increase the lipid and caloric content of an infant's diet.[41] This is an option when the mother's milk supply exceeds the infant's needs. She can be instructed to fractionalize the milk by separating from the hindmilk the milk expressed during the first 2-3 minutes after letdown. Foremilk can be frozen for later use and fresh hindmilk brought to the hospital. Hindmilk may provide as much as 30 kcal/oz.[41] A thorough evaluation of the infant's intake and nutritional status should be conducted, especially if hindmilk supplementation continues for more than a few weeks.

An estimation of the caloric content of human milk, including hindmilk, can be made using the creamatocrit technique. The creamatocrit is the length of the cream column separated from milk by centrifugation and expressed as a percentage of the total milk column.[69] The technique, described in detail elsewhere,[70,71] is as follows:

- Fill glass capillary tube(s) with about 75 µl milk
- Seal tube(s) at one end with clay
- Centrifuge at 3000 rpm for 15 minutes
- Measure both the length of cream column and total milk column using a ruler marked in mm or a microhematocrit reader
- Express creamatocrit as the percentage of the cream to the total milk column

The energy content of the milk can be estimated using a table[72] or calculated[69] as follows:

- Fresh sample: Energy (kcal/dl) = 5.99 x creamatocrit (%) + 32.5
- Frozen sample: Energy (kcal/dl) = 6.20 x creamatocrit (%) + 35.1

The creamatocrit estimation of energy content correlates strongly with actual measurement of milk energy.[69-71]

Preferably, infants should receive only their own mother's milk, which is specially suited to their nutritional and immunological needs. However, the survival and quality of life of a small group of infants may depend on banked human milk. In 1985, the Human Milk Banking Association of North American (Appendix M) was formed to improve communication between milk banks and assure uniform operational guidelines.

Initiation of Breast-feedings

In the past, breast-feeding was considered too stressful for small preterm infants. Guidelines for initiating breast-feedings stated that the infant should weigh at least 1,500 g, be 34 weeks' gestational age, and be able to bottle-feed without stress. Following these guidelines often led to breast-feeding failure as infants learned bottle-feeding techniques and mothers' milk supplies diminished with prolonged pumping.

Research shows that infants can breast-feed as early as 32 weeks' gestation and as small as 1,300 g.[42,43] During breast-feeding, small preterm infants showed better suck and swallow coordination and breathing patterns, more stable temperatures, and absence of bradycardia than during bottle feedings.[42,43,67]

Infants should be introduced to the breast as soon as they are stable, on minimal O_2 support, and able to maintain their body temperatures double-wrapped for 5-10 minutes out of the isolette.[44,45] Allowing the VLBW infant to suck on the "emptied" breast is useful not only in stimulating sucking, but also in promoting maternal milk flow and prolonged laxtation.[46] These first breast-feedings are practice sessions, and the infant should not be expected to breast-feed nutritively. The infant may lick the nipple or latch on and suck once or twice. This may be done during nasogastric (NG) feedings, so that the infant will begin to associate the breast with feelings of satiety. These sessions are important for promoting a good milk supply and encouraging early feeding behaviors. The infant should continue to receive NG feedings until he/she begins to consistently latch on and suck nutritively for at least five minutes.

Bottle feedings should be postponed until the infant is breast-feeding nutritively at least once or twice a day. The breast-feeding care plan needs to be individualized for each mother/baby dyad, depending on the mother's availability to the infant and the infant's ability to suckle effectively.[67]

Institutions that do not routinely offer bottle feeds to hospitalized breast-fed infants have documented significantly longer duration and exclusivity of breast-feeding.[44,47] Breast-feeding ICU infants are not given routine bottle feedings. Introduction to breast-feeding begins when the infant is of at least 30 weeks' gestation and stable. When discharge is imminent (two to three days), mothers room in with their infants on the postpartum unit. When the transition from tube-feeding to breast-feeding is managed this way, 70% of mothers who initially choose to breast-feed in the neonatal ICU are breast-feeding at discharge.[44] Kliethermes et al[47] studied the transition of tube-fed preterm infants to exclusive breast-feeding. They found that nasogastric supplemented preterm infants who were learning to breast-feed were more likely to be breast-feeding at discharge, at three days, and at three months and six months posthospital discharge than were preterm infants offered bottles during the transition period.[47]

Kangaroo Care

Kangaroo care, a method of skin-to-skin care for premature infants, has gained acceptance in hospitals in the United States.[73] The infant is placed skin-to-skin in an upright position on the mother's or father's chest for one to several hours daily in the neonatal ICU setting. Mothers are encouraged to breast feed ad lib in response to infant cues. During kangaroo care, infants' O_2 saturations may be higher, and mothers may have more stable milk production and continue to breast-feed longer than with traditional contact.[48] Other advantages include earlier discharge of the baby, earlier breast-feeding success, and increased parental confidence.[19-21]

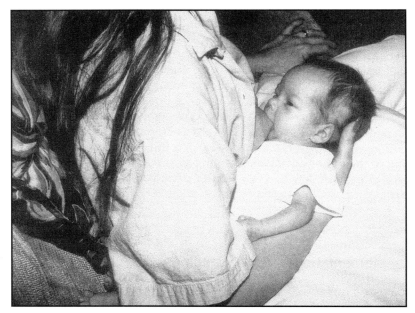

Figure 17.1. Clutch, or football, hold.

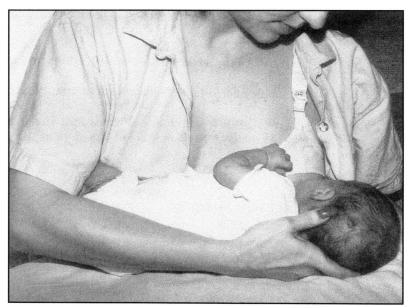

Figure 17.2. Modified cradle hold.

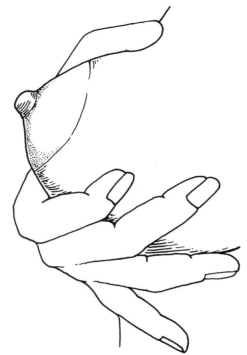

Figure 17.3. C-cup hold.

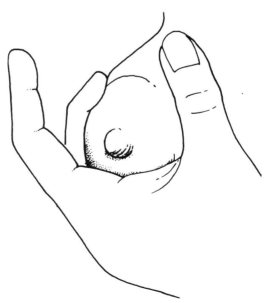

Figure 17.4. For additional support, the mother can use her index finger to support the infant's chin, or the thumb and index finger can come forward to support the jaw.

Breast-feeding Techniques

Instruction and support for the mother during initial feeding sessions is important in promoting optimally effective breast-feeding. Progress toward exclusive breast-feeding is often slow, and parents may become discouraged if the infant's progress does not match the parents' expectations. Patience and calm persistence is imperative, as the infant often takes "three steps forward, two back" throughout the hospital stay. The mother should be seated in a comfortable high-backed chair, with pillows to support herself and her baby. The infant should be held in a flexed position, with body in straight alignment facing the breast. Poor positioning during feeding can lead to poor suck and swallow coordination.[4,73] Both the clutch, or football hold (Figure 17.1), and modified cradle hold (Figure 17.2) work well with the preterm infant. The breast should be supported during the entire feeding using the C-cup hold (Figure 17.3). If the infant needs additional support, the mother can use her index finger to give support under the chin, or the thumb and index finger can come forward to support the jaw (Figure 17.4). The infant may go to breast more than once in a three-hour feeding schedule, according to the infant's demand. Feedings may take 20 to 45 minutes.

Signs that the infant is breast-feeding effectively include rhythmical, sustained suckling, audible swallowing, softening of the maternal breast, and maternal signs of milk ejection.[45] Knowledge of infant behavioral cues are important to prevent overstimulation and to increase feeding success. The preterm infant has short periods of awake, alert behavior during which the infant is most receptive to learning and mastering new skills. Sensitivity to infant cues of tiring and overstimulation will optimize attempts to master breast-feeding. The Newborn Individualized Developmental Care and Assessment Program (NIDCAP) has been developed by Als et al.[49,50] It is a model to assess infant behavior, especially in the ICU. NIDCAP has been effective in assisting ICU staff and parents in recognizing preterm infant behavior in response to environmental stimulation. Modification of the environment, timing of breast-feedings to coincide with infant readiness, and proper handling of the infant can have an impact on the degree of breast-feeding competence.[51]

Supplementation of Early Feedings

During early breast-feedings, the preterm infant may not be able to obtain a full feeding at the breast. Some experts suggest test-weighing before and after feedings to determine milk intake. This method has been shown to be reliable when the electronic scales being used have high concurrent validity.[45] When close approximation of actual intake is necessary, as in the case of the preterm baby, use of clinical indexes to assess breast milk intake may not be accurate enough to ensure adequate growth.[52] Test-weighing can increase maternal reassurance and help staff individualize human milk supplementation.[53] Supplements can be given through the nasogastric tube following the feeding, or the total amount can be divided up over the next several feedings. More mature hospitalized infants may be observed during the breast-feeding session and supplemented as follows:

- No supplement is given when the infant breast-feeds effectively for longer than five minutes.
- Half the volume is supplemented by NG tube when the infant feeds for five minutes effectively.
- The total volume is given if the infant does not breast-feed effectively.
- Daily weight measurements need to be monitored closely to assure adequate growth.[44]

Supplementation of Later Feedings

When the mother's milk supply is low or the infant's sucking at the breast is insufficient to sustain adequate growth, additional supplementation may be necessary. Using devices other than bottles with breast-feedings has two advantages: The infant receives all nourishment at the breast, stimulating an improved milk supply, and the infant avoids bottle-feedings, which can reinforce poor feeding patterns and confuse an infant learning to breast-feed.[54] Some babies appear able to easily switch between bottle and breast-feeding, while others may begin to prefer the bottle. It is nearly impossible to predict these preferences. It is ideal to strictly limit, as much as possible, the exposure to bottles during the transition from tube-feeding to established breast-feeding.

A device such as the Medela Supplemental Nutrition System (Medela Inc.) or Lact-Aid (Lact-Aid International, Athens, Tenn.) can be used to supply additional expressed human milk or formula during breast-feedings. Cup feeding to supplement babies in the NICU can be a safe and helpful alternative feeding method. Several articles in the literature discuss the advantages of cup feeding of preterm and term infants and describe "how to" safely cup feed.[4,55,56] Finger-feeding can be used to supplement breast-feeding. After scrupulous handwashing, a 5-French feeding tube attached to a 30 cc syringe of milk or a supplementer with tubing is attached to the parent's finger. The infant receives milk while sucking on the parent's finger.[57] Other supplementation techniques, such as syringe, eyedropper, and spoon

Table 17.2. Discharge Planning

	Good attachment, effective suckling	Poor attachment, Ineffective suckling
Sufficient milk supply	• Discharge breast-feeding every 1½-3 hr or on demand, at least 8 feeding/24° • Check weight 1 wk • Monitor voids/stools • Pump after most feeds for 2 wks	• Consult with lactation specialist • Offer breast frequently • Offer supplements with cup, spoon, finger-feeding, or bottle • Pump every 3 hr to maintain supply • Skin-to-skin contact • Check weight 4-5 d
Poor milk supply	• Offer breast every 1½-3 hr • Use nursing supplementer at breast with minimal supplement • Check weight 4-5 d • Rest with baby • Pump after most feeds until milk supply adequate • Consider use of fenugreek or metoclopramide	• Consult with lactation specialist • Offer breast frequently • Offer full supplements • Pump every 2-3 hr • Reassess situation frequently • Consider use of fenugreek or metoclopramide • Check weight 2-3d

feeding, have been used successfully with breast-feeding premature infants.[4]

Several breast-feeding assessment tools have been developed for use by parents and staff to determine breast-feeding competency. They have been used with full-term breast-fed infants[58-60] and may have limited value in the NICU. Two documentation tools, The Preterm Infant Breastfeeding Behavior Scale (PIBBS)[61] and the NICU Breastfeeding Record[62] assess parameters unique to the preterm infant and can assist staff and parents in identifying lactation difficulties and emerging infant breast-feeding competence.

Discharge Planning

Throughout the time of transition from tube-feeding to breast-feeding, the health care professional should discuss breast-feeding management at home with the breast-feeding mother and support person. As the day of discharge approaches, the mother should be encouraged to visit more frequently for additional breast-feedings, or room-in if facilities are available. An individualized care plan that considers the mother's milk supply and the infant's feeding capabilities should be discussed. With earlier discharge, mothers can expect that they may need to continue to pump after breast-feedings for the first two to four weeks at home, offering expressed milk to the infant after breast-feeding according to the infant's need.

Table 17.2 outlines an approach to discharge planning from the NICU for the breast-feeding mother and baby. Good attachment/effective suckling coupled with sufficient milk supply is the best scenario; poor attachment/ineffective suckling coupled with poor milk supply is the worst. Fenugreek is an herb with a reputation as a galactagogue that is widespread but undocumented.[63] The dose used is variable, but many recommend about 2-3 capsules three times a day.[63] Maple syrup odor in urine and sweat may occur, as well as diarrhea, hypoglycemia, and dyspnea.[63] Metoclopramide (brand name Reglan) is used to stimulate prolactin release from the pituitary and enhance breast milk production.[63] A dose of 10-15 mg three times a day is most effective.[63] Response is variable. Side effects include nausea, gastric cramping, and diarrhea.[63] Use beyond two to four weeks is not recommended.[63]

The first few weeks at home with a preterm infant is a very vulnerable period. Mothers have a profound concern about infant growth and breast milk intake.[64] They report that they are unable to use clinical observation as an effective means of assessing intake during the first two weeks postdischarge.[64] The use of the Medela Baby Weigh Scale (Appendix M), which is available for rent in some community pharmacies, can provide reassurance for parents immediately after discharge.[67]

A breast-feeding diary can be a valuable tool for the parents and health care provider in assessing breast-feeding progress. Parents may want to keep a daily record of feedings (including duration and frequency), wet diapers, and bowel movements to assure adequacy of intake. Less than six wet diapers and two bowel movements in 24 hours signals a need for more frequent breast-feedings or supplements.[65] Frequent weight checks are important when breast-feeding is not going well. Weight gain after the first week home is about one ounce/day.[65]

Many clients need a referral to a lactation consultant for follow-up. An infant with a poor suck may need to be referred to a therapist with neurodevelopmental training (see Chapter 19). Some mothers may decide to express milk for offering in a bottle or to wean to formula. Others returning to work or school may want to offer an occasional bottle once breast-feeding is established to prepare the baby for her absence. A traumatic birth experience followed by a poor breast-feeding experience can undermine a woman's self-esteem. Mothers are supported for what they are able to do and reassured that good mothering can be practiced regardless of feeding method.

A list of breast-feeding resources available to parents and health care professionals caring for a high-risk newborn can be found in Appendix M.

To summarize this chapter, providing human milk for the hospitalized neonate allows parents the opportunity to both nourish and nurture their infant. Mothers need support and information about pumping to maintain lactation and techniques for breast-feeding their newborn. Research-based breast-feeding protocols should be established in neonatal ICUs in order to facilitate and promote breast-feeding. Health care professionals need to be knowledgeable about the breast-feeding process and supportive of the breast-feeding mother and infant.

References

1. Bines J, Walker WA. Human milk: Carrier of biochemical messages to the nursing infant. Breastfeeding Abstracts 10(4): 1991.
2. Lucas A, Cole TJ, et al. Breastmilk and subsequent intelligence quotient in children born preterm. Lancet. 339:261, 1992.
3. Lucas A, Cole TJ. Breastmilk and neonatal necrotizing entercolitis. Lancet 336:1519, 1990.
4. Walker M. Breastfeeding premature babies. Lactation consultant series unit 14. La Leche League International, 1990.
5. Ehrenkranz RA, Acherman B, Mezger J. Breastfeeding and premature infants: Incidence and success, abstracted. Pediatr Res 19:99A (abstr 530), 1985.
6. Richards M, Larg M, McIntosh C, et al. Breastfeeding the vlbw infant: Successful outcome and maternal expectations. Pediatr Res 20:383A (abstr 1385), 1986.
7. Kaufman K, Hall L. Influences of the social network on choice and duration of breastfeeding in mothers of preterm infants. Res Nurs Health 12:149, 1989.
8. Akre J, ed. Infant feedings: The physiological basis. Geneva: World Health Organization, 1990; 21.
9. Mulford C. Subtle signs and symptoms of the milk ejection reflex. J Hum Lact 6(4):177, 1990.
10. Akre J, ed. Infant feeding: The physiologic basis. Geneva: World Health Organization, 1990; 22.
11. Hopkinson J, Schanler J, Garga C. Milk production by mothers of premature infants. Pediatrics 81(6):816, 1988.
12. Riordan R, Auerbach K. Breastfeeding and human lactation. 2nd ed. Boston: Jones and Bartlett Publishers, 1999; 399.
13. Lawrence R. Breastfeeding: A guide for the medical profession. 5th ed. St. Louis: Mosby, 1999; 696.
14. Zinaman M, Hughes V, Queenan J, et al. Acute prolactin and oxytocin responses and milk yield to infant suckling and artificial methods of expression in lactating women. Pediatrics 89(3):437, 1992.
15. Groh-Wargo S, Toth A, Mahoney K, et al. The utility of a bilateral breast pumping system for mothers of premature infants. Neonatal Network 14 (8):31, 1995.

16. Hill P, Aldag J, Chatterton R. The effect of sequential and simultaneous breast pumping on milk volume and prolactin levels: A pilot study. J Hum Lact 12(3):193, 1996.

17. Stutte P, Bowles B, Morman G. The effects of breast massage on volume and fat content of human milk. Genesis 10:22, 1988.

18. Feher S, Berger L, Johnson J, et al. Increasing breast milk production for premature infants with a relaxation/imagery audio tape. Pediatrics 83(1):57, 1989.

19. Anderson GC. Skin-to-skin: Kangaroo care in Western Europe. Am J Nurs May 1989; 662.

20. Whitelaw A. Kangaroo baby care: Just a nice experience or an important advance for preterm infants? Pediatrics 85(4):604, 1990.

21. Anderson GC. Current knowledge about skin to skin (Kangaroo) care for preterm infants. J Perinatol 11(3):216, 1991.

22. Ehrenkranz R, Ackerman B. Metoclopramide effect on faltering milk production by mothers of premature infants. Pediatrics 78(4):614, 1986.

23. Gunn AJ, Gunn TR, Rabone DL. Growth hormone increases breast milk volumes in mothers of preterm infants. Pediatrics 98(2):279, 1996.

24. Costa K. A comparison of colony counts of breast milk using two methods of breast cleansing. J Obstet Gynecol Neonatal Nurs 18:231, 1989.

25. American Academy of Pediatrics Committee on Fetus and Newborn. Guidelines for perinatal care, 4th ed. American Academy of Pediatrics and American College of Obstetricians and Gynecologists, 1997; 289.

26. Garza C. Johnson C, Harrist R, et al. Effects of methods of collection and storage on nutrients in human milk. Early Hum Dev 6:295, 1982.

27. Paxson CL, Cress CC. Survival of human milk leukocytes. J Pediatr 94:127, 1979.

28. Lawrence R. Breastfeeding: A guide for the medical profession. 5th ed. St. Louis: Mosby, 1999; 684.

29. Larson E, Zuill R, Zier V, et al. Storage of human milk. Infect Control 5(3):127, 1986.

30. Pierce K, Tully MR. Currents in human milk banking. Mother's own milk: Guidelines for storage and handling. J Hum Lact 8(3):159, 1992.

31. McCoy R, Kadowski C, Wilko S, et al. Nursing management of breastfeeding for preterm infants. J Perinatol Neonatal Nurs 2(1):45, 1988.

32. Sigman M, Burke K, Swarner O, et al. Effects of microwaving human milk: Changes in IgA content and bacterial count. J Am Diet Assoc 89(5):690, 1989.

33. Jocson MA, Mason EO, Schanler RJ. The effects of nutrient fortification and varying storage conditions on host defense properties of human milk. Pediatrics 100(2):240, 1997.

34. Meier P, Wilks S. The bacteria in expressed mothers milk. MCN 12:420, 1987.

35. Botsford K, Weinstein R, Boyer K, et al. Gram-negative bacilli in human milk feedings: Quantitation and clinical consequences for premature infants. J Pediatr 109(4):707, 1986.

36. Siimes M, Hallman J. A perspective on human milk banking. J Pediatr 94(1):173, 1979.

37. Carroll L, Davies DP, Osman M, et al. Bacteriological criteria of feeding raw breast-milk to babies in neonatal units. Lancet Oct 6, 1979; 732.

38. Meier P, Wilks S. The bacteria in expressed mothers' milk. MCN 12:420, 1987.

39. Stocks RJ, Davies DP, Allen F, et al. Loss of breast milk nutrients dur-
     ing tube feedings. Arch Dis Child. 60:165, 1985.

40. Lemons P, Miller K, Eitzen H, et al. Bacterial growth in human milk
     during continuous feedings. Am J Perinatol 1(1):76, 1983.

41. Valentine CJ, Hurst NM, Schanler RJ. Hind milk improves weight gain
     in low-birth-weight infants fed human milk. J Pediatr Gastroenterol
     Nutr 18(4):474, 1994.

42. Meier PP, Anderson GC. Responses of small preterm infants to bottle
     and breastfeeding. MCN 12:97, 1987.

43. Meier PP. Bottle and breastfeeding: Effects on transcutaneous oxygen
     pressure and temperature in preterm infants. Nurs Res 37:36, 1988.

44. Stine MJ. Breastfeeding the premature newborn: A protocol without
     bottles. J Hum Lact 6(4):167, 1990.

45. McCoy R, Kadowski C, Wilks S, et al. Nursing management of breast-
     feeding for preterm infants. J Perinatol Neonatal Nurs 2(1):46, 1988.

46. Narayahan I, Mehta R, Choudhury D, et al. Sucking on the 'emptied'
     breast: non-nutritive sucking with a difference. Arch Dis Child 66:241,
     1991.

47. Kliethermes PA, Cross ML, Lanese MG, et al. Transitioning preterm
     infants with nasogastric tube supplementation: Increased likelihood of
     preterm breastfeeding. JOGNN 28:264, 1999.

48. Bier AB, Ferguson AE, Morales Y, et al. Comparison of skin-to-skin
     contact with standard contact in low-birth-weight infants who are
     breastfed. Arch Pediatr Adolesc Med 150:1265, 1996.

49. Als H, Lester BM, Tronick EC, Brazelton TB. Manual for the assess-
     ment of preterm infants' behavior. In Fitzgerald AE, Lester BM,
     Yogman MW, eds. Theory and research in behavioral pediatrics, vol 1.
     New York: Plenum Press, 1992; 64-133.

50. Als H. Manual for the naturalistic observation of newborn behavior.
     Newborn individualized developmental care and assessment program
     (NIDCAP). Rev. Boston: Harvard Medical School, 1995.

51. Nyqvist K, Ewald U, Sjoden P. Supporting a preterm infant's behavior
     during breastfeeding: A case report. J Hum Lact 12(3):221, 1996.

52. Meier PP Engstrom JL, Fleming B, et al. Estimating milk intake of hos-
     pitalized preterm infants who breastfeed. J Hum Lact 12(1):21, 1996.

53. Meier PP, Engstrom JL, Crichton CL. A new scale for in-home test-
     weighing for mothers of preterm and high risk infants. J Hum Lact
     10(3):163, 1994.

54. Walker M. Breastfeeding the premature infant. NAACOG's Clinical
     Issues in Perinatal and Women's Health Nursing: Breastfeeding.
     Philadelphia: JP Lippincott, vol 3:4;624.

55. Lang S, Lawrence CJ, Orme R. Cup-feeding: An alternative method of
     infant feeding. Arch Dis Child. 71:365, 1994.

56. Kuehl J. Cup feeding the newborn: What you should know. J Perinatol
     Neonatal Nurs 11(2):56, 1997.

57. NAACOG Committee on Practice. OGN nursing practice resource:
     Facilitating breastfeeding. Nurse's Association of the American
     College of Obstetricians and Gynecologists, 1991.

58. Jensen D, Wallace S, Kelsay P. LATCH: A breastfeeding charting sys-
     tem and documentation tool. JOGNN. 23(1):27, 1994.

59. Mulford C. The mother-baby assessment (MBA): An "Apgar Score" for
     breastfeeding. J Hum Lact 8(2):79, 1992.

60. Tobin D. A breastfeeding evaluation and education tool. J Hum Lact 12(1):47, 1996.

61. Nyqvist K, Rubertsson C, Ewald U, et al. Development of the preterm infant breast-feeding behavior scale (PIBBS): A study of nurse-mother agreement. J Hum Lact 12(3):207-20, 1996.

62. Baker BJ, Rasmussen TW. Organizing and documenting lactation support of NICU families. JOGNN 26(5):515-20, 1997.

63. Hale T. medications and mothers' milk. 7th ed. Amarillo,Texas: Pharmasoft Medical Publishing, 1998.

64. Hall W, Shearer K, Kavanaugh R. Comparison of confidence between mothers who breastfed and formula-fed their preterm infants. J Perinatol Neonatal Nurs 11(2):44, 1997.

65. Huggins K. The Nursing Mother's Companion. 4th ed. Boston: Harvard Common Press, 1999; 80.

66. Schanler RJ, Shulman RJ, Lau C. Feeding strategies for premature infants: Beneficial outcomes of feeding fortified human milk versus preterm formula. Pediatrics 103:1150, 1999.

67. Schanler RJ, Hurst NM, Lau C. The use of human milk and breast-feeding in premature infants. Clin Perinatol 26(2):379, 1999.

68. Atkinson SA. Human milk feeding of the micropremie. Clin Perinatol 27(1):235, 2000.

69. Wang CD, Chu PS, Mellen BG, Shenai JP. Creamatocrit and the nutrient composition of human milk. J Perinatol 19(5):343, 1999.

70. Lucas A, Gibbs JAH, Lyster RLJ, Baum JD. Creamatocrit: simple clinical technique for estimating fat concentration and energy value of human milk. Br Med J 1:1018, 1978.

71. Lemons JA, Schreiner RL, Gresham EL. Simple method for determining the caloric and fat content of human milk. Pediatrics 66:626, 1980.

72. Kirsten D, Bradford L. Hindmilk feedings. Neonatal Network 18(3):68, 1999.

73. Lau C, Hurst N. Oral feeding in infants. Curr Prob Pediatr 29(4):105-124, 1999.

74. Arnold L. Recommendations for collection, storage, and handling of a mother's milk for her own infant in the hospital setting. 3rd Edition. Denver, CO: Human Milk Banking Association of North America, 1999.

Nutritional Care for High-Risk Newborns (Rev. 3d. Ed.)
S. Groh-Wargo, M. Thompson, J. Cox, editors
© 2000, Precept Press, Inc., Chicago

18

FEEDING METHODOLOGIES

Jacqueline Jones Wessel, MEd, RD, LD, CNSD

ENTERAL FEEDING IS THE preferred method of nutritional support when possible, even in the premature infant. The G.I. tract is structurally complete by 20 weeks' gestation, but its functioning gradually matures throughout gestation and early infancy.

Bottle- and breast-feeding require a coordinated G.I. response:

- Established sucking and swallowing
- Efficient gastric emptying and motility
- Regulated salivary, gastric, pancreatic, and hepatobiliary secretions
- Effective absorption, secretion, and mucosal protection provided by appropriate enterocyte function
- Economic utilization of the products of digestion and absorption
- Effective expulsion of undigested and waste products[1]

Premature infants may have difficulties with suck and swallow coordination, gastroesophageal reflux, gastric retention, and poor motility that may affect which feeding method is chosen for enteral feeding.[2-4]

Initiation and Progression of Feedings

First feedings are usually sterile water, human milk, or formula. If used as the initial feeding, 5% glucose water has been shown to be as deleterious to the lungs as formula if aspirated directly.[5] Traditional practice is to use sterile water to check for patency and to rule out some types of tracheoesophageal fistula. Feedings are then advanced to human milk or formula.

Although enteral feedings are important to the adaptation of the neonatal gut, the risk of necrotizing enterocolitis (NEC) may make one hesitate to initiate enteral feedings. Although the exact etiology of NEC is unknown, it occurs predominately in enterally-fed premature infants (see Chapter 25).[6,7] Delaying the onset of enteral feedings has not been shown to decrease the incidence of NEC; in fact, the delayed feeding groups had an increased incidence of the disease.[8,9]

Some investigators have linked a decrease in the incidence of NEC in their nurseries with the use of a "slow" feeding regimen, advancement by about 20 cc/kg/day. An increase in NEC was associated with a "fast" feeding regimen, i.e., advancement by about 60 cc/kg/day.[10] Other studies have linked NEC with high volumes of formula.[11-13] Until more is learned about the etiology of NEC, slow, cautious advancement of feedings by about 15-35 cc/kg/day seems justified for infants thought to be at highest risk for developing NEC .[12-15,101] This group would include premature infants of < 1.5 kg as well as larger infants with a compromised G.I. tract as a result of asphyxia.[102]

The safety of feeding preterm infants while an umbilical artery catheter (UAC) is in place is controversial. A prospective, randomized trial in preterm infants did not show an increased incidence of feeding problems, including NEC, in infants fed with a low UAC in place,[16] but the practice of feeding with any type (low or high) of UAC in place remains controversial.[17]

Many intensive care nurseries have developed feeding guidelines for use in initiating and advancing enteral feedings (Table 18.1). Although these guidelines are useful, they do not take the place of clinical expertise in assessing the infant's tolerance to feedings. The infant's clinical status; abdominal examination; tolerance to previous feedings; and stooling characteristics, including pattern, guaiac testing, and the presence or absence of reducing substances, should be considered prior to the advancement of feedings.[18] Gastric residuals are often checked to assess tolerance, keeping in mind that the stomach is a secretory organ that may always contain some fluid.[103] Guidelines for intermittent feedings suggest withholding feedings if residuals are greater than half of the previous feeding. For continuous infusions, feedings are withheld if the residual is greater than the previous hour's feeding volume.[19]

Positioning of the infant in the right lateral or prone position is traditionally thought to facilitate stomach emptying.[20] More recent evidence suggests left lateral or prone positioning may be preferred.[104] After the first few days of life, however, body position may not affect stomach emptying.[21,22] Prone positioning may be beneficial before and after feedings for the ventilated very low birthweight (VLBW) infant.[23]

The issue of whether to use full- or half-strength formula, if human milk is not available, in the initiation and advancement of

Table 18.1. Enteral Feeding Guidelines*

Hypocaloric (priming) feeds: For infants < 1,250 g birth weight; 10 cc/kg/d PF12[†] or MBM[†]

Progressive feeds:

Birth weight (g)	Feeding (type)[†]	Schedule (C or I)[‡]	Initial rate (cc/kg/d)	Volume increase (cc/kgld)	Full feedings (cc/kg/d)
< 750	PF24/MBM	C/q 2 hr	10	15	150
750-1,000	PF24/MBM	C/q 2 hr	10	15/20	150
1,001-1,250	PF24/MBM	C/q 2 hr	10	20	150
1,251-1,500	PF24/MBM	q 3 hr	20	20	150
1,501-1,800	PF24/MBM	q 3 hr	30	30	150
1,801-2,500	NEF/MBM	q 3 hr	40	40	165
> 2,500	T20/MBM	q 3 hr	50	50	180

* From MetroHealth Medical Center, Cleveland, OH
† MBM = Maternal breast milk; Fortify MBM for < 1,500 g birth-weight infants
  PF = Premature formula; PF12 = 12 kcal/oz; PF24 = 24 kcal/oz
  T = Term formula, 20 kcal/oz; NEF = Nutrient enriched formula, 22 kcal/oz
‡ C = Continuous, not recommended when MBM is used; I = Intermittent

enteral feedings continues to be debated. Two small studies used half-strength formula at double volume.[24,25] Infants on double-volume, half-strength formula achieved 100 kcal/kg faster than those on full-strength formula. No strong evidence from larger studies presently exists to support one method over the other.

Minimal Enteral Nutrition (MEN)

MEN, also called hypocaloric or priming feedings, consists of very low volume feedings (10-20 cc/kg/day) initiated to acclimate the G.I. tract to feedings, stimulate gut hormones, and promote G.I. maturation.[26] Full- or half-strength premature infant formula or full-strength human milk can be used. Feedings may be started at 48 hours and are held at the priming level for the first one to two weeks. Priming feedings have been shown to be well tolerated, to decrease indirect hyperbilirubinemia and cholestatic jaundice, and to improve bone mineralization in VLBW infants.[27,28] MEN feeding groups tend to achieve full feedings sooner, sustain improved growth, experience fewer episodes of sepsis, and be discharged home earlier than groups who are kept NPO.[29,30,105] Related positive effects include increased release of gastrin and other enteric hormones, and maturation of the duodenal motor response.[30-35] MEN does not appear to increase the risk of NEC although this is not universally accepted.[106] MEN studies have varied in day of feeding initiation, caloric density and type of feeding, and initial volume and rate of feeding advancement. This limits the ability to generalize the results. Clinically, MEN is widely accepted as a positive feeding option if used in carefully selected individual infants.[107]

Feeding Methods

The optimal method of feeding of premature infants is difficult to determine. Infants will often require two or more methods during their stay in the nursery. Coordinated suck and swallow doesn't usually develop until about 32-34 weeks' gestational age (GA).[36] Very sick infants or those mechanically ventilated will be unable to nipple-feed. Alternative methods of feeding have been devised with varying results (Table 18.2).

Nasogastric and Orogastric Feedings

Nasogastric (NG) feedings are delivered by inserting a feeding gavage tube from the nose to the stomach. Orogastric (OG) feedings are given by passing a gavage tube through the mouth to the stomach. NG or OG feedings can be administered either continuously or intermittently (bolus). Nasal or oral gavage to the stomach has been used for the initiation of feedings in infants who cannot as yet nipple-feed, who do not have an adequate gag reflex, and who have high respiratory rates. Infants between 32 and 36 weeks' GA often are fed with a combination of bottle or breast feedings and gavage feedings until they are able to take adequate feedings by nipple.

Tube placement should be carefully checked prior to each feeding to assure correct placement. The feeding tube may be removed between feedings to reduce the risk of gastroesophageal reflux (GER). There is increased risk of GER because the tube partially opens the lower esophageal sphincter. In some infants, however, the tube is left in because of their intolerance of tube passage and removal. Changing the tube is associated with vagal stimulation, which may increase the frequency of apnea and bradycardia.[37] A study evaluating the effects of indwelling versus intermittently placed feeding tubes on weight gain, apnea, and bradycardia, however, showed no difference in either episodes of apnea and bradycardia, or in rates of weight gain.[38] Feeding tube size is selected according to body weight: 3.5- or 5-French for infants weighing < 1,000 g and 5- or 8-French for infants > 1,000 g.[39]

Drawbacks to gavage feedings are intolerance of tube passage, risk of inappropriate tube placement, and risk of gastric perforation (rarely seen).[40] Damage to the palate with palatal grooves has been seen with the long-term use of indwelling oral feeding tubes.[41] OG tubes are not easy to secure and may be prone to dislodgement.[39] OG placement may be preferred, however, in infants with respiratory distress, as most neonates are primarily nose breathers.[37,42] Nasal feeding tubes can increase upper airway resistance, may cause nasal septum erosion, and may increase the incidence of purulent rhinitis and otitis media.[18] Indwelling NG tubes may allow for easier progression to nipple feedings without having to pull/replace the tube every feeding. However, some infants attempting to bottle feed with an indwelling NG tube in place have more difficulty with sucking and breathing than those without an NG tube.[43]

Transpyloric Feedings

In transpyloric feedings, the feeding tubes are passed through the pylorus into the small intestine. Transpyloric feedings are given continuously; bolus feedings are not recommended with this feeding method because the small intestine does not have the same capacity for expansion as the stomach. Infants to be considered for transpyloric feedings include those (1) intolerant to NG/OG feeding, (2) at risk for aspiration, (3) experiencing greater than usual problems with gastric emptying, (4) diagnosed with pylorospasm, or (5) receiving nasal continuous positive airway pressure (CPAP). CPAP may distend the stomach, sometimes decreasing tolerance to gastric feedings.[44] The transpyloric feeding tubes may be nasoduodenal (ND), oroduodenal (OD), nasojejunal (NJ), or orojejunal (OJ). Tube placement may be done in the nursery, but for patients whose tube passage is difficult, placement may be done using fluoroscopy in the radiology department.

A drawback to continuous transpyloric feedings is the possibility of intestinal perforation; however, the use of Silastic tubes has eliminated the morbidity related to the stiffening of polyvinyl tubes, thus decreasing the incidence of intestinal perforation.[37,40] Long-term use of transpyloric feedings may predispose infants to late pyloric stenosis.[45] The potential for fat malabsorption exists, as lingual and gastric lipase secretions are bypassed. Fat malabsorption is more likely with NJ than ND feedings because of the potential of the NJ feedings for decreased pancreatic enzyme contact.[46,47]

Several researchers have observed increased growth in infants given transpy-loric feedings,[48,49] although more recent studies have shown no advantage of transpyloric feedings over intermittent gavage feedings.[50,51] Most studies have shown that transpyloric feedings are safe and can be used for infants otherwise unable to tolerate

Table 18.2.   Comparison of Feeding Techniques

Methodology	Indications	Contraindications	Potential Problems	Advantages
Nipple- /breast-feeding	Infant 32-34 wk gestational age with coordinated suckling, swallowing and gag reflex	Acute illness	Aspiration	Allows for physiologic feedings
		High respiratory rate (> 80)	Fluid overload with ad lib feedings	Inexpensive
	Infant free of stress (i.e. no significant problems with apnea, bradycardia)	Inadequate sucking, swallowing, and gagging reflexes	Poor weight gain due to increased caloric expenditure while sucking	Suitable for infant at home
		Vomiting		Establishes a normal pattern of hunger and satiety
	Respiratory rate < 60/min	Cyanosis	Breast-feeding—unable to quantitate intake	
		Distended abdomen		
		Upper G.I. anomalies (i.e., large cleft palate or trachoesophageal fistula)		
		Change in stool composition or frequency; diarrhea		
		Maternal use of contraindicated drugs, certain maternal illnesses, if breast feeding		
Nasogastric/orogastric (NG/OG)	Infant in stable condition but does not have ability to coordinate suck, swallow, and gag reflexes	Acute illness	Reflux and aspiration	Provide enteral feeds to infants unable to nipple-feed.
		Vomiting	Bleeding	Relatively easy procedure
		Cyanosis	Perforation	Can be used at home after careful instruction and warning of risks
		Distended abdomen	Obstruction	
		Change in stool composition or frequency; diarrhea	Nasal erosion (NG)	
		Anomalies (i.e., tracheoesophageal fistula)	Palatal grooves (OG)	
		Inexperienced personnel	Bradycardia due to vagal stimulation	

Table 18.2. Comparison of Feeding Techniques (continued)

Methodology	Indications	Contraindications	Potential Problems	Advantages
Transpyloric (nasojejunal, orojejunal, nasoduodenal, oroduodenal	Infant exhibits repeated apnea and/or stomach distention from other types of tube feeding	Bolus feeding	Perforation	Way of providing enteral feeds to infant unable to nipple feed
		Acute illness	Bleeding	Less risk of aspiration than feedings into the stomach
	Infant shows continued gastric residuals without ileus	Vomiting	Obstructions	
		Cyanosis	Alterations in flora	
	Infant requires prolonged continuous positive airway pressure (CPAP) requiring gastric decompression	Distended abdomen	Intussusception	
		Changes in stool frequency; diarrhea	Dumping syndrome	
	Infant with pylorospasm		Diarrhea	
	Infant with severe gastroesophageal reflux	Anomalies of G.I. tract	Decreased cyclic enteric hormone response	
		Inexperienced personnel	Feeds less well digested, especially fat, as contact with various enzymes is decreased	
Gastrostomy/jejunostomy	Infant with neurological damage or anatomical malformation who requires long-term tube feeding	Ability to tolerate nipple feed within a short period of time	Infection	Allows for easier care of selected infants
			Dumping syndrome from improper feeding techniques	Suitable for infant at home or other type of facility
	Infant requires long-term continuous feeds (i.e., > 2 mo)	Changes in stool frequency; diarrhea		
			Tube displacement resulting in leakage and/or obstruction	

enteral feedings.[44,48,49,51] Surveys of the transpyloric feeding practices of level III nurseries showed no consensus on the technique or on the guidelines for when this feeding method should be used.[51,52]

Manometry has been used to assess the intestinal motor activity responses of preterm infants given intragastric or transpyloric feedings in small (4 ml/kg) or large (10 ml/kg) volumes. There were similar differences as compared with the prefed state with either method or volume. The use of dilute formula (⅓ strength), however, did not change motor activity from the fasting state. Only ¾ to full-strength 20 cal/oz formula changed motor activity. This suggests that either gastric or transpyloric feedings in small volume can be used to elicit a preterm motility response, but dilute formula may not be the optimal choice for this stimulation.[53] At this point, it would appear that transpyloric feedings should be reserved for infants who have been unable to tolerate gastric feedings.

Gastrostomy Tubes

Gastrostomy feedings are delivered via a gastrostomy tube (GT) from the abdomen directly into the stomach. For infants with severe GER, a fundoplication may be done at the same time as a surgically inserted G-tube; however, this is not mandatory. Feedings may be delivered continuously or intermittently (bolus). GT feedings are useful for:

- Infants whose progression to all-nipple feedings is expected to be prolonged (i.e., greater than two months)
- Infants with short bowel syndrome (to promote gut adaptation in the transition from TPN to enteral feedings)
- Infants who are neurologically impaired and unable to nipple-feed adequately.

Freedom from the continued use of OG or NG feeding tubes may decrease oral aversion and help in the transition to nipple-feeding in some infants. Gastrostomy/jejunostomy (GJ) tubes are also available; they may have two ports, one for gastric decompression and the other for jejunal feedings. GJ feeding may be used for the postoperative surgical neonate after gastric surgery. For example, after a procedure such as the Nissan fundoplication, a two-port GJ feeding tube may be used, with the gastric port being used for drainage of the stomach and the jejunal port used for continuous feedings.

Both types of tubes, GT and GJ, may be inserted either surgically or percutaneously. The surgical method is usually the Stamm gastrostomy procedure, in which a catheter is directly inserted into the anterior wall of the stomach and secured by a purse string suture. The catheter has a balloon or mushroom tip to help anchor the tube in the stomach.[37] The percutaneous endoscopic gastrostomy (PEG) or jejunostomy (PEJ) is inserted percutaneously using endoscopy.

Techniques for insertion, as well as management issues, are described elsewhere.[54-56] Although the insertion of percutaneous tubes does not require general anesthesia and avoids the surgical paralytic ileus that may involve the stomach and large intestine,[37] it is still an invasive procedure; a decision for each infant should be carefully made.

Button-type gastrostomy tubes may be used for the larger infant. The smallest size available at this time is 16-French, which can be used to replace a 14-French gastrostomy tube.[57] These tubes are designed to have a flatter profile against the stomach, and some have a snap-in mechanism for feedings. The button tubes may be used to replace the original tube in an established gastrostomy tract, two to three months postprocedure, and are often inserted in an outpatient setting.[58]

True long-term jejunostomies are rarely used in the neonate. For infants with extensive abdominal surgery and multiple ostomies, continuous feedings may be given through the stomach. Drainage from the ostomy(ies) may be refed through a mucous fistula or jejunostomy to try to feed the entire remaining intestine. Some clinicians have considered the use of jejunostomy feedings in severe bronchopulmonary dysplasia (BPD). This would allow enteral feedings to be continued through severe respiratory difficulties.

Continuous Versus Intermittent Feedings

Intermittent (bolus) feedings cause cyclical bursts of G.I. hormones, including insulin, in the preterm infant.[59] The baseline concentrations of insulin are higher in the continuously fed than in the bolus-fed infant.[59] Some consider bolus-feeding to be more physiological, although others argue that the current practice of presenting the premature infant's gut with bolus feedings of large volume (a total of 150-180 cc/kg) at about two weeks of age is not physiological either.[59] Animal studies suggest that bolus feedings may stimulate a greater gastrointestinal hormonal response than continuous feedings, resulting in increased small intestinal mucosal mass and enzyme activity.[60] In infant studies, however, slow, continuous infusion of feedings over two hours enhanced duodenal motor responses and gastric emptying more than bolus feeding over 15 minutes.[61]

Continuous NG feedings are sometimes used with an indwelling NG tube. This method of feeding is used for (1) very small infants, (2) infants who have not tolerated bolus feedings, (3) infants who have malabsorption problems with bolus feedings, or (4) infants who have not tolerated intermittent tube placement. Continuous feedings are always used with transpyloric and GJ feeding, and are often used with GT feeding. Continuous feedings are given via a pump at a steady slow rate. In the nursery, pumps intended for I.V. fluids are often used because of their accuracy at smaller volumes. Economical enteral pumps may be used at home, when feeding volumes are generally larger.

Some reports have shown greater weight gain and decreased energy expenditure with continuous feedings than with intermittent feedings.[62-65] Others have shown VLBW infants to have similar growth, equal episodes of feeding intolerance, similar macronutrient retention rates, and comparable lengths of stay whether they are fed continuously or intermittently.[66,67] Still others have reported less feeding intolerance and greater rates of weight gain with bolus feedings than with continuous feedings.[28]

Continuous feedings may facilitate respiratory stability in small premature infants recovering from respiratory distress syndrome.[68] In infants with intestinal problems, absorption may be improved by using continuous feedings, because the amount of substrate presented to the gut at one time is decreased. One crossover study of infants with intestinal disease showed greater absorption of fat, nitrogen, copper, zinc, and calcium.[64]

Continuous feeding regimens are associated with nutrient delivery problems. Human milk is particularly affected, because its fat is not homogenized.[39] The adherence of fat to feeding tubing and syringes results in a significant loss of fat as well as protein.[69,70] The rate of infusion of human milk correlates inversely with the degree of fat loss.[71] More lipid is lost during infusion of previously frozen milk than fresh, but more lipid is lost from fresh milk than refrigerated milk.[72,73] A method of minimizing the loss of fat by tilting the delivery syringe with a wooden wedge is described by Narayan and by Schanler.[74,75]

Human milk fortifiers, added to increase the energy, macronutrients, vitamin, mineral, and trace element concentrations in human milk, have been found to have losses when delivered continuously. The losses of calcium and phosphorus are the largest and are greater with fat-free powdered than liquid fortifier.[76] The liquid fortifier contains lipid, and use of continuously fed human milk with a liquid fortifier results in greater lipid delivery; however, most of the lipid delivered is from the fortifier, not the milk.[73] Bacterial growth in continuous feedings does not increase significantly over a 12-hour period in either human milk or formula.[77]

Medium-chain triglycerides (MCT) added to formulas or human milk separate from the formula or milk and/or adhere to the feeding apparatus. In either case, the risk of a fat bolus at the end of each infusion period increases.[78] Caloric supplementation through the use of concentrated formulas or emulsified fat products may be warranted as an alternative means for decreasing fat loss. Some of the lipid losses can be attenuated by the use of shorter tubing, complete emptying of the feeding bag or syringe, and progression to intermittent bolus feeding as soon as the clinical course indicates the transition.[74]

Early studies showed greater loss of calcium and other minerals when premature formulas were given continuously than when these formulas were used for intermittent feedings.[79,80] Since that time, premature infant formulas have been reformulated. The delivery of minerals when feeding continuously has improved significantly and is no longer considered to be a problem.[81]

In summary, the choice between continuous and intermittent feedings for PT infants remains controversial. Continuous feeding may afford benefit to some PT infants, but others do well with bolus feeding. The choice should follow an assessment of the individual infant's clinical status. In practice, intermittent feeding may be the most common method, with continuous feeding used for the smallest and sickest.

Transition to Nipple-Feeding

Nipple feedings are attempted in stable infants of at least 32-34 weeks' gestation who have coordinated suck-swallow-breathe patterns and respiratory rates of < 60 per minute.[82] Prolonged nipple-feedings may increase energy expenditure. If feedings take over 30 minutes, alternative feeding methods may need to be considered. Alternatives might include use of a higher calorie formula to decrease volume needed to meet calorie goals or use of some intermittent gavage feedings.

The transition to nipple-feedings from gavage feedings is accomplished gradually. It can be done according to the infant's condition or based on a schedule-for example, once per day-then once a shift, every third, every other, then every feeding. Nipple-feedings are often introduced in a continuously fed infant once a day, turning the pump off for an hour and allowing the infant to nipple-feed the amount of the hourly rate during that time. This is often more successful than feeding "on top" of the drip rate.

Progression to all-nipple feedings from continuous feedings depends on tolerance. The reason that the continuous feedings were originally started should also be considered. Infants with malabsorption problems due to short gut syndrome, etc., often make the transition slowly, with one nipple-feeding at the hourly rate, then two, then three, etc. By combining a two-hour "window" off the continuous feedings and nippling, that amount can be fed, and then a transition to a three-hour schedule can be made. Some infants are fed by mouth in the daytime and tube-fed at night, using a continuous drip or intermittent gavage for not only nighttime feedings but also making up any deficit from the day's feedings.

Some infants become overwhelmed with nipple feeding and need help pacing or controlling the feeding. Techniques for facilitating nipple feedings are described in Chapter 19 and in the literature.[83,84,108] Nurses and parents who feed preterm infants need to observe the infant's cues and changes in sucking patterns during a feeding.[85,109] The continuous sucking period results in a greater volume of intake, but has more detrimental effects on breathing pattern and oxygenation than intermittent sucking.[85]

Nonnutritive sucking (NNS) is the practice of using pacifiers for infants to suck on during gavage feedings. Some studies have shown that NNS improves weight gain and results in earlier discharge in premature infants who were tube-fed,[86-88,110] but others have found no significant change in weight gain.[89,90] NNS has not been found to increase gastric emptying,[91] and only one study has shown decreased intestinal transit time.[88] Because NNS facilitates the maturation of the sucking reflex,[88] a plan for oral motor stimulation by its use should be considered as clinically indicated for the transition from tube-feeding to nipple- or breast-feeding. In one study, 10 minutes of NNS prior to a preterm infant's first nipple feeding promoted neurological organization and feeding success.[92] Heart rates did not increase during nippling in this study, suggesting that energy expenditure during feeding is not as excessive as has been assumed for all infants.[92]

The transition from nipple- to breast-feeding is usually attempted when the infant is about 34 weeks' GA, has established tolerance and growth on enteral feedings, has a coordinated suck-swallow-breathe pattern, and can maintain body temperature.[42] This is a conservative approach, and some professionals may feel comfortable allowing breast-feeding earlier. Highly successful lactation programs in a very low birth weight population (< 1,500 g) have been reported.[93,111] Syringe-type feeding devices with soft, very small tubing to bypass bottle feeds for the potentially breast-fed infant are available; however, these feeding techniques call for a skilled feeder because of the risk of aspiration (see Chapter 17).[94]

Feeding Equipment

A variety of nipples are available for term and premature infants. Nipples designed for use by premature infants are softer, smaller, and allow for greater flow at lower sucking pressures. Flow rates of various types of nipples and the differences between nipples of the same kind are discussed in detail elsewhere.[95] The high rate of milk flow during feedings may contribute to the ventilatory depression, feeding-related apnea, and/or bradycardia sometimes observed in premature infants during bottle feedings.[96] Premature infants may be more prone to aspirate when a high-flow nipple is used because of immature suck and swallow coordination. Because of its flow rate, a standard-size nipple may be more appropriate than a premature nipple.[83] Some term infants with a very weak suck may use a premature high-flow nipple successfully; also, milk flow may be altered by the tightness of seal on the bottle. There needs to be individual consideration in the choice of nipple regardless of whether the infant is premature. Occasionally, at discharge infants may prefer the special size or flow of a nipple for prematures. These nipples may be ordered for home use by contacting the supplier.

Pacifiers are used for offering nonnutritive sucking during tube-feeding, and for use between breast- or bottle-feeding. Commercial pacifiers are constructed to meet safety standards set by the U.S. Consumer Products Safety Commission (personal communication, Children's Medical Ventures, 1999). Pacifiers are available in both term and preterm size. Mam and MiniMam (Sassy, Inc., Kentwood, MI), and Soothie, Wee Thumbie, and Wee Soothie (Children's Medical Ventures, S. Weymouth, MA) are names of some commercially available pacifiers. Use of homemade pacifiers is strongly discouraged. These makeshift pacifiers are sometimes constructed from nipples stuffed with cotton or gauze that is taped to the plastic collar. A case of an infant who died when the nipple of a makeshift pacifier came off and was aspirated has been reported.[97] Overuse of pacifiers is discouraged especially for the breast-fed infant. Some breast-fed babies use pacifiers without problems, but they may interfere with breast-feeding for others.[98,112] Guidelines for use of pacifiers, criteria for an effective pacifier, and descriptions of selected pacifiers are available.[99]

Discharge and Follow-up

Some infants may require feeding assistance at discharge. Continued use of tube feedings may be needed for some infants who have not fully made the transition to nipple feedings, including

- Infants who have marked oral aversion
- Infants who are neurologically impaired
- Infants unable to take sufficient volume of nipple feedings
- Infants unable to sustain growth on all nipple feedings
- Infants with intestinal problems resulting in malabsorption with all-nipple feedings

Some infants are discharged from the hospital prior to achieving full nipple- or breast-feedings. Parents need to receive detailed training in feeding techniques appropriate for their infant, and coordination of discharge teaching with all disciplines involved is important. Home-based care needs a supportive multidisciplinary home care team. A description of a home gavage program and clinic is provided elsewhere.[100] Infants who are discharged on tube feedings need close monitoring and follow-up (see Appendix N).

Each of the feeding techniques described above has advantages and disadvantages. Successful enteral feeding of the high-risk infant often demands creativity and flexibility. An infant may need multiple feeding methods during the transition to oral feedings. The team approach, including input of the nutritionist, nurse, occupational therapist, speech pathologist, lactation consultant, and physician, can facilitate choosing successful feeding regimens for infants at different stages in their development and clinical course.

References

1. Weaver LT, Lucas A. Development of gastrointestinal structure and function. In: Hay WW, ed. Neonatal nutrition and metabolism. St. Louis: Mosby, 1991; 71-90.
2. Berseth CL. Gestational evolution of small intestine motility in preterm and term infants. J Pediatr 115:646, 1989.
3. Carlos MA, Babyn PS. Changes in gastric emptying in early postnatal life. J Pediatr 130:931, 1997.
4. Dumont RC, Rudolph CD. Development of gastrointestinal motility in the infant and child. Gastroenterol Clin North Amer 23:655, 1994.
5. Olson M. The benign effects on rabbit's lungs of the aspiration of water compared with 5% glucose or milk. Pediatrics 46:538, 1970.
6. Kliegman RM, Fanaroff AA. Necrotizing enterocolitis. N Engl J Med 310:1093, 1984.
7. Neu J. Necrotizing enterocolitis: The search for a unifying pathogenic theory leading to prevention. Pediatr Clin North Amer 43:409, 1997.
8. LaGamma EF, Ostertag SG, Birenbaum H. Failure of delayed oral feedings to pre-vent necrotizing enterocolitis. Am J Dis Child 139:385, 1985.
9. Ostertag S, LaGamma EF, Reisen CE, et al. Early enteral feeding does not affect the incidence of necrotizing enterocolitis. Pediatrics 77:275, 1986.
10. Goldman HI. Feeding and necrotizing enterocolitis. Am J Dis Child 134:553, 1980.
11. Brown EG, Sweet AY. Preventing necrotizing enterocolitis in neonates. JAMA 240:2452, 1978.
12. Anderson DM, Kliegman RM. The relationship of neonatal alimentation practices to the occurrence of endemic necrotizing enterocolitis. Am J Perinatol 8:62, 1991.
13. Zabielski PB, Groh-Wargo SL, Moore JJ. Necrotizing enterocolitis: Feeding in endemic and epidemic periods. J Parenter Enter Nutr 13:520, 1989.
14. Book LS, Herbst JJ, Jung AI. Comparison of fast- and slow-feeding rate schedules to the development of necrotizing enterocolitis. J Pediatr 89:463, 1976.

15. Ruyyis SF, Ambalavanan N, Wright L, Carlo WA. Randomized trial of "slow" versus "fast" feed advancements on the incidence of necrotizing enterocolitis in very low birth weight infants. J Pediatr 134:293, 1999.

16. Davey AM, Wagner CL, Cox C, et al. Feeding premature infants while low umbilical artery catheters are in place: A prospective randomized trial. J Pediatr 124:795, 1994.

17. Heird WC, Gomez MR. Total parenteral nutrition in necrotizing enterocolitis. Clin Perinatol 21(2):389, 1994

18. Kaempf J. Techniques of enteral feeding in the preterm infant. In: Hay WW, ed. Neonatal nutrition and metabolism. St. Louis: Mosby, 1991; 335-48.

19. Hendricks KM, Walker WA. Manual of pediatric nutrition. Toronto: Decker, 1990; 104.

20. Yu VY. Effect of body position on gastric emptying in the neonate. Arch Dis Child 50:500, 1975.

21. Blumenthal I, Ebel A, Pildes R. Effect of posture on the pattern of stomach emptying in the newborn. Pediatrics 63:532, 1979.

22. Siegel M, Lebenthal E. Development of gastrointestinal motility and gastric emptying during the fetal and newborn periods. In: Lebenthal E, ed. Human gastrointestinal development. New York: Raven Press, 1989; 285.

23. Mizuno K, Itabushi K, Okuyama K. Effect of body positioning on the blood gases and ventilation volume of infants with chronic lung disease before and after feeding. Am J Perinatol 12:275, 1995.

24. Currao WJ, Cox C, Shapiro DL. Diluted formula for beginning the feeding of premature infants. Am J Dis Child 142:730, 1988.

25. Sarna MS, Sali A, Pandey KK, et al. Premature infant feeding: The role of diluted formula. Ind Pediatr 27:829, 1990.

26. Slagle TA, Gross SJ. Effect of early low volume enteral substrate on subsequent feeding tolerance in very low birthweight infants. J Pediatr 113:526, 1988.

27. Dunn L, Hulman S, Weiner J, et al. Beneficial effects of early hypocaloric enteral feeding on neonatal gastrointestinal function: Preliminary report of a randomized trial. J Pediatr 112:622, 1988.

28. Schanler RJ, Shulman RJ, Lau C, et al. Feeding strategies for premature infants:Randomized trial of gastrointestinal priming and tube-feeding method. Pediatrics 103:434, 1999.

29. Troche B, Harvey-Wilkes K, Engle WD, et al. Early minimal feedings promote growth in critically ill premature infants. Bio Neonate 67:172, 1995.

30. Meetze WH, Valentine C, McGuigan JE, et al. Gastrointestinal priming prior to full enteral nutrition in very low birth weight infants. J Pediatr Gastroenterol Nutr 15:163, 1992.

31. Lucas A, Bloom SR, Aynsley-Green A. Postnatal surges in plasma gut hormones in term and preterm infants. Biol Neonate 41:63, 1982.

32. Lucas A, Bloom SR, Aynsley-Green A. Gut hormones and 'minimal enteral feeding.' Acta Paediatr Scand 75:719, 1986.

33. Berseth CL. Effect of early feeding on maturation of the preterm infant's small intestine. J Pediatr 120:947, 1992.

34. Berseth CL. Minimal enteral feedings. Clin Perinatol 22(1):195, 1995.

35. al Tawil Y, Berseth CL. Gestational and postnatal maturation of duodenal motor responses to intragastric feeding. J Pediatr 129:374, 1996

36. Gryboski JD. Suck and swallow in the premature infant. Pediatrics 43:96, 1969.
37. Pereira GR, Ziegler MM. Nutritional care of the surgical neonate. Clin Perinatol 16:233, 1989.
38. Symington A, Ballantyne M, Pinelli J, et al. Indwelling versus intermittent feeding tubes in premature neonates. J Obstet Glynecol Neonatal Nurs 24:321, 1995.
39. Schanler RJ. Special methods in feeding the preterm infant. In: Tsang RC, Nichols BL, eds. Nutrition during infancy. Philadelphia: Hanley and Belfus, 1988; 314-25.
40. Cox MA. Nutrition. In: Cloherty JP, Stark AR, eds. Manual of neonatal care. Boston: Little, Brown, 1985; 423-58.
41. Neal P, Bull MJ, Jansen RD, et al. Palatal grooves secondary to oral feeding tubes. J Perinatol 5:41, 1988.
42. Miller MJ, Carlo WJ, Strohl KP, et al. Determination of oral breathing in premature infants. Pediatr Res 19:354a, 1985.
43. Shiao SPK, Youngblut JM, Anderson GC, et al. Nasogastric tube placement: Effects on breathing and sucking in very-low-birth-weight infants. Nurs Res 44:82, 1995
44. Pereira GR, Lemons JA. Controlled study of transpyloric and intermittent gavage feeding in the small preterm infant. Pediatrics 67:68, 1981.
45. Latchaw LA, Jacir NN, Harris BH. The development of pyloric stenosis during transpyloric feedings. J Pediatr Surg 24:823, 1989.
46. Minoli I, Coppalini B, Galli C, et al. Essential fatty acid status in premature newborns fed by nasoduodenal technique. Pediatrics 67:73, 1981.
47. Roy RN, Pollnitz RP, Hamilton JR, et al. Impaired assimilation of nasojejunal feeds in healthy low-birth-weight newborn infants. J Pediatr 90:431, 1977.
48. Wells DH, Zachman RD. Nasojejunal feedings in low-birth-weight infants. J Pediatr 87:276, 1975.
49. Callie MV, Powell GK. Nasoduodenal versus nasogastric feeding in the very low birthweight infant. Pediatrics 56:1065, 1975.
50. Laing IA, Laing MA, Callahan O, et al. Nasogastric compared with nasoduodenal feeding in low birthweight infants. Arch Dis Child 61:138, 1986.
51. Dryburgh E. Transpyloric feeding in 40 infants undergoing intensive care. Arch Dis Child 55:879, 1980.
52. Chan J, Ferraro AR. The use of transpyloric feedings in the NICU: A national survey. Neonatal Network 10:37, 1991.
53. Koenig WJ, Amarnath RP, Hench V, et al. Manometrics for preterm and term infants: A new tool for old questions. Pediatrics 95:203, 1995.
54. Gauderer MW, Stellato TA. Gastrostomies: Evolution, techniques, indications, and complications. Curr Prob Surg 23:658, 1986.
55. Deveney KE. Endoscopic gastrostomy and jejunostomy. In: Rombeau JL, Caldwell MD, eds. Enteral and tube feeding. Philadelphia: Saunders, 1990; 217-29.
56. Neal J, Slayton D. Neonatal and pediatric PEG tubes. MCN 17:184, 1992.
57. Huddleston KC, Palmer KL. A button for gastrostomy feedings. MCN 15:315, 1990.

58. Gauderer MW, et al. The gastrostomy "button"-a simple, skin-level nonrefluxing device for long-term enteral feedings. J Pediatr Surg 19:803, 1984.

59. Aynsley-Green A, Adrian TE, Bloom SE. Feeding and the development of enteroinsular hormone secretion in the preterm infant: Effect of continuous gastric infusion of human milk compared to intermittent bolus. Acta Paediatr Scand 71:379, 1982.

60. Shulman RJ, Redel CA, Stathos TH. Bolus versus continuous feedings stimulate small-intestinal growth and development in the newborn pig. J Pediatr Gastroenterol Nutr 18:350, 1994.

61. de Ville K, Knapp E, Al-Tawil Y, Berseth CL. Slow infusion feedings enhance duodenal motor responses and gastric emptying in preterm infants. Am J Clin Nutr 68:103, 1998.

62. Krishnan V, Satish M. Continuous vs. intermittent nasogastric feeding in very low birthweight infants. Pediatr Res 15:537, 1981.

63. Toce SS, Keenan WJ, Homan SM. Enteral feeding in very-low birth weight infants. Am J Dis Child 141:439, 1987.

64. Parker P, Stroop S, Greene H. A controlled comparison of continuous versus intermittent feeding in the treatment of infants with intestinal disease. J Pediatr 99:360, 1987.

65. Grant J, Denne SC. Effect of intermittent versus continuous enteral feeding on energy expenditure in premature infants. J Pediatr 118:928, 1991.

66. Silvestre MA, Morbach CA, Brans YW, et al. A prospective randomized trial comparing continuous versus intermittent feeding methods in very low birthweight neonates. J Pediatr 128:748, 1996.

67. Atkintorin SM, Kamat M, Pildes RS, et al. A prospective randomized trial of feeding methods in very low birth weight infants. Pediatrics 100:716, 1997.

68. Blondheim O, Abasi S, Fox WW, et al. Effect of enteral gavage feeding rate on pulmonary functions of very low birth weight infants. J Pediatr 122:751, 1993.

69. Stocks RJ, Davies DP, Allen E Loss of breast milk nutrients during tube feeding. Arch Dis Child 60:164, 1985.

70. Brennan-Behm M, Carlson G-E, Meier P, Engstrom J. Caloric loss from expressed mother's milk during continuous gavage infusion. Neonatal Network 13:27, 1994.

71. Greer FR, McCormick A, Loker J. Changes in fat concentration of human milk during delivery by intermitent bolus and continuous mechanical pump infusion. J Pediatr 105:745, 1984.

72. Lemons PM, Miller K, Eitzen H, et al. Bacterial growth in human milk during continuous feeding. Am J Perinatol 1:76, 1983.

73. Lavine M, Clark RM. The effect of short-term refrigeration of milk and the addition of breast milk fortifier on the delivery of lipids during tube feeding. J Pediatr Gastroenterol Nutr 8:496, 1989.

74. Narayan I, Singh B, Harvey D. Fat loss during feeding of human milk. Arch Dis Child 59:475, 1984.

75. Schanler RJ, Garza C, Nichols BL. Fortified mother's milk for very low birth weight infants: Results of growth and nutrient balance studies. J Pediatr 107:437, 1985.

76. Bhatia J, Rassin DK. Human milk supplementation: Delivery of energy, calcium, phosphorus, magnesium, copper, and zinc. Am J Dis Child 142:445, 1988.

77. Dodd V, Froman R. A field study of bacterial growth in continuous feedings in a neonatal intensive care unit. Neonatal Network 9:17, 1991.
78. Mehta NR, Hamosh M, Bitman J, et al. Adherence of medium-chain fatty acids to feeding tubes during gavage feeding of human milk fortified with medium chain triglycerides. J Pediatr 112:474, 1988.
79. Bhatia J, Fomon SJ. Formula for premature infants: Fate of calcium and phosphorus. Pediatrics 72:37, 1983.
80. Antonson DL, Smith JL, Nelson RD, et al. Stability of vitamin and mineral concentrations of a low birthweight infant formula during continuous enteral feeding. J Pediatr Gastroenterol Nutr 2:617, 1983.
81. Bhatia J. Ltr to ed. Pediatrics 75:800, 1985.
82. Gomella N. Neonatology. Norwalk, Conn.: Appleton and Lange, 1991; 61-81.
83. Shaker CS. Nipple feeding premature infants: A different perspective. Neonatal Network 8:9, 1990.
84. Jordan S. The controlled or paced bottle feeding. Mother Baby J 3:21, 1998.
85. Shiao SY. Comparison of continuous versus intermittent sucking in very-low-birth-weight infants. J Obstet Gynecol Neonatal Nurs 26:313, 1997.
86. Measel CP, Anderson GC. Non-nutritive sucking during tube feedings: Effect upon clinical course in premature infants. J Obstet Gynecol Neonatal Nurs 8:265, 1979.
87. Field T, Ignatoff E, Stringer S, et al. Non-nutritive sucking during tube feedings: Effects on preterm neonates in an intensive care unit. Pediatrics 70:381, 1982.
88. Bernbaum JC, Pereira GR, Watkins JB, et al. Non-nutritive sucking during gavage feeding enhances growth and maturation in premature infants. Pediatrics 71:41, 1983.
89. DeCurtis M, McIntosh N, Ventura V, et al. Effect of non-nutritive sucking on nutrient retention in preterm infants. J Pediatr 109:888, 1986.
90. Ernst JA, Rickard KA, Neal PR, et al. Lack of improved growth outcome related to nonnutritive sucking in very low birthweight premature infants fed a controlled nutrient intake: A randomized prospective study. Pediatrics 83:706, 1989.
91. Szabo JS, Hellemeier AC, Oh W. Effect of non-nutritive and nutritive suck on gastric emptying in premature infants. J Pediatr Gastroenterol Nutr 4:348, 1985.
92. McCain GC. Promotion of preterm infant nipple feeding with nonnutritive sucking. J Pediatr Nurs 10:3, 1995.
93. Yu VY, Jamieson J, Bajuk B. Breast milk feeding in very low birth weight infants. Aust Paediatr J 17:186, 1981.
94. Medela Inc., McHenry, Ill.
95. Mathew OP. Nipple units for newborn infants: A functional comparison. Pediatrics 81:688, 1988.
96. Mathew OP. Breathing patterns of preterm infants during bottle feedings: Role of milk flow. J Pediatr 119:960, 1991.
97. Millunchick EW, McArtor RD. Fatal aspiration of a makeshift pacifier. Pediatrics 77:369, 1986.
98. Lawrence RA, ed. Breastfeeding: A Guide for the medical profession. 5th ed. St. Louis: Mosby, 1999; 289-90.

99. Morris SE, Klein MD, eds. Pre-feeding skills: A comprehensive resource for feeding development. Tucson, Ariz: Therapy Skill Builders, 1987; 356-59.

100. Evanochko C, Jancs-Kelly S, Boyle R, et al. Facilitating early discharge from the NICU: The development of a home gavage program and neonatal outpatient clinic. Neonatal Network 15:44, 1996.

101. Kennedy KA, Tyson JE, Chamnanvanakij S. Rapid versus slow rate of advancement of feedings for promoting growth and preventing necrotizing enterocolitis in parenterally fed low-birth-weight infants. (Cochrane Review). In: The Cochrane Library, 10/28/99. Oxford: Update Software.

102. Kamitsuka MD, Horton MK, Williams MA. The incidence of necrotizing enterocolitis after introducing standardized feeding schedules for infants between 1250 and 2500 grams and less than 35 weeks of gestation. Pediatrics 105:379, 2000.

103. Ziegler EE. Trophic feeds. In: Ziegler EE, Lucas A, Moro G. Nutrition of the Very Low Birthweight Infant. Nestle Nutrition Workshop Series, Paediatric Programme, Vol. 43. Philadelphia: Nestec Ltd., Vevey/Lippincott Williams and Wilkins, 1999; 233-244.

104. Ewer AK, James ME, Tobin JM. Prone and left lateral positioning reduce gastroesophageal reflux in preterm infants. Arch Dis Child Fetal Neonatal Ed 81:F201, 1999.

105. McClure RJ, Newell SJ. Randomised controlled study of clinical outcome following trophic feeding. Arch Dis Child Fetal Neonatal Ed 82:F29, 2000.

106. Tyson JE, Kennedy KA. Minimal enteral nutrition in parenterally fed neonates. (Cochrane Review). In: The Cochrane Library, 7/24/97. Oxford: Update Software.

107. Thureen PJ. Early aggressive nutrition in the neonate. NeoRev September, 1999:e45.

108. Lau C, Hurst N. Oral feeding in infants. Curr Prob Pediatr 29(4):105-124, 1999.

109. Shaker CS. Nipple feeding preterm infants: An individualized, developmentally supportive approach. Neonatal Network 18(3):15, 1999.

110. Pinelli J, Symington A. Non-nutritive sucking for the promotion of physiologic stability and nutrition in preterm infants. (Cochrane Review). In: The Cochrane Library, 11/24/98. Oxford: Update Software.

111. Kliethermes PA, Cross ML, Lanese MG, et al. Transitioning preterm infants with nasogastric tube supplementation: Increased likelihood of breastfeeding. JOGNN 28(3):264, 1999.

112. Aarts C, Hornell A, Kylberg E, et al. Breastfeeding patterns in relation to thumb sucking and pacifier use. Pediatrics 104(4):e50, 1999.

Nutritional Care for High-Risk Newborns (Rev. 3d. Ed.)
S. Groh-Wargo, M. Thompson, J. Cox, editors
© 2000, Precept Press, Inc., Chicago

19

ASSESSMENT AND TREATMENT OF FEEDING PROBLEMS/ DYSFUNCTION

Jacquelyn L. Chamberlin, MA, OTR/L

TYPICAL FULL-TERM NEWBORNS HAVE reflexive behaviors enabling them to suck and swallow and to coordinate sucking bursts with pauses to breathe. This remarkably efficient oral-motor development is an important beginning of the nutritional process for the human infant. As the infant matures during the first few months of life, these early reflexive behaviors disappear, and eating becomes a learned behavior.[1] As reflexive feeding is replaced by voluntary, controlled eating, the typical infant begins to associate eating with interactive pleasure and satiety. Feeding is one of the first social contacts between parent and child. Infants born prematurely or critically ill are at risk for having problems in establishing behaviors required for successful oral feeding and weight gain.[1] This chapter will discuss some of the problems observed and offer suggestions for overcoming them.

Typical Development

In order to understand the most common problems of premature infants, it is important to know something about the early developmental process of the oral-motor mechanism. Function of the infant's oral-motor mechanism is present long before oral feeding is feasible.[2] The reflexive behaviors of rooting, sucking, and swallowing

Table 19.1.   Normal Oral-Motor Development

Preterm

Gestational age	Reflexive behavior	Oral-motor development
28 wk	Rudimentary rooting present in the form of yawning and some delayed lip movement	Nonnutritive suck may be possible with a pacifier. Lips rarely engage the nipple. No neck or shoulder stability for feeding posture
30 wk	Rooting reflex involves head movements of extension and rotation. Synchronization of sucking and swallowing begins	Nonnutritive suck stronger and may assist tube feedings. Lips may engage the nipple for longer periods during nonnutritive sucking
32 wk	Rooting reflex consistent, especially before feedings. Gag reflex is present and consistent. Respiratory effort can be modified to accommodate swallowing, but is still precarious and exerted efforts may cause apnea	Sucking becomes more prolonged and rhythmic. Some stripping action of the tongue can be seen/felt. Lips and tongue engage nipple with fair strength but tire quickly
34 wk	Reflexes of rooting, sucking, swallowing and gagging are mature	Maturity of reflexive behaviors allow more consistent, prolonged effort at sucking. Infant should be "safe" to feed with close attention to physiological stress signals. Endurance for oral feeding may be brief, requiring "time-outs" and/or partial tube feedings. Strengthening of the lips and tongue over time will improve endurance
35-38 wk		Reflexive oral-motor mechanism is mature

undergo a systematic maturation process from early fetal life.[3] Table 19.1 describes typical development of reflexive behaviors and the oral-motor function at various gestational ages.

Another important developmental element, physiologic flexion, is present in the typical term infant. This strong flexor posture of the infant provides additional body support for efficient nipple-feeding.[5,6] Premature infants are mechanically different from typical term infants. Physiologic flexion is weak or totally absent, depending on the infant's gestational age at birth. Therefore, the premature infant is at a mechanical disadvantage in feeding posture.[5,6] Buccal fat pads, which also assist nipple-feeding in the typical term infant, are diminished or absent in the premature infant.[5,6]

Table 19.1. Normal Oral-Motor Development (continued)

Term

Postterm age	Reflexive behavior	Oral-motor development
0-2 mo	Reflexes of gagging, rooting, sucking, swallowing, phasic bite, and tongue protrusion are present	Reflexive sucking pattern (sometimes referred to as suckling pattern) for nutritive sucking gradually changes over period to controlled negative pressure sucking pattern. Infant develops association between hunger/satiety and nutritive/nonnutritive sucking
2-4 mo	Reflexes of rooting, sucking (reflexive) and phasic bite are inhibited by control of voluntary muscle groups. Tongue protrusion reflex is diminishing. Point of activation of the gag reflex is moving further back on the tongue	Voluntary control of oral-motor structures and neck musculature enables infant to control eating behaviors by turning away from bottle and care-giver
4-6 mo	Tongue protrusion reflex is inhibited by control of voluntary muscle groups. Gag reflex is reduced to typical adult level	Infant can suck solids from a spoon, form bolus with tongue and swallow. Vertical, one-plane chewing appears (sometimes referred to as munching)

References: Saint-Anne Dargassues,[2] Jain,[3] McBride and Danner,[4] Morris[5]

Common Developmental Feeding Problems

Premature infants who have attained the age at which typical oral-motor maturation supports oral feeding continue to be at a disadvantage. Intra-oral observations of premature infants' suck/swallow/breathe patterns by real-time ultrasound compared with observations of term infants' patterns suggest that this sequential coordination is less efficient even when the premature infant reaches term.[7] The infant's ability to maintain physiologic stability may still be tenuous, contributing to disorganization of the suck/swallow/breathe coordination. Weak physiologic flexion and the imbalance of muscle strength (extension > flexion) provide a weak basis for feeding behaviors. The exertion of effort to complete a feeding may cost more energy than the infant has available.[3] Critically ill term infants also may have diminished strength and endurance for full oral feedings.[8,9] Recovery from a life-threatening event takes time. During recovery, the infant may need to be sup-

(TEXT CONTINUED ON PAGE 352)

Table 19.2. Feeding Problems Common to Many Infants

Problem	Probable cause	Prevention/intervention strategies
Decreased strength of lip closure and flat tongue action, resulting in decreased strength of suck	Loss of physiologic flexion as a result of premature birth; the earlier the birth, the less the strength of the flexor groups	Provide nonnutritive sucking during period before infant can be orally fed When oral feedings are begun, use preemie-style nipple to establish nippling without fatiguing infant. As strength of sucking increases, use regular nipple early in oral feeding to "make the muscles work hard" and finish feeding with preemie-style nipple (It is a good idea to use the same shape for the entire feeding—e.g., use the Ross standard [yellow] and switch to the Ross premature [red]) Stroking the infant's cheeks and lips prior to nipple-feeding may increase oral sensitivity and improve initial muscle strength During feeding, supporting the infant's cheeks can assist the infant's sucking efficiency in the same way term infant's buccal pads would. Support at the base of the infant's tongue will assist nipple compression (be sure that the support is to the base of the tongue and not to the chin or jaw)
Decreased endurance with oral feedings	Loss of physiologic flexion, requiring greater muscle work to maintain flexed feeding position. Immaturity of the neurobehavioral and neuromuscular systems and/or recovery phase for the neurobehavioral and neuromuscular systems. Lack of experience with oral feedings	Support the infant in a flexed, semiupright position during feeding (swaddling and containment) Allow the infant short time-out periods when it appears that the infant is becoming fatigued or disorganized (sucking stops, jaw drops, eyes glaze) Keep extraneous interaction and stimulation to a minimum Look for quality of feeding behavior (active feeding) and discontinue feeding at 20-30 min or when the infant is no longer able to actively feed (gavage the rest)
Difficulty coordinating sucking and swallowing with pauses for breathing and recovery	Immaturity of the neurobehavioral and neuromuscular systems and/or recovery phase for the neurobehavioral and neuromuscular systems. Lack of experience with oral feedings	Keep the environmental stimulation to a minimum. If the environment is busy, the infant, processing so much sensory information, may lose the intrinsic coordination of the sensory and motor components of feedings "Pacing" may be used to assist the infant with sensory cues to stop sucking. The care-giver may assist the infant to pause for breathing by lifting the nipple off of the tongue after a series of 1-2 bursts of sucking and swallowing, thereby "pacing" the infant's coordination of nutritive sucking behaviors

References: Morris,[5] Shaker,[6] Harris,[10] Mathew,[12] Bernbaum[13]

Table 19.3. Feeding Problems Common to Infants with Prolonged Respiratory Problems

Problem	Probable cause	Prevention/intervention strategies
Increased oral defensiveness as evidenced by aversive behaviors	Prolonged and frequently noxious simulation of the oral and nasal areas, such as endotracheal intubation and suctioning, placement of nasogastric or orogastric tube for feedings	DURING ACUTE PHASES OF TREATMENT:
		Prevent, as possible, the need to change and reposition tubes
		Provide, as tolerated, pleasurable facial and oral stimulation, such as firm facial stroking with bathing and after tube changes, and nonnutritive sucking during awake periods, especially with tube feedings
		DURING RECOVERY PHASES OF TREATMENT:
		Provide extra-oral stimulation with slow, firm stroking of lips, chin and cheeks prior to oral feeding
		Establish a baseline of what textures and quantities are tolerated and make *very* gradual transitions in texture (thickness and chunkiness) and quantities
		If prolonged tube feeding is anticipated (x months vs. x weeks), gastrostomy tube should be considered to provide feeding volumes and avoid frequent replacement of nasogastric tubes
	Shortness of breath (dyspnea) and increased rate of breathing (tachypnea)	Keep environmental stimulation to a *minimum* (for a fragile infant with respiratory problems, this is a must)
		Monitor infant for signs of readiness (e.g., quiet, alert state) and/or fatigue (glazed expression and floppy muscle tone)
		Increase oxygen flow during feeding. If infant is not on oxygen, suggest using oxygen during feeding
		Allow more quiet, minimal interaction, time-out periods as the infant becomes disorganized and fatigued

(CONTINUED ON NEXT PAGE)

Table 19.3. Feeding Problems Common to Infants with Prolonged Respiratory Problems (continued)

Problem	Probable cause	Prevention/intervention strategies
Frequent vomiting of feedings	Increased oral/nasal/bronchial secretions	Coordinate feeding with pulmonary treatments, i.e., feed infant after a brief rest period following respiratory treatment and suctioning to clear bronchial secretions
	Increased intake of air with feedings due to inefficient oral-motor coordination	Burp the infant frequently. Consider holding infant in a supported sitting position in care-giver's lap and gently rub infant's back in an upward direction toward infant's left shoulder
	Prolonged use of NG or OG tube resulting in persistent insufficiency of gastroesophageal sphincter	Position infant in reflux position (prone with head elevated 45°) after feeding
	Altered sensory perception and awareness in the oropharyngeal area	Initiate a team discussion about the long-term medical, physical, and behavioral needs of the infant. Consideration of gastrostomy tube placement, while a medical decision, is often initiated by an experienced care-giver who feeds the infant frequently
		Develop a feeding program that incorporates gradual changes in texture and quantity of food as tolerated by the infant and behavior modification interventions that are carried out with consistency by caregivers.
Rumination	Lack of attachment to primary caretaker	Establish a primary care team as early as possible, but by at least 3-4 mo corrected age. Include the family in all planning as they desire and as possible
	Inappropriate environment and/or lack of developmentally appropriate environment/activities	Provide age-appropriate developmental intervention through primary care team
		At typical feeding times, promote normal social and developmental behaviors, such as allowing infant to explore food with fingers, as the infant's condition allows
	Decreased communication with care-givers resulting in feelings of lack of control	Provide age-appropriate social and language behaviors and choices, using "signs" and/or augmentative communication as needed
		Feed "on demand"

Table 19.3.   Feeding Problems Common to Infants with Prolonged Respiratory Problems (continued)

Problem	Probable cause	Prevention/intervention strategies
Impaired ability to tolerate spoon feeding	Delayed exposure to spoon-feeding	Offer strained foods by spoon at 4-6 mo corrected age, as infant's condition allows. Hold infant or place in infant seat for support and provide appropriate social interaction with oral feedings. Allow infant to explore food with fingers and the spoon
	Poor appetite due to fatigue, prolonged illness, and/or psychosocial deprivation	Do not attempt feeding immediately after stressful care procedures (i.e., suctioning and bagging, blood draw); allow for physiological and psychosocial recovery. Do not overstimulate before, during or after feeding; maintain calm, quiet, social atmosphere
		Begin spoon/solid feedings slowly and maintain calm, quiet atmosphere, accepting and praising infant's success. Keep "mealtime" calm, positive, interactive, happy. *Do not force feed*
		Provide consistent exposure to others eating and drinking

References: Morris,[5] Harris[10] Martin and Pridham,[11] Kavalhuna and Malnight,[14] Vohr et al.,[15] Sheagren et al.,[16] Blackman and Nelson,[17] Geertsma, et al.[18] Handen et al.,[19] Palmer and Heyman[20]

Table 19.4. Unusual Feeding Problems of Infants

Problem	Probable cause	Prevention/intervention strategies
Absent gag reflex	Central nervous system (CNS) compromise. May be, but less likely, medication reaction	Do not feed infant orally. If an infant does not have sufficient CNS function to respond to gag stimulus, the risk of aspiration of fluid is too great to risk oral feeding
		Provide nonnutritive sucking until infant is consistent in responding to gag stimulus
Hyperactive gag reflex	Disorganized, immature CNS	Provide extra-oral stimulation before attempting to place nipple in infant's mouth
	CNS compromise	
	Prolonged and frequently noxious oral stimulation	Allow infant to draw nipple into mouth using rooting reflex and/or slowly and gently insert nipple into infant's mouth, keeping gentle downward pressure on tongue from tip to comfortable position. If infant begins to gag, nipple can be rolled to the side of the infant's mouth, and often this action will allow the infant to reorganize and recover sufficiently to engage the nipple again
		If after several attempts at several feedings behaviors do not decrease, consider asking for a modified barium swallow with a technician or therapist present who is trained in oral-motor videofluoroscopy
Altered level of consciousness, usually hyporeactive	CNS compromise	Attempt to arouse infant by uncovering (monitor skin temperature for cooling), bringing to a supported semiupright position and gently rocking the infant up and down. Do not feed a sleeping infant
	Medication reaction	Check with care-givers (nurse from previous shift, physician, etc.) for causes for hyporeactivity (i.e., new or changed medication)
		If arousal is not evident over several hours/feedings, check with physician for suspected CNS compromise
		Continue to attempt to arouse infant with each feeding and monitor progress

Table 19.4.   Unusual Feeding Problems of Infants (continued)

Problem	Probable cause	Prevention/intervention strategies
Chewing action by infant rather than true sucking; may be accompanied by gagging and crying	CNS compromise and/or disorganized CNS	Attempt to feed infant with caution
		Provide extra-oral stimulation, especially lip and cheek stimulation, prior to attempting to place nipple in infant's mouth
		Monitor infant for evidence of swallowing fluid and discontinue feeding if infant seems to be having difficulty
		Report behaviors to and check with physician for suspected CNS compromise
Repeated and prolonged choking, gagging, and/or vomiting with oral feeding attempts	CNS compromise and/or disorganized CNS	Provide extra-oral stimulation prior to attempting to place nipple in infant's mouth
		Allow infant to draw nipple into mouth using rooting reflex and/or slowly and gently insert nipple into infant's mouth, keeping gentle downward pressure on tongue from tip to comfortable position. If infant begins to gag, nipple can be rolled to the side of the infant's mouth, and often this action will allow the infant to reorganize and recover sufficiently to engage the nipple again
	Moderate to severe gastroesophageal reflux	Gently burp the infant frequently, with the supported sitting/back rubbing method
		After feeding, place infant in supported semireclined prone position (reflux position with approximately 45° incline)
		If after several attempts at several feedings vomiting continues, consider asking for a modified barium swallow with a technician or therapist present who is trained in oral-motor videofluoroscopy

References: McBride and Danner;[4] Morris;[5] Harris[10]

Table 19.5. Special Problems Common to Infants with Cleft Lip, Cleft Palate or Cleft Lip and Palate

Problem	Probable cause	Prevention/intervention strategies
Inadequate lip seal	Cleft lip	Use a nipple with a large base. A cross-cut nipple may work well. If the infant is not successful with a typical nipple, a preemie-style nipple or a special elongated nipple may be needed
		For breast-feeding, it may be helpful for mother to hold her infant with the cleft lip side next to her breast to allow her breast to fill the defect. This will necessitate a different hold for each breast (i.e., cradling infant on one side and using the "football" hold for the other side)
Inefficient or weak negative pressure sucking	Cleft palate	In addition to using a special elongated nipple with a large base, a plastic bottle that can be squeezed to assist liquid delivery into the infant's mouth may be needed. The bottle should be squeezed rhythmically with the infant's sucking rhythm to avoid overfilling the mouth and/or filling the mouth during respiratory recovery phase of coordination
		The use of a cup to deliver liquid to the infant's lips and allow "lapping" of the liquid by the infant is another method that may be tried. This method, described completely in the article by Lang et al.,[23] is more commonly used in countries other than the United States.
		For breast-feeding, it may be helpful to use a warm washcloth on the breast to begin the let-down process just before placing the infant to the breast. Holding the nipple in infant's mouth throughout feeding and assisting flow by expressing milk into infant's mouth can help compensate for decreased negative pressure. It may be useful to use a special supplementary device (see Chapter 17)
		Some infants may be fitted with a special plate or prosthesis to assist with palatal alignment, and this plate may assist sucking

Table 19.5. Special Problems Common to Infants with Cleft Lip, Cleft Palate or Cleft Lip and Palate (continued)

Problem	Probable cause	Prevention/intervention strategies
Regurgitation of fluid through the nose	Fluid flowing into the nasal cavity during sucking and swallowing	Positioning for feeding an infant with a cleft palate or cleft lip and palate is very important. The infant should be fed in a semiupright position (45-60°) to allow gravity to assist the flow of liquid down into the pharynx and away from the nasal cavity. If a plastic bottle is being used to assist infant's suck, avoid overfilling the infant's mouth. This may take some experimentation to adjust the care-giver's assistance with the infant's needs, and this "fit" may change over time
Choking and/or gagging during feedings	Swallowing problems; may be from transient, mechanical or coordination difficulties	Avoid overfilling the infant's mouth with fluid from enlarged holes and/or assistance with a plastic bottle. Check the infant's feeding position. Choking or gagging usually indicates a problem with swallowing that may be from ineffective feeding techniques. If problems persist, a swallowing study may be needed to check the infant's ability to coordinate swallowing
Decreased endurance with oral feedings and poor weight gain	Inefficient feeding due to oral defect resulting in infant's tiring before an adequate amount of milk can be ingested	Look for quality of feeding behavior (active feeding) and interaction with the feeding situation. Discontinue feeding after 20-30 min, conserving the energy of the infant and the care-giver for subsequent feedings. Gavage supplementation should be considered if the infant's volumes are consistently low

References: Morris,[5] Clarren et al.,[22] Lang et al.,[23] Choi et al.,[24] Cox,[25] Weatherly-White[26] ported nutritionally by other than oral feedings. The delicate balancing of enteral feedings by nasogastric tube (NG), orogastric tube (OG), or by mouth requires both an understanding of what is theoretically possible (based on gestational age) and of what is practical (based on the present condition of the infant).[10] Table 19.2 describes the most common problems encountered with oral feedings of stable, growing premature and recovering term infants.

Prolonged and Unusual Developmental Feeding Problems

Some infants cared for in the neonatal intensive care unit (NICU) will develop chronic respiratory problems requiring longer than usual convalescence. These infants may spend several months or years in the hospital and present many challenges to the staff and to their families.[10,11,14,15] Among these challenges is supporting the infants' oral feedings within the limitations of their respiratory problems. These infants have many of the same problems described in Table 19.2 over the convalescent period. In addition, other feeding problems can be encountered (Table 19.3). (See Chapter 21 for discussion of the disease state and nutritional problems of infants with bronchopulmonary dysplasia.)

There are signs that identify infants who are having significant problems establishing oral feeding.[4,5,10,21] These signs, along with their probable causes and prevention/intervention measures, are displayed in Table 19.4. When any of these signs is present and persists, the professional team may need to consider alternative means of providing enteral nutrition.

Infants born with a cleft lip, cleft palate, or cleft lip and palate pose a different set of problems in establishing adequate oral feeding. In general, the smaller and less complicated the infant's defect, the easier and less complicated the feeding adaptations. These infants usually have difficulty with sucking efficiency and yet have adequate swallowing coordination.[22] Feeding intervention for these infants may require adaptations to positioning, nipples, and bottles, or even introduction of early cup drinking[23] to "mechanically" assist milk delivery to the oropharyngeal area for swallowing.[5,22] The trick is to support normal infant and care-giver behaviors during the period that the "mechanical" assistance is needed. Some of the special problems and intervention strategies for infants with cleft lip and/or palate are described in Table 19.5.

General Considerations for Successful Oral Feedings

Success in establishing oral feeding and weight gain is an *important* prerequisite for the infant's discharge from the NICU.[6,10,11,21] Professional care-givers, as well as parents, can assist the infant in gaining skill in feeding behaviors.[11] Care and attention should be given to environmental, behavioral, and equipment adaptations that can optimize the infant's maturing behaviors.

Environmental distractions should be minimized. Strong lights and extraneous noise can disorient the immature infant.[5,6,16,17,20] The care-giver can also be distracted by a busy environment. A quiet room with a controlled light source is the best place to begin feeding an immature infant orally. When this "luxury" is not available, a quiet corner with the infant facing away from the main area of the room may be used.

The infant should be in a quiet-alert state for optimal feeding behavior.[6] Premature infants have shorter, less durable quiet-alert periods. Although it is not always possible to arouse the infant to quiet-alert, lightly swaddling the infant and bringing him to a semi-upright position (45-60°) may result in a more aroused state for feeding. Cradling the swaddled infant in one arm and using a lightweight, graduated 2 oz feeding cylinder can free the care-giver's hand for supporting the infant's chin and cheeks if necessary.[5] Supporting the infant in this slightly flexed, semiupright position will enhance the efficiency of sucking and swallowing.[6] Soft talking or singing can help the infant to attain and/or maintain an arousal state for feeding. Slow, rhythmic rocking may help the infant establish a rhythmic sucking pattern.[6] For some infants, however, any extraneous sensory stimulation is disorganizing.[14,16,20]

Choosing an appropriate nipple is *important*. Consideration must be given by the care-giver to problems identified by a preliminary assessment.[6,20] If the infant is premature, a "preemie" style nipple may be a good beginning.[12] If the infant has difficulty with lip closure, an "orthodontic" nipple with a larger, flatter circumference does not require as much lip approximation. There is no prescription, however, for which nipple will work with which infant. Once the primary care-giver has determined the "best" choice of nipple, it is important to be consistent over a period of time rather than try more than one nipple in several consecutive feedings. (Chapter 18 discusses issues of early enteral feedings and methods, including selecting equipment.)

Mothers who choose to breast-feed their infants (premature, recovering, or anatomically different) need support from professional care-givers.[5,10,14,22,23,24,26] Many of the intervention strategies described above can be adapted to assist the mother and infant.

(Chapter 17 gives specific guidance regarding when and how to introduce breast-feeding.)

The most important thing to remember during oral feedings is to monitor the infant's behaviors at all times.[5,10,14,20,22] Fragile, immature, recovering infants tell the care-giver with subtle signs when they are ready for and capable of oral feedings. A relaxed feeding posture when aroused indicates readiness. A flaccid posture, gaze aversion, and splayed fingers indicate the infant is fatigued. If the care-giver ignores these subtle signs, the infant may demonstrate more serious symptoms of physiologic instability and compromise.[5,10,14,21] Quality of oral feeding in the beginning is much more important than quantity (unfinished volumes can be fed by a gavage tube). An individualized, developmentally supportive approach to feeding that involves the family can promote earlier hospital discharge.[27,28]

References

1. Illingsworth RS, Lister J. The critical or sensitive period, with special reference to certain feeding problems in infants and children. J Pediatr 65:839, 1964.
2. Saint-Anne Dargassues S. Neurological development in the full-term and premature neonate. Amsterdam: Excerpta Medica, 197-224, 1977.
3. Jain L, Sivieri E, Abbasi S, et al. Energietics and mechanics of sucking in the preterm and term neonate. J Pediatr 111:894, 1987.
4. McBride MC, Danner SC. Sucking disorders in neurologically impaired infants: Assessment and facilitation of breastfeeding. Clin Perinatol 14:109, 1987.
5. Morris SE, Klein MD. Pre-feeding skills. Tucson: Therapy Skill Builders, 1987.
6. Shaker CS. Nipple feeding premature infants: A different perspective. Neonatal Network 8:9, 1990.
7. Harris MB. Oral-motor management of the high-risk neonate. Phys Occup Ther Pediatr 6:231, 1986.
8. Stevenson RD. Feeding and nutrition in children with developmental disabilities. Pediatr Ann 24:255, 1995.
9. Taminiau JAJM, Kinderziekenhuis E. Energy expenditure in congenital heart disease. J Pediatr Gastroenterol Nutr 21:322, 1995.
10. Harris MB. Oral-motor management of the high-risk neonate. Phys Occup Ther Pediatr 6:231, 1986.
11. Martin RJ and Pridham KF. Early experiences of parents feeding their infants with bronchopulmonary dysplasia. Neonatal Network 11:23, 1992.
12. Mathew OE. Nipple units for newborn infants: A functional comparison. Pediatrics 81:688, 1988.
13. Bernbaum JC, Perira GR, Watkins JB, et al. Non-nutritive sucking during gavage feeding enhances growth and maturation in premature infants. Pediatrics 71:41, 1983.
14. Kavalhuna R, Malnight M. Meeting the needs of the extended care NICU patient. Neonatal Network 2:19, 1984.

15. Vohr BR, Bell EF, Oh W. Infants with bronchopulmonary dysplasia-Growth patterns and neurologic and developmental outcome. Am J Dis Child 136:443, 1982.
16. Sheagren TG, Mangurten HH, Brea F, et al. Rumination-A new complication of neonatal intensive care. Pediatrics 66:551, 1980.
17. Blackman JA, Nelson C. Rapid introduction of oral feedings to tube-fed patients. J Dev Behav Pediatr 8:63, 1987.
18. Geertsma MA, Hyams JS, Pelletier JM, et al. Feeding resistance after parenteral hyperalimentation. Am J Dis Child 139:255, 1985.
19. Handen BL, Mandell F, Russo DC. Feeding induction in children who refuse to eat. Am J Dis Child 140:52, 1986.
20. Palmer MM and Heyman MB. Assessment and treatment of sensory-versus motor-based feeding problems in very young children. Inf Young Child 6:67, 1993.
21. Bazyk S. Factors associated with the transition to oral feeding in infants fed by nasogastric tubes. Am J Occ Therapy 44:1070, 1990.
22. Clarren SK, Anderson B, Wolf LS. Feeding infants with cleft lip, cleft palate, or cleft lip and palate. Cleft Palate J 24:244, 1987.
23. Lang S, Lawrence CJ, Orme RL'E. Cup feeding: An alternative method of infant feeding. Arch Dis Child 71:365, 1994.
24. Choi BH, Kleinheinz J, Joos U, et al. Sucking efficiency of early orthopaedic plate and teats in infants with cleft lip and palate. Int J Oral Maxillofac Surg 20:167, 1991.
25. Cox BG. Looking forward-A guide for parents of the child with cleft lip and palate. Evansville, Ind.: Mead Johnson, 1991.
26. Weatherley-White RC. Surgical timing and postoperative feeding in the cleft lip child. In: Kernahan DA, Rosenstein SW, eds. Cleft lip and palate: A system of management. Baltimore: Williams & Wilkins, 1990; 33-36.
27. Shaker CS. Nipple feeding preterm infants: An individualized, developmentally supportive approach. Neonatal Network 18(3):15, 1999.
28. Lau C and Hurst N. Oral feeding in infants. Current Problems in Pediatrics 29(4):105, 1999.

MEDICAL/ SURGICAL PROBLEMS

Nutritional Care for High-Risk Newborns (Rev. 3d. Ed.)
S. Groh-Wargo, M. Thompson, J. Cox, editors
© 2000, Precept Press, Inc., Chicago

20

RESPIRATORY PROBLEMS

Gerri Keller, MEd, RD, LD

R ESPIRATORY PROBLEMS ARE COMMON in the prematurely born neonate but are less frequent in the full-term neonate. Pulmonary problems may be due to immaturity (causing respiratory distress syndrome or apnea), infection, aspiration (intrauterine, intrapartum, or postnatal), transient tachypnea, or persistent pulmonary hypertension. Respiratory symptoms may also be associated with severe metabolic acidosis, some central nervous system disorders, or surgical problems such as tracheoesophageal fistula and diaphragmatic hernia.[1]

Respiratory Distress Syndrome

Respiratory distress syndrome (RDS) is the most common neonatal respiratory problem among preterm infants and the fourth leading cause of infant mortality in the United States in 1997.[2] Because RDS is the result of lung immaturity, its incidence generally increases with decreasing birth weight and gestational age. More than 60% of infants of < 30 weeks' gestation have some degree of RDS.[3] This figure drops to 0.05% for term infants.[3] The clinical signs of RDS are cyanosis in room air, expiratory grunting, sternal and intercostal retractions, nasal flaring and tachypnea which typically occur within the first 6 hours of life and increase in severity until about 48-72 hours. Clinical, physiological and biochemical improvement may begin to occur at this time, and recovery may be rapid over the following three to four days. If symptoms of respiratory distress require delivery of high concentrations of oxygen, or if work of breathing suggests actual or potential respiratory failure, especially if chest X-ray shows typical changes of decreased lung aeration, ventilatory support and exogenous surfactant are commonly used. In some cases, progression to chronic lung disease may occur (see Chapter 21).

Characteristics of lung immaturity that contribute to RDS include inadequate pulmonary surfactant synthesis and a smaller pulmonary capillary bed in contact with an inadequate surface area for gas diffusion.[1] The fetus begins to synthesize and store surfactant at around 24 weeks' gestation, but its appearance in alveolar fluid may occur much later.[5] Surfactant reduces alveolar surface tension, maintains alveolar stability, decreases opening pressure, and protects the epithelial cell surface. Without surfactant, the alveoli may completely collapse at the end of each expiration instead of remaining slightly inflated. Normally, at around 35 weeks' gestation pulmonary cells are capable of producing adequate surfactant. At this stage, the pulmonary capillary bed is adequately developed, and cells capable of gas diffusion adequately cover the alveolar surface area. Several intrauterine (placental insufficiency, maternal oversedation) and postnatal factors (acute hypoxia, hypovolemia, systemic hypotension, uncorrected metabolic acidosis, extreme hyothermia) may enhance or delay this course of maturation; these factors are discussed elsewhere.[1]

Prevention of RDS may include the inhibition of premature labor in conjuction with maternal glucocorticoid therapy. Several studies have shown that there is a decrease in the mortality, morbidity, and incidence of RDS with maternal glucocorticoid therapy.[6-8] The mechanism by which glucocorticoid hormones function is not completely understood, but it is hypothesized that they mobilize surfactant into fetal lung alveoli.[9]

After delivery, several medical treatments may be used alone or in various combinations, depending on the gestational age of the infant and the severity of RDS. Some of these treatments include supplemental oxygen, continuous positive airway pressure (CPAP), mechanical ventilation, exogenous surfactant therapy, maintenance of adequate pulmonary toilet, prevention of metabolic or respiratory acidosis, and prevention of hypovolemia and hypotension.

Infants who require assisted ventilation beyond the first 10 days to two weeks of life may be at an increased risk for progression to chronic lung disease. Some studies have supported the use of dexamethasone in these infants to decrease pulmonary edema, decrease the inflammatory response, increase surfactant synthesis, and increase antioxidant activity.[10] These effects would, it is hoped, decrease the incidence or severity of chronic sequellae. Dexamethasone has been shown to improve pulmonary compliance, decrease mean airway pressure required for ventilation, and hasten weaning from mechanical ventilation.[11,12]

Several nutrition-related side effects of dexamethasone use have been reported (see Appendix E). Infants who receive this steroid during the first six weeks of life may experience greater amounts of weight loss, take longer to regain birth weight, and display an overall pattern of slow weight gain and linear growth when compared with infants who do not receive steroids.[12] Nephrocalcinosis, osteoporosis, fractures, sodium retention, hypertension, and hyperlipidemia also have been reported.[10]

Apnea

In the newborn, apnea (the cessation of breathing) may be due to immature neuronal control of respiratory rate and rhythm and immature response to chemoreceptors that are sensitive to changes in arterial carbon dioxide pressure. Apnea may also occur as a symptom of infection, electrolyte imbalance, gastroesophageal reflux, overstimulation, or hyperthermia. If apnea is mild, gentle tactile or proprioceptive stimulation, stroking, or patting may be all that is required. Theophylline or caffeine may be used to treat persistent apnea (see Appendix E). Severe apnea may require CPAP or assisted ventilation.[1,9]

Meconium Aspiration Syndrome

Meconium aspiration syndrome (MAS) results when meconium is excreted by the fetus into the amniotic fluid and aspirated into the lung. Meconium consists of desquamated fetal cells, undigested portions of amniotic fluid, and various fetal intestinal secretions. Meconium is normally retained by the G.I. tract of the fetus until after delivery. There is passage of meconium in utero in about 8-20% of all deliveries, occurring most frequently in term, postterm and small-for-gestational-age (SGA) infants.[13] The percentage of infants who actually aspirate meconium is small. The most severe form of meconium aspiration occurs in the infant who has been exposed to chronic placental insufficiency. Successful treatment relies on promptly removing meconium from the airway and providing adequate pulmonary toilet, supplementary oxygen, and/or mechanical ventilation as needed.[14] Hypoxia as a result of aspiration places the neonate at risk for neurologic and psychomotor insult.

Other Aspiration Syndromes

Weak or immature swallowing or cough reflex in the preterm infant or infant with respiratory or neurologic compromise may allow aspiration of feedings or regurgitated stomach contents. This aspiration may cause an obstructed airway and acute apnea that may progress to respiratory distress and pneumonia.[1]

Transient Tachypnea of the Newborn

Transient tachypnea of the newborn (TTN) results from the delayed resorption of fetal lung fluid. This disorder is often seen in premature infants or following birth by cesarean section or breech presentation because the thorax does not experience the normal compression encountered during a term vaginal cephalic delivery. Although the course of TTN is initially difficult to distinguish from RDS, most infants will recover in 12-24 hours if symptoms are mild. Recovery may take > 72 hours in severe cases.[9,13] Usual neonatal supportive care and supplemental oxygen are generally all that are needed. Fluid overload may increase symptoms.

Persistent Pulmonary Hypertension

Persistent pulmonary hypertension (PPHN) refers to the condition that once was called persistent fetal circulation (PFC), or persistent transitional circulation. In PPHN, the high pulmonary vascular resistance present during fetal life continues after birth, diminishing pulmonary blood flow, supporting a right-to-left shunting of blood flow through the foramen ovale and the ductus arteriosus, which causes hypoxemia and cyanosis.[1] Although the etiology of PPHN is unknown, it occurs mainly in term and postterm infants associated with placental insufficiency, hypoxia, and ischemia in utero. PPHN may also occur with MAS, RDS, congenital diaphragmatic hernia, or sepsis; in these cases, medical treatment of PPHN is adjunct to overall treatment of the underlying problem.

Medical treatment of PPHN is aimed at increasing pulmonary blood flow by decreasing pulmonary vascular resistance. Vasodilators such as tolazoline have been used to reduce pulmonary vascular resistance, but their effectiveness is limited due to the associated systemic vasodilation. Potent vasodilators include supplemental oxygen, inhaled nitrous oxide (NO), and hyperventilation.[15] Hyperventilation may require paralyzing, sedative, or analgesic drugs. Systemic blood pressure and cardiac output must be adequately maintained and may require expanding intravascular volume and use of drugs such as dopamine and/or dobutamine.

The use of hyperventilation remains controversial.[16] Hyperventilation has been associated with impairment in neurological outcome, possibly due to decreased cerebral blood flow, although there is no clear evidence that hyperventilation directly causes brain injury.[17] A more conservative approach to care employs more conventional modes of respiratory therapy, but allows modest hypercapnia, acidosis, and hypoxemia to avoid the possible adverse effects of hyperventilation, which may include barotrauma, lung hyperinflation, impaired venous blood return, and decreased cardiac output. There is also concern that hypercapnia may cause cerebral vasodilatation and predispose infants to intracranial bleeding, although the latter is uncommon in term infants.[16,17]

When either mode of therapy is not successful, specialized ventilatory techniques such as high-frequency ventilation and/or extracorporeal membrane oxygenation (ECMO) may be used. Extracorporeal membrane oxygenation (ECMO), a form of cardiopulmonary bypass, may be indicated for a select group of infants in which other conventional treatments have failed; this technique is described in detail elsewhere.[19-21] Arteriovenous access for ECMO requires at least temporary ligation of the right common carotid artery. Although collateral circulation seems to maintain adequate cerebral perfusion, right carotid blood flow may remain subnormal long after ECMO is discontinued.[20,22] How this affects an infant's risk for cerebral vascular accident later in life, particularly when there is a family history of atherosclerosis, is unknown. At some centers, surgical repair of the right carotid artery is done at the time of decannulation, a measure that may improve long-term patency.[23] Venovenous vascular access is now being used for ECMO. Although venovenous access may be technically more difficult than arteriovenous access and requires that the infant have adequate cardiac function, it does not require ligation of the carotid artery.

Preventive Nutrition

Nutrition plays an indirect role in preventing respiratory problems in the neonatal period in that adequate prenatal nutrition supports full-term gestation, which allows full development and maturation of fetal lung tissue. Several nutrition factors may be linked to the prevention of the progression to chronic lung disease (see Chapter 21). Although adequate hydration is necessary to prevent hypovolemia and maintain the adequate systemic vascular resistance that prevents PPHN, total fluid intake should be individualized. A 10-20% loss from birth weight during the first week of life allows contraction of extracellular fluid volume and elimination of lung edema associated with RDS. Overhydration may lead to edema, patent ductus arteriosis, or congestive heart failure.[24] It has been suggested that a delay in the diuretic phase that normally occurs within the first four to five days of life may be linked to the development of bronchopulmonary dysplasia (BPD).[25,26] This seems to be true also for infants who experience a net weight gain during the first week of life as opposed to a loss from birth weight that represents fluid loss.[27] Interstitial edema may cause a decrease in lung compliance and increase the need for ventilator support. Mechanical ventilation increases the risk of barotrauma and oxygen toxicity, which can lead to chronic lung disease.[25,26]

Treatment Nutrition

Fluid and electrolyte management of the neonate with respiratory problems is determined by renal maturation, metabolic processes affected by respiratory failure, and medications used (see Chapter 10). When pulmonary insufficiency occurs, excretion of extracellular fluid and sodium are decreased, thus fluid and sodium administration may be limited, particularly during the initial oliguric phase.[53] Subsequently, during the diuretic phase, or when diuretic medications are used, hyponatremia may occur if sodium losses exceed fluid losses. This diminishes further effects of diuretic medications and may inhibit growth.[24,28] Sodium supplementation may be needed to maintain normal serum sodium levels.[29] Chloride and potassium balance may be affected by diuretics in the same way and require supplementation.

Inadequate nutrition may play a role in decreased lung growth and alveolar development, reduced lung connective tissue and lung tissue repair, reduced synthesis of surfactant, increased susceptibility to tissue damage from hyperoxia, and increased susceptibility to pulmonary infection.[30] Suboptimal nutrition can deplete energy reserves of the respiratory muscles and subsequently may inhibit weaning from mechanical ventilation.[31] Reduced bone mass of the ribcage due to inadequate mineral intake reduces support of lung tissue and chest wall compliance.[32]

Parenteral nutrition is usually initiated within the first 24-48 hours of life if the infant is medically unable to receive enteral feedings (see Chapters 8-11). Initially providing at least 1.0-1.5 g protein/kg/d and 35-65 nonprotein kcal/kg/day improves nitrogen retention and may improve regulation of glucose metabolism and transport, especially for the ventilated extremely low birth weight infant.[24,33] Parenteral fat may be started at doses of 0.5 to 1.0 g/kg/day as early as day 1 without affecting pulmonary status, although serum triglyceride levels may be significantly increased with early use of steroids.[34,35] Lipids provide a concentrated source of energy, which may be particularly advantageous when fluid tolerance is limited. Use of parenteral lipid during ECMO has been controversial. Reports regarding lipid interference with gas exchange in the artificial lung are not consistent.[36] This may not present a serious problem, because infants eligible for ECMO generally are at least 2,000 g birth weight, 35 weeks' gestation, and receive ECMO for an average duration of only five to eight days.[18] Although infants receiving ECMO may experience profound catabolism, providing excess energy does not prevent protein loss and may contribute to increased CO_2 retention. Recommendations for parenteral nutrition are 80-100 kcal/kg/d and 2.5 gm protein/kg/d.[54]

The influence of carbohydrate and fat proportions as sources of energy on the overall effect of respiratory gas exchange in infants with respiratory problems is not clear. Higher fat regimens appear to reduce carbon dioxide production without increasing oxygen consumption or impairing growth.[37] Higher carbohydrate regimens increase carbon dioxide production, but may not be associated with significantly increased carbon dioxide retention, possibly because energy needs are high during the neonatal period, particularly when respiratory compromise is present.[38] Initiation of enteral feedings can begin when bowel sounds are present, the respiratory pattern is stabilized, and the abdomen is soft and not distended, even if the neonate is receiving mechanical ventilation.[32] In the first few days of life, feeding low-volume, hypocaloric feedings of human milk or formula has been shown to stimulate G.I. function and improve subsequent tolerance of enteral feedings.[39,40] As enteral feedings are advanced, parenteral nutrition can be reduced (see Chapters 15 and 18).

Severe respiratory distress has been shown to increase caloric expenditure by 25 to 40%, probably due more to hypermetabolism than to increased work of breathing.[41-46] Enteral caloric requirements necessary to support growth for the infant with respiratory problems are individualized, usually ranging from 120 to 160 kcal/kg/day. Providing adequate calories may be difficult, especially for an infant who requires fluid restriction. Concentrating enteral formulas and using human milk fortifiers may be helpful (see Chapters 16 and 21 and Appendix K).

Initially, nipple-feedings may be withheld and enteral feedings provided by an orogastric or nasogastric tube. Intermittent bolus gastric tube feedings may exaggerate respiratory problems, especially if vomiting or gastroesophageal reflux with aspiration is present.[47] In some cases, continuous tube feedings or transpyloric tube feedings may be better tolerated.

Effective sucking and swallowing may be impaired by immaturity, lack of energy, the presence of an endotracheal tube, or an increased respiratory rate. Infants whose respiratory rate is > 60 breaths/minute may require careful evaluation and monitoring during attempts to nipple-feed to prevent increased risk of aspiration.[48]

Slower-flow nipples and allowing the infant to pause frequently may help the infant to maintain stability and control during nipple-feeding. Tachypnea may increase the difficulty of coordinating the suck and swallow sequence. Nipple-feedings may be started in infants with mild elevations in respiratory rate, dyspnea, or supplemental oxygen needs if they are adequately monitored for signs of distress or fatigue (see Chapters 18 and 27).

Prolonged use of feeding and endotracheal tubes can confuse oral function and impair sucking ability.[49] When the endotracheal tube is removed, allowing nonnutritive sucking (NNS) during tube feedings has been shown to (1) enhance the maturation of the sucking reflex, allowing a more rapid transition to oral feeding; (2) decrease intestinal transit time; and (3) improve weight gain.[50] Although a more recent study does not support these findings,[51] NNS allows the neonate to associate satiety with sucking, which is positive feedback for the development of oral motor skills.

Follow-up Issues

Most of the respiratory problems described in this chapter resolve without special long-term nutrition problems other than those associated with prematurity, neurological compromise, or other neonatal conditions that require nutrition follow-up. Exceptions are infants whose RDS has progressed to chronic lung disease. The type and severity of respiratory illness has been shown to affect growth and cognitive outcomes more than birth weight or gestational age alone.[52] Many infants with BPD appear to have slower rates of growth and lower developmental scores at two-year follow-up than infants with a history of RDS alone.[52] Specific areas of nutrition assessment in follow-up may include growth, nutrient intake, ability to bottle-feed, readiness for semisolid foods, acceptance of different food textures, fluid tolerance, and interest in self-feeding.

Infants treated with arteriovenous vascular access for ECMO, particularly without carotid artery repair, may continue to have diminished right common carotid artery blood flow.[20,22] It is unknown whether these infants should eventually modify dietary fat and cholesterol intake after two years of age, particularly when there is a family history of atherosclerosis.

Case Study

NK was born at 23 5/7 weeks on 3/30/98. Mother presented with complete cervical dilation and delivered the baby vaginally. Maternal glucocorticoid therapy could not be given. Birth weight, length, and head circumference were 610 g, 30.5 cm, and 21 cm respectively. Apgars were 2 at 1 minute and 6 at 5 minutes. She initially had a positive respiratory effort, and was easily intubated and placed on a conventional ventilator. She received two doses of surfactant. At 3 days of life, she was changed from a conventional ventilator to a high-frequency ventilator. Her respiratory status deteriorated and she was placed back on a conventional ventilator. NK had an excellent response to a 14-day course of dexamethasone to help decrease oxygen requirement and wean ventilator settings. She received two doses of indomethacin to close her large patent ductus arteriosis (PDA) but on day 13 surgical ligation was necessary. She was extubated to continuous positive airway pressure (CPAP) on day 54 of life. CPAP was discontinued on day 59. NK was discharged on day 99 with a diagnosis of mild bronchopulmonary dysplasia and supplemental oxygen (1/8 liter) by nasal cannula. Fluids were initiated on day 1 (dextrose and water) at 70 ml/kg/d. A Broviac catheter was placed on day 2 and central hyperalimentation begun to provide 4 mg glucose/kg/min, 0.5 g pro/kg/day, electrolytes, vitamins, and minerals. Lipids were added on day 4 at 0.6 g fat/kg/day. She required 11 days of double phototherapy which greatly increased insensible water losses, so that fluids were advanced to 175 ml/kg/day by day 6. Dextrose concentration was limited throughout hospitalization due to hyperglycemia, but protein and lipids were advanced over the first several days to provide 2.7 g/kg/day and 3 g/kg/day respectively. Total calories were advanced to 80 kcal/kg/day. Continuous enteral feedings of human milk were started on day 8 (10 ml/kg/day) but subsequently discontinued on day 9 due to severe atelectasis, respiratory acidosis and possible sepsis. Continuous enteral feedings of human milk (10 ml/kg/day) were successfully restarted on day 17. Enfamil Human Milk Fortifier (Mead Johnson Nutritionals, Evansville, Ind.) was added to human milk on day 26 and full enteral feedings (150 ml/kg/day, 120 kcal/kg/day) were reached by day 29. Bolus feedings were achieved at 2 months of life. The first oral feed was offered on day 66 at 32 weeks' postmenstrual age. NK reached full oral feedings on day 95 at 36.5 weeks' postmenstrual age. By discharge, NK was taking ad libidum feedings every three hours of Similac NeoSure (Ross Products Division, Abbott Laboratories, Columbus, Ohio) 24 kcal/oz or human milk fortified to 24 kcal/oz with NeoSure formula powder, providing an average energy intake of 130 kcal/kg/day. Her discharge weight, length, and head circumference were 2610 g, 47 cm and 32.5 cm respectively, all between the 25-50th percentile on the Lubchenco intrauterine growth chart.

References

1. Stahlman MT. Acute respiratory disorders in the newborn. In: Avery GB, ed. Neonatology: Pathophysiology and management of the newborn, 3d ed. Philadelphia: Lippincott, 1987; 418.
2. Guyer B, MacDorman MF, Martin JA et al. Annual summary of vital statistics--1997. Pediatr 102:1333, 1998.
3. Usher RH, Allen AC, McLean FH. Risk of respiratory distress syndrome related to gestational age, route of delivery and maternal diabetes. Am J Obstet Gynecol 111:826, 1971.
4. Nugent J. Acute respiratory care of the newborn. J Obstet Gynecol Neonatal Nurs 12:31s, 1983.
5. Hansen T, Corbet A. Lung development and function. In: Taeuch HW, Ballard RA, Avery ME, eds. Schaffer and Avery's diseases of the newborn, 6th ed. Philadelphia: Saunders, 1991.
6. Liggins GC, Howie RN. A controlled trial of antepartum glucocorticoid treatment for prevention of the respiratory distress syndrome in premature infants. Pediatrics 50:515, 1972.
7. Papageorgiou AN, Doray JL, Ardila R et al. Reduction of mortality, morbidity, and respiratory distress syndrome in infants weighing less than 1,000 grams by treatment with betamethasone and ritodrine. Pediatrics 83:493, 1989.
8. Kwong MS, Egan EA. Reduced incidence of hyaline membrane disease in extremely premature infants following delay of delivery in mother with preterm labor: Use of ritodrine and betamethasone. Pediatrics 78:767, 1986.
9. Hagedorn MI, Gardner SL, Abman SH. Respiratory distress. In: Merenstein GB, Gardner SL, eds. Handbook of neonatal intensive care, 2d ed., St. Louis: Mosby, 1989; 365.
10. Yoder MC, Chua R, Tepper R. Effect of dexamethasone on pulmonary inflammation and pulmonary function of ventilator-dependent infants with broncho-pulmonary dysplasia. Am Rev Respir Dis 143:1044, 1991.
11. Yeh TF, Torre JA, Rastogi A, et al. Early postnatal dexamethasone therapy in premature infants with severe respiratory distress syndrome: A double-blind, controlled study. J Pediatr 117:273, 1990.
12. Mammel MC, Johnson DE, Green TP, et al. Controlled trial of dexamethasone therapy in infants with bronchopulmonary dysplasia. Lancet 1:1356, 1983.
13. Fanaroff AA, Martin RJ. Neonatal-perinatal medicine. Diseases of the fetus and infant, 4th ed. St. Louis: Mosby, 1987.
14. Cleary GM and Wiswell TE. Meconium-stained amniotic fluid and the meconium aspiration syndrome. Pediatr Clin North Amer 45:511, 1998.
15. Kinsella JP and Abman SH. Controversies in the use of inhaled nitric oxide therapy in the newborn. Clin Perinatol 25:203, 1998.
16. Walsh-Sukys MC, Cornell DJ, Houston LN, et al. Treatment of persistent pulmonary hypertension of the newborn without hyperventilation: an assessment of diffusion of innovation. Pediatr 94:303, 1994.

17. Sahni R, Wung JT, James LS. Controversies in management of persistent pulmonary hypertension of the newborn. Pediatr 94:307, 1994.

18. Engle WA, Peters EA, West KW. Neonatal extracorporeal membrane oxygenation. Indiana Med 5:50, 1989.

19. Short BL, Miller MK, Anderson KD. Extracorporeal membrane oxygenation in the management of respiratory failure in the newborn. Clin Perinatol 14:737, 1987.

20. Voorhies TM, Tardo CL, Starrett AL, et al. Evaluation of the cerebral circulation in neonates following extracorporeal membrane oxygenation. Ann Neurol 18:390, 1985.

21. Kanto WP and Bunyapen C. Extracorporeal membrane oxygenation: controversies in selection of patients and management. Clin Perinatol 25:123-136, 1998.

22. Lott IT, McPherson D, Towne B, et al. Long-term neurophysiologic outcome after neonatal extracorporeal membrane oxygenation. J Pediatr 116:343, 1990.

23. Taylor BJ, Seibert JJ, Glasier CM, et al. Evaluation of the reconstructed carotid artery following extracorporeal membrane oxygenation. Pediatrics 90:568, 1992.

24. Adamkin DH. Issues in the nutritional support of the ventilated baby. Clin Perinatol 25:79-96, 1998.

25. Brown ER, Stark A, Sosenko I, et al. Bronchopulmonary dysplasia: Possible relationship to pulmonary edema. J Pediatr 92:982, 1978.

26. Van Marter LJ, Leviton A, Allred EN, et al. Hydration during the first days of life and the risk of bronchopulmonary dysplasia in low birth weight infants. J Pediatr 116:942, 1990.

27. Shaffer SG, Quimiro CL, Anderson JV, et al. Postnatal weight changes in low birth weight infants. Pediatrics 79:702, 1987.

28. Brem AS. Electrolyte disorders associated with respiratory distress syndrome and bronchopulmonary dysplasia. Clin Perinatol 19:223-232, 1992.

29. Vanpee M, Herin P, Broberger U, et al. Sodium supplementation optimizes weight gain in preterm infants. Acta Paediatr 84:1312-4, 1995.

30. Sosenko IRS, Frank L. Nutritional influences on lung development and protection against chronic lung disease. Semin Perinatol 15:462, 1991.

31. Bell EF, Oh W. Nutritional care. In: Goldsmith JP, Karatkin EH, eds. Assisted ventilation of the neonate. Philadelphia: Saunders, 1981.

32. Cohen IT, Meunier KM, Hirsh MP. Effects of lipid emulsion on pulmonary function in infants. In: Kinney JM, Borum PR, eds. Perspectives in clinical nutrition. Baltimore: Urban and Schwarzenberg, 1989; 415.

33. Thureen PJ, Anderson AH, Baron KA, et al. Protein balance in the first week of life in ventilated neonates receiving parenteral nutrition. Am J Clin Nutr 68:1128-35, 1998.

34. Sentipal-Walerius, Dollberg S, Mimouni F, et al. Effect of pulsed dexamethasone therapy on tolerance of intravenously administered lipids in extremely low birth weight infants. J Pediatr 134:229-232, 1999.

35. Brown RL, Wessel J, and Warner BW. Nutrition considerations in the neonatal extracorporeal life support patient. Nutr Clin Pract 9:22-27, 1994.

36. Piedboeuf B, Chessex P, Hazan J, et al. Total parenteral nutrition in the newborn infant: Energy substrates and respiratory gas exchange. J Pediatr 118:97-102, 1991.

37. Chessex P, Belanger S, Peidboeuf, et al. Influence of energy substrates on respiratory gas exchange during conventional mechanical ventilation of preterm infants. J Pediatr 126:619-624, 1995.
38. Niermeyer S. Nutritional and metabolic problems in infants with bronchopulmonary dysplasia. In: Bancalari E, Stocker JT, eds. Bronchopulmonary dysplasia. Washington, D.C.: Hemisphere Publishing, 1988; 313-36.
39. Slagle TA, Gross SJ. Effects of early hypocaloric enteral feeding on neonatal gastrointestinal function: Preliminary report of a randomized trial. J Pediatr 112:622, 1988.
40. Dunn L, Hulman S, Weiner J, et al. Beneficial effects of early hypocaloric enteral feeding on neonatal gastrointestinal function: Preliminary report of a randomized trial. J Pediatr 112:622, 1988.
41. Billeaud C, Piedboeuf B, Chessex P. Energy expenditure and severity of respiratory disease in very low birth weight infants receiving long-term ventilatory support. J Pediatr 120:461, 1992.
42. Yeh TF, McClenan DA, Ajayi OA, et al. Metabolic rate and energy balance in in- fants with bronchopulmonary dysplasia. J Pediatr 114:448, 1989.
43. Weinstein MR, Oh W. Oxygen consumption in infants with bronchopulmonary dysplasia. J Pediatr 99:958, 1981.
44. Kurzner SI, Bautista DB, Sargent CW, et al. Growth failure in bronchopulmonary dysplasia: Elevated metabolic rates and pulmonary mechanics. J Pediatr 112:73, 1988.
45. Hazan J, Chessex P, Piedboeuf B, et al. Energy expenditure during synthetic surfactant replacement therapy for neonatal respiratory distress syndrome. J Pediatr 120:S29, 1992.
46. Kao LC, Durand DJ, Nickerson BG. Improving pulmonary function does not decrease oxygen consumption in infants with bronchopulmonary dysplasia. J Pediatr 112:615, 1988.
47. Topper WH. Enteral feeding methods for compromised neonates and infants. In: Lebenthal E, ed. Textbook for gastroenterology and nutrition in infancy. New York: Raven Press, 1981.
48. Morris SE, Klein, MD. Pre-feeding skills: A comprehensive resource for feeding de-velopment. Tucson: Therapy Skill Builders, 1987; 96.
49. Lemons JA, Brady MS, Rickard K, et al. Considerations in feeding the very-low- birth-weight infant. Perinatol Neonatol May/June 1982.
50. Bernbaum JC, Pereiar GR, Watkins JB, et al. Nonnutritive sucking during gavage feeding enhances growth and maturation in premature infants. Pediatrics 71:41, 1983.
51. Ernst JA, Rickard KA, Neal PR, et al. Lack of improved growth outcome related to nonnutritive sucking in very low birth weight premature infants fed a controlled nutrient intake: A randomized prospective study. Pediatrics 83:706, 1989.
52. Meisels SJ, Plunkett JW, Roloff DW, et al. Growth and development of preterm in-fants with respiratory distress syndrome and bronchopulmonary dysplasia. Pediatrics 77:345, 1986.
53. Baumgart S and Costarino AT. Water and electrolyte metabolism of the micropremie. Clin Perinatol 27:131, 2000.
54. Shew SB, Keshen TH, Jahoor F, et al. The determinants of protein catabolism in neonates on extraco oreal membrane oxygenation. J Pediatr Surg 34:1086, 1999.

Nutritional Care for High-Risk Newborns (Rev. 3d. Ed.)
S. Groh-Wargo, M. Thompson, J. Cox, editors
© 2000, Precept Press, Inc., Chicago

21

BRONCHOPULMONARY DYSPLASIA

Janice Hovasi Cox, MS, RD

BRONCHOPULMONARY DYSPLASIA (BPD) WAS originally described in 1967 as a chronic pulmonary disorder developing in some premature infants with severe respiratory distress syndrome (RDS) who were treated with intermittent positive pressure ventilation (IPPV)—the active inflation of the lungs during inspiration under positive pressure from a cycling valve—and supplemental oxygen.[1] BPD was classified according to the degree of severity into four stages of progression. These stages were specifically described based on age, radiographic changes in the lung, pulmonary function tests, and the need for IPPV and/or supplemental oxygen.

More recently, diagnostic criteria for BPD have been described as the need for assisted ventilation for at least three days during the first two weeks of life, with clinical signs of respiratory compromise, and the need for supplemental oxygen, and radiologic evidence of pulmonary changes characteristic of BPD persisting beyond 28 days of age.[2,3] With increased survival rates of infants born at < 28 weeks' gestation, this definition may not be as useful in distinguishing the group of infants whose lungs are quite immature and meet the criteria at 28 days of age from infants who will progress to chronic lung disease (CLD) and continue to have compromised respiratory health throughout childhood. Some investigators have suggested the term "chronic lung disease of infancy" to describe infants who meet the criteria for BPD beyond 36 weeks' postmenstrual age and whose disease is more likely to progress.[3,4] "Atypical," "Type I," or "developmental" CLD are terms used to describe CLD which occurs later—typically appearing between days 6 and 10 and resolving before hospital discharge.[82]

The diagnosis of BPD, or chronic lung disease, is used to identify a broad spectrum of chronic pulmonary changes. The pathologic changes that characterize BPD are progressive. The immature lung produces inadequate amounts of pulmonary surfactant to maintain alveolar stability and protect the epithelial cell surface. The pulmonary capillary bed and epithelial cells capable of gas diffusion are not fully developed. When these immature tissues must perform the task of adequately oxygenating the newborn, supplemental oxygen and assisted ventilation are often needed to support life. Necrosis of alveolar and bronchial epithelium occur in the immature lung when exposed to high concentrations of oxygen and increased pressures and/or volumes associated with assisted ventilation. Regeneration and proliferation of damaged tissues may include bronchial squamous metaplasia and interstitial fibrosis.[4] A review of factors associated with BPD has recently been published.[4]

Because of varied reporting methods, the incidence of BPD is difficult to define. Reported incidence varies from 2.5% among neonates requiring assisted ventilation to 38% in infants of < 1,000 g birth weight.[5] Significant advances in respiratory management, including improved technology for assisted ventilation, more precise delivery of supplemental oxygen, better evaluation of blood gases, and the use of exogenous surfactant, have diminished the incidence and severity of BPD in infants of > 1,000 g birth weight. These same advances have also allowed the increased survival of infants of < 1,000 g birth weight who now present with the most challengig problems associated with BPD.

The original radiographic descriptions of the four-stage progression of BPD are still seen in more severe cases, but more commonly, radiographic findings are more subtle and clinical symptoms are less severe, although lung pathology is that of BPD.[6] It is now recognized that BPD may follow other primary lung problems, such as meconium aspiration pneumonia, neonatal pneumonia, congestive heart failure, hypoplastic lungs, pulmonary air leaks, Wilson-Mikity syndrome, or any other primary lung problem requiring prolonged use of assisted ventilation and supplemental oxygen.[6]

The etiology of BPD is not completely settled, although many factors may be involved. Immature lungs, increased concentrations of inspired oxygen, assisted ventilation, volutrauma, barotrauma, endotracheal intubation, excess fluid administration, patent ductus arterious, and sepsis are the major predisposing factors.[4,83] Pulmonary edema may also play an important role. Maternal glucocorticoid therapy used to enhance lung maturation before birth may decrease the risk for BPD. Exogenous surfactant may be given after birth to support alveolar stability and protect the epithelial cells of the immature lung. Increased concentrations of inspired oxygen may damage lung tissues by providing oxygen-free radicals that surpass the infant's antioxidant enzyme system or by altering the pulmonary inflammatory process.[4]

Very low birth weight infants who develop BPD may have decreased cortisol synthesis and relative adrenal insufficiency during the first week of life compared with infants who do not develop BPD.[7,8] Early administration of exogenous steroids have been shown to hasten weaning from mechanical ventilation, to decrease the incidence of BPD, and/or to reduce the severity of progression to chronic lung disease.[9-12] Steroids decrease pulmonary edema and the inflammatory response and increase both surfactant synthesis and antioxidant activity.[9,13] Weaning from steroids may sometimes be prolonged. Steroids may be associated with several nutritional side effects (see Treatment Nutrition section and Appendix E, dexamethasone).

BPD encompasses a wide spectrum of illness. Infants may die or begin to convalesce or recuperate during any stage of progression. Most studies reporting altered growth or nutrition refer to infants who have had precursor respiratory illness, whose clinical signs of respiratory compromise (e.g., tachypnea, carbon dioxide retention, need for supplemental oxygen, steroids, and/or diuretics) persist beyond 36 weeks' postconceptual age, and who have radiologic evidence of BPD.

Nutritional Implications

Growth Failure

Documented studies of growth in patients with BPD show reduced rates of growth and reduced percentile ranking during the first one to two years of life when compared to normal term infants of same postmenstrual age.[14-19] Mean weight, length, and head circumference for children with chronic severe BPD have been plotted against the Stuart grids in Figures 21.1, 21.2, and 21.3. During acute RDS, patients may take longer to regain birth weight. Increments in length and head circumference also may lag during this period. Although percentile rankings of weight and length for patients with BPD continue to fall below norms at 1-2 years of age,[14-19] the growth velocity of length and head circumference may approach the norm within a few weeks of reaching term.[15] Formula that is enriched with greater amounts of protein, minerals, and electrolytes than standard formula has been shown to support linear catch-up growth in patients with BPD when fed at 37-44 weeks' postmenstrual age.[20] The rate of gain in weight may approach the norm later, at 6-8 months postterm age.[14,15] Long-term follow-up studies indicate that catch-up growth may occur by age 3 or by ages 7-10.[16,21,22]

Although infants with BPD grow less well than their term-born peers of the same postmenstrual age, it is not clear whether infants with BPD grow less well than infants of comparable birth weight and gestational age at birth. These differences may be difficult to identify clearly because of the variation in the severity of the disease, even when standard diagnostic criteria are used. Several recent studies have reported that infants of low birth weight, especially < 1,250 g, with or without BPD, are lighter and shorter during the first one to two years than postmenstrual-age-matched infants born at term.[14,15,18,23] Infants having severe BPD requiring supplemental oxygen beyond 36 weeks' postconceptual age or having increased resting metabolic expenditures may grow less well than their peers of similar birth weight and postpostmenstrual age for up to 8 years of age.[14,15,21-24]

It is not clear what causes this variation in growth, although recurrent illness, increased metabolic needs, and/or lower nutrient intakes may be contributing factors.[15,24-27] Use of medications such as methylxanthines and beta-agonists may increase metabolic rate and energy requirements.[28] Maintaining adequate levels of tissue oxygenation has been shown to improve growth.[31-33] Supplemental oxygen may be needed, particularly during feedings or other medical procedures when transient episodes of hypoxemia may occur.[34] Weight gain is diminished during the first week of steroid administration, but improves dramatically as the dose is tapered. Steroids also affect linear growth by decreasing length velocity. Rebound linear growth usually occurs once steroids are discontinued, but there is some concern that weight gain may exceed that expected for linear growth.[4,29,30] Other risk factors for growth failure in patients with BPD include low socioeconomic status, feeding problems, and difficult temperament.[35]

Feeding Problems

Infants surviving with severe BPD may exhibit a decreased ability to suck and swallow efficiently. Endotrachial tube placement for mechanical ventilation may preclude oral feedings or pleasant oral stimulation. Tachypnea or palatal grooves associated with prolonged endotracheal tube placement may make the suck and swallow sequence tiring or difficult. The ability to initiate self-feeding or to tolerate spoon-feedings may be impaired. Infants with BPD may experience many noxious stimuli in or near the mouth during the first few months of life; examples are endotracheal tube placement, feeding tube positioning, suctioning, and taping. These infants may later demonstrate aversion to feedings by pulling away from the nipple, arching, gagging, and vomiting.[3] Gastroesophageal reflux, rumination, or recurrent vomiting may compromise nutritional intake.[36] (See Chapter 19 for a detailed discussion of feeding problems, causes, preventive measures, and treatment for infants with prolonged respiratory problems.)

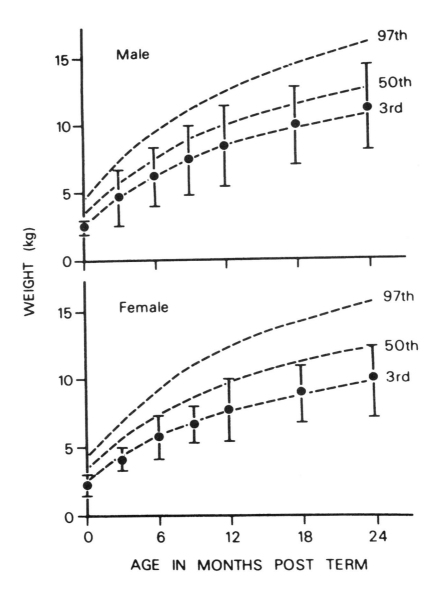

Figure 21.1. Weight measurements from term.

The mean ±2 SD for the study sample are plotted against the Stuart graph.[14]
(Reprinted with permission of Mosby Year Book, 1981)

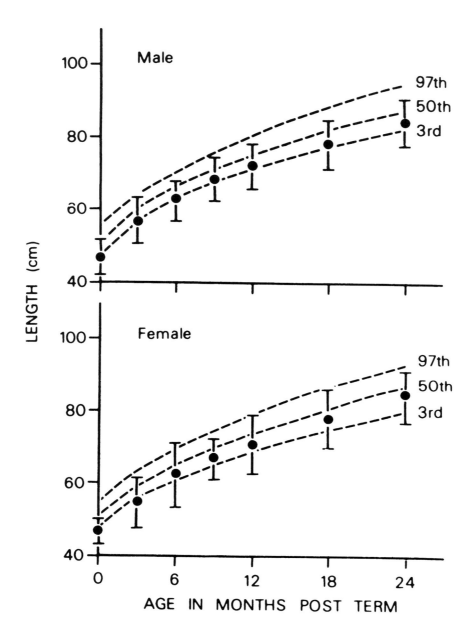

Figure 21.2. Crown-heel measurements from term.

The mean ±2 SD for the study sample are plotted against the Stuart graph.[14] (Reprinted with permission of Mosby Year Book, 1981)

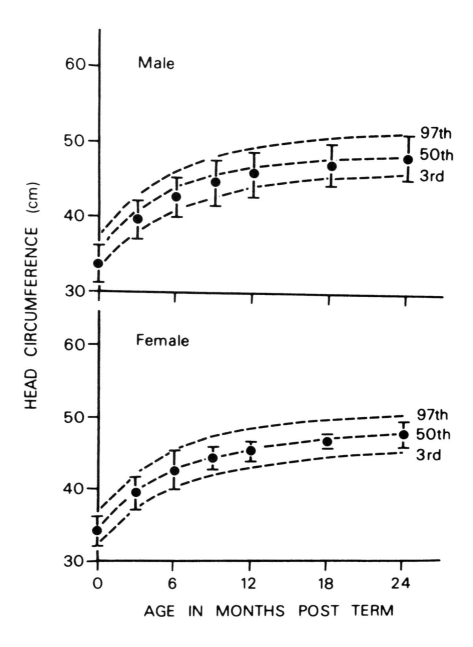

Figure 21.3. Head circumference measurements from term.

The mean ± SD for the study sample are plotted against the Nelihaus graph.[14]
(Reprinted with permission of Mosby Year Book, 1981)

Fluid and Electrolyte Balance

Fluid and electrolyte tolerance changes as kidney function matures and respiratory disease progresses. Fluid and sodium tolerance may be decreased as pulmonary hypertension and/or cor pulmonale develops. Left ventricular hypertrophy may also be present.[3] Diuretics are used frequently to prevent fluid retention, pulmonary edema, and allow adequate administration of fluids to meet nutrient needs. Furosemide and thiazide diuretics have been associated with hyponatremia, hypokalemia, hypochloridemia, and metabolic alkalosis.[37] Spironolactone may be used to counteract secondary hyperaldosteronism induced by the volume depletion and associated sodium loss caused by active diuretic therapy. It also inhibits the exchange of sodium for potassium in the distal renal tubule, thus preventing potassium loss.

Mineral Balance

Infants at greater risk of developing BPD are often those also at greater risk of developing osteopenia and nephrocalcinosis (see Chapters 29 and 30). Calcium and phosphorus intake may be limited by fluid restriction, especially during parenteral nutrition or when human milk is given without mineral fortification.

Respiratory effort may be impaired by a compliant rib cage that may occur with osteopenia and/or the intercostal muscle weakness associated with phosphorus depletion.[38] Drug nutrient interactions may further compromise mineral balance. Furosemide, a potent diuretic, is associated with hypercalciuria, osteopenia, and renal calculi, although the last may be more closely related to the severity and duration of respiratory disease and other aspects of medical management.[39,41] Although thiazide diuretics are associated with electrolyte losses, they have less effect on mineral balance. Sodium supplementation during thiazide diuretic therapy enhances calciuria and may be a contributing factor in osteopenia and nephrocalcinosis.[42] Steroids may decrease absorption of calcium and phosphorus.

Preventive Nutrition

Primary

Early excessive fluid administration may be associated with the development of BPD.[43,44] It may be that an inadequate endogenous handling of fluids precludes the normal diuresis and weight loss of 10-20% of birth weight during the first three to four days of life.[31] Fluid needs may vary greatly due to insensible losses, depending on treatments and environment, so that patients must be monitored closely to provide adequate fluid without overhydration. Initial fluid tolerance may be as low as 55-70 ml/kg/day, increasing to 80-150 ml/kg/day during the first week.[45]

Undernutrition may play a general role in the development of BPD, in that the body's natural defenses and ability to repair tissues may be impaired by deficient or depleted nutrient stores. Premature birth deprives the infant of nutrient stores that accrue primarily during the last trimester. Limited fluid tolerance and immature absorptive and metabolic capabilities limit nutrient delivery during initial extrauterine life with respiratory compromise. Of particular interest are overall energy and protein intake as well as essential fatty acids, zinc, copper, iron, selenium, and vitamins A and E.[46,48] Early administration of parenteral nutrition supports positive nitrogen balance and may prevent nutrient depletion (see Chapters 9-11). Early introduction of small-volume enteral feedings may enhance G.I. tract adaptation, earlier transition from parenteral to enteral feedings, and ultimately improved nutritional status (see Chapters 14 and 15).

Because vitamin E functions as an antioxidant, it has been the subject of several studies in its relationship to reduction of oxygen-free radicals and the development of BPD. Although no dose/benefit relationship has been clearly identified, review of the literature would suggest that a goal of achieving normal term serum levels of vitamin E (1.0-3.5 mg/dl) is reasonable.[4,49,50] This can be accomplished with standard pediatric parenteral multivitamin doses or, if parenteral nutrition is not being administered, orally supplementing with 5-25 mg vitamin E/day in divided doses during the first two to four weeks and 5 mg/day thereafter.[51-54] An infant must take at least 150-200 ml of a premature infant formula, 250-500 ml of a standard infant formula or 1 ml of a standard enteral liquid multivitamin preparation to receive 5 mg of vitamin E.

Vitamin A plays an important role in epithelial tissue repair. Because the newborn, particularly the premature infant of < 1,000 g birth weight, has a relatively low vitamin A status, supplementation would seem logical.[55] In a small but well-designed study, a supplemental dose of 2,000 IU vitamin A as water-miscible retinyl palmitate was administered intramuscularly every other day until establishment of enteral feedings. When at least 75% of energy intake was given enterally, 1 ml of a standard liquid multivitamin preparation containing 1,500 IU vitamin A was added to the feeding. Significantly lower incidence of BPD was seen in the vitamin A-supplemented group when compared with a control group.[56] A smaller, but still significant reduction in the incidence of BPD was found in a larger and more recent study using doses of 5,000 IU given intramuscularly three times a week for four weeks. Despite these higher doses, low serum retinol levels were evident in 24% of the infants studied, perhaps indicating the need to study even higher doses.[48] Two significant notes of caution are the risks of toxicity with this fat-soluble vitamin and the difficulty presented by intramuscular injections in this population, although enteral administration may be efficacious. Definitive dose/response studies have not yet been reported.[57]

Inositol, a component of membrane phospholipids, may serve as a substrate enhancing the synthesis and secretion of pulmonary surfactants. In a well-designed European study, a dose of 80 mg/kg inositol given I.V. to premature infants with RDS was associated with an increased survival without development of BPD.[58] Inositol, part of the vitamin B complex, is essential for some animals, but its significance in human nutrition has not been fully established. Although human colostrum has relatively high levels of inositol, parenteral nutrition solutions generally do not include it. Inositol supplementation in surfactant-treated infants deserves further study.[4]

Secondary

Prevention of nutritional problems in patients with BPD include:

- Administering adequate protein, calories, vitamins, and minerals to support normal growth while maintaining fluid and sodium balance (This indicates the need for an increased understanding of caloric needs and growth potential during the acute and chronic phases of lung disease and during convalescence)
- Providing comprehensive care through an interdisciplinary team approach, including the patient's family, physician, primary care nurse, occupational or physical therapist, developmental specialist or psychologist, and nutritionist

Treatment Nutrition

Fluid and Electrolytes

Fluid tolerance may be limited to 75-90 ml/kg/day during the antecedent respiratory illness, when pulmonary edema and reduced cardiac output may be present.[43,44] Fluid tolerance may be modified by other factors in the clinical condition or the environment (see Chapter 9). Fluid may be increased to 95-150 ml/kg/day as the acute phase of illness resolves.[44,59] During continued convalescence, fluid may be increased as tolerated. Sodium tolerance is generally 1.5-3.5 mEq/kg/day, depending on cardiac output and the use and effectiveness of diuretics. If sodium loss exceeds water loss with diuretic therapy, as may occur with immature kidney function, sodium supplementation of 4-10 mEq/kg/day may be necessary to prevent hyponatremia and improve response to diuretics.[42,60,81] Potassium and chloride must often be supplemented, depending upon the use of diuretics.[61,62]

Calories and Protein

Initially, the patient should be provided with at least 70 (parenteral) or 95 (enteral) kcal/kg/day and 2.0 g/kg/day of protein, increasing to 120-130 kcal/kg/day and 2.5-3.5 g/kg/day of protein.[45,59] During convalescence, calories may be increased as necessary to support growth or catch-up growth, often 130-180 kcal/kg/day.[4,24,63] Adequate calories and protein can be provided while limiting fluid intake by using infant formula concentrated up to 30 kcal/oz (1 kcal/ml). Although these formulas should not provide an excessive renal solute load, particularly if the infant is growing, urine specific gravity or osmolarity should be monitored when fluids are restricted to < 100 ml/kg/day. If human milk is used, human milk fortifiers can be added to increase protein, mineral, and caloric intake. (See Appendix J for examples and indications for use of concentrated formulas and human milk fortifiers.) Concentrating formula alone does not ensure adequate growth unless adequate volumes are prescribed and given and adequate nutrient intake is actually achieved.[64] Improved linear growth, lean tissue accretion, and improved bone mineral density has been shown when infants with BPD are fed formula enriched in protein and mineral content.[20] Complete liquid nutrition products (30 kcal/oz) that are designed for children over 1 year of age may also be used for older infants, although supplemental intake of some nutrients (e.g., iron, vitamins A and D) may be needed to achieve adequate intake.[84]

Increasing caloric density of formulas to 30 kcal/oz by increasing fat or carbohydrate has also been studied.[65] Adding fat decreased carbon dioxide production, but was associated with lower weight gain. Fat provided 67% of the total energy intake and 64% of total energy absorption. This exceeds the usual recommendation of < 60%. Ketosis was not reported, but the trial period was only one week and may not have been of long enough duration to induce ketosis. Adding carbohydrate did not increase carbon dioxide production over that observed with standard formula. Weight gain was within normal limits with carbohydrate supplementation, but increases in arm fat area may indicate a tendency to increase fat mass rather than lean tissue accretion. The formula used in this study was specially formulated to include higher nutrient intake than what can be achieved simply by adding fat or carbohydrate to commercially available premature infant formulas.

If energy requirement and fluid tolerance indicate the need for added fat (0.25 to 1 g/oz of formula) and/or carbohydrate (0.25 to 2 g/oz of formula), the final concentration of protein, fat, and carbohydrate should remain within recommended guidelines of 7-18% protein, 30-55% fat, and 35-65% carbohydrate.[66] Fat contributing > 60%

of the total energy intake is not generally recommended.[45] Other nutrients may require supplementation to achieve recommended intake when fluid restriction is required.

Emulsified oil products are more practical than nonemulsified oils when the patient is fed a continuous drip of formula, inasmuch as it is less likely to separate from the formula solution. As fat separates to the top of the water-based formula, it frequently remains in the holding chamber or coats both chamber and tubing. Thus, it may never reach the patient, or it may be administered as a bolus, possibly reducing absorption efficiency or delaying gastric emptying.[67] Problems associated with separation of nonemulsified fats can be minimized if the formula and oil mixture is blended adequately.

Steroid administration increases endogenous muscle protein catabolism but does not suppress protein synthesis.[29,68] Monitoring protein intake to ensure adequacy may be needed during steroid administration, particularly when steroid doses are maximized or when repeated courses of treatment are needed. Protein intake should be optimal even if energy intake must be limited to prevent excessive weight gain during periods of poor linear growth or if carbohydrate and fat are added to increase the caloric density of formulas.

Vitamins

Standard vitamin supplementation is recommended based on gestational age, weight, feeding route, and product (see Chapters 11 and 15). Adequate vitamin D intake (400 IU/day) may be particularly important, because immobility, lengthy hospitalization (and lack of exposure to sunlight), and medications (dexamethasone and/or diuretics) may compromise calcium and phosphorus metabolism (see Appendix E).[67A] Folic acid may be supplemented if chronic diarrhea or chronic antibiotic therapy is present.[39] Folic acid, not included in standard infant multivitamin supplements, must be given separately.

Minerals

Calcium and phosphorus supplements may be needed to achieve normal recommended intakes, particularly if the need for parenteral nutrition is prolonged and/or fluid restriction is necessary.[69] Human milk fortifiers may be helpful in providing adequate mineral intake for the infant receiving human milk. Specific attention must be paid to mineral content when concentrating formulas or supplementing calories. When calcium and phosphorus supplements are used, they should be given in divided doses to maximize absorption and avoid wide fluctuations in serum levels.[70] The urine calcium-creatinine ratio may be monitored to ensure the safety of calcium supplementation.[42,71] Iron supplements may be needed to maintain nor-

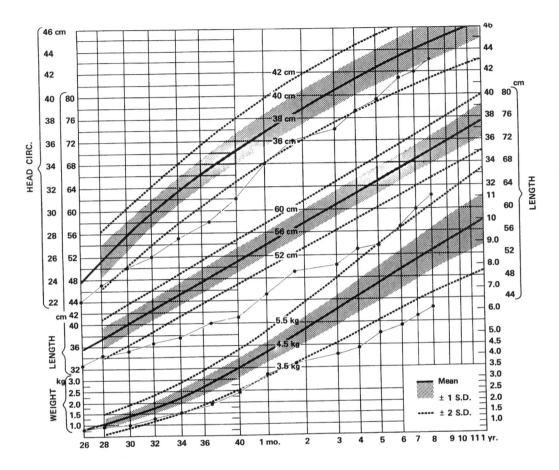

Figure 21.4. Growth of brochopulmonary dysplasia case study
patient DC.

Growth chart used is the Oregon Growth Record. Used with permission.[79]

mal red blood cell formation and hemoglobin levels, thereby maximizing tissue oxygenation and minimizing oxygen consumption.[39]
Trace minerals, which are involved in lung tissue integrity and
repair, should be adequately provided.[72]

Drug/nutrient interactions

Drugs most commonly used in the treatment of BPD include
furosemide, chlorothiazide, spironolactone, theophylline, albuterol,
dexamethasone, cromolyn sodium, and antibiotics. (See Appendix E

and growth and nutrient sections above for information regarding drug/nutrient interactions.)[58]

Foods

Foods given by spoon are often tolerated more easily than liquids given by nipple. Spoon-feeding may begin as early as 3-4 months' corrected chronological age, depending on clinical condition and developmental progress. At 6-8 months' corrected chronological age, infants may be at a critical stage for learning to take foods from a spoon and to chew.[73,74] Omitting the introduction of spoon-feeding at or before this time may contribute to subsequent feeding problems. Oral control and swallowing may be more easily accomplished when foods with a thicker consistency are given. If oral defensiveness or oral motor delay is present, or if respiratory status remains compromised, oral feedings should be initiated under supervision of an occupational therapist or other qualified professional.[75,76] Foods recommended are those low in fluid and sodium content and rich in calories, protein, and minerals. These include cereal, fruit-flavored yogurt, pudding, white or sweet potato (pureed), ice cream, sherbet, and similar foods.

Other Corrective and Preventive Measures

Providing access to adequate nutrition is not the sole responsibility of the nutritionist. Many feeding problems associated with chronic lung disease require the expertise of an experienced occupational, speech, or physical therapist (see Chapter 19). Similarly, provision of optimal nutrition and development of physical abilities may be futile if the patient is unwilling to eat. Many feeding problems may be the product of psychosocial problems and maladaptive behaviors that require therapy. The institutional setting is an adequate but not optimal substitute for the family home, and the rotation of care-givers with eight-hour shifts, five-day weeks, vacations, and holidays often hinders or prohibits emotional attachment of the infant to a primary care-giver. Exposure to normal eating behaviors is often limited or absent, and although discharge to the family may be complex, it may be highly cost-effective and directly associated with improvement in the child's developmental progress and social interaction.[76,77]

Meeting the psychosocial needs of the patient may be difficult in the hospital setting, but it is not impossible. Gentle handling during all procedures and routine care should be consistently provided, along with additional comforting, and pleasant or gentle touching to counteract painful stimuli. Staff members should observe, respect, and respond to signals the patient gives regarding states of receptiveness to stimulation. These signals may include changes in pulse, respirations, or color; hand halt; finger splays; changes in muscle

Table 21.1.   Daily Nutrient Intake of Case Study Subject with Bronchopulmonary Dysplasia

Age	Weight (kg) Length (cm) Head (cm)	Ponderal index* percentile	Formula and Supplements	Fluid ml/kg/d	Energy‡ kcal/kg/d	Protein g/kg/d	Weight gain vs. norm g/d	Length gain vs. norm mm/d	Steroid§
32-36 wk	1.78 kg 40 cm length 29 cm head	2.8 80th %ile	Similac Special Care 24 kcal/oz†	170	135 (145)	3.7	20 (28)	1.25 (1.7)	on
	Birth weight is regained within 2 wk. Parenteral nutrition is started day 1 and increased to meet full nutrient needs by day 7. Trophic feeds are started day 3. Feedings are gradually increased and parenteral nutrition weaned, then discontinued on day 17. Weight gain follows -2 S.D. on Oregon Growth Record; length is well below -2 S.D.; head growth is slightly below -2 S.D. Weight for length increases. Decrease energy intake; begin feeding therapy to decrease oral defensiveness								
36 wk to term	2.463 kg 41 cm length 31 cm head	3.6 >95th %ile	Similac Special Care 24 kcal/oz iron 2 mg/kg/d	160	125 (172)	3.4	24 (30)	0.3 (0.9)	weaning
	Weight gain is not excessive, but linear growth is well below normal, causing weight for length status to increase well above the norm. Further decrease energy intake. Change to Similac NeoSure 22 kcal/oz and decrease volume. Add protein to ensure adequate intake while receiving catabolic steroid. Add water to provide adequate fluid intake and decrease risk of nephrolithiasis. Continue feeding therapy								
term to 1 mo corrected	3.152 kg 45 cm length 34 cm head	3.5 >95th %ile	Similac NeoSure 22 kcal/oz† ProMod†, water iron 2 mg/kg/d	155	105 (140)	3.4	23 (30)	1.3 (1.1)	off
	Linear growth begins to increase as steroids are weaned and discontinued, but weight is still excessive for length. Adipose tissue in chin and neck area have increased and may start to interfere somewhat with respiratory management, as patient will likely need tracheostomy due to long-term ventilator dependence. Support continued linear growth, but decrease rate of weight gain to support a more normal weight-to-length ratio. Decrease calories, but maintain adequate protein and fluid intake								
1-2 mo corrected	3.580 kg 49 cm length 36 cm head	3.0 85th %ile	Similac NeoSure 22 kcal/oz ProMod, water iron 2 mg/kg/d	145	80 (95)	3.0	14 (35)	1.3 (1.1)	off
	Head circumference catches up to 5th %ile IHDP or -2S.D. Oregon Growth Record. Linear growth continues at same rate. Rate of weight gain decreased. Weight for length ratio back within normal limits. Increase energy intake. Continue feeding therapy								
2-3 mo corrected	4.083 kg 50 cm length 37 cm head	3.3 90th %ile	Similac NeoSure 22 kcal/oz ProMod, water iron 2 mg/kg/d	150	95 (120)	3.2	17 (27)	0.3 (1.1)	on
	To improve mechanical ventilatory management during acute exacerbation of respiratory disease, steroid burst given with plan to wean over 2-3 wk. Weight gain as expected, but linear growth slows dramatically, so weight for length increases somewhat. Continue same nutrition, as steroids should be weaned soon								

Table 21.1. Daily Nutrient Intake of Case Study Subject with Bronchopulmonary Dysplasia (continued)

Age	Weight (kg) Length (cm) Head (cm)	Ponderal Index# Percentile	Formula and Supplements	Fluid ml/kg/d	Energy kcal/kg/d	Protein g/kg/d	Weight gain vs. norm g/d	Length gain vs. norm mm/d	Steroid
3-4 mo corrected	4.298 kg 53 cm length 38.5 cm head	2.9 80th %ile	Similac NeoSure 22 kcal/oz ProMod, water iron 2 mg/kg/d	165	100 (115)	3.3	7 (20)	0.9 (0.7)	weaning
	Steroid dose decreased. Linear growth improves. Weight gain slows so that weight for length ratio improves. Continue same nutrition								
4-5 mo corrected	4.989 kg 53.5 cm length 39.5 cm head	3.3 90th %ile	10% Dextrose I.V. Similac NeoSure 22 kcal/oz iron 2 mg/kg/d	150	85 (106)	2.0	23 (17)	0.25 (0.7)	weaning
	Tracheostomy and gastrostomy surgically placed this month, with several days of I.V. fluids. Feedings restarted and up to full volume within 1 wk, but protein supplement not restarted, so average intake of energy and protein are below expected needs. As expected, linear growth slows in spite of decreased steroid dose. Restart supplemental protein. Provide adequate nutrition to support normal linear growth but maintain energy intake to support only modest weight gain								
5-6 mo corrected	5.300 kg 56.3 cm length 41.3 cm head	3.0 85th %ile	Similac NeoSure 22 kcal/oz ProMod, water iron 2 mg/kg/d	150	90 (103)	3.0	10 (16)	0.9 (0.7)	off
	Modest weight gain. Head circumference continues catch-up growth; length begins catch-up phase. Increase intake to support catch-up growth								
6-7 mo corrected	5.691 kg 60 cm length 42 cm head	2.6 50th %ile	Similac NeoSure 22 kcal/oz ProMod, water iron 2 mg/kg/d	150	110 (110)	3.5	13 (13)	1.25 (0.5)	off
	Rate of weight gain is normal. Rate of linear growth is well above normal. Weight for length is at the mean. Head growth continues catch-up. Continue to increase intake as needed to support continued catch-up growth								
7-8 mo corrected	6.116 kg 62 cm length 43 cm head	2.6 50th %ile	Similac NeoSure 22 kcal/oz	165	120 (120)	3.2	14 (13)	0.67 (0.5)	off
	Rate of weight gain is normal. Rate of linear growth continues catch-up. Head growth achieves 25th %ile on IHDP or -1 S.D. on Oregon Growth Record								

* Ponderal Index = [weight in grams x 100] ÷ [length in cm]^3
† Similac formulas and ProMod Protein Supplement are manufactured by Ross Products Division of Abbott Laboratories, Columbus, Ohio.
‡ Energy intake is given in kcal/kg/d of actual body weight; energy intake per kg of ideal weight (50th percentile ponderal index) is given in parentheses.
§ Dexamethasone

tone; gaze aversion or tracking; lip smacking; tongue protrusion; bite reflex; and many others.

A consistent primary care team should be in place that includes the patient's family and small group or "family" of nurses who are committed to providing "hands-on" care consistently throughout the hospitalization. The function of the primary care team in relation to nutrition concerns is to establish a consistent method or pattern for feedings and to allow the patient to form an emotional attachment to (and develop a trusting relationship with) a person or persons providing daily care.[78]

The patient should be encouraged to actively initiate exploration of the environment and to develop purposeful and socially appropriate communication skills. If a patient can learn that ringing a bell or making a noise with a rattle can elicit attention from a loving caregiver, he or she may not have to resort to vomiting or ruminating or disconnecting ventilator tubing to get attention.

Routines should be established, but variety should be provided within the routines. When developmentally appropriate, the patient should be given opportunities to routinely observe and participate in settings in which primary care persons are eating and drinking.

Case Study

DC was born at 26 weeks' gestation with Apgars 1 at one minute and 5 at five minutes. He was intubated and resuscitated with 100% oxygen. Exogenous surfactant was administered. Birth weight was 648 g; length was 32.5 cm and head circumference was 22 cm. Weight and head circumference plotted at the 10th percentile with length at the twenty-fifth percentile on the Lubchenco Intrauterine Growth Chart.[80] Initial weight loss was 10% of birth weight by day 8; birth weight was regained by day 14. Parenteral nutrition was started on day 1 and was maintained until full enteral feedings were established. Trophic enteral feedings of premature infant formula were started on day 3 and gradually increased to provide 120 kcal/kg/day by day 17. Feedings were subsequently increased to establish a more normal rate of weight gain, although linear growth continued to lag, probably because of a continued need for dexamethasone.

By 36 weeks' postmenstrual age, DC continued to require mechanical ventilation and supplemental oxygen. Pulmonary changes characteristic of BPD were evident on chest x-ray. Medications at this time included dexamethasone, diuril, aldactone, caffeine, albuterol, intal, sodium chloride, and potassium chloride. Growth is documented in Figure 21.4. Growth assessment, nutritional intake and nutritional care plans throughout hospitalization are documented in Table 21.1.

DC was discharged at 8 months' corrected age with mechanical ventilation, supplemental oxygen, flovent, and enriched formula. Weight and length were below -2 S.D. on the Oregon Growth Record with head circumference at -1 S.D.

Weight plotted at the 5th percentile on the Infant Health and Development Program (IHDP) growth chart with length slightly below the 5th percentile and head circumference at the 25th percentile. Head growth and weight gain were increasing at a normal rate for corrected age, while linear growth continued to catch up. The nutrition plan at discharge included use of enriched formula until 1 year corrected age and to continue feeding therapy to decrease oral defensiveness and increase tolerance of oral feedings.

References

1. Northway WH Jr, Rosan RC, Porter DY. Pulmonary disease following respirator therapy by hyaline membrane disease: Bronchopulmonary dysplasia. n Engl J Med 276:357, 1967.
2. Bureau of Maternal and Child Health and Resources Development. Guidelines for the care of children with chronic lung disease: Bronchopulmonary dysplasia. Pediatr Pulmonol 6 (suppl 3):3, 1989.
3. Farrell PA, Fiascone JM. Bronchopulmonary dysplasia in the 1990s: A review for the pediatrician. Curr Probl Pediatr 27:133, 1997.
4. Barrington KJ, Finer NN. Treatment of bronchopulmonary dysplasia: A review. Clin Perinatol 25:177, 1998.
5. Escobedo MB, Gonzalez A. Bronchopulmonary dysplasia in the tiny infant. Clin Perinatol 13:315, 1986.
6. Northway WH. Bronchopulmonary dysplasia: Twenty-five years later. Pediatrics 89:969, 1992.
7. Watterberg KL, Gerdes JS, Cook KL. Impaired glucocorticoid synthesis in preterm infants who develop chronic lung disease (CLD) (1364). Pediatr Res 45:232A, 1999.
8. Watterberg KL, Gerdes JS, Gifford KL, et al. Prophylaxis against early adrenal insufficiency to prevent chronic lung disease in premature infants (1365). Pediatr Res 45:232A, 1999.
9. Ng PC. The effectiveness and side effects of dexamethasone in preterm infants with bronchopulmonary dysplasia. Arch Dis Child 68:330, 1993.
10. Durand M, Sardesai S, McEvoy C. Effects of early dexamethasone therapy on pulmonary mechanics and chronic lung disease in very low birth weight infants: a randomized, controlled trial. Pediatrics 95:584, 1995.
11. Rastogi A, Akintorin SM, Bez ML, et al. A controlled trial of dexamethasone to preventbronchopulmonary dysplasia in surfactant-treated infants. Pediatrics 98:204, 1996.
12. Tapia JL, Ramirez R, Cifuentes J, et al. The effect of early dexamethasone administration on bronchopulmonary dysplasia in preterm infants with respiratory distress syndrome. J Pediatr 132:48, 1998.

13. Yeh TF, Torre JA, Rastogi A et al. Early postnatal dexamethasone therapy in premature infants with severe respiratory distress syndrome: A double-blind, controlledstudy. J Pediatr 117:273, 1990.
14. Bozinski MEA, Albert JM, Ushanalini V, et al. Bronchopulmonary dysplasia and postnatal growth in extremely premature black infants. Early Human Develop 21:83, 1990.
15. Davidson S, Schrayer A, Wielunsky E, et al. Energy intake, growth, and development in ventilated very-low-birth-weight infants with and without bronchopulmonary dysplasia. Am J Dis Child 144:553, 1990.
16. Meisels SJ, Plunkett JW, Roloff DW, et al. Growth and development of preterm infants with respiratory distress syndrome and bronchopulmonary dysplasia. Pediatrics 77:345, 1986.
17. Yu VYH, Orgill aa, Lim SB, et al. Growth and development of very low birthweight infants recovering from bronchopulmonary dysplasia. Arch Dis Child 58:791, 1983.
18. Vohr BR, Bell EF, Oh W. Infants with bronchopulmonary dysplasia: Growth pattern and neurologic and developmental outcome. Am J Dis Child 136:443, 1982.
19. Markestad T, Fitzhardinge PM. Growth and development in children recovering from bronchopulmonary dysplasia. J Pediatr 98:597, 1981.
20. Brunton JA, Saigal S, Atkinson SA. Growth and body composition in infants with bronchopulmonary dysplasia up to 3 months corrected age: A randomized trial of a high-energy nutrient-enriched formula fed after hospital discharge. J Pediatr 133:340, 1998.
21. Robertson CMT, Etches PC, Goldson E, et al. Eight-year school performance, neurodevelopmental, and growth outcome of neonates with bronchopulmonary dysplasia: A comparative study. Pediatrics 89:365, 1992.
22. Blayney M, Kerem E, Whyte H, et al. Bronchopulmonary dysplasia: Improvement in lung function between 7 and 10 years of age. J Pediatr 118:201, 1991.
23. Vrlenich LA, Bozynski EA, Shyr Y, et al. The effect of bronchopulmonary dysplasia on growth at school age. Pediatrics 95:855, 1995.
24. Kurzner SI, Bautista DB, Sargent CW, et al. Growth failure in bronchopulmonary dysplasia: Elevated metabolic rates and pulmonary mechanics. J Pediatr 112:73, 1988.
25. Yeh TF, McClenan DA, Ajayi OA, et al. Metabolic rate and energy balance in infants with bronchopulmonary dysplasia. J Pediatr 114:448, 1989.
26. Wilson DC, McClure G, Halliday HL, et al. Nutrition and bronchopulmonary dysplasia. Arch Dis Child 66:37, 1991.
27. Billeaud C, Piedboeuf B, Chessex P. Energy expenditure and severity of respiratory disease in very low birth weight infants receiving long-term ventilatory support. J Pediatr 120:461, 1992.
28. Davis JM, Sinkin RA, Aranda JV. Drug therapy for bronchopulmonary dysplasia. Pediatr Pulmonol 8:117, 1990.
29. Gibson AT, Pearse RG, Wales JKH. Growth retardation after dexamethasone administration: assessment by knemometry. Arch Dis Child 69:505, 1993.
30. Gilmore CH, Senipal-Walerius JM, Jones JG, et al. Pulse dexamethasone does not impair growth and body composition of very low birth weight infants. J Am Coll Nutr 14:455, 1995.

31. Groothuis JR, Rosenberg aa, Zerbe GO. Home oxygen promotes weight gain in infants with bronchopulmonary dysplasia. Pediatr Res 20:227A, 1986.

32. Cox MA, Cohen AJ, Slavin RE, et al. Improved growth in infants with bronchopulmonary dysplasia treated with nasal cannula oxygen. Pediatr Res 18:492, 1984.

33. Moyer-Mileur LJ, Nielson DW, Pfeffer KD, et al. Eliminating sleep-associated hypoxemia improves growth in infants with bronchopulmonary dysplasia. Pediatrics 98:779, 1996.

34. Patel BD, Dinwiddie R, Kumar SP, et al. The effects of feeding on arterial blood gases and lung mechanics in newborn infants recovering from respiratory disease. J Pediatr 90:435, 1977.

35. Johnson DB, Cheney C, Monsen ER. Nutrition and feeding in infants with bronchopulmonary dysplasia after initial hospital discharge: Risk factors for growth failure. J Am Diet Assoc 98:649, 1998.

36. Schlagren RG, Mangurten HH, Grea F, et al. Rumination-a new complication of neonatal intensive care. Pediatrics 66:551, 1980.

37. Davis JM, Sinkin RA, Aranda JV. Drug therapy for bronchopulmonary dysplasia. Pediatr Pulmonol 8:117, 1990.

38. Toffolo A, Trevisanuto D, Meneghetti S, et al. Non-furosemide-related renal calcification in premature infants with bronchopulmonary dysplasia. Acta Paediatr Jpn 39:433, 1997.

39. Southall DP, Samuels MP. Bronchopulmonary dysplasia: A new look at management. Arch Dis Child 65:1089, 1990.

40. Hufnagle KG, Khan SN, Penn D, et al. Renal calcifications: A complication of long-term furosemide therapy in preterm infants. Pediatrics 70:360, 1982.

41. Robinson CM, Cox MA. The incidence of renal calcification in low birthweight infants on lasix for bronchopulmonary dysplasia. Pediatr Res 20:359A, 1986.

42. Campfield T, Braden G, Flynn-Valone P, et al. Effect of diuretics on urinary oxalate, calcium, and sodium excretion in very low birth weight infants. Pediatrics 99:814, 1997.

43. Brown E, Stark A, Sosenko L, et al. Bronchopulmonary dysplasia: Possible relationship to pulmonary edema. J Pediatr 92:982, 1978.

44. Van Marter LJ, Leviton A, Allred EN, et al. Hydration during the first days of life and the risk of bronchopulmonary dysplasia in low birthweight infants. J Pediatr 116:942, 1990.

45. Lund CL, Collier SB. Nutrition and bronchopulmonary dysplasia. In: Lund CH, ed. Bronchopulmonary dysplasia strategies for total patient care. Petaluma, Calif.:Neonatal Network, 1990; 75.

46. Frank L, Sosensko IRS. Undernutrition as a major contributing factor in the pathogenesis of bronchopulmonary dysplasia. Am Rev Respir Dis 725, 1988.

47. Darlow BA, Inder TE, Graham PJ, et al. The relationship of selenium status to respiratory outcome in the very low birth weight infant. Pediatrics 96:314, 1995.

48. Tyson JE, Ehrenkranz RA, Stoll BJ, et al. Vitamin A supplementation to increase survival without chronic lung disease in extremely low birth weight (ELBW) infants: a 14-center randomized trial (1161). Pediatr Res 45:199A, 1999.

49. Ehrenkranz RA, Bonta BW, Ablow RC, et al. Amelioration of bronchopulmonary dysplasia after vitamin E administration. N Engl J Med 299:564, 1978.

50. Watts JL, Milner R, Zipursky A, et al. Failure of supplementation with vitamin E to prevent bronchopulmonary dysplasia in infants less than 1,500 g birth weight. Eur Respir J 4:188, 1991.

51. Jansson L, Lindroth M, Työppönen J. Intestinal absorption of vitamin E in low birthweight infants. Acta Paediatr Scand 73:329, 1984.

52. Hittner HM, Speer ME, Rudolph AJ, et al. Retrolental fibroplasia and vitamin E in the preterm infant—Comparison of oral versus intramuscular: oral administration. Pediatrics 73:238, 1984.

53. Greene HL, Moore MEC, Phillips B, et al. Evaluation of a pediatric multivitamin preparation for total parenteral nutrition. II. Blood levels of vitamins A, D and E. Pediatrics 77:539, 1986.

54. Gutcher GR, Farrell PM. Early intravenous correction of vitamin E deficiency in premature infants. J Pediatr Gastroenterol Nutr 4:604, 1985.

55. Denny LC, Carlson SE, Gupta I, et al. Vitamin A status at birth in relation to respiratory distress syndrome, the need for mechanical ventilation, and the development of chronic lung disease in very low birth weight (vlbw) infants. J Am Diet Assoc 91 suppl:A-115, 1991.

56. Shenai JP, Rush MG, Stahlman MT, et al. Plasma retinol-binding protein response to vitamin A administration in infants susceptible to bronchopulmonary dysplasia. J Pediatr 116:607, 1990.

57. Lawson EE, Stiles AD. Vitamin A therapy for prevention of chronic lung disease in infants. J Pediatr 111:247, 1987.

58. Hallman M, Bry K, Hoppu K, et al. Inositol supplementation in premature infants with respiratory distress syndrome. n Engl J Med 326:1233, 1992.

59. Oh W. Nutritional management of infants with bronchopulmonary dysplasia. In: Bronchopulmonary dysplasia and related chronic respiratory disorders: Report of the 90th Ross Conference on Pediatric Research. Columbus, Ohio: Ross Laboratories, 1986; 96.

60. Vanpee M, Herin P, Broberger U, et al. Sodium supplementation optimizes weightgain in preterm infants. Acta Paediatr 84:1312, 1995.

61. Perlman JM, Moore V, Seigel MJ, et al. Is chloride depletion an important contributing cause of death in infants with bronchopulmonary dysplasia? Pediatrics 77:212, 1986.

62. Brem AS. Electrolyte disorders associated with respiratory distress syndrome and bronchopulmonary dysplasia. Clin Perinatol 19:223, 1992.

63. Kalhan SC, Denne SC. Energy consumption in infants with bronchopulmonary dysplasia. J Pediatr 116:662, 1990.

64. Fewtrell MS, Adams C, Wilson DC, et al. Randomized trial of high nutrient density formula versus standard formula in chronic lung disease. Acta Paediatr 86:577, 1997.

65. Pereira GR, Baumgart S, Bennett MJ, et al. Use of high-fat formula for premature infants with bronchopulmonary dysplasia: Metabolic, pulmonary, and nutritional studies. J Pediatr 124:605, 1994.

66. American Academy of Pediatrics Committee on Nutrition. Commentary on breast feeding and infant formulas, including proposed standards for formulas. Pediatrics 57:278, 1976.

67. Chudley AE, Brown DR, Holzman IR, et al. Nutritional rickets in two very low birthweight infants with chronic lung disease. Arch Dis Child 55:687, 1980.

67A. Cavell B. Effect of feeding an infant formula with high energy density on gastric emptying in infants with congenital heart disease. Acta Paediatr Scand 70:513, 1981.

68. Ng PC. The effectiveness and side effects of dexamethasone in preterm infants with bronchopulmonary dysplasia. Arch Dis Child 68:330, 1993.

69. American Academy of Pediatrics Committee on Nutrition. Calcium requirements in infancy and childhood. Pediatrics 62:826, 1978.

70. Koo WWK, Antony G, Stevens LH. Continuous nasogastric phosphorus infusion in hypophosphatemic rickets of prematurity. Am J Dis Child 138:172, 1984.

71. Ghazali S, Barratt, TM. Urinary excretion of calcium and magnesium in children. Arch Dis Child 49:97, 1974.

72. Sosenka IRS, Frank L. Nutritional influences on lung development and protection against chronic lung disease. Semin Perinatol 15:462, 1991.

73. Dowling S. Seven infants with esophageal atresia: A developmental study. Psychoanalytic study child 32:215, 1977.

74. Coyner AB, Zelle RS. Habilitative approaches to facilitate more adaptive oral patterns related to eating and expressive language. In: Developmentally disabled infants and toddlers: Assessment and intervention. Philadelphia: FA Davis, 1983; 443.

75. Leib SA, Benfield G, Guidubaldi J. Effects of early intervention and stimulation of the preterm infant. Pediatrics 66:83, 1978.

76. Koops BL, Abman SH, Accurso FJ. Outpatient management and follow-up of bronchopulmonary dysplasia. Clin Perinatol 11:101, 1984.

77. Stein RE, Jessop DJ. Does pediatric home care make a difference for children with chronic illness? Findings from the pediatric ambulatory care treatment study. Pediatrics 73:845, 1984.

78. Kavalhuna R, Malnight M. Meeting the needs of the extended care nicu patient. Neonatal Network Feb:19, 1984.

79. Babson SG, Benda GI. Growth graphs for the clinical assessment of infants of varying gestational age. J Pediatr 89:815, 1976.

80. Lubchenco LO, Hansman C Boyd E. Intrauterine growth in length and head circumference as estimated from live births at gestational ages from 26 to 42 weeks. Pediatrics 37:403, 1966.

81. Baumgart S and Costarino AT. Water and electrolyte metabolism of the micropremie. Clin Perinatol 27:131, 2000.

82. Charafeddine L, D'Angio CT, and Phelps DL. Atypical chronic lung disease patterns in neonates. Pediatrics 103:759, 1999.

83. Marshall DD, Kotelchuck M, Young TE, et al. Risk factors for chronic lung disease in the surfactant era: A North Carolina population-based study of very low birth weight infants. Pediatrics 104:1345, 1999.

84. Puangco MA, Schanler RJ. Clinical experience in enteral nutrition support for premature infants with bronchopulmonary dysplasia. J Perinatol 2:87, 2000.

Nutritional Care for High-Risk Newborns (Rev. 3d. Ed.)
S. Groh-Wargo, M. Thompson, J. Cox, editors
© 2000, Precept Press, Inc., Chicago

22

PATENT DUCTUS ARTERIOSUS

Elaine Poole-Napp, MS, RD, LD

THE DUCTUS ARTERIOSUS IS a fetal circulatory pathway through which blood from the right ventricle and pulmonary arterial system flows into the descending aorta for delivery to the placenta. The ductus is important in fetal circulation because it diverts blood away from the fluid-filled lungs toward the aorta and placenta, where oxygen exchange will occur (see Figure 22.1 for a diagram of the infant heart). The ductus normally constricts and functionally closes within a few hours to several days after birth, although the potential to reopen may last throughout the first week.[1]

In the term infant, delayed patency of the ductus arteriosus (PDA) beyond the first few days is usually permanent, and represents an anatomic defect if it is not found in association with persistent pulmonary hypertension (PPHN).[1] The incidence of PDA in term infants is one in 2,500-5,000 live births. When it occurs in association with PPHN, the ductus usually closes when PPHN resolves. If PDA occurs as an anatomic defect, it may occur in isolation or be associated with other cardiac anomalies such as coarctation of the aorta and ventricular septal defect. If present in isolation, PDA may not be detected unless or until pulmonary vascular resistance drops and there is a significant increase in left-to-right shunting of blood flow and volume overload of the left ventricle. This may result in congestive heart failure, pulmonary edema, progressive development of pulmonary vascular resistance, and failure to thrive. Medical management includes fluid restriction, diuretics, and/or digitalis. Surgical repair usually occurs within the first year of life.[1]

A small asymptomatic PDA usually requires no intervention and often closes spontaneously within the first year. If spontaneous closure does not occur, the child may later experience easy fatigability or dyspnea with exertion. Pulmonary hypertension and congestive heart failure may not occur until the third or fourth decade of life if the PDA is allowed to remain.[2]

When PDA occurs with nonreactive pulmonary vessel obstruction, patency of the ductus is needed to limit the severity of pulmonary hypertension. Perfusion of these infants may be dependent on the flow of blood from the subpulmonary ventricle to the aorta through the patent ductus, which is sustained by administration of prostaglandin E.[3]

Patency of the ductus among preterm infants is a reflection of immaturity. The occurrence rate of PDA in preterm infants is inversely proportional to gestational age and birth weight, and may be as high as 80% in infants < 1,000 g birth weight.[4-6] If the PDA is detectable only as a murmur and is not associated with respiratory distress or significant left-to-right shunting of blood flow, these infants may be monitored clinically, as spontaneous closure may occur up to several months of age.[1] PDA in preterm infants, particularly those < 750 g birth weight and those with respiratory distress syndrome, may cause significant left-to-right shunting, increased need for assisted ventilatory support, and can eventually lead to pulmonary damage. PDA in these patients is also associated with central nervous system ischemia, necrotizing entercolitis, and bronchopulmonary dysplasia.[1]

PDA among ventilator-dependent infants or those with related cardiorespiratory symptoms is treated promptly. Indomethacin, a prostaglandin synthetase inhibitor thought to be most effective during the first 7-10 days of life, may be used to medically induce closure of the PDA.[7] Dosing regimens may vary depending upon gestational age and postnatal age. If symptoms remain after two courses of indomethacin, surgical ligation is performed.[1]

Preventive and Therapeutic Nutrition

A nutrition-related factor thought to contribute to failure of the PDA to close is fluid overload, usually exceeding 180 ml/kg/day, in very low birth weight infants during the first few days of life.[6,8] General recommendations to prevent prolonged patency of the ductus include careful management of fluid balance during the first week of life (see Chapter 8). Initial management of symptomatic PDA includes fluid restriction, usually 120-130 ml/kg/day.[9] Adequate nutrition is a priority, particularly in the very low birth weight infant, but even in the more mature preterm or term infant, as the symptoms of the PDA may not fully resolve for more than a week. Adjustment of the nutrient density of parenteral nutrient solutions may be needed to provide adequate nutrition during fluid restriction.

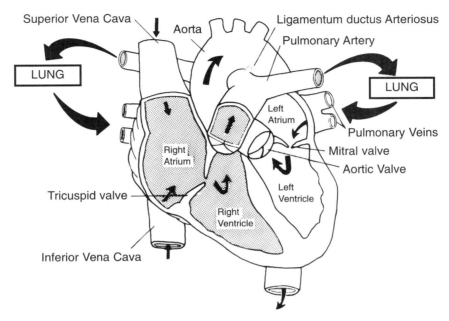

Figure 22.1. Anatomy of the normal heart.

Fortifiers can be added to human milk, and formula can be concentrated to 24-30 kcal/oz to provide recommended levels of calories and nutrients in smaller volumes. The potential renal solute load and osmolality of the feeding is increased when formula is concentrated. The infant's renal status and G.I. tolerance should be considered (see Appendix H for calculation of renal solute load and Appendix I for higher calorie formula recipes.) Diuretics may also be administered and may create a need for electrolyte replacement. (See Appendix E for drug/nutrient interactions.)

Indomethacin, used to medically induce closure of the PDA, may be associated with several complications that are related to the nutritional status of the infant, including bowel perforation.[10-15] Studies have suggested that blood flow patterns and cytoprotective barriers in the G.I. tract are altered by indomethacin, whether administered parenterally or enterally. The disturbance in midgut perfusion appears to be made worse when indomethacin is infused rapidly. Enteral administration of indomethacin is associated with a higher reported incidence of G.I. perforation than I.V. administration. Enteral feedings may be held during indomethacin administration. Indomethacin may cause transient oliguria, contraindicating its use for infants with renal insufficiency. Modest fluid restriction may be needed temporarily.[1,4,6,11-14]

Case Study

A female infant of 25 weeks' gestation was born weighing 700 g. She was delivered to a primigravida mother with a six-hour history of backache. Delivery occurred within 30 minutes of hospital arrival due to incompetent cervix. Although the infant tried to cry in the delivery room, she required intubation, ventilatory support, and exogenous surfactant for clinical symptoms of respiratory distress syndrome (RDS).

Parenteral nutrition was begun on day 2 of life at 100 ml/kg/day, providing protein intake of 1 g/kg/day and energy intake of 48 kcal/kg/day. Trophic feedings of a 20 kcal/oz premature infant formula were started on day 3. On day 4 of life, she developed a loud systolic murmur. Her resting heart rate rose from 140 to 170 beats per minute and her ventilator and oxygen needs increased. Patency of the ductus arteriosus was confirmed by echocardiogram. No other cardiac lesions were noted. Urine output was 3.5 ml/kg/hour and serum creatinine was 0.9 mg/dl, indicating adequate renal function for treatment with indomethacin. A dose of 0.14 mg (0.2 mg/kg) of indomethacin was administered. Her enteral feedings were held and total fluids were maintained at 100 ml/kg/day as her urine volume fell to 1 ml/kg/hour. The murmur became inaudible. She received additional doses of indomethacin at 12 and 24 hours after the initial dose.

From days 5 to 10, she tolerated a gradual increase in parenteral nutrition to 150 ml/kg/day and trophic enteral feedings of her mother's milk at 2 ml every three hours. On day 10, her ventilator and oxygen needs increased as her murmur returned. A repeated course of indomethacin was administered. Enteral feedings were interrupted and parenteral feedings were decreased during the course of drug therapy. Her murmur resolved and ventilatory needs returned to baseline values. Her parenteral fluid intake was gradually advanced to provide 150 ml/kg/day, a protein intake of 3 g/kg/day and an energy intake of 86 kcal/kg/day. Trophic feedings were restarted and gradually advanced as parenteral nutrition was gradually weaned.

Nutrient	Concentration	Daily intake
Amino acids	2.2 %	3.3 g/kg
Dextrose (hydrous)	12.0 %	18.0 g/kg
Lipid	1.4 %	2.1 g/kg
Nonprotein energy	55 kcal/dl	82 kcal/kg
Total energy	64 kcal/dl	95 kcal/kg
Sodium	3.0 mEq/dl	4.5 mEq/kg
Potassium	2.4 mEq/dl	3.6 mEq/kg

Nutrient	Concentration	Daily intake
Chloride	3.0 mEq/dl	4.5 mEq/kg
Calcium	2.0 mEq/dl	3.0 mEq/kg
Phosphorus	0.8 mM/dl	1.2 mmol/kg
Magnesium	0.2 mEq/d	0.3 mEq/kg
Pediatric trace minerals	0.13 mL/dl	0.2 ml/kg
Pediatric multivitamin	0.25 dose/dl	0.3 dose/day
Water		150 ml/kg

References

1. Clyman RI. Patent ductus arteriosus in the premature infant. In: Taeusch HW, Ballard RA, eds. Avery's diseases of the newborn. 7th ed. Philadelphia:Saunders, 1998.
2. Driscoll DJ. Left-to-right shunt lesions. Pediatr Clin North Am 46:355, 1999.
3. Day RW, Tani LY, Minich L, et al. Congenital heart disease with ductal-dependent systemic perfusion: Doppler ultrasound flow velocities are altered by changes in fraction of inspired oxygen. J Heart Lung Transplant 14:718, 1995.
4. Dooley K. Management of the premature infant with patent ductus arteriosus. Pediatr Clin North Am 31:1159, 1984.
5. Ellison RC, Peckham GJ, Lang P, et al. Evaluation of the preterm infant for patent ductus arteriosus. Pediatrics 71:364, 1983.
6. Page GG. Patent ductus arteriosus in the preterm neonate. Heart Lung 14:156, 1985.
7. Kumar RK, Yyh YU. Prolonged low-dose indomethacin therapy for patent ductus arteriosus in very low birth weight infants. J Pediatr Child Health 33:38, 1997.
8. Bell EF, Warburton D, Stonestrut BS, et al. Effect fluid administration has on the development of symptomatic patent ductus arteriosus and congenital heart failure in preterm infants. N Engl J Med 302:598, 1980.
9. Gersony WM. Patent ductus arteriosus in the neonate. Pediatr Clin North Am 33:545, 1986.
10. Gersony WM, Peckham GJ, Ellison RC, et al. Effects of indomethacin in premature infants with PDA: Results of a national collaborative study. J Pediatr 102:895, 1983.
11. Romagnoli C, Zecca E, Papacci P, et al. Furosemide does not prevent indomethacin-induced renal side effects in preterm infants. Clin Pharmacol Ther 62:181, 1997.
12. Coombs RC, Morgan MET, Durbin GM, et al. Gut blood flow velocities in the newborn: Effects of patent ductus arteriosus and parenteral indomethacin. Arch Dis Child 65:1067, 1990.
13. Furzan JA, Reisch J, Tyson JE, et al. Incidence and risk factors for symptomatic patent ductus arteriosus among inborn very-low-birth-weight infants. Early Hum Dev 12:39, 1985.

14.   Knight DB. Patent ductus arteriosus: How important to which babies? Early Hum Dev 29:287, 1992.
15.   Shorter NA, Liu JY, Mooney DP, et al. Indomethacin-associated bowel perforations: A study of possible risk factors. J Pediatr Surg 24:442, 1999.

Nutritional Care for High-Risk Newborns (Rev. 3d. Ed.)
S. Groh-Wargo, M. Thompson, J. Cox, editors
© 2000, Precept Press, Inc., Chicago

23

CONGENITAL HEART DISEASE

Susan J. Carlson, MMSc, RD, LD, CNSD,
and Jean M. Ryan, RD, LD, CNSD

CONGENITAL HEART DISEASE (CHD) is estimated to occur in 10 of 1,000 live births each year.[1] The effect of the cardiac defect on growth, development, and nutritional status depends on the particular lesion and its severity. Cardiac disease of infancy is often classified as cyanotic or acyanotic. Cyanotic defects are associated with right-to-left shunts, cyanosis, and growth retardation. Acyanotic defects associated with large left-to-right shunts and/or left-sided cardiac obstruction may result in congestive heart failure, dyspnea, poor feeding, and poor weight gain.[2] Figure 23.1 provides an illustration of normal heart anatomy. A description of some common congenital cardiac defects, symptoms, treatment, and effects on growth is given in table 23.1.[1,3-6] More complete explanations and illustrations of cardiac defects may be found elsewhere.[7] Patent ductus arteriosus is discussed in Chapter 22.

Infants with CHD are at risk for malnutrition and growth failure. The incidence of both acute and chronic malnutrition has been estimated at 80% in hospitalized infants with CHD.[8] The precise cause of growth failure is uncertain but is thought to be multifactorial.[9-11] Many infants with CHD have extracardiac congenital anomalies or intrauterine growth retardation, which may limit growth potential.[10] Pulmonary hypertension, particularly if the heart defect is cyanotic, is an important factor associated with malnutrition and growth failure.[54] Additional medical conditions that include congestive heart failure, reduced cardiac output, recurrent respiratory infections, tachypnea, acidosis, and cyanosis may contribute to slow growth rates as well. These symptoms are often associated with increased

The contributions of Coleen Greecher, MS, RD, CNSD to this chapter in the previous edition of this book are gratefully acknowledged.

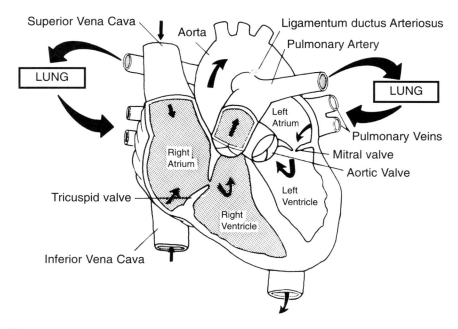

Figure 23.1. Anatomy of the normal heart.

fatigue during oral feedings, abdominal distention, and delayed gastric emptying. Anorexia and inadequate intake may result.

Hypermetabolism has been noted in some infants with cardiac disease.[12,13] Specific tissues such as the cardiac and respiratory muscles may have increased metabolic demands associated with increased rigidity of the lungs; extra caloric expenditure is required for physical activity and the work of breathing.[14,55] Hypermetabolism may also be related to the degree of malnutrition.[15] The high proportion of lean body mass in the malnourished child increases the amount of metabolically active tissue per kilogram of actual weight.

Malabsorption may play a role in growth failure in this population. Mild protein malabsorption and significant fat malabsorption have been reported in infants with congestive heart failure (CHF) and with transposition of the great arteries with cyanosis.[16] Fat malabsorption, found to be > 20 kcal/kg/day, could not be explained by G.I. abnormalities or bile salt concentrations. Additionally, lipid metabolism may be impaired in infants with CHD.[56]

Growth failure associated with CHD is frequently due to inadequate energy intake.[4,15,17] A significant number of children with CHD manifest lack of appetite and food aversions.[18] Prior to corrective operation, infants were found to consume, on average, only 82% of estimated energy needs.[12] After surgery for cardiac repair or palliation, many infants demonstrate catch-up growth,[57] first in weight and then in length. Despite improvement in growth, growth failure and

Table 23.1. Common Congenital Cardiac Defects

Defect	Description	Symptoms/treatment	Growth implications
Patent ductus arteriosis	Failure of contraction of ductus arteriosis that connects the PA and aorta	Heart murmur/fluid restriction, pharmacologic closure, ligation or division	Weight negatively affected prior to duct closure. Growth acceleration following closure
Ventricular septal defect (VSD)	Communication between ventricles allowing blood flow between them	Congestive heart failure/primary closure	Large VSD associated with severe growth failure
Transposition of the great arteries (TGA)	Two parallel and separate circulatory systems exist, one pulmonary and one systemic	Cardiomegaly, cyanosis/arterial switch	Growth retardation in a third to half of patients
Pulmonary stenosis	Obstruction to right ventricular outflow	Variable presentation/valvectomy	Normal growth unless lesion is severe
Aortic stenosis	Obstruction to left ventricular outflow	Variable presentation/valvotomy	Growth failure noted in 16% of patients
Tricuspid atresia	Absent atrioventricular connection failure	Slightly increased heart size/Staged surgical repair	40% of children have marked weight and height growth retardation
Atrial septal defect (ASD)	Communication between 2 atria persists after birth	Asymptomatic or mild respiratory symptoms/direct closure of defect, patch graft	Normal growth unless lesion is severe; then weight gain is poor
Coarctation of the aorta	Narrowing of aorta beyond left subclavian artery	Elevated upper extremity blood pressure, congestive failure/medical management, balloon angioplasty or surgical repair	Growth normal with simple defect
Tetrology of Fallot	Right ventricular outflow obstruction, VSD	Cyanosis, dyspnea/primary repair	Moderate growth failure, primarily in weight
Hypoplastic left heart syndrome	Absence or severe hypoplasia of some or all left-sided heart structures	Respiratory distress, pallor, congestive failure/ Norwood's procedures, cardiac transplantation, or nontreatment (controversial)	Unknown; early mortality (before recent surgical procedures) precluded observations of growth

malnutrition can continue into childhood and adolescence.[8] Aggressive nutritional management should be attempted to maximize growth potential.

Preventive Nutrition

CHD cannot be prevented by diet, but its medical complications can be prevented or attenuated by appropriate nutritional management. For the infant with some forms of CHD, a higher sodium intake combined with excess fluid intake may result in fluid retention, an increased workload for a compromised heart, and the development of CHF. Signs of CHF include rapid breathing, changes in behavior, irritability, periorbital edema, and diaphoresis.[19] Control of fluid and sodium intakes in infants with CHD may help prevent CHF.

Treatment Nutrition

Nutritional treatment for infants with CHD should focus on supplying adequate energy and protein to support growth and limiting fluid and sodium in order to prevent fluid retention.[20] The method of feeding to meet this goal should be determined on an individual basis to maximize oral motor and psychosocial development.

Nutritional Assessment

Nutritional assessment for infants with CHD should follow general guidelines, including standard anthropometric, clinical, intake, and biochemical data.[21] Growth should be assessed by plotting on standardized weight and length charts. Most infants with cardiac disease are born near term at a weight appropriate for gestational age. Within the first several weeks, growth rates slow significantly. Weight for age and rate of growth tend to be lower in infants with CHD than in age-matched controls.[17] Growth problems are suspected if weight is below the 5th percentile on National Center for Health Statistics (NCHS) growth charts, if weight is disproportionately low for length, or if the rate of weight gain followed serially is less than the 25th percentile for babies of similar weight.[22] It may be difficult to distinguish between growth failure attributable to the cardiac lesion and growth failure secondary to inadequate calorie intake, particularly when hypermetabolism and malabsorption are present. Average weight gain for age can be obtained from growth velocity tables.[23] A month-old infant may average 20-40 g of weight gain/day. Weight alone may not be a reliable indicator of growth secondary to fluid retention and diuretic use. Daily weight gain of > 50 g is considered excessive and is likely due to fluid accumulation.[24] Serial anthropometric measurements such as triceps skinfold thickness and arm circumference may be helpful in assessing changes in body muscle and energy stores.

Clinical assessment may provide information regarding edema, respiratory rate, tolerance of enteral feedings, and ability to feed orally. Observation of a meal will help identify dysfunctional feeding behaviors.[25] A review of current medications may delineate potential drug-nutrient interactions.[26] Careful monitoring of input and output can provide information about fluid balance, G.I. function, and tolerance of feedings. Calculation of fluid, calorie, and protein intake per kilogram per day should be performed at least weekly and evaluated in light of growth trends. Intake of iron should also be analyzed.

Electrolyte levels, in conjunction with weight changes, are used to monitor fluid status and calibrate proper diuretic doses. Serum electrolytes should be monitored daily during acute phases of the disease and weekly once the infant is stable. Low serum sodium and potassium levels may indicate a dilutional process. If edema is not present, low levels likely reflect increased losses secondary to aggressive diuretic therapy. High serum electrolyte levels may indicate dehydration (relative concentration).

In general, infants with CHD demonstrate adequate visceral protein status.[27] However, serum protein imbalance may play a role in the development of edema; it is therefore important to assure protein adequacy in infants with CHD. Serum albumin or prealbumin values may provide information regarding protein status (see Chapter 5). Blood urea nitrogen (BUN) levels may serve as an indicator of adequacy of protein intake if renal function is normal.

Iron deficiency has been demonstrated in infants with cyanotic CHD and may further compromise systemic oxygenation by reducing the oxygen-carrying capacity of the red blood cell.[28] Cyanotic CHD induces erythropoiesis, thereby increasing hemoglobin (Hb), hematocrit (Hct), and red blood cell (RBC) counts independent of iron status. Severe cyanotic CHD may result in high Hct and increased blood viscosity. Indicators of iron deficiency in this population include: increased Hct relative to Hb (Hct/Hb > 3), significantly reduced mean corpuscular volume (MCV) < 72.7 Fl, and an excessive rate of erythropoiesis (RBC > 6.88 x 10^{12}/L).[29]

Fluid Intake

Fluid balance is a key factor in the medical management of most infants with CHD. Insensible fluid losses may be increased as much as 10-15% above normal.[30] Fluid losses occur secondary to high ambient temperature, fever, diuretic therapy, and tachypnea.[31] Despite increased fluid losses, most infants with CHD show symptoms of fluid overload and are fluid-restricted to prevent excess fluid accumulation.[32] In the early postoperative period, infants are at significant risk for fluid overload due to high fluid volumes given intraoperatively, fluids administered with cardiac medications, and reduced cardiac and renal function. Fluid restriction to 30-50 ml/kg/day is common. In addition, to control edema, most infants will receive diuretics such as thiazides, furosemide, spironolactone, or a combination of these medications (see Appendix E for drug/nutrient interactions). Infants sensitive to fluid intakes and placed on strict fluid restrictions may have difficulty achieving nutritional goals.[30] During the postoperative period, fluid conservation strategies include concentrating I.V. medications to limit excess fluid administration. Compounding I.V. medications in high dextrose concentrations ($D_{25}W$) can improve energy intake. Other nutritional management strategies include liberalizing fluid intake to the maximum volume tolerated without medical compromise and increasing nutrient density of feedings to meet nutritional goals.

Energy Intake

Setting energy intake goals is extremely important. A reasonable initial goal may be to achieve calorie intake comparable to that of healthy infants of similar size.[22,31] Infants who show poor growth or those with severe cardiac disease may need an extra 30-60 kcal/kg/day over the Recommended Dietary Allowances (RDA) in order to maintain normal growth.[33,34]

Human milk or standard infant formula should be the primary energy source. However, if an infant is hypermetabolic, tires easily, is tachypneic, or has other symptoms affecting the ability to take in an adequate volume of formula, the standard 20 kcal/oz (67 kcal/100 ml) concentration may not deliver adequate energy for growth. Increasing the nutrient density of feedings can improve energy intake and enhance growth.[35-37] Formulas supplying higher nutrient densities can safely be fed if fluid intake and output and urine specific gravity or osmolality are carefully monitored.[31] As formula concentration increases, the concentration of protein and electrolytes also increases, raising the renal solute load (see Appendix H). This increases the risk of dehydration, which is identified by an elevated urine specific gravity or osmolality. In general, 24-30 kcal/oz (80-100 kcal/100 ml) formula concentrations are well tolerated and pose minimal risk for dehydration.[38] Increasing the caloric density of formula to levels > 30 kcal/oz may best be achieved by adding carbohydrate or fat to avoid increasing the renal solute load. Use of carbohydrate or fat modulars to increase caloric density of 20-24 kcal/oz (67-80 kcal/100 ml) formula will dilute protein and nutrient concentrations and are, therefore, not generally recommended. (See Appendices I and J for specific examples of concentrated formulas and modular use.)

Expressed human milk, combined with formula concentrates or powders, may be required to deliver adequate energy for the term infant. Commercially available human milk fortifiers as energy and protein sources are indicated only in the preterm infant and should not be used to concentrate human milk feedings for term infants with CHD. When concentration of breast milk or formula is necessary, advancing the concentration and volume in a stepwise fashion is advised to prevent side effects of diarrhea, abdominal pain, malabsorption, and, in certain high-risk infants, necrotizing enterocolitis.

Protein Intake

Protein requirements in the infant with CHD should equal those of the healthy infant. Infants with growth failure may have increased protein requirements in relation to their need for catch-up growth. Feedings of high caloric density made from concentrated formulas or breast milk mixed with concentrated formulas are likely to meet protein needs. Protein intake should be carefully evaluated when infants are fed high-caloric-density feedings made by the addition of carbohydrate or fat to breast milk or 20 kcal/oz formulas. Protein content of feedings should be maintained at 8-10% of total calories.

Vitamin, Mineral, and Electrolyte Intakes

Additional vitamins are not required for formula-fed infants with CHD. Breast-milk-fed infants should receive an A, D, and C vitamin supplement. Iron deficiency and iron deficiency anemia have been documented in some infants with cyanotic CHD.[28] Iron-fortified formulas are recommended for formula-fed infants, while breast-milk-fed infants should receive an iron supplement.[39] Electrolyte supplementation is a frequent requirement for infants with CHD. Chronic use of diuretics results in increased urinary excretion of sodium, potassium, chloride, magnesium and calcium. The degree of supplementation required depends on the type and amount of diuretics used and serum electrolyte values.

Feeding Methods

If the mother of an infant with CHD wishes to breast-feed her infant, it is possible to do so. Breast-fed infants with CHD have been found to maintain oxygen saturations better than their formula-fed counterparts.[40] Growth in infants at least partially breast-fed has been found to equal or exceed that of infants receiving formula alone.[41] Breast massage to stimulate letdown and milk flow prior to putting the infant to the breast may decrease the effort required by the infant to nurse. If the infant appears to tire easily and does not empty the breasts, or fails to gain adequate weight from breast-feeding, it is possible to use a supplemental nursing device to allow the infant to suck concentrated formula from a tube taped close to the mother's nipple.

This allows stimulation of the mother's milk production as well as delivery of concentrated formula to foster growth of the infant.

Concentrating breast milk or formula is often the first nutritional treatment for poor growth in infants with cardiac disease. If a trial of 24-30 kcal/oz formula does not facilitate growth, or results in excessive G.I. losses, a trial of nasogastric tube feeding may be helpful.[15,17,20,30,42,43] Continuous enteral feeding, at a rate of 120-169 kcal/kg/day, has been shown to promote weight gain with minimal effect on respiratory rate, heart rate, and fluid retention.[42-44] Infants who tire easily during feeding, have rapid respiratory rates, or are catabolic may benefit most from continuous feeding. It appears that continuous enteral feeding may also be advantageous preoperatively or during periods of infection in promoting continued growth. Older infants may be able to tolerate larger volumes of bolus feedings during the day and benefit from nighttime continuous tube feeding. This can be provided by a 10-12-hour nighttime tube feeding (to allow a normal daytime routine).

Solid foods may be introduced when the infant is at the physically and developmentally appropriate stage. Dry cereal may be mixed with high-caloric-density formula or breast milk to enhance energy intake. Avoidance of presalted baby foods and table foods limits excessive sodium intake.[20] If oral and enteral nutrition are inadequate or impossible, parenteral nutrition (PN) is indicated. (See Chapters 8-13 for specific information on initiation and management of PN.)

Infants with CHD may be delayed in basic motor skills as a result of prolonged illness and hospitalization.[45,46] A physical or occupational therapist can recommend feeding, positioning, and routine activities that may greatly enhance development in these infants (see Chapter 19).

Other Nutritional Conditions Associated with CHD

Left-sided cardiac obstruction or cardiopulmonary bypass during cardiac surgery may result in decreased perfusion of the G.I. tract.[47] Reduced G.I. perfusion has been associated with protein-losing enteropathy, necrotizing enterocolitis (NEC) or mesenteric ischemia, cow's milk protein sensitivity, and gluten induced enteropathy. NEC and other gastrointestinal ischemias have been reported in approximately 7-8% of term infants with CHD.[48,49] Cow's milk protein sensitization has been documented in a small sample of infants with CHD.[50] Gluten-induced enteropathy, responsive to gluten-free diet, has also been reported in 6/2,500 cases of children with CHD. The incidence of celiac disease in the general population is about 1 in 2,000.[51] In addition, prostaglandin use has been associated with gastric distention and may contribute to feeding intolerance.[52] Given these findings, studies to rule out gastrointestinal disease should be performed in infants who do not gain weight on concentrated formula or who have significant G.I. symptoms. Gastroesophageal reflux

(GER), associated with neurological impairment, has been documented in children with CHD.[53] If an infant with CHD presents with recurrent respiratory symptoms, pneumonia, and FTT, a diagnostic workup for pathologic GER may be warranted (see Chapter 27).

In summary, the nutritional care of infants with CHD presents many challenges to the health care team. Providing adequate, but not excessive, fluids, with appropriate energy and nutrient intake is the cornerstone of nutritional management. Creative use of available feeding modalities can result in the provision of optimal nutrition to promote growth.

Case Study

KB was born at 41 3/7 weeks' gestation weighing 3,460 g and measuring 50 cm in length. Physical examination revealed a cardiac murmur and features consistent with trisomy 21. She was admitted to the neonatal intensive care unit for a genetic workup. An echocardiogram showed a common AV canal, large PDA, left-to-right shunt, and increased pulmonary artery pressures. The infant was started on 24 kcal/oz cow's milk formula with iron and discharged to home within the first week of life. Cardiac repair was planned for 6 months of age.

At four months of age, the infant returned for a routine cardiology clinic appointment, including a repeat echocardiogram. At that time, the infant was consuming 3-4 oz feedings of 24 kcal/oz cow's milk formula with iron every 3-4 hours. No symptoms of CHF or feeding difficulties were noted and growth was acceptable. Results of the echocardiogram revealed AV canal with increased pulmonary vascular resistance, and mitral and tricuspid valve regurgitation. Due to concerns about increasing pulmonary hypertension, plans were made for surgery within two weeks for AV canal repair.

The infant was admitted to the pediatric intensive care unit postoperatively. Preoperatively, the infant weighed 5.4 kg (50th percentile weight for age on the Down syndrome growth chart) and 59 cm (50th percentile length for age on the Down syndrome growth chart). Medications, including epinephrine, dobutamine, furosemide, milrinone, morphine, fentanyl, and nipride were started. The infant's weight on postoperative day (POD) 1 was 6.1 kg. The infant was placed on a fluid restriction of 40 cc/kg/day. Serum glucose was elevated to 150-160 mg/dl until the epinephrine was weaned on POD 3. After weaning the epinephrine, medications were infused into a central line with a $D_{25}W$ solution. In addition, parenteral nutrition was started using $D_{25}W$, 5% AA at 3 ml/hour and 1 g/kg/day of 20% intravenous fat emulsion (IFE). Over the next few days, fluids were liberalized, urine output increased, and parenteral nutrition was advanced to provide 2 g protein/kg/day and 2 g fat/kg/day. Energy intake from parenteral nutrition, IFE, and dextrose in medication drips averaged 60-70 kcal/kg/day. By POD 5, fluids were liberalized to 100 cc/kg/day and enteral feedings were initiated using 5 ml/hour of 24 kcal/oz cow's milk formula with iron. Over the next week, drip feedings were gradually advanced as parenteral nutrition was weaned. On POD 8, the infant was extubated and enteral feedings were transitioned to oral feedings with nasogastric (NG) bolus supplements. Fluids remained restricted and oral intake was limited; therefore, formula concentration was advanced to 27 kcal/oz. Oral intake gradually improved and NG supplements were discontinued. The infant was discharged home consuming approximately 120 kcal/kg/day from 27 kcal/oz cow's milk formula with iron feedings. The infant continues to be monitored at outpatient clinic visits to evaluate growth and feeding.

References

1. Hoffman JJE. Incidence of congenital heart disease: I. Postnatal incidence. Pediatr Cardiol 16:103, 1995.
2. Nouri S. Congenital heart defects: Cyanotic and acyanotic. Pediatr Ann 26:92, 1997.
3. Feldt RH, Strickler GB, Weidman WH. Growth of children with congenital heart disease. Am J Dis Child 117:573, 1969.
4. Rosenthal A, Castaneda AR. Growth and development after cardiovascular surgery in infants and children. Prog Cardiovasc Dis 18:27, 1975.
5. Sacksteder S, Gildea JH, Dassy C. Common congenital cardiac defects. Am J Nurs 78:266, 1978.
6. Fanaroff AA, Martin RJ, eds. Neonatal-Perinatal Medicine. 5th ed. St. Louis: Mosby Year Book, 1992; 916-17.
7. Hurst JW, Nugent EW, Anderson RH, et al. Congenital heart disease. In: Hurst JW, Anderson RH, Becker et al., eds. Atlas of the Heart. New York: Gower Medical Publishers, 1988; 31.
8. Cameron JW, Rosenthal A, Olson AD. Malnutrition in hospitalized children with congenital heart disease. Arch Pediatr Adolesc Med 149:1098, 1995.
9. Mitchell IM, Logan RW, Pollock JCS, et al. Nutritional status of children with congenital heart disease. Br Heart J 73:277, 1995.
10. Poskitt EME. Food, growth, and congenital heart disease. Nutr Health 5:153, 1987.
11. Forchielli ML, McColl R, Walker WA, et al. Children with congenital heart disease: A nutrition challenge. Nutr Rev 52:348, 1994.
12. Barton JS, Hindmarsh PC, Scrimgeour CM, et al. Energy expenditure in congenital heart disease. Arch Dis Child 70:5, 1994.
13. Mitchell IM, Davies PSW, Day JME, et al. Energy expenditure in children with congenital heart disease, before and after cardiac surgery. J Thorac Cardiovasc Surg 107:374, 1994.
14. Pittman JG, Cohen P. The pathogenesis of cardiac cachexia. New Engl J Med 271:403, 1964.

15. Yahav J, Auigad S, Frand M, et al. Assessment of intestinal and cardiorespiratory function in children with congenital heart disease on high caloric formulas. J Pediatr Gastroenterol Nutr 4:778, 1985.

16. Sondheimer JM, Hamilton JR. Intestinal function in infants with severe congenital heart disease. J Pediatr 92:572, 1978.

17. Menon G, Poskitt EME. Why does congenital heart disease cause failure to thrive? Arch Dis Child 60:1134, 1985.

18. Thommessen M, Heiberg A, Kase BF, et al. Feeding problems, height and weight in different groups of disabled children. Acta Paediatr Scand 80:527, 1991.

19. Clare MD. Home care of infants and children with cardiac disease. Heart Lung 14:218, 1985.

20. Greecher C. Congenital heart disease: A nutrition challenge. Nutr Focus 5:1, 1990.

21. American Dietetic Association Quality Assurance Committee Practice Group of Dietitians in Pediatric Practice. Congenital heart disease in quality assurance criteria for pediatric nutrition conditions: A model. Chicago: ADA, 1988.

22. Rickard K, Brady MS, Gresham EL. Nutritional management of the chronically ill child. Pediatr Clin North Am 24:157, 1977.

23. Guo S, Roche AF, Fomon SJ, et al. Reference data on gains in weight and length during the first two years of life. J Pediatr 119:355, 1991.

24. Hazinski MF. Congenital heart disease in the neonate. III. Congestive heart failure. Neonatal Network 1(6):8, 1983.

25. Norris MKG, Hill CS. Nutritional issues in infants and children with congenital heart disease. Crit Care Nurs Clin North Am 6:153, 1994.

26. Abdulla R, Young S, Barnes SD. The pediatric cardiology pharmacopoeia. Pediatr Cardiol 18:162, 1997.

27. Salzer HR, Hascke, F, Wimmer M, et al. Growth and nutritional intake of infants with congenital heart disease. Pediatr Cardiol 10:17, 1989.

28. West DW, Scheel JN, Stover R, et al. Iron deficiency in children with cyanotic congenital heart disease. J Pediatr 117:266, 1990.

29. Oleay L, Ozer S, Gurgey A, et al. Parameters of iron deficiency in children with cyanotic congenital heart disease. Pediatr Cardiol 17:150, 1996.

30. Heymsfield SB, Andrews JS, Hood R, et al. Nutrition and the heart. In: Grand RJ, Sutphen JL, Dietz WH, eds. Pediatric nutrition. Stoneham, Mass.: Butterworth, 1987; 597.

31. Fomon SJ, Ziegler EE. Nutritional management of infants with congenital heart disease. Am Heart J 83:581, 1972.

32. Mitchell IM, Davies PSW, Pollock JCS, et al. Total body water in children with congenital heart disease before and after cardiac surgery. J Thorac Cardiovasc Surg 110:633, 1995.

33. Huse DM, Feldt RH, Nelson RA, et al. Infants with congenital heart disease. Am J Dis Child 129:65, 1975.

34. Krieger I. Growth failure and congenital heart disease. Am J Dis Child, 120:497, 1970.

35. Balluff M. Nutritional management of the high risk infant. Nebr Med J 67:57, 1982.

36. Cavell B. Effect of feeding an infant formula with high energy density on gastric emptying in infants with congenital heart disease. Acta Paediatr Scand 70:513, 1981.

37. Jackson M, and Poskitt EME. The effects of high-energy feeding on energy balance and growth in infants with congenital heart disease and failure to thrive. Br J Nutr 65:131, 1991.
38. Saigal S, Sinclair JC. Urine solute excretion in growing low-birth-weight infants. J Pediatr 90:934, 1977.
39. Gidding SS, Rosenthal A. Iron supplementation in cyanotic congenital heart disease. Clin Pediatr 27:261, 1988.
40. Marino BL, O'Brien P, LoRe H. Oxygen saturations during breast and bottle feedings in infants with congenital heart disease. J Pediatr Nurs 10:360, 1995.
41. Combs VL, Marino BL. A comparison of growth patterns in breast and bottle-fed infants with congenital heart disease. Pediatr Nurs 19:175, 1993.
42. Vanderhoof JA, Hofschire PJ, Baluff MA, et al. Continuous enteral feedings. Am J Dis Child 136:825, 1982.
43. Schwarz SM, Gewitz MH, See CC, et al. Enteral nutrition in infants with congenital heart disease and growth failure. Pediatrics 86:368, 1990.
44. Bougle D, Iselin M, Kahyat A, et al. Nutritional treatment of congenital heart disease. Arch Dis Child 61:799, 1986.
45. Loeffel M. Developmental considerations of infants and children with congenital heart disease. Heart Lung 14:214, 1985.
46. O'Brien P, Boisvert JT. Discharge planning for children with heart disease. Crit Care Nurs Clin North Am 1:297, 1989.
47. Booker PD, Romer H, Franks R. Gut mucosal perfusion in neonates undergoing cardiopulmonary bypass. Br J Anaesth 77:597, 1996.
48. Leung MP, Chen K, Hui P, et al. Necrotizing enterocolitis in neonates with symptomatic congenital heart disease. J Pediatr 113:1044, 1988.
49. Hebra A, Brown MF, Hirschl RB, et al. Mesenteric ischemia in hypoplastic left heart syndrome. J Pediatr Surg 28:606, 1993.
50. Ventura A, Canciani GP, Tamburlini G. Congenital heart disease and cow's milk intolerance. Helv Paediat Acta 39:269, 1984.
51. Congdon PJ, Fiddler GI, Littlewood JM, et al. Coeliac disease associated with congenital heart disease. Arch Dis Child 57:78, 1982.
52. Kriss VM, Desai NS. Relation of gastric distention to prostaglandin therapy in neonates. Radiology 203:219, 1997.
53. Wessner KM, Rosenthal A. Gastroesophageal reflux in association with congenital heart disease. Clin Pediatr 22:424, 1983.
54. Varan B, Tokel K, Yilmaz G. Malnutrition and growth failure in cyanotic and acyanotic congenital heart disease with and without pulmonary hypertension. Arch Dis Child 81:49, 1999.
55. Ackerman IL, Karn CA, Denne SC, et al. Total but not resting energy expenditure is increased in infants with ventricular septal defects. Pediatr 102:1172, 1998.
56. Lundell K-H, Sabel K-G, Eriksson BO. Plasma metabolites after a lipid load in infants with congenital heart disease. Acta Paediatr 88:718, 1999.
57. Schuurmans FM, Pulles-Heintzberger CFM, Gerver WJM, et al. Long-term growth of children with congenital heart disease: A retrospective study. Acta Paediatr 87:1250, 1998.

Nutritional Care for High-Risk Newborns (Rev. 3d. Ed.)
S. Groh-Wargo, M. Thompson, J. Cox, editors
© 2000, Precept Press, Inc., Chicago

24

HYPERBILIRUBINEMIA

John V. Hartline, MD

JAUNDICE IS FREQUENTLY FOUND during the physical examination of newborn infants. It is probably the most perplexing among newborn findings in that it is most often normal, i.e., physiological, but it may be the harbinger of more serious underlying problems, or the bilirubin itself may become elevated to toxic levels. This chapter will highlight some of the basic concepts regarding various types of neonatal jaundice and will address their nutritional ramifications. Jaundice is the clinical reflection of elevated levels of bilirubin. Although serum bilirubin increases above the normal childhood and adult level (1 mg/dl) in virtually all neonates, clinical jaundice generally will be noticed when bilirubin levels exceed 7-8 mg/dl. In dark-skinned individuals, jaundice may not be evident until higher levels are reached.

Metabolism

Bilirubin is a waste product of the metabolism of the heme moiety of the hemoglobin molecule. In the normal neonate, bilirubin is produced at 6-8 mg/kg/day. This rate is about twice the adult rate on a per-kilogram basis. Factors contributing to the increased bilirubin load are the high neonatal hematocrit, the increase in heme degradation as hematopoietic function ceases (temporarily) at birth, decreased life span of the neonatal red blood cell, and the frequent occurrence of localized blood breakdown associated with focal bruising and/or blood accumulations (subgaleal clot, cephalohematoma, or ecchymosis of the buttocks or perineum in breech presentations).

Bilirubin is transported in the blood in its unconjugated, lipid-soluble "indirect" form bound to albumin. Hepatic uptake of the unconjugated bilirubin is mediated through binding proteins in the liver cell. Once in the liver, the glucuronyl transferase enzyme system conjugates bilirubin with glucuronide to form bilirubin monoglucuronide and diglucuronide, which constitute the water-soluble, nontoxic "direct" bilirubin that is later excreted into the bile. Because of the immaturity of the bilirubin glucuronosyltransferase system, the neonate produces a greater proportion of monoglucuronide and a smaller proportion of diglucuronide than does the adult.[1] Conjugated bilirubin may be acted upon by intestinal glucuronidases, resulting in the reformation of unconjugated bilirubin, which may be absorbed back into the blood, the "enterohepatic circulation of bilirubin." Four factors combine to potentiate intestinal absorption of bilirubin in the newborn period. First, monoglucuronide is more easily converted to bilirubin than is diglucuronide. Second, significant levels of beta-glucuronidase are found in the neonatal intestine. Third, neonates lack the intestinal flora needed to convert to stercobilin. Fourth, meconium accumulated within the intestine has both bilirubin and beta-glucuronidase. These factors also play a significant role in the jaundice associated with lower intestinal anatomic obstruction or cystic fibrosis. With adequate intestinal motility, bilirubin is transported to the large intestine, where intestinal bacteria irreversibly convert the bilirubin to stercobilin, the form excreted in stools.

Physiological elevation of bilirubin occurs in virtually all newborns. Physiological elevation of bilirubin has two phases. Phase 1 is associated with decreased hepatic glucuronosyltransferase activity in the presence of an increased bilirubin load. Hepatic uptake and excretion are also low, but the enzyme activity is rate-limiting in phase 1. Race affects the pattern of neonatal jaundice.[2] Among white or black infants, the mean peak bilirubin is 5-6 mg/dl occurring at 60-72 hour of age. East Asian infants experience a higher peak (10-14 mg/dl) occurring at 72-120 hours of age. Phase 2 is associated with the gradual decline in bilirubin due to diminished hepatic uptake. Mean bilirubin levels among black or white infants will have declined to < 2mg/dl by day 5, whereas levels < 2 mg/dl occur at 7-10 days of age among the Asian infants.

Bilirubin may have an as yet unidentified role as a natural antioxidant. Plasma antioxidant levels have been shown to vary directly with bilirubin concentration. Levels of other antioxidants are not large enough to account for differences in antioxidant activity.[3] Antioxidant activity of bilirubin may play a protective role at a time when other antioxidants are lacking.[4]

As long as the ratio of unconjugated bilirubin molecules-to-albumin molecules is < 1:1, bilirubin is tightly bound and is not free to enter lipid-laden tissues such as the brain. If bilirubin levels exceed the ability of the serum albumin to bind bilirubin, due either to high levels or to conditions decreasing the binding capacity of the serum albumin, bilirubin may enter the brain tissue. Neurotoxicity of bilirubin may be manifested initially by subtle signs such as lethargy, irritability, changes in muscle tone, or poor feeding. These signs and symptoms are not specific and usually are not due to elevated bilirubin. True bilirubin neurotoxicity, known as kernicterus, is manifested by opisthotonus, seizures, fever, high-pitched cry, apnea and/or death. Infants surviving kernicterus are at high risk for motor delay, choreoathetosis, asymmetric spasticity, dental dysplasia, mental retardation, cognitive dysfunction and/or sensorineural hearing loss.[1]

Early Hospital Discharge and Neonatal Jaundice

Earlier discharge from the hospital has been associated with increased readmission to the hospital for hyperbilirubinemia.[5] Clinical features associated with increased risk for subsequent hyperbilirubinemia include maternal diabetes mellitus, East Asian heritage, lower gestational age, oxytocin use during labor, male sex, breast-feeding, glucose-6-phosphate dehydrogenase deficiency, and history of jaundice in a sibling. Universal bilirubin screening at 20-28 hours of age has been proposed as a means to predict the risk for subsequent hyperbilirubinemia.[6] Fifty-two percent of newborns will have a bilirubin < 5 mg/dl at 24 hours and none of these will be expected to develop a level > 17 mg/dl by day 5 of life. If the 95th percentile value of < 8 mg/dl is used, the risk for a subsequent rise to > 17 mg/dl is 2%. Hour-specific bilirubin percentile curves have been generated that relate the early-obtained bilirubin level to the predicted course over the first week of life. Use of these data may help to identify higher risk infants who need diagnostic evaluation, earlier treatment and/or follow-up bilirubin levels after discharge. Nutritional considerations play an important role, in that most of the affected infants have been breast-fed and many of the readmitted infants have had excessive weight loss with dehydration at readmission. In some infants, clinical kernicterus has occurred. Strategies available to prevent the risks of severe hyperbilirubinemia among early-discharged infants are application of risk screening, universal bilirubin determinations at 24 hours of age plotted for risk of subsequent hyperbilirubinemia, appropriate diagnostic testing and breast-feeding support while in the hospital, and outpatient clinical evaluation at 48 to 72 hours after hospital discharge.

Jaundice Among Breast-Fed Infants: Breast-Feeding and Breast Milk

Breast-fed infants as a group experience higher levels of bilirubin in the first days of life.[7] This has been called breast-feeding jaundice. Breast-feeding jaundice occurs when breast milk intake is inadequate; it perhaps could aptly be termed "lack-of-breast milk jaundice."[11] Breast-fed infants show no increase in bilirubin systhesis when compared with formula-fed infants; the increased bilirubin load results from greater enterohepatic circulation of bilirubin. When the incidence of jaundice has been analyzed according to breast-feeding practices, hyperbilirubinemia correlates with less frequent breast-feeding, higher weight loss, and decreased number of stools.[8] The more often breast-feeding occurs and the more milk that is taken, the lower the peak bilirubin level. In one study, bilirubin on day 3 was lower in breast-fed infants than among controls.[9] Another study compared three groups of infants: 605 infants who were breast-fed on demand; 623 infants who received a combination of breast and formula feeding; and 226 infants who were formula-fed. Neither the percentage of infants with bilirubin level > 12.9 mg/dl on day 3 nor weight loss were significantly different among the three groups.[10] Breast-feeding jaundice should be considered a preventable condition. Mothers encouraged to breast-feed early and frequently (9-12 times/day) generally will have infants with lower bilirubin levels. Use of lactation consultants and the avoidance of water supplements also have been advocated.

Breast-fed infants may present with a second form of jaundice: prolonged unconjugated hyperbilirubinemia noted beyond the first or second week of life, which occurs in 30-60% of breast-fed infants. This has been called breast milk jaundice.

The etiology of breast milk jaundice is uncertain. Studies of components of human milk initially suggest that hormonal residues (pregnane-3-alpha, 20-beta diol) interfere with bilirubin metabolism. Subsequent studies refute that claim. Breast milk given to infants with prolonged jaundice shows similar levels of beta-glucuronidase activity when compared with controls.[12,13] Breast milk given to jaundiced infants promotes bilirubin absorption and also inhibits hepatic glucuronosyltransferase activity, although the specific constituent responsible has yet to be identified. Of note, colostrum does not have these effects; they become active in transitional and mature milk. High fatty acid content of the breast milk given to affected infants may enhance enterohepatic circulation, resulting in a persistently high bilirubin load. Because enhanced enterhepatic circulation results in the higher bilirubin pool among babies with breast-feeding jaundice and in prolonged bilirubin elevation among babies with breast milk jaundice, an etiologic link may be present. Optimal breast-feeding practices may serve to decrease breast milk jaundice and, by reducing the bilirubin pool size, reduce the impact of breast milk jaundice.[7]

The diagnosis of breast milk jaundice is usually one of exclusion. The infant with breast milk jaundice has elevated unconjugated bilirubin. The baby's appearance is healthy and robust. Hemolysis, enclosed bleeding, hypothyroidism, and other pathological conditions have been ruled-out.

Management of breast milk jaundice should first emphasize more frequent breast-feeding. If bilirubin levels rise to > 20 mg/dl, feeding supplementation with formula (not water), with or without phototherapy may be instituted. Temporary discontinuance of breast-feeding for one or two days should be reserved for infants with unusually high or resistant hyperbilirubinemia. With a pause in breast-feeding, bilirubin levels drop quickly and rebound only slightly after resumption of breast-feeding. Bilirubin levels reported among infants fed a casein hydrolysate formula, which inhibits beta-glucuronidase, are lower than among standard infant formula-fed or breast-fed infants.[14] Aggressive counseling to promote resumption of breast-feeding should be part of the therapeutic plan. When jaundice is associated with other identified etiologies, breast-feeding should be continued and more frequent feedings encouraged.

Unconjugated Hyperbilirubinemia

Pathological elevations of unconjugated ("indirect") bilirubin result from either increased production of bilirubin, decreased excretion, or a combination of the two. Increased production of bilirubin results from conditions of increased red blood cell (RBC) breakdown. Hemolysis may result from blood group incompatibility between the mother and infant due to maternal antibodies crossing the placenta and coating the fetal RBC. These antibodies may be due to isoimmunization, i.e., antibodies formed due to exposure to RBC antigens at the time of an earlier pregnancy (as commonly was the case with Rh hemolytic disease) or mismatched blood transfusion (rare). Natural antibodies such as anti-A or anti-B (normally present in nontype AB individuals) may occasionally be of the IgG variety, small molecules able to cross the placenta and cause ABO hemolytic disease if the infant is type A, B, or AB. Hemolysis may also be associated with incompatibility in the so-called minor blood groups. In these antibody-mediated conditions, maternal screening should detect the antibody; testing of the neonatal RBCs for attached antibody (Coombs' test) should make the diagnosis in most cases. Structural RBC abnormalities such as sphero-cytosis or enzymatic deficiencies such as glucose-6-phosphate dehydrogenase (G6PD) deficiency may also lead to neonatal hemolysis. G6PD is usually not associated with early jaundice, in that the hemolysis is not rapid. Recent studies show that G6PD infants presenting with hyperbilirubinemia also have a deficiency in the hepatic glucuronosyltransferase system (Gilbert syndrome), resulting in inhibited metabolism of bilirubin.[15] G6PD heterozygotes, who would test as normal on screening for G6PD, are also at risk for significant hyperbilirubinemia if they have the Gilbert gene.[16] An increased bilirubin load may be associated with an initial high hematocrit (polycythemia) or with the breakdown of extra-vascular blood.

Decreased excretion of bilirubin also contributes to the physiological bilirubin elevation, as noted above. Pathological conditions associated with prolonged unconjugated hyperbilirubinemia include congenital absence of glucuronyl transferase enzyme (e.g., Crigler-Najjar syndrome) or the presence of inhibitors of the enzyme system (e.g., Lucey-Driscoll syndrome), which can interfere with bilirubin metabolism. Persistent levels of unconjugated bilirubin may also herald neonatal hypothyroidism, as patients with hypothryoidism have diminished bilirubin conjugation.[17] Conditions associated with decreased intestinal motility or intestinal obstruction may lead to enhanced enterohepatic circulation and persistent jaundice.

Elevated bilirubin in the neonate raises concern regarding two areas: the underlying cause and the level of the unconjugated bilirubin. When unconjugated bilirubin levels fall outside of the physiologic range, diagnostic evaluation should be undertaken. Hyperbilirubinemia is a symptom, not a disease in itself. In general, jaundice occurring early (evident at < 24 hours of age) indicates hemolysis. Peak levels above the physiological range may be due to hemolysis; degradation of enclosed blood from caput, cephalohematoma, or cutaneous bruising; or high enterohepatic circulation. Prolonged or persistent jaundice suggests inhibition of bilirubin metabolism or unusually high enterohepatic circulation. Diagnosis of underlying hemolysis is necessary in order to be aware of present or future concerns with anemia. Some immune-mediated disorders require exchange transfusion, and hypothyroidism mandates prompt replacement therapy. Sepsis in the neonate, which may also be associated with pronounced or prolonged jaundice, requires appropriate antibiotic therapy. It is very unusual for sepsis to present as jaundice in an otherwise well-appearing child. Jaundice with sepsis is often combined (indirect and direct) and is not often "early." The workup for pathologic jaundice includes a CBC, which should be evaluated for hematologic features of sepsis: neutropenia, neutophilia, increased immature to total neutrophil fraction (> 0.2), and/or thrombocytopenia. Negative C-reactive protein studies correlate highly with absence of sepsis.

The second concern, the level of the bilirubin, is another controversial issue.[1,18] Initial studies of Rh hemolytic disease (erythroblastosis fetalis) related bilirubin levels in excess of 20 mg/dl to increasing risk of neurotoxicity. Although the treatment of Rh negative mothers with anti-Rh antibodies has nearly eliminated Rh hemolytic disease, these data led to the "vigintiphobia" (fear of 20) that has dictated much of the treatment of jaundice associated with other conditions. The degree to which bilirubin is toxic to newborn infants whose bilirubin elevation is due to causes other than Rh disease is an area of great controversy. Among term infants, bilirubin toxicity is rarely noted at levels of < 25 mg/dl, and many clinicians have seen infants present with much higher levels who demonstrate no acute nor chronic consequences. Preterm infants have lower levels of serum albumin and less effective binding of bilirubin to albumin. For these reasons, phototherapy and/or exchange transfusion are recommended at lower bilirubin levels among preterm infants. Jaundiced infants on lipid-containing parenteral infusions present the potential for free fatty acids to compete with bilirubin for albumin binding sites. With lipid infusions of ≤ 2g/kg/24 hours and with bilirubin < 12 mg/dl, there is no need to interrupt lipid administration for this reason.[19]

Conjugated Hyperbilirubinemia

Elevation of conjugated "direct" bilirubin (> 1.5-2.0 mg/dl) suggests disruption in the excretion of the conjugated bilirubin from the liver, either by obstruction to bile flow or due to hepatocellular injury. Although conditions resulting in conjugated hyperbilirubinemia are less common than the unconjugated variety, many of these conditions have nutritional consequences. Detailed reviews of conditions causing cholestatic jaundice have recently been published.[20,21]

The two most common causes of cholestatic jaundice are extrahepatic biliary atresia and idiopathic neonatal cholestasis. These account for 60-80% of cases in most series. Distinction of these two entities is often quite difficult, but nevertheless is extremely important. Clay-colored stools suggest biliary obstruction. Ultrasound of the gallbladder may be helpful in that biliary atresia is commonly (but not always) associated with absence of the gallbladder. Bile secretion into the intestine can be assessed by hepatobiliary scintigraphy. After five days' treatment with phenobarbital (5 mg/kg/day) to stimulate bile flow, technetium-labeled iminodiacetic acid is administered. Scanning of the abdomen can show whether bile is present in the intestine. Absence of G.I. excretion on a single scan is not diagnostic of atresia, in that some patients with intrahepatic cholestasis will fail to demonstrate excretion. Spivak et al. found a second scan to be helpful in differentiating biliary atresia from neonatal hepatitis and inspissated bile syndrome.[22] On the other hand, they noted no excretion among five of six infants with a paucity of intrahepatic bile ducts, two of six with stasis associated with parenteral nutrition, and one with cholangiolitis. If biliary atresia is diagnosed, early attempts to establish bile flow by hepatic portoenterostomy is essential if success is to be expected. Surgery done at less than two months of age results in 90% chance for bile flow. Surgery at more than three months of age is associated with only 20% chance for intestinal bile flow.[21]

Hepatocellular diseases such as hepatitis due to congenital infections with cytomegalovirus, herpes virus, rubella, toxoplasmosis, syphilis, and hepatitis B can present with elevated conjugated bilirubin in the neonatal period. Bacterial infections of the neonate also may be associated with cholestasis. Some metabolic diseases may present with elevated "direct" bilirubin. Alpha-l-antitrypsin deficiency (the third most frequent cause, 5-10% of cases), galactosemia, fructosemia, tyrosinemia, glycogen storage disease IV, Niemann-Pick disease, Gaucher's disease, Wolman disease, cystic fibrosis, and peroxisomal disorders should be considered in cases in which other causes are not evident. A small series of newborn infants with perinatal asphyxia have been reported to have cholestasis and other findings similar to neonatal hepatitis.[23] After search for identifiable etiologies has failed, the diagnosis of idiopathic neonatal hepatitis may be made.

Cholestatic jaundice may be seen in the newborn in association with parenteral nutrition of greater than two weeks' duration. This jaundice is more common among parenterally fed premature infants, with an incidence of > 50% in infants of < 1,000 g.[21] The exact precipitating factors are unknown, but present wisdom suggests that prematurity; prolonged fasting, with its effects on intestinal mucosa (atrophy), bile flow (reduced), bile salts (decreased pool size) and bacterial flora; and composition of the parenteral solution all may contribute. Phenobarbital has been given as a choleretic, but its value is not yet confirmed. In most cases, the discontinuation of parenteral feeding and resumption of enteral feedings is associated with the gradual resolution of the cholestasis over several weeks to months.

Treatment of Jaundice

Unconjugated Hyperbilirubinemia

Treatment of infants with elevated unconjugated bilirubin has nonspecific and specific components. Nonspecific treatment includes the treatment of the underlying cause (e.g., antibiotics for sepsis) and promotion of the normal metabolic pathways by frequent feedings and adequate hydration to promote intestinal motility. If breast-feeding, mothers should be encouraged to breast-feed early and frequently (9-12 times/day) and to avoid supplementing their infants' feedings with water.

The most common treatment specific for bilirubin is phototherapy. Light in the visible blue (and perhaps green) spectrum has been shown to affect bilirubin in two ways.[24] Photo-oxidation results in polar, water-soluble products. This process is quite slow and is probably not the clinically significant effect. Photo-isomerization produces both a labile (geometric) and a stable (structural) isomer, with the former constituting the majority of the clinical effect. Both of these are efficiently secreted into the gut without need for conjugation in the liver. In infants with intestinal obstruction, the rebound hyperbilirubinemia following discontinuation of phototherapy is thought to be associated with the reversion of the labile photoisomer to native bilirubin and subsequent resorption into the circulation. Phototherapy is associated with loose stools and also with increased insensible water losses. Fluids may be increased by 10-20 ml/kg/day (0.5 ml/kg/hour for infants < 1,500 g and by 1 ml/kg/hour for infants > 1,500 g).

Phototherapy is generally indicated when the infant is felt to be at risk for developing a potentially toxic bilirubin level. The effectiveness of phototherapy depends on four factors: wavelength (420-500 nm), irradiance as measured in microwatts/cm²/nm; amount of surface area exposed, and time. Because the blue color of the light is noxious to caregivers and makes observation for other conditions difficult, most phototherapy is given using white light. Measurement of the irradiance in the blue spectrum can be used to measure the intensity of the therapy. Phototherapy using green light has been found to be less effective than when blue light is used.[25] Irradiance is highest with halogen lights and least with the fiberoptic blankets. Instruments are available to measure irradiance. Bilirubin degradation is proportional to irradiance up to 50 mW/cm²/nm. Although time of exposure is significant, periods off phototherapy of up to one hour do not detract from clinical efficacy. Taking advantage of this feature can allow for adequate breast-feeding. Use of the light blanket during feeding can maintain some phototherapy during feeding periods. With documented hemolytic disease, phototherapy is often started early, followed by frequent bilirubin level determinations to assess its effect. Because the theoretical toxicity of bilirubin involves bilirubin level, factors affecting binding, gestational age, and presence or extent of other conditions, phototherapy is often initiated when bilirubin levels reach about 5 mg/dl less than the level at which an exchange transfusion would be considered. If jaundice is noted early, the rise is rapid, or if the patient is expected to have unusually excessive bilirubin load (e.g., lots of bruising), phototherapy may be started earlier.

The development of the exchange transfusion led to a marked reduction in the incidence of bilirubin-associated neurotoxicity. Subsequently, the use of phototherapy has decreased the number of exchange transfusions needed for affected infants. With excessively high bilirubin levels or with evidence of neurotoxicity on clinical examination, exchange transfusion is indicated. It is the only treatment documented to affect long-term outcome in these situations. (Exchange transfusion is also indicated if profound hemolytic anemia is present at birth). Using umbilical vessels, small volumes of the baby's blood are repeatedly exchanged for equal volumes of bank blood to effect a lowering of bilirubin levels. Using a total volume equal to two times the estimated blood volume of the infant, about 85% of the infant's blood will be replaced. Exchange transfusion has been associated with an increased risk for necrotizing enterocolitis. Feeding tolerance and abdominal examinations are followed closely after exchange.

The American Academy of Pediatrics has published a practice parameter as a general guide to the management of jaundice in the term or near-term infant.[26] The practice parameter sets guidelines for the consideration and/or use of phototherapy and recommended levels for performing an exchange transfusion. Re-evaluation at 48 to 72 hours after discharge of the infant discharged at < 48 hours of age is also recommended so as to pick up jaundice, excessive weight loss, difficulties with breast-feeding and other conditions not showing symptoms in the first two days of life.

Four other therapeutic approaches have been applied to newborn jaundice: (1) binding of bilirubin in the gut to block enterohepatic circulation; (2) interventions directed at increasing intestinal motility; (3) stimulation of the hepatic glucuronosyltransferase system by pharmacological agents; and (4) blocking the action of heme oxygenase, the first enzyme in the degradation of heme to bilirubin. Agar, cholestyramine, and activated charcoal have been used to bind intestinal bilirubin. Rectal stimulation[27] and frequent feeding[9] enhance motility and thereby allow less time for bilirubin absorption. Phenobarbital given to the mother or to the infant after birth will activate the transferase system and result in lower bilirubin levels. Clofibrate, a medication studied in France, also activates the enzyme system.[28] Tin-Mesoporphyrin given orally is an effective inhibitor of bilirubin production and clinically lowers bilirubin synthesis in term and near-term newborns[29], preterm newborns[30], and infants who are G6PD deficient.[31]

Conjugated Hyperbilirubinemia

In that conjugated bilirubin is not toxic per se, treatment is related to the underlying condition and to the nutritional consequences of cholestasis. Infants with inborn errors of metabolism should be treated as soon as possible with the appropriate limitation and/or supplementation of the nutrients specifically related to their condition.

Infants with cholestasis associated with parenteral nutrition may benefit from small "trophic" feedings of breast milk or dilute infant formula to enhance the development of G.I. function. Enteral feedings should be established as soon as they are tolerated. For infants on prolonged parenteral feeding, some advocate cyclic administration. In that copper and manganese are excreted through the bile, and normal losses would be decreased, they may be deleted from the parenteral feeding solution.[32]

In addition to the specific treatments related to their primary condition, dietary modifications are helpful to promote optimal nutrition and growth in patients with chronic cholestasis. Steatorrhea may be expected, due to the decreased presence of bile acids in the intestine. Decreased fat absorption also can be expected, and fat-soluble vitamin deficiencies may result. Medium-chain triglycerides will provide fat intake that does not require bile salts for micelle formation to allow absorption. Essential fatty acid deficiency may occur when infants who malabsorb fat due to hepatobiliary disease are given formula containing predominantly MCT oil as a fat source (Portagen, Mead Johnson, Evansville, Ind.) and only 3% of total calories from linoleic acid. Higher intakes of linoleic acid are recommended, either by supplementation or by the use of infant formulas containing MCT oil but with greater linoleic acid content (e.g., Pregestimil, Mead Johnson; or Alimentum, Ross Laboratories, Columbus, Ohio).[33]

Fat-soluble vitamins A and E can be provided in their water-soluble forms. Vitamin A should be given at 10,000-25,000 I.U./day. Vitamin E should be given orally at 50-400 I.U./day as d-alpha-tocopherol or at 15-25 lu/day as d-alpha-tocopheryl polyethylene glycol 1,000 succinate. Vitamin D should be given at 5,000-8,000 lu/day of D2 or at 3-5 µg/kg/day of 25-hydroxyvitamin D. Vitamin K (2.5 mg) can be given every other or every third day. Levels of these vitamins and prothrombin time should be monitored; if sufficient levels are not maintained, intramuscular injections may be necessary.[34] Optimal intake of calcium, phosphorus, and zinc should be maintained. Water-soluble vitamin deficiency has been reported. Recommended intake of water-soluble vitamins is twice the Recommended Dietary Allowance.[35]

Hypercholesterolemia may develop in patients with cholestasis. Phenobarbital may lower the level by stimulating the catabolism of cholesterol to bile acids. Cholestyramine may be successful by binding bile acids and increasing cholesterol metabolism, thereby removing the feedback inhibition of the bile acids. If cholestyramine is used, the patient should be monitored for metabolic acidosis due to chloride release. Trace element loss may be enhanced due to loss of enterohepatic circulation.

Case Study

History. A two-day old, 3.5 kg, term, white male breast-fed infant presents with jaundice first noted at 18 hours of age, at which time the bilirubin measures (12.0 total, 11.8 indirect). The mother is O, Rh positive with a negative antibody screen. The infant is B, Rh positive, with negative Coombs test. The ABO test detects some circulating anti-B in the infant's serum. The CBC shows a hematocrit of 36 with normal WBCs and platelets, and 20 nucleated RBCs per 100 WBCs. The child has been placed on a fiberoptic "biliblanket." The child is taking breast milk well and the physical examination is negative. The mother's first baby had been "under the light" for a while. Family history is negative for any known hematological diseases. There is no Mediterranean ancestry.

At 48 hours of age, the baby's bilirubin has risen to 19.3 (18.9 indirect). The baby continues to thrive, having lost only 60 g since birth. Neither bruising nor cephalohematoma is evident.

Diagnostic Considerations. The early rise in bilirubin ("early jaundice") indicates significant blood breakdown resulting in excess bilirubin production. Although the shortened life span of the fetal RBC and larger proportion of ineffective erythropoiesis causes bilirubin production of the newborn to exceed that of the older child or adult, jaundice due to these physiologic mechanisms does not cause visible icterus in the first 24 hours of life. Hemolysis is the major consideration in early jaundice. Because jaundice requiring treatment was seen in the mother's first-born, isoimmunization is less likely because sensitization would not be evident in a first pregnancy. The rapidity of bilirubin rise suggests hemolysis to a degree more than one typically should attribute to direct Coombs-negative BO incompatibility. Antibodies attached to the RBC due to sensitization to one of the rare blood types would cause the direct Coombs to be positive.

Abnormalities of the shape of the RBC can cause hemolysis. Hereditary spherocytosis is a dominant condition and could affect a first-born infant. This family presents with no history of anemia and no family member has had a splenectomy, which is often needed among patients with spherocytosis. Eliptocytosis can also present with hemolysis. Both of these present morphological changes evident on the blood smear not seen in this baby's blood.

Abnormalities of RBC enzymes can lead to neonatal hemolysis. The child was white and not of Mediterranean extraction, making G6PD deficiency less likely. Also, babies with G6PD tend to become icteric after the first 24 hours of life, since abnormal bilirubin conjugation is part of the pathogenesis of jaundice in this condition. These babies are especially susceptible to pathologic jaundice after early discharge from the hospital. Some foods such as fava beans trigger hemolysis among G6PD patients. Breast-feeding mothers of G6PD babies should avoid such foods, since acute hemolysis in the breast-fed infant has been documented.[32]

Familial recurrence could suggest conditions such as the Lucey-Driscoll syndrome, due to a maternal serum inhibitor of bilirubin metabolism, but inhibition more often results in pronounced peak levels or prolonged jaundice. As noted, there was no evidence of enclosed bleeding. Babies with significant bruising can develop hyperbilirubinemia, which is more likely to be pronounced and/or prolonged hyperbilirubinemia rather than the early-onset variety noted in this baby.

Because the rapid rise in bilirubin and the unusually low hematocrit strongly suggest hemolysis and the usual, more common entities discussed above were not found, enzymatic studies of the red blood cell were done. These studies ultimately showed that the baby had pyruvic kinase deficiency. Tests on the older sibling confirmed the condition in him as well.

Therapeutic Considerations. A rising bilirubin in the term infant at this level could be treated by more intense phototherapy, but it is possible that light alone would not contain the rise. If the bilirubin is not controlled by more light, then exchange could be needed. In the otherwise healthy, jaundiced term infant, many neonatologists would recommend exchange with the bilirubin approaching 25 mg/dl. More intense phototherapy can be done using two or more bilirubin "spotlights," fluorescent lights, a fiberoptic blanket under the infant, or a combination. Note that the light intensity in the blue spectrum can deteriorate with bulb use. Monitoring the intensity of blue spectrum light can be useful. If testing materials are not available and the treatment is not as effective as expected, try using new bulbs. The AAP Practice Parameter gives guidance for when exchange transfusion should be considered.[26] If the baby is in a unit in which personnel are not experienced in the technique of exchange transfusion, transfer to an appropriate facility should occur.

Nutritional Considerations. Encourage frequent breast-feedings. In the presence of adequate oral intake, interruption of breast-feeding is not wise in these cases, because breast milk is not causing the problem. More frequent feeding may enhance intestinal motility. Brief periods out from under the lights do not diminish the effectiveness of phototherapy. If desired, the fiberoptic blanket can be used during feedings. If transfer is necessary, lactation support should be provided for the mother to promote return to breast-feeding.

Long-term Planning. Late anemia can follow chronic hemolysis. Patients with hereditary spherocytosis may need splenectomy at some time. Families should be educated regarding recurrence risk when jaundice is due to conditions with likelihood of repetition. Genetic counseling should be offered in cases of familial hereditary conditions, such as pyruvic kinase deficiency.

References

1. Gourley GR. Bilirubin Metabolism and Kernicterus. Adv Pediatr 44:173, 1997.
2. Hodgman J and Edwards N. Racial differences in neonatal jaundice. Clin Pediatr 31:719, 1992.
3. Belanger S, Lavoie JC, Chessex P. Influence of bilirubin on the antioxidant capacity of plasma in newborn infants. Biol Neonate 71(4):233 , 1997.
4. Hegyi T et al. The protective role of bilirubin in oxygen radical diseases of the preterm infant. J Perinatol 14(4):296, 1994.
5. Maisels MJ, Newman TB. Jaundice in full-term and near-term babies who leave the hospital within 36 hours. Clin Perinatol 25(2):295, 1998.
6. Johnson L, Bhutani VK. Guidelines for management of the jaundiced term and near-term infant. Clin Perinatol 25(3):555, 1998.
7. Gartner LM, Lee KL. Jaundice in the breastfed infant. Clin Perinatol 26(2):431, 1999.
8. Tudehope D, Bayley G, Munro D, et al. Breast feeding practices and severe hyperbilirubinemia. J Pediatr Child Health 27:240, 1991.
9. De Carvalho M, Klaus M, and Merkatz M. Frequency of breastfeeding and serum bilirubin concentration. Amer Dis Child 136:747, 1982.
10. Rubaltelli FF. Unconjugated and conjugated bililrubin pigments during perinatal development. IV. The influence of breast-feeding on neonatal hyperbilirubinemia. Biol Neonate 64:104, 1993.
11. Neifert, M. The optimization of breast-feeding in the perinatal period. Clin Perinatol 25(2):303, 1998.
12. LaTorre A, Targioni G, Rubaltelli FF. Beta-glucuronidase and hyperbilirubinemia in breast-fed infants. Biol Neonate 75:82, 1999.
13. Ince Z, Coban A, Peker I, et al. Breast milk beta-glucuronidase and prolonged jaundice in the neonate. Acta Paediatr 84:237, 1995.
14. Gourley GR, Kreamer B, Cohnen M, Kosorok M. Neonatal jaundice and diet. Arch Pediatr Adolesc Med 153:184, 1999.
15. Kaplan M, Rubaltelli FF, Hammerman C, et al. Conjugated bilirubin in neonates with glucose-6-phosphate dehydrogenase deficiency. J Pediatr 128:695, 1996.
16. Kaplan M, Beutler E, Vreman HJ, Hammerman C, Levy-Lahad E, Renbaum P, Stevenson D. Neonatal Hyperbilirubinemia in glucose-6-phosphate dehydrogenase-deficient heterozygotes. Pediatr 104:68, 1999.
17. LaBrune P, Myara A, Huguet P, Folliot A, Vial M, Trivin F, Odievre M. Bilirubin uridine diphosphate glucuronosyl transferase hepatic activity in jaundice associated with congential hypothryoidism. J Pediatr Gastroenterol Nutr 14(1):79, 1992.
18. Newman TB, Maisels MJ. Does hyperbilirubinemia damage the brain of healthy full-term infants? Clin Perinatol 17:331, 1990.

19. Spear ML et al. Effect of heparin dose and infusion rate on lipid clearance and bilirubin binding in premature infants receiving intravenous fat emulsions. J Pediatr 112:94, 1988.

20. Heubi JE, Daugherty CC. Neonatal Cholestasis: An approach for the practicing pediatrician. Curr Prob Pediatr 20:235, 1990.

21. Haber BA, Lake AM. Cholestatic jaundice in the newborn. Clin Perinatol 17:483, 1990.

22. Spivak W, Sarkar S, Winter D, et al. Diagnostic utility of hepatobiliary scintigraphy with 99m-Tc-DISIDA in neonatal cholestasis. J Pediatr 110:885, 1987.

23 Vajro P, Amelio A, Stagni A, Paludetto R, Genovese E, Giuffre M. Cholestasis in newborn infants with perinatal asphyxia. Acta Pediatr 86(8):895-8, 1997.

24. Tan KL. Phototherapy for newborn jaundice. Clin Perinatol 18:429, 1991.

25. Myara A, Sender A, Valette V, et al. Early changes in cutaneous bilirubin and serum bilirubin isomers during intensive phototherapy of jaundiced neonates with blue and green light. Biol Neonate 71(2):75, 1997.

26. American Academy of Pediatrics Provisional Committee for Quality Improvement and Subcommittee on Hyperbilirubinemia. Practice parameter: management of hyperbilirubinemia in the healthy term newborn. Pediatr 94(4):558, 1994.

27. Cottrell BH, Anderson GC. Rectal or axillary temperature measurement: effect on plasma bilirubin and intestinal transit of meconium. J Pediatr Gastroenterol Nutr 3:734, 1984.

28. Galiban JC, Benattar C, Lindenbaum A. Clofibrate treatment of neonatal jaundice. Pediatrics 86:647, 1990.

29. Kappas A, Drummond GS, Henschke C, Valaes T. Direct comparision of sn-mesoporphyrin, an inhibitor of bilirubin production, and phototherapy in controlling hyperbilirubinema in term and near-term newborns. Pediatrics 95:468, 1995.

30. Valaes T, Petmezaki S, Henschke C, Drummond GS, Kappas A. Control of jaundice in preterm newborns by an inhibitor of bilirubin production: studies with tin-mesoporphyrin. Pediatrics 93:1, 1994.

31. Valaes T, Drummond GS, Kappas A. Control of hyperbilirubinemia in glucose-6-phosphate dehydrogenase-deficient newborns using an inhibitor of bilirubin production, sn-mesoporphyrin. Pediatrics 101:1, 1998.

32. Triplett WC. Clinical aspects of zinc, copper, manganese, chromium and selenium metabolism. Nutr Int 1:60, 1985.

33. Pettei MJ, Daftary S, Levine JJ. Essential fatty acid deficiency associated with the use of a medium-chain-triglyceride formula in pediatric hepatobiliary disease. Am J Clin Nutr 53:1217, 1991.

34. Sippel CJ, Balistreri WF. Bile acid secretion and cholestasis. In: Hay WW, ed. Neonatal nutrition and metabolism. St. Louis: Mosby Year Book, 1991; 451.

35. Sokol RJ, Heubi JE, Butler-Simon N, et al. Treatment of vitamin E deficiency during chronic childhood cholestasis with oral d-alpha-tocopheryl polyethylene glycol-1000 succinate. Gastroenterol 93:975, 1987.

36. Kaplan M, Hammerman C. Severe neonatal hyperbilirubinemia: a potential complication of glucose-6-phosphate dehydrogenase deficiency. Clin Perinatol 25(3):575, 1998.

Bibliography

Gourley GR. Breastfeeding, diet, and hyperbilirubinemia. NeoReviews 1:e25-e31, 2000.

Hammerman C and Kaplan M. Recent developments in the management of neonatal hyperbilirubinemia. NeoReviews 1:e19-e24, 2000.

25

NECROTIZING ENTEROCOLITIS

Pamela T. Price, PhD, RD, CNSD

NECROTIZING ENTEROCOLITIS (NEC) IS an acquired gastrointestinal disease that in its mildest form appears as feeding intolerance and in its extreme form is characterized by diffuse or patchy areas of necrotic small and/or large bowel with or without perforation.[1] Mortality is high, and morbidity related to NEC contributes to prolonged or recurrent hospitalization, delayed growth, and neurodevelopmental impairment.[2-7]

The overall incidence of NEC is 1.0-7.7% of all neonatal intensive care unit (NICU) admissions.[8,9] Although NEC is predominantly a disease of stressed preterm infants, 7-10% of patients are full-term infants.[5,7-9] In a large multicenter study, infants with gestational age of < 28 weeks accounted for only 33% of the cases of NEC occurring during the first seven days of life but 78% of cases occurring after 29 days of life. Median age of onset was 19 days for infants < 0.9 kg, 11 days for infants 0.9-1.3 kg, and 7 days for infants 1.3-1.5 kg. The overall incidence of NEC in infants ≤ 1.5 kg is 6.0-8.8%.[10-11]

Recent advances in NICU care have resulted in increased survival of smaller infants. Additionally, the introduction of exogenous surfactant therapy in the early 1990s has been correlated with a decrease in mortality. As a result, the rate of NEC increased from 11.5 deaths per 100,000 live births in the presurfactant period (1983-85), to 12.3 deaths per 100,000 live births in the postsurfactant period (1990-92). During 1990 and 1991, 91% of deaths due to NEC were low-birth-weight (LBW) infants. Most occurred after the first week of life. Death was inversely related to birth weight; therefore, the improvement in survival of the small, very immature infants, who are at the greatest risk of developing NEC, may account for the increase in NEC-associated infant mortality.[12]

The etiology of NEC remains unknown, but is felt to be a complex, multifactorial event (see Figure 25.1). Intestinal ischemia, the presence of pathogenic bacteria, and the availability of a metabolic substrate (i.e., formula) are seen in most diseased infants.[13,14,77] In addition, antenatal indomethacin therapy for preterm labor and intrauterine cocaine exposure have been identified as risk factors for the development of NEC.[15-17] Although not yet proven, it has been hypothesized that magnesium and copper deficiency may contribute to NEC by impairing the antioxidant defense through a decrease in synthesis of glutathione and reduced activity of Cu/Zn superoxide dismutase.[18] On the other hand, antenatal maternal steroid therapy appears to result in a significantly decreased incidence of NEC, possibly due to acceleration of intestinal maturity induced by corticosteroids.[19-21] Postnatal steroid administration does not decrease the incidence of NEC as effectively as prenatal treatment but may improve clinical outcome.[22]

NEC may occur as an endemic or sporadic disease with 0-2 cases every month and is often related to feeding; it may also occur as intermittent epidemics in which affected infants are related in space and time or have the same microbiological organism.[5,7,23] NEC is suspected as a result of G.I. signs and symptoms (see Table 25.1). Radiographic findings of pneumatosis intestinalis or intrahepatic venous gas are specific to NEC and are useful in confirming the diagnosis.[8,23,24]

A system of classification has been developed by Walsh and Kliegman:[7]

Stage I. Stage I NEC includes infants who have suspected NEC. They may manifest feeding intolerance, mild abdominal distention, increased gastric residuals, and guaiac-positive stools; radiologic signs are those of a normal intestine, mild ileus, or intestinal dilation. Often these infants have feeding intolerance, which is common in LBW infants.

Stage IIA. In stage IIA, diagnosis of NEC is confirmed by radiologic evidence of pneumatosis intestinalis; abdominal tenderness is often present along with the symptoms seen in stage I.

Stage IIB. This stage includes all of the above signs as well as acidosis and thrombocytopenia, portal venous gas, and possibly abdominal cellitis or right lower quandrant mass. The infant is moderately ill.

Stage III. Stage III, the more advanced NEC, is marked by clinical instability, with progressive deterioration of vital signs, respiratory failure, disseminated intravascular coagulation, and shock. This stage is divided into stage IIIA, where the bowel is intact, and Stage IIIB, where intestinal perforation has occurred.

The most common late complication of NEC is intestinal stricture.[25] This is seen in 25-35% of survivors (see Table 25.2). Many of

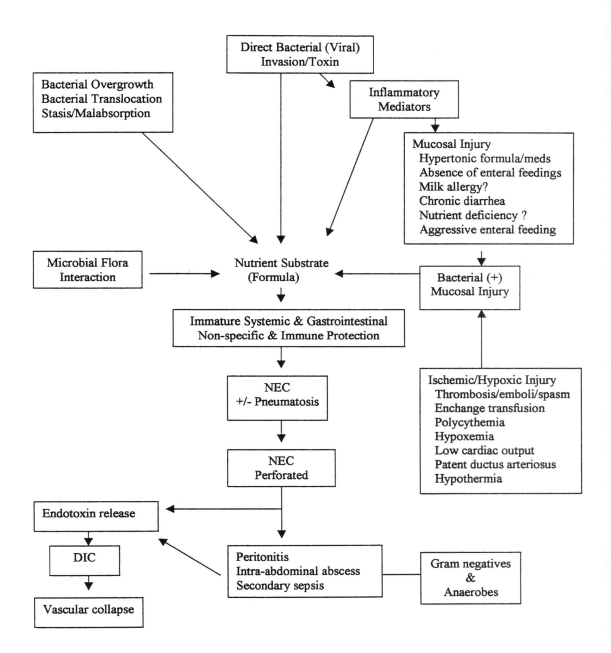

Figure 25.1. A schema of factors important in the pathogenesis of NEC.[21,23,24]

the complications seen post-NEC are related to the development of short bowel syndrome (see Chapter 28) or as a result of infection or metabolic complications of parenteral nutrition (PN) (see Chapter 8). Several excellent reviews have been published.[8,21,24]

Preventive Nutrition

Although NEC has been reported to occur in infants who have never been fed,[14,26-28] over 95% of all infants who develop the disease have been fed enterally.[8] The theory is that if infants are fed before developing adequate intestinal function or before adequate function returns following an ischemic episode, bacteria will proliferate in a nutrient-rich environment of undigested material, increasing the risk of developing NEC.

Concerns over risks associated with feedings (e.g., aspiration pneumonia, NEC) have resulted in a more cautious approach of delaying feedings for several days to weeks. However, this practice has not resulted in a lower incidence of NEC and, in fact, may promote its occurrence.[29,30]

When PN is used exclusively for the provision of nutrients, morphologic and functional changes occur in the gut, with a significant decrease in intestinal mass, a decrease in mucosal enzyme activity,[31-33] and an increase in gut permeability.[27] The changes, perhaps due primarily to the lack of luminal nutrients rather than the PN per se, result in impaired barrier function, potentially leading to bacterial translocation from the gut lumen to the systemic circulation.[34-37] It is possible that inflammatory mediators that are released after endotoxin or bacterial invasion across the mucosal barrier may result in vasoconstriction and tissue hypoxia resulting in NEC.[21]

It has been demonstrated that early feedings, even the provision of very small enteral feedings, may impart certain benefits as a result of providing luminal nutrients to the enterocytes and by stimulating the release of enteric hormones, which exert a trophic effect on the proliferative cells of the gut.[38,39] Studies of early hypocaloric enteral feedings in sick very low birth weight (VLBW) infants have shown that infants given 12-24 ml of formula/kg/day (4-20 kcal/kg/day) starting during the first one to eight days of life, when compared to infants who remain fasted during the same period of time have:

- Better weight gain[40-43]
- A greater decline in serum bilirubin levels with less time spent under phototherapy[44]
- Less cholestasis[44]
- Lower serum concentrations of alkaline phosphatase[44]
- More rapid functional maturation of the intestine[40]

Table 25.1. Clinical Manifestations of Neonatal Necrotizing Enterocolitis[7,8,66]

Specific	Nonspecific
Abdominal distention	Apnea and bradycardia
Bloody stools	Shock
Abdominal tenderness	Acidosis
Gastric retention	Lethargy
Guaiac-positive stool	Temperature instability
Bilious emesis	Cyanosis
Diarrhea	Frequent or seedy stools
Right lower quandrant mass	
Abdominal wall erythema	

- Increased serum gastrin[40,41]
- Increased subsequent feeding tolerance[40,41,45]
- Faster attainment of full enteral feedings[40,43-45]

None of the early feeding studies demonstrated any complications of early feeding, including NEC. However, minimal enteral feeding does not appear to decrease the incidence of NEC.[46]

The composition of feedings and rate of administration have been viewed as important factors in the potential for the development of NEC.[27,47-51] Hypertonic feedings and hyperosmolar medications have been associated with an increased risk of NEC.[51,52] Theoretically, circulating blood volume could be seriously reduced if a hypertonic feeding is given, for the reason that fluid shifts from the vascular compartment into the intestinal lumen to render the feeding isotonic and thus reduce mesenteric perfusion. In one prospective study, 87% of the infants developed NEC when fed a hypertonic formula (650 mOsm/L), compared to 25% of infants fed a standard cow's milk formula (359 mOsm/L).[51] Although most infant formulas are isotonic to blood, the addition of certain medications and supplements or the concentration of formula may significantly increase the osmolality.[53,54] (See Appendix H.)

It is generally agreed that enteral feedings should be initiated slowly and advanced over several days. Establishing standardized feeding guidelines for the NICU may decrease the incidence of

Table 25.2. Complications of Neonatal Necrotizing Enterocolitis

Immediate

Shock	Gastrointestinal perforation
Sepsis	Intra-abdominal abcess
Acute tubular necrosis	Neutropenia-thrombocytopenia
Disseminated intravascular coagulation	

Delayed

Short bowel syndrome	Enterocyst
Malabsorption syndrome	Polyposis
Cholestasis	Anastomotic leak
Recurrent NEC	Anastomotic stenosis
Stricture	Chronic salt and water depletion
Atresia	Sepsis
Aganglionosis	Growth failure
Enterocolic fistula	Treatment complications

Adapted from Kliegman and Fanaroff[23]

NEC.[74] The use of dilute versus full-strength formula is an issue of debate. To date, no well-controlled studies have been reported demonstrating an advantage of dilute formulas. Early introduction of 24 cal/oz isotonic premature infant formula has been shown to be well tolerated.[55]

Acid is an effective barrier to many potentially pathogenic microorganisms. However, the stomach of preterm infants may not respond with rapid production of gastric acid and peptic proteases as older children and adults do when ingesting food. One study showed a decreased incidence of NEC in infants receiving a formula supplemented with acid to achieve a pH of 3-4 compared with infants fed a regular formula.[75] However, more studies are needed before applying this to routine practice.[21]

The contribution enteral feeding makes to the occurrence of NEC remains unclear; however, if the carbohydrate in the formula is malabsorbed, it may provide substrate for colonic bacterial flora.[50,56] The substrate ferments, producing hydrogen gas-the gas often found in pneumatosis intestinalis.[8] Ischemia of the gut due to perinatal asphyxia, respiratory distress syndrome, patent ductus arteriosis, hypotension, and exchange transfusion may injure the G.I. mucosa, rendering it more susceptible to bacterial translocation and damage due to proteolytic enzyme activity.

The presence of a low umbilical arterial catheter has been purported to increase the risk of NEC, especially if the infant is fed during the period of catheterization. However, a prospective, randomized clinical trial did not support this association.[57]

Although no interventions have proven to be effective in preventing NEC in all cases, several preventive measures have been proposed. These should be considered for LBW infants and for those who have had an intrauterine or neonatal episode that may have resulted in potentially poor perfusion of the gut.

Early introduction of hypocaloric feedings. In infants with birth weight ≤ 1,500g, feedings of 12-24 kcal/oz premature infant formula at the rate of 12-24 ml/kg/day begun during the second to third day of life will provide gut stimulation in preparation for an advanced feeding schedule when the infant is more stable.[41-45,58,73]

Slow rate of feeding increase. Increases in formula intake of about 10-20 ml/kg/day are considered safe; greater volume increments may be associated with an increased incidence of NEC, although the upper limit that can be safely advanced is not known.[47-49,59,74]

Use of human milk. Human milk, with its many immunoprotective properties, has been suggested as the feeding of choice to prevent the development of NEC.[60,61,76,77] However, NEC has been reported in preterm infants fed human milk exclusively.[61-65] Although the issue of the use of fresh versus frozen or heat-treated human milk is a confounding variable, in one study pasteurized donor milk seemed to be as protective as raw maternal milk.[61] At least two cases of NEC have been reported in infants fed only fresh human milk.[65] Therefore, infants fed human milk should have their feedings advanced as slowly as infants fed formula.

Low-osmolality formulas. Although most infant formulas are isotonic to blood plasma, the addition of medications or nutritional supplements and the concentrating of the formulas increases their osmolality. Highly osmolar feedings should be avoided in the effort to decrease the risk of NEC (see Appendix H).[51]

Low-lactose formulas. Use of formulas with a reduced lactose load, such as the premature infant formulas, effectively decreases the amount of lactose presented to the gut for hydrolysis; the remainder of the carbohydrate is in the form of glucose polymers, which are well tolerated and easily digested by the premature infant, with serum glucose and insulin responses similar to those of a lactose feeding.[66] Theoretically, this modified carbohydrate formula reduces the undigested carbohydrate in the gut, thereby reducing the amount available for bacterial fermentation.[56]

Observation of signs of feeding intolerance. Abdominal distention, guaiac-positive stools, or excessive gastric residuals signal the need to either decrease or stop enteral feedings. More frequent stools and seedy stools have been reported in infants who developed NEC (see Table 25.1).[8,67]

Treatment Nutrition

Early and aggressive treatment of NEC includes vigorous I.V. fluid resuscitation, bowel rest with nasogastric decompression, correction of hematocrit and thrombocytopenia, and empiric I.V. antibiotic therapy. Serial abdominal radiographs are performed to detect pneumatosis intestinalis and possible perforation.[8]

The following nutrition and feeding measures are initiated:

- Cessation of feeding, removal of gastric residuals, continued gastric emptying, and decompression with a nasogastric tube
- Total parenteral nutrition during the period of bowel rest and slow feeding progression
- Careful attention to calorie and protein intake (infants who have had NEC have increased needs secondary to gut injury and/or surgery)[68]
- If bowel resection takes place, attention to nutrients that may be malabsorbed and type of feeding required (see Chapter 28)
- Gradual reintroduction of enteral feedings as outlined above with either a protein hydrolysate infant formula or a premature infant formula

After a diagnosis of NEC is made, enteral feedings are withheld for 10-21 days. As feedings are gradually reintroduced, parenteral support is withdrawn. After the period of gut injury and bowel rest, secondary lactose intolerance and other enzyme deficiencies may occur. Human milk is generally well tolerated but if human milk is not available and formula must be used, a low-lactose (including premature infant formula), lactose-free, or protein hydrolysate infant formula is used until full enteral feedings are established and well tolerated. Although some centers use a protein hydrolysate infant formula after NEC, no well-controlled studies have demonstrated that they are more effective than premature infant formula. The lower calcium concentration of the protein hydrolysate infant formulas, compared to the high needs of the premature infant, may increase the risk of osteopenia if used over an extended period.[69-71] Once tolerated, a lactose-containing formula should be used. Tests for reducing substances in the stool should be routinely conducted; if reducing substances are found in the stool, the use of a protein hydrolysate infant formula or other lactose-free formula should be considered for one to two weeks.[8,72] The reappearance of clinical signs of NEC must continue to be monitored (Table 25.1).

Follow-up Issues

Infants who have recovered from NEC and are discharged from the hospital require careful follow-up. Anthropometric parameters should be followed and plotted to identify deviations in growth. G.I. disturbances that may indicate stricture formation, such as abdominal distention, diarrhea, obstipation, or bloody stools, need to be described to the care-giver, and the infant should be closely assessed if symptomatic.[5,23,25]

If the infant is on a special formula, such as a protein hydrolysate infant formula, a feeding challenge, with a milk-based formula or, if lactose intolerance is present, with a soy-based formula, should be conducted after four to six weeks to assess feeding tolerance.

Case Study

RJ is a former 1,100 g, 28 weeks' gestational age, appropriate-for-gestational-age infant who was born to a mother who used cocaine regularly during her pregnancy. His Apgar scores were 4 at one minute and 8 at five minutes. On day of life (DOL) 1, he developed grade II respiratory distress syndrome, for which he received supplemental oxygen but did not require assisted ventilation; on DOL 2 he developed hyperbilirubinemia, for which he was treated with phototherapy. He was started on parenteral nutrition on DOL 3 and was given 20 kcal/oz premature infant formula at a rate of 16 ml/kg/day (1.5 ml every 2 hours). On DOL 5 his feedings were advanced by 16 ml/kg/day (1.5 ml every 2 hours) to 32 ml/kg/day (3.0 ml every 2 hours). On DOL 8 he was receiving premature infant formula at a rate of 82 ml/kg/day (7.5 ml every 2 hours) when he passed a bloody stool and, subsequently, developed abdominal tenderness and distention with a gastric residual of 6 ml, for which feedings were stopped; a no. 8-French nasogastric tube was placed for gastric decompression and drainage. Blood, urine, stool, and cerebral spinal fluids were cultured and he was started on antibiotics empirically. Pneumatosis intestinalis was identified on X-ray; there was no portal or free peritoneal air. The infant was placed on NPO for 14 days, and PN was started. Serial radiographic findings demonstrated resolution of the pneumatosis intestinalis. The infant was diagnosed as having NEC stage IIA. After 14 days, feedings of a premature infant formula were started at a rate of 20 ml/kg/day and advanced slowly at 15 ml/kg/day. On the third day of feedings, the stool was positive for reducing substances. Although one approach would have been to continue the premature infant formula and continue to observe the infant, in this case the formula was changed to a protein hydrolysate infant formula. No further feeding problems were encountered. The infant reached feedings of 150 ml/kg/day after 10 days. Due to the potential risk of osteopenia of prematurity while on the protein hydrolysate formula, the serum phosphorus and alkaline phosphatase levels were closely monitored. He was subsequently challenged with a premature infant formula, which he tolerated well.

References

1. Crissinger KD, Ryckman FC, Flake AW, et al. Necrotizing enterocolitis. In: Fanaroff aa, Martin RJ, eds. Neonatal-perinatal medicine: Diseases of the fetus and infant, 5th ed. St. Louis: Mosby Year Book, 1992; 1068.
2. Walsh MC, Kliegman RM, Hack M. Severity of necrotizing enterocolitis: Influence on outcome at 2 years of age. Pediatrics 84:808, 1989.
3. Pokorny WJ, Garcia-Prats JA, Barny YN. Necrotizing enterocolitis: Incidence, operative care and outcome. J Pediatr Surg 21:1149, 1986.
4. Kanto WP Jr, Wilson R, Richetts RR. Management and outcome of necrotizing enterocolitis. Clin Pediatr 24:79, 1985.
5. Kliegman RM, Fanaroff aa. Neonatal necrotizing enterocolitis: A nine-year experience. Am J Dis Child 135:603, 1981.
6. Hack M, DeMonterice D, Merkatz IR, et al. Rehospitalization of the very low birthweight infant: A continuum of perinatal and environmental morbidity. Am J Dis Child 135:263, 1981.
7. Walsh MC, Kliegman RM. Necrotizing enterocolitis: Treatment based on staging criteria. Pediatr Clin North Am 33(1):179, 1986.
8. Kliegman RM, Walsh MC. Neonatal necrotizing enterocolitis: Pathogenesis, classification, and spectrum of illness. Curr Probl Pediatr 17(4):213, 1987.
9. Kosloske AM. Epidemiology of necrotizing enterocolitis. Acta Paediatr Suppl 396:2, 1994.
10. Uauy R, Fanaroff A, Korones S, et al. Necrotizing enterocolitis (nec) in vlbw infants: Biodemographic and clinical correlates. Pediatr Res 27:228A, 1990.
11. The Vermont-Oxford Trials Network: very low birth weight outcomes for 1990. Investigators of the Vermon-Oxford Trials Network Database Project. Pediatrics 91:540, 1993.
12. Holman RC, Stoll BJ, Clarke, MJ, Glass RI. The epidemiology of necrotizing enterocolitis infant mortality in the United States. Public Health Briefs 87:2026, 1997.
13. Kosloske AM. Pathogenesis and prevention of necrotizing enterocolitis: A hypothesis based on personal observation and a review of the literature. Pediatrics 74:1086, 1984.
14. Ballance WA, Dahms BB, Shenker N, et al. Pathology of neonatal necrotizing enterocolitis: A ten-year experience. J Pediatr 117:S6, 1990.
15. Norton ME, Merrill J, Cooper BA, et al. Neonatal complications after the administration of indomethacin for preterm labor. N Engl J Med 329:1602, 1993.
16. Klein JF, Shahrivar F. Effects of intrauterine cocaine exposure on the perinatal morbidity of preterm infants. Pediatr Res 27:211A, 1990.

17. Downing gj, Horner SR, Kilbride HW. Characteristics of perinatal cocaine-exposed infants with necrotizing enterocolitis. Am J Dis Child 145:26, 1991.

18. Caddell JL. A review of evidence of a role of magnesium and possibly copper deficiency in necrotizing enterocolitis. Magnesium Res 9:55, 1996.

19. Bauer CR, Morrison JC, Poole WK, et al. A decreased incidence of necrotizing en- terocolitis after prenatal glucocorticoid therapy. Pediatrics 73:682, 1984.

20. Morriss FH Jr, Moore M, Weisbrodt NW, et al. Ontogenic development of gastrointestinal motility: IV. Duodenal contractions in preterm infants. Pediatrics 78:1106, 1986.

21. Neu J. Necrotizing enterocolitis: the search for a unifying pathogenic theory leading to prevention. Pediatr Clin North Am 43:409, 1996.

22. Halac E, Halac J, Begue EF, et al. Prenatal and postnatal corticosteroid therapy to prevent neonatal necrotizing enterocolitis: A controlled trial. J Pediatr 117:132, 1990.

23. Kliegman RM, Fanaroff aa. Necrotizing enterocolitis. N Engl J Med 310:1093, 1984.

24. Kliegman RM. Pathophysiology and epidemiology of necrotizing enterocolitis. In: Fetal and Neonatal Physiology. 2nd ed. Philadelphia: Saunders, 1998.

25. Janik JS, Ein SH, Mancer K. Intestinal stricture after necrotizing enterocolitis. J Pediatr Surg 16:438, 1981.

26. Gregory JR, Campbell JR, Harrison MW, et al. Neonatal necrotizing enterocolitis: A ten year experience. Am J Surg 141:562, 1981.

27. Goldman HI. Feeding and necrotizing enterocolitis. Am J Dis Child 134:553, 1980.

28. Marchildon MB, Buck BE, Abdenour G. Necrotizing enterocolitis in the unfed infant. J Pediatr Surg 17:620, 1982.

29. LaGamma EF, Ostertag SG, Birenbaum H. Failure of delayed oral feedings to prevent necrotizing enterocolitis: Results of study in very-low birth-weight neonates. Am J Dis Child 139:385, 1985.

30. Ostertag SG, LaGamma EF, Reisen CE, et al. Early enteral feeding does not affect the incidence of necrotizing enterocolitis. Pediatrics 77:275, 1986.

31. Cameron IL, Pavlat WA, Urban E. Adaptive responses to total intravenous feeding. J Surg Res 17:45, 1974.

32. Castro GA, Copeland EM, Dudrick SJ, et al. Intestinal disaccharidase and peroxidase activities in parenterally nourished rats. J Nutr 105:776, 1975.

33. Johnson LR, Copeland EM, Dudrick SJ, et al. Structural and hormonal alterations in the gastrointestinal tract of parenterally fed rats. Gastroenterology 68:1177, 1975.

34. Zeigler TR, Smith RJ, O'Dwyer ST, et al. Increased intestinal permeability associated with infection in burn patients. Arch Surg 123:1313, 1988.

35. Alverdy JC, Aoys E, Moss GS. Total parenteral nutrition promotes bacterial trans- location from the gut. Surgery 104:185, 1988.

36. Deitch EA. The role of intestinal barrier failure and bacterial translocation in the development of systemic infection and multiple organ failure. Arch Surg 125:403, 1990.

37. Deitch EA. Role of bacterial translocation in necrotizing enterocolitis. Acta Paediatr suppl 396:33, 1994.
38. Adrian TE, Lucas A, Bloom SR, et al. Growth hormone response to feeding in term and preterm neonates. Acta Paediatr Scand 72:251, 1983.
39. Lucas A, Bloom SR, Aynsley-Green A. Gut hormones and 'minimal enteral feeding'. Acta Paediatr Scand 75:719, 1986.
40. Berseth CL. Early hypocaloric enteral feedings induce functional maturation of preterm intestine. Pediatr Res 29:291A, 1991.
41. Meetze W, Valentine C, McGuigan JE, et al. Gastrointestinal priming prior to full enteral nutrition in very low birth weight infants. J Pediatr Gastroenterol Nutr 15:163, 1992.
42. Troche B, Harvey-Wilkes K, Nielsen HC, et al. Early minimal feedings promote growth in critically ill premature infants. Pediatr Res 27:292A, 1990.
43. Troche B, Harvey-Wilkes K, Engles WD, et al. Early minimal feedings promote growth in critically ill premature infants. Biol Neonate 67:172, 1995.
44. Dunn L, Hulman S, Weiner J, et al. Beneficial effects of early hypocaloric enteral feeding on neonatal gastrointestinal function: Preliminary report of a randomized trial. J Pediatr 112:622, 1988.
45. Slagle TA, Gross SJ. Effect of early low-volume enteral substrate on subsequent feeding tolerance in very low birth weight infants. J Pediatr 113:526, 1988.
46. Heird WC, Gomez MR. Total parenteral nutrition in necrotizing enterocolitis. Clin Perinatol 2:389, 1994.
47. McKeown RE, Marsh D, Amarnath U, et al. Role of delayed feeding and feeding increments in necrotizing enterocolitis. J Pediatr 121:764, 1992.
48. Anderson DM, Kliegman RM. The relationship of neonatal alimentation practices to the occurrence of endemic necrotizing enterocolitis. Am J Perinatol 8:62, 1991.
49. Zabielski PB, Groh-Wargo SL, and Moore JJ. Necrotizing enterocolitis: Feeding in endemic and epidemic periods. J Parenter Enter Nutr 13:520, 1989.
50. Book LS, Herbst JJ, Jung AL. Comparison of fast- and slow-feeding rate schedules to the development of necrotizing enterocolitis. J Pediatr 89:463, 1976.
51. Book LS, Herbst JJ, Atherton SO, et al. Necrotizing enterocolitis in low-birth- weight infants fed an elemental formula. J Pediatr 87:602, 1975.
52. Willis DM, Chabot J, Radde IC, et al. Unsuspected hyperosmolality of oral solu- tions contributing to necrotizing enterocolitis in very-low-birth-weight infants. Pediatrics 60:535, 1977.
53. Ernst JA, Williams JM, Glick MR, et al. Osmolality of substances used in the intensive care nursery. Pediatrics 72:347, 1982.
54. White KC, Harkavy KL. Hypertonic formula resulting from added oral medications. Am J Dis Child 136:931, 1982.
55. Melnick G, Crouch JB, Cakackkas HL, et al. Tolerance of LBW infants to early and late introduction of two 24 kcal formulas. Pediatr Res 23:488A, 1988.

56. Kien, CL. Colonic fermentation of carbohydrate in the premature infant: Possible relevance to necrotizing enterocolitis. J Pediatr 117:S52, 1990.

57. Davey AM, Wagner CL, Cox C, Kendig JW. Feeding premature infants while low umbilical artery catheters are in place: a prospective, randomized trial. J Pediatr 124:795, 1994.

58. LaGamma EF, Browne LE. Feeding practices for infants weighing less than 1500 g at birth and the pathogenesis of necrotizing enterocolitis. Clin Perinatol 21:271, 1994.

59. Rayyis SF, Ambalavanan N, Wright L, Carlo WA. Randomized trial of "slow" versus "fast" feed advancements on the incidence ofnecrotizing enterocolitis in very low birth weight infants. J Pediatr 134:293, 1999.

60. Barlow B, Santulli TV, Heird WC, et al. An experimental study of acute neonatal enterocolitis: The importance of breast milk. J Pediatr Surg 9:587, 1974.

61. Lucas A, Cole TJ. Breast milk and neonatal necrotizing enterocolitis. Lancet 336:1519, 1990.

62. Eyal F, Sagi E, Arad I, et al. Necrotizing enterocolitis in the very low birthweight infant: Expressed breast milk feeding compared with parenteral feeding. Arch Dis Child 57:274, 1982.

63. Moriartey RR, Finer NN, Cox SF, et al. Necrotizing enterocolitis and human milk. J Pediatr 94:295, 1979.

64. Kliegman RM, Pittard WB, Fanaroff aa. Necrotizing enterocolitis in neonates fed human milk. J Pediatr 95:450, 1979.

65. Reisner SH, Garty B. Necrotising enterocolitis despite breast feeding. Lancet 2:507, 1977.

66. Cicco R, Holzman IR, Brown DR, et al. Glucose polymer tolerance in premature infants. Pediatrics 67:498, 1981.

67. Andrews JD, Krowchuk HV. Stool patterns of infants diagnosed with necrotizing enterocolitis. Neonatal Network 16:51, 1997.

68. Shulman RJ, DeStefano-Laine L, Petitt R, et al. Protein deficiency in premature in- fants receiving parenteral nutrition. Am J Clin Nutr 44:610, 1986.

69. Giles MM, Fenton MH, Shaw B, et al. Sequential calcium and phosphorus balance studies in preterm infants. J Pediatr 110:591, 1987.

70. Greer FR, Tsang RC. Calcium, phosphorus, magnesium, and vitamin D requirements for the preterm infant. In: Tsang RC, ed. Vitamin and mineral requirements in preterm infants. New York: Marcel Dekker, 1985; 99.

71. Ziegler EE, O'Donnell AM, Nelson SE, et al. Body composition of the reference fetus. Growth 40:329, 1976.

72. Book LS, Herbst JJ, Jung AL. Carbohydrate malabsorption in necrotizing enterocolitis. Pediatrics 57:201, 1976.

73. McClure RJ, Newell SJ. Randomised controlled study of clinical outcome following trophic feeding. Arch Dis Child Fetal Neonatal Ed 82:F29, 2000.

74. Kamitsuka MD, Horton MK, Williams MA. The incidence of necrotizing enterocolitis after introducing standardized feeding schedules for infants between 1250 and 2500 grams and less than 35 weeks of gestation. Pediatrics 105 (2):379, 2000.

75. Carron V, Egan EA. Prevention of necrotizing enterocolitis. J Pediatr Gastroenterol Nutr 11:317, 1990.

76. Schanler RJ, Shulman RJ, Lau C. Feeding strategies for premature infants: Beneficial outcomes of feeding fortified human milk versus preterm formula. Pediatrics 103 (6):1150, 1999.
77. Neu J, Weiss MD. Necrotizing enterocolitis: Pathophysiology and prevention. JPEN 23 (5):S13, 1999.

Nutritional Care for High-Risk Newborns (Rev. 3d. Ed.)
S. Groh-Wargo, M. Thompson, J. Cox, editors
© 2000, Precept Press, Inc., Chicago

26

CONGENITAL ANOMALIES OF THE ALIMENTARY TRACT

Christina J. Valentine, MS, RD, LD

IT HAS BEEN ESTIMATED that a congenital anomaly will occur in around four of every 100 live births.[1] This chapter will review the nutritional implications for a select number of defects involving the oral, esophageal, and gastrointestinal areas.

Cleft Lip/Palate

A cleft lip and/or palate, one of the most common birth defects, occurs in one in 700 births in the United States.[1,2] They are most prevalent in white, male infants and are often associated with other anomalies. These babies thus should be examined carefully for associated anomalies.[1] The etiology has not been identified but is thought to be associated with both environmental and genetic factors.[3]

Clefts occur due to failure of embryonic fusion of the lip and/or mouth during the sixth week of gestation, when the maxillary, premaxillary, and lateral nasal process normally unite.[4] A cleft lip can involve separation of one or both sides of the upper lip and can also include the upper dental ridge.[3,4] A cleft palate can be associated with or without a cleft lip and affect the soft and hard palate on one or both sides.[3] Alteration in the growth of the palate may occur postnatally from long-term use of orogastric tubes causing a palatal groove.[5] Infants with cleft defects may have difficulty with sucking, swallowing, breathing, hearing, and talking.[3] The site and extent of the cleft determines the severity of the feeding difficulty.[2,6]

Management of clefts may involve several surgical repairs.[2] The timing of the first repair is controversial, but typically depends on the infant's age, weight, and specifics of the anatomy of the lesion.[7] Early primary repair has been associated with improved weight gain, shorter hospital stay, and decreased cost.[7]

Treatment Nutrition

Infants with clefts often experience feeding difficulties and slow weight gain due to poor sucking and prolonged nippling time.[2] Knowledge of sucking mechanics, milk flow characteristics, and the anatomical involvement of the cleft are helpful when determining feeding method.[6,8] Correction of the defect may require more than one surgical procedure; thus, maintenance of optimal nutrient intake by I.V. or tube feedings may be necessary pre- and postoperatively.[2]

Adequate sucking is generated by negative intraoral pressure and effective muscular movement.[6,9] Negative pressure is generated by good lip and velopharynx seal, along with expansion of the intraoral cavity by contraction of the tongue or mandible movement.[6] Breast-fed infants accomplish this by stabilizing the nipple against the palate while tongue movement strips milk from the breast.[6] Bottle-fed infants use their tongues and palates less, relying primarily on their gums to hold the nipple.[6]

Sucking can be influenced by the type of nipple used, something that should be considered in the assessment of feeding the infant with cleft lip and/or palate.[8,9] Nipple size and shape affect the infant's ability to close his mouth and form a good seal around the nipple. Size also determines how far back milk will be delivered into the infant's throat. Firmness of the nipple and the size of the nipple hole will require variable strength in the infant's suck and will influence milk flow. Several small holes in the nipple have been recommended instead of one large hole as a means of helping to regulate the rate of milk flow.[8,9] All of these factors play a role in determining how to feed an infant with a cleft defect.

A cleft lip can cause an air leak around the infant's seal on the nipple, preventing development of adequate negative pressure.[6] Plugging the air leak caused by the cleft can be accomplished by breast-feeding with the cleft side against the breast. Infants with small, isolated cleft palates can usually breastfeed.[6] A regular hold in an upright position can be used on one breast, and in order to keep the cleft against the other breast when switching sides, a "football hold" may be necessary, with the infant held facing the mother and curled under her arm. The use of a large, soft-base nipple is often effective if the infant is bottle-feeding.[3,6] Regular bottle nipples do not work as well.

Positioning of the infant when feeding is important. A semisitting position is recommended in order to direct milk into the pharynx and away from the cleft and nasal cavity.[3] Slow, direct delivery of milk

Table 26.1.   Recommended Nipples or Feeding Techniques for Infants With Cleft Defects

Defect	Suggested nipples/feeding techniques
Isolated cleft lip	Breast-feeding or large, soft-base nipples
Cleft of soft palate	Breast-feeding or nipples with long shafts
Cleft palate*	Breast-feeding or nipples with large openings, cross-cuts, or a preemie nipple
Cleft lip and palate	Manual breast expression into infant's mouth
	Cleft palate nipples
	Cleft palate feeders

Adapted from Morris and Klein[3] and Clarren et al.[6]

* A wide cleft palate may require cleft lip and palate intervention techniques.

into the infant's mouth may be necessary if the cleft palate is wide or if the infant has both a cleft lip and palate.[3,6] Infants with these defects are unable to seal their lips or their velopharynx and are unable to position and compress the nipple to regulate milk flow.[6] Manual expression of the breast and the use of a supplemental nursing device are often successful.[3,6] Bottle-feeding should be attempted with special cleft palate feeders.[3,6] Suggested nipples for feeding infants with cleft lip and/or palate are listed in Table 26.1. Regardless of the defect, infants should be encouraged to suck in order to strengthen the oral-facial muscles.[10] After surgery, the infant's ability to seal the nipple and create adequate intraoral pressure is improved, and nipple feedings by breast or bottle can resume immediately.[3,6,7] Growth and feeding difficulties are often seen early on, so it is imperative that these children be managed by a registered dietitian.[11]

Several resources on cleft defects are available for parents to provide support and information.[12-14]

Esophageal Atresia and Tracheoesophageal Fistula

Esophageal atresia (EA) and tracheoesophageal fistula (TEF) are congenital defects that occur in one in 3,000 live births.[15] More than half of infants with TEF also will have other anomalies (e.g., VATER,

VACTER, or CHARGE syndromes).[15] Atresia, the incomplete continuity of the esophagus, with or without fistula, can occur. The most common (87%) is the Vogt type 3, in which a blind upper pouch is present (proximal esophageal atresia), with a fistula from the trachea to the lower esophagus.[15,16] The etiology of EA and/or TEF is unknown. It has been suggested that an EA is caused by a vascular accident in utero. Fistula formation may be the result of excessive epithelia that forms a septum between the trachea and esophagus.[17]

Treatment Nutrition

The immediate goal in medical management of EA is surgical repair by a direct, end-to-end anastomosis of the esophageal segments.[18] If the segments are too short to be connected, a staged repair is conducted, the segments being stretched until they can be attached.[16,17] Another approach involves making a flap from the upper pouch to bridge the gap to the lower esophagus.[18] Surgical ligation is performed if a fistula is present. Endoscopic laser coagulation also has been shown to be successful in eliminating a fistula and can be an alternative to surgery.[19]

Continuous salivary suction is important both pre- and postoperation in the patient with EA.[20] A gastrostomy tube is also placed to decompress the stomach, drain the secretions, and feed the infant until the esophagus is repaired and healed.[15,16] For infants with severe hyaline membrane disease, a gastrostomy tube may complicate ventilator management by creating air leaks, so use of a transanastomotic tube has been recommended.[21]

After birth, the infant with EA or TEF should be given I.V. fluids with dextrose and electrolytes, and once renal function is apparent (good urine output, normal serum electrolytes), parenteral nutrition (PN) should begin.[16] Full PN should contain about 90-100 kcal/kg with 3 g pro/kg and 3-4 g fat/kg daily.[22] Forty-eight hours after primary repair, the infant can be fed through the gastrostomy or transanastomotic tube.[15] If no signs of an anastomotic leak appear, oral feedings can begin about one week after repair.[23] To prevent aspiration, the infant should be placed in a prone, propped position by elevating the bed. Feedings may need to progress slowly and be supplemented with PN if disordered peristalsis occurs or if a staged repair is necessary.[15]

A suggestion for progression of enteral feedings is to begin at 20 cc/kg/day and increase by 20 cc/kg/day to a goal minimum of 150 cc/kg/day. Human milk, fortified human milk, standard infant formulas, or premature formulas can be fed, depending on fluid intake. When nipple-feedings are adequate (> 180 cc/kg/day, nippled within 20 minutes at eight divided feedings), the gastrostomy or transanastomotic tube can be removed and human milk or standard formulas can be used.[15] Human milk or formula may be supplemented or concentrated to allow for adequate intake at smaller volumes (see Chapter 16).

Anastomosis leakage, recurring fistulas, esophageal dysmotility, gastroesophageal reflux, and vomiting are a few of the potential complications following surgery.[15] In one study, all of the infants with EA had significant reflux and 85% required esophageal dilation for stenosis.[17] In contrast, only 13% of infants with fistulas had episodes needing antireflux surgery. It is estimated that two thirds of the infants repaired will experience respiratory problems, esophageal dysmotility, and gastroesophageal reflux.[15] Poor weight gain and faltering growth can occur with vomiting. Reflux treatment with medications or surgery may be warranted. (See Chapter 27).[24,25] Long-term outcome is favorable, although approximately one-third of patients will continue to experience respiratory and various gastrointestinal symptoms.[70,71]

Pyloric Stenosis

Pyloric stenosis is the most common anomaly producing emesis in the newborn period.[26] It occurs in one in 300 births, with a predominance among white males.[26] Seven percent of children with pyloric stenosis have associated esophageal or inguinal hernias. The etiology is multifactorial, resulting in thickened circular muscle fibers obstructing the pyloric channel. Postnatal feedings subsequently exacerbate the problem by causing edema and inflammation and projectile vomiting.[26] In addition, "gastric waves" and/or an olive-sized mass can be found on abdominal exam. A classic "string sign" is witnessed by upper G.I. examination reflecting a distended stomach and narrowed pyloric canal.[27] Abdominal ultrasounds are not recommended for use in diagnosis.[26,28]

Treatment Nutrition

Intravenous fluids and electrolytes may be necessary before surgery, due to prolonged and/or extensive vomiting.[26] Individual examination as to hydration status should be made. Serum and urine electrolytes should be monitored along with a careful clinical examination to titrate fluids and electrolytes. A *nothing per os* (NPO) status is necessary until after surgical correction with pyloromyotomy.[26] After surgery, I.V. fluids should be used until full enteral nutrition is achieved. Successful enteral feeding has been documented 8-12 hours after surgery;[26] thus, parenteral nutrition is usually not necessary. Feeding tolerance, growth, and development should continue to be monitored, but long-term problems are rare.

Omphalocele

Omphalocele, a defect that occurs in one in 6,000 births, is often associated with other congenital anomalies (e.g., tetralogy of Fallot, diaphragmatic hernias, trisomy syndromes, Beckwith-Wiedemann syndrome).[29-32] It is defined as the herniation of intra-abdominal contents into the base of the umbilical cord. The contents are covered with a translucent, avascular sac consisting of peritoneum and amniotic membrane.[29,32] The defect can vary in size from 4 cm, containing only small loops of bowel, to very large defects (5-20 cm), which can consist of all of the small and large intestine, the liver, the pancreas, the spleen, and the bladder.[29,31,32] The umbilical cord may be attached either at the apex or at the inferior margin of the sac.[31] Mortality can be as high as 30% with large omphaloceles. Generally, function of the G.I. tract is normal, and anomalies of the intestine are rare.[29,31,33] The etiology is uncertain, but is thought to be genetic in origin because the incidence of recurrence is high in affected families.[29]

Treatment Nutrition

Immediately after birth, the protruding sac is kept moist with antiseptic pads.[29,31] Feedings are withheld, nasogastric aspiration is begun to decompress the intestine, and I.V. glucose is administered at standard volumes. PN should be started by day 1 or 2. Primary surgical closure is the preferred treatment, but it can be impossible if the sac is too large for the abdominal cavity.[29,31] With giant omphaloceles, staged closures with or without prosthesis may be necessary.[34,35] The first state of repair involves attachment of a Silastic "silo" to the skin-amnion junction, which is suspended over the abdomen.[34] The intestinal contents are then gradually returned to the abdomen by plicating the sac on alternative days, a process that can take up to 10-14 days.[31]

Infusion of a dextrose/electrolyte solution may be required if these patients develop third space fluid losses.[34] PN and, sometimes, mechanical ventilation are required throughout this process. PN and I.V. fat emulsion (IFE) with 90-100 kcal/kg, 3 g pro/kg and 3-4 g fat/kg daily appear to be well tolerated.[22] Once the defect is closed and nasogastric drainage is no longer bilious, enteral feedings can begin.[34] Infection at the surgical sites of closure can be a problem.[31] Other postoperative complications include pyloroduodenal and other adhesive bowel obstructions.[30,35] More than 80% of these obstructions occur within the first two years. Most long-term survivors have small-to-moderate ventral hernias.[29]

Gastroschisis

Gastroschisis occurs in fewer than one in 10,000 live births.[36] It is the congenital protrusion of abdominal contents through a defect in the abdominal wall, usually to the right of the umbilicus.[37] The etiology is unknown, but the condition could be caused by environmental factors that result in the herniation of the umbilical cord at 10 weeks' gestation.[29,31] Mortality can approximate 13%.[36] Unlike the omphalocele, gastroschisis is rarely associated with other congenital anomalies, but can have associated intestinal defects, such as intestinal atresia or volvulus.[36-38]

The exact cause for intestinal atresia is unknown, but may be the result of the abdominal defect pinching the prolapsed intestine or from vascular accidents with intrauterine volvulus.[37] Further differences between gastroschisis and omphalocele include the location of the gastroschisis to the right of the umbilicus, the absence of a sac with a gastroschisis, and exposure of the protruded intestine to amniotic fluid in utero. The gastroschisis often appears thick and has foreshortened gut. Finally, the gastroschisis has a noneviscerated liver when compared to the omphalocele.

Treatment Nutrition

Medical treatment is similar to that for omphalocele. Nasogastric suction is used to decompress the bowel, and sterile packs are used to wrap the protruding contents.[31,39] Enemas are sometimes given to facilitate evacuation. I.V. fluids and PN on day 1 or 2 support the infant pre- and postoperatively. Three main surgical options are available to repair the defect: (1) primary fascial repair, (2) closure with skin flaps, and (3) use of a "silo."[36] Primary repair, possible in 90% of cases, results in less morbidity.[36] The abdominal wall is often stretched manually to accommodate the bowel.[29,31,32] When the abdomen is still too small for the intestines, it can be laterally stretched and then closed over the bowel.[36] If most of the intestinal contents can be reduced into the cavity, some surgeons then cover the defect with an umbilical patch, avoiding the need for multiple operations.[36] Finally, if complete closure fails, a Silastic "silo" pouch can be applied, as in the treatment of omphalocele.[31] The entire intestine is examined during surgery for gangrene, perforations, or atresia, and if indicated, resection and anastomosis or temporary ileostomy is done.[29,31,32] Some have reported healthier intestines if the intestine is replaced in the abdomen with neither exteriorization nor anastomosis.[37]

In the postoperative period, bowel motility is delayed.[38] The etiology of dysmotility and malabsorption is unknown, but a recent animal study has speculated that nitric oxide synthetase activity is elevated, causing smooth muscle relaxation and hypoperistalsis.[40] PN with IFE is often essential for nutrition support until adequate enteral feedings are tolerated. The bowel is kept decompressed by continuous nasogastric suction. Basic daily requirements for PN are 90-100 kcal/kg, 3 g pro/kg, with IFE providing 3-4 g fat/kg.[41] Protein losses may be increased, so additional amounts to provide 3-4 pro/kg/day may need to be added in the PN.[32] When G.I. function returns, malabsorption or dumping can occur with feeding.[32] Expressed human milk, fortified human milk, or premature formulas containing half lactose and half glucose polymers and 40-60% MCT oils with increased nutrients per volume compared to the elemental "predigested" formulas often are well tolerated. If these are malabsorbed, lactose-free or elemental formulas often are recommended.[32] Advancement of feedings should be gradual; increasing the enteral feeding by 20 cc/kg/day, with concurrent decreases in PN, has been successful. Changes in gastric residuals, emesis, and stool output should be carefully monitored. Infants who have had bowel resections may experience decreased absorption and increased nutrient losses (see Chapter 28).[42]

Congenital Diaphragmatic Hernia

Congenital diaphragmatic hernia (CDH), which has an estimated incidence of 0.45 per 1,000 live births, is caused by a failure in the closure of the pleuroperitoneal canal.[43] The entire small bowel, along with portions of the colon, stomach, spleen, and kidney, can occupy the space of the left pleural cavity.[43] This affects the growth of lung and often results in hypoplastic lung(s) having low air capacity and poor compliance. A fatal outcome is usually secondary to increased pulmonary vascular resistance and persistent pulmonary hypertension.[44] A mortality rate of 30-50% is expected, despite surgical treatment of the defect within 24 hours.[44] Associated anomalies include the cardiac, gastrointestinal, nervous, and genitourinary systems.

Treatment Nutrition

In the medical management of the infant with CDH, the first step recommended is to provide warmth and adequate ventilation and to achieve acid/base balance.[43] A gastric tube is passed to prevent gastric or intestinal distention into the chest. The next step is to reduce the hernia and repair the defect.[45] After a vertical incision is made to open the peritoneal cavity, the loops of bowel, spleen, and other viscera can be drawn into the abdomen.[43] The normal contour of the diaphragm is carefully recreated, after which the abdominal wall can be closed with sutures. If intra-abdominal pressure is high, a

Silastic sheet similar to that used for the omphalocele or gastroschisis is created around the surgical wound.[46]

After repair of the defect, ventilator management, pharmacologic support, and I.V. nutrition are necessary. Extracorporeal membrane oxygenation (ECMO) has been suggested as the way to treat persistent pulmonary hypertension associated with CDH.[44,47] Mortality rates are high: 43% do not survive.[48] Infants who survive are supported with full PN (see above). With the bowel repaired, enteral tube feedings can begin as soon as the pulmonary condition allows. Enteral feeding advancement at 20 cc/kg/day should be slow to allow for often limited gastric emptying times. Nipple-feedings should not begin until the infant has a respiratory rate of < 60.[49] Transpyloric feedings may be necessary if severe limitations are evident with gastric emptying. Lower volume (130 ml/kg/day) and higher caloric density (27-30 kcal/oz) formulas may also be warranted to promote weight gain without exacerbating reflux. Enteral long-chain triglycerides should be avoided if the infant has chylothorax.[72]

Congenital Obstruction

Congenital obstruction may present as a result of intestinal atresia, malrotation, and/or volvulus.[50-54] Intestinal atresia is the congenital failure of the gut lumen to recanalize following the normal period of hyperplasia of the endoderm.[55] Atresias can occur at the duodenum, jejunum, or ileum. Malrotation, an abnormal rotation of the gut occurring in utero, may or may not be symptomatic. Volvulus occurs in 40-80% of infants with malrotation.[53] Volvulus is the strangulation (twist or knot) of the bowel, producing variable degrees of ischemic necrosis and resulting in single or multiple sites of atresia.[53]

Intrauterine volvulus without malrotation can also cause disturbances of growth and function of the developing bowel.[52,53] Infants with any one of these defects often fail to pass meconium and present with bilious emesis and abdominal distention.[50] Maternal polyhydramnios and other congenital anomalies are often associated with these obstructions. In one center, 64% of infants with obstructions had accompanying anomalies, with Down syndrome the most predominant.[50] If no severe associated anomalies are present, the prognosis for infants with congenital obstructions is excellent.[51]

After diagnosis, all infants should receive I.V. fluids and nasogastric suction.[51,52] PN with 90-100 kcal/kg, 3 g pro/kg/day and 3-4 g fat/kg/day should be the goal once renal function is established. Surgical treatment can involve resection of the necrotic bowel and ileostomy, or resection and primary end-to-end re-anastomosis.[53,56] Primary anastomosis may eliminate the need for further surgery to close the enterostomy and thus decrease hospital stay and morbidity. Trophic enteral feeding should begin gradually to allow for gut adaptation.[52] A small, continuous drip of 10-20 cc/kg/day of expressed human milk or half-strength premature formula appears to work well. Even in the full-term infant, premature formulas with 40-50% glucose polymers and 40-60% MCT are well tolerated and provide increased vitamins and minerals per volume. If the bowel has had large areas resected, the infant may be left with a short gut and its associated nutritional problems (see Chapter 28).

Congenital Megacolon (Hirschsprung's Disease)

Congenital megacolon, or Hirschsprung's disease, which happens in one in 5,000 live births, occurs as a result of autosomal dominant, autosomal recessive, or polygenic forms.[57] New genetic evidence links specific human chromosomes to these mutations.[57] A male-to-female ratio has been found to be 4:1. As the length of the involved mucosa increases, however, this ratio decreases to 1:1.[58] Congenital megacolon is characterized by the absence of ganglion cells in a distal intestinal segment.[59,60] Generally, the affected area is the rectosigmoid, but it can include the entire colon.[61,62] Short-segment aganglionosis accounts for about 70% of the cases.[58] The aganglionic bowel has an increased number of adrenergic and cholinergic nerve fibers, and the concentration of acetylcholine is two to nine times higher than in the normal colon.[63] The autonomic imbalance leads to a constant state of contraction without propulsion. As a result, the colon hypertrophies and there is enormous dilation proximal to the contracted area. Feces can accumulate in large quantities, leading to ulceration, perforation, and peritonitis. Associated anomalies include Down syndrome, defects in cardiac septation, tetralogy of Fallot, and Dandy-Walker syndrome.[58]

Treatment Nutrition

Infants with Hirschsprung's disease usually present in the newborn period with abdominal distention, vomiting, and failure to pass meconium.[63] Diagnosis is made by rectal wall biopsy that shows no ganglion cells. During this time, the infant is supported by I.V. nutrition and rectal irrigants to decompress the bowel.[63] A colostomy is generally performed in the neonate, and surgical resection with anastomosis is completed when the infant weighs 15-20 lb.[63] Various surgical options are reported, with the goal of treatment to resect the aganglionic bowel and then pull bowel with normal ganglion cells down to the distal rectum.[61] Nipple- or tube-feedings can begin two or three days postoperatively.[63] Feedings can be advanced as tolerated, using human milk, preterm, or standard infant formulas. PN support may be needed during feeding advancement. Symptoms of diarrhea, incontinence, abdominal distention, or enterocolitis can recur in 30%

of cases postoperatively, so signs of feeding tolerance should be discussed with the family and monitored closely (see Chapter 3).[61,64]

Meconium Plug Syndrome

Meconium plug syndrome is a rare, benign condition of intestinal obstruction by a stringy or rubbery meconium plug; it is not generally associated with cystic fibrosis.[65] It may be caused by decreased colonic motility, which allows excessive water absorption and inspissation of intestinal contents, or it may be the first sign of Hirschsprung's disease. The plug can be passed by barium enema or a saline rectal irrigation, and ileostomy is usually unnecessary.[65,66] The infant is well thereafter, unless Hirschsprung's disease is present.

Meconium Ileus

Meconium ileus consists of thick, viscous meconium obstructing the distal ileum.[65] About 15% of infants born with cystic fibrosis will present with this defect.[65] Dilation and hypertrophy of the proximal bowel usually occurs, and complications include volvulus, perforation, and meconium peritonitis.[66]

Treatment Nutrition

Most infants who have uncomplicated meconium ileus can be treated with hypertonic enemas.[65] Fluid balance must be carefully monitored when hypertonic contrast is used. Infants are placed on NPO status and given an orogastric tube and I.V. fluids before the enema. Full PN should begin by the second or third day of life. Gastrografin enemas are given until the meconium is passed and abdominal distention is relieved.[66] Perforation is a complication of this technique. It has been suggested that manometric monitoring be done during the enema procedure to record pressure and possibly prevent a perforation.[67]

If the enema fails, a laparotomy is usually necessary.[66] The dilated loop of bowel is resected and meconium is removed from the proximal bowel. An ileostomy is done, which is generally closed within one month. An alternative method that avoids resection of the bowel involves appendectomy and Gastrografin injection into the meconium through the appendix stump.[68] The meconium is then expressed by gentle manipulation of the bowel, and the appendix stump ligated and closed. Postoperatively, Gastrografin is given through a nasogastric tube until all meconium is passed by the rectum. Enteral feedings are usually withheld until the meconium is passed. Full PN should continue until full enteral feedings are established. If the infant has had a large part of the ileum removed, a short bowel may be present with its related nutritional problems (see Chapter 28).

Case Studies

Infants with congenital anomalies can have difficulties with nutrition both pre- and postoperatively. Nutrition plans must be individually designed and flexible enough to adapt to ongoing problems that may result from treatment or surgery or from the nature of the disease state. The following cases present examples of how nutrition support can be involved. They are not intended to dictate how infants must be fed, but rather to give some insight into what can be done. Further research is warranted in this area to provide a more definite approach to care.

Case A

A 3,560 g, 36 weeks' gestation, large-for-gestational-age girl was born to a diabetic mother by elective cesarean section. Apgar scores were 6 at one minute and 8 at five minutes. She was diagnosed with a left diaphragmatic hernia, which was repaired on the first day of life. The infant was intubated at birth and required maximal ventilator support (100% FiO_2). PN began on day of life (DOL) 2, with 80 cc/kg/day of 12.5% dextrose and 2.2% crystalline amino acids. I.V. fat emulsion (IFE), using a 20% solution running over 24 hours, provided 1 g/kg/day of fat. Triglycerides, checked four hours after IFE initiation, were normal at 46 mg/dl. PN and IFE were progressed to a full volume of 130 cc/kg and 20 cc/kg, respectively, by DOL 5. The infant was able to start enteral feedings with expressed human milk on DOL 10. Feedings, given at 20 cc/kg through an orogastric tube, progressed daily by 20 cc/kg, with a concurrent decrease in the PN and IFE. When the infant was on 100 cc/kg/day of human milk, two packets of Enfamil Human Milk Fortifier (Mead Johnson, Evansville, IN) were added to each 100 cc. After 24 hours, this fortification increased to four packets per 100 cc of human milk (full-strength dose). Fortification was necessary because her volume was restricted to 150 cc/kg/day. Throughout her feeding progression, records were reviewed for urine output, prefeed residual, stool output, and emesis. Diuretic treatment with Lasix began on DOL 12 to assist in weaning the infant from mechanical ventilation. The infant reached full enteral feedings by DOL 17. Residuals were frequent (n = 8/24 hours) but small (< 7 cc per feeding). Supplemental potassium chloride at 1 mEq/100 cc of fortified human milk began on DOL 18, secondary to the hypokalemia caused by the Lasix treatment. Nutrition laboratory values, monitored every other week, included serum calcium, phosphorus, alkaline phosphatase, BUN, and albumin. These values were normal at each screen. The infant's weight gain and head circumference were averaged weekly and were 25-30 gm/day and 0.5 cm/week, respectively. Fer-In-Sol (Mead Johnson) supplementation to provide 2 mg/kg/day elemental iron began on DOL 30.

The infant's medical course became complicated on DOL 90 by left pulmonary branch stenosis and a patent foramen ovale; her volume was restricted to 130 cc/kg/day. She also began experiencing increased reflux when nipple-feedings were attempted. The mother's milk supply, meanwhile, had diminished. The infant was placed on Similac concentrated to 27 kcal/oz (Ross, Columbus, OH), inasmuch as this would provide increased calories and protein at her volume restriction. A multivitamin supplement at 1 cc/day was also started to provide 100% of the RDA for vitamins. On DOL 115, a gastrostomy tube was placed and a Nissen fundoplication was performed secondary to unmanageable reflux and risk of aspiration. After the gastrostomy and prior to discharge, the infant was allotted a volume of 150 cc/kg/day and given Similac 24 with Iron (Ross). Fer-In-Sol was discontinued. The infant was discharged on DOL 158 and the mother was instructed in how to mix 24-cal/oz formula from powder or concentrate. At discharge, the infant weighed 6,850 g. (25%ile weight for age).

Case B

A 36-weeks' gestation, 2,110 g, appropriate-for-gestational-age girl was born via cesarean due to fetal distress. She had been prenatally diagnosed with gastroschisis. Orogastric suction began immediately after delivery, and 10% dextrose was administered I.V. at 65 cc/kg/day. Sterile gauze was applied to the exposed bowel. Surgery was performed on DOL 2. Reduction and repair of the gastroschisis was accomplished and a neoumbilicus created. No atresia or other anomalies were noted, and there was minimal tension with closure. Nasogastric drainage was noted postoperatively. PN providing 95 kcal/kg, 3 g pro/kg, and 2 g fat/kg daily was started on DOL 3. Triglycerides were normal, and potassium was low when laboratory values were screened. IFE was increased to 3 g/kg and then progressed to 4 g/kg/day by DOL 5. Additional potassium chloride was added to the PN. The infant remained NPO and had about 85 cc/day of gastric drainage. This gastric drainage was replaced daily with additional I.V. fluids containing normal saline.[69] Feedings began on DOL 16, when bilious drainage had stopped. Nipple-feedings of expressed human milk were initiated at 20 ml/kg/day. They were well-tolerated and were advanced by 20 ml/kg/day up to full enteral feedings of 150 ml/kg/day. (PN and IFE were decreased accordingly.) Breast-feedings went well when the mother came to visit, and the infant gained weight at 20 g/day. She was discharged on DOL 30 on full breast-feeding. A multivitamin with iron was also given at 1 cc/day because her total volume of intake, still at less than a quart, could not provide recommended amounts of vitamins or iron.

References

1. Nadler HL, Sacks AJ, Evans MI. Genetics in surgery and prenatal diagnosis. In: Raffensperger JG, ed. Swenson's Pediatric Surgery. 5th ed. New York: Appleton and Lange, 1990; 56.
2. Wellman CO, Coughlin SM. Preoperative and postoperative nutritional management of the infant with cleft palate. J Pediatr Nurs 6:154, 1991.
3. Morris SE, Klein MD. Prefeeding issues for children with cleft palate. In: Prefeeding Skills, a Comprehensive Resource for Feeding Development. Tucson: Therapy Skill Builders, 1987; 337.
4. Harris JWS. Clefts of the lip and palate. In: Dobbing, J, Davis JA, eds. Scientific Foundations in Pediatrics. 2nd ed. Baltimore: University Park Press, 1981; 686.
5. Arens R, Reichman B. Grooved palate associated with prolonged use of orogastric feeding tubes in premature infants. J Oral Maxillofac Surg 50:64, 1992.
6. Clarren SK, Anderson B, Wolf LS. Feeding infants with cleft lip, cleft palate, or cleft lip and palate. Cleft Palate J 24:244, 1987.
7. Weatherly-White RCA, Kuehn DP, Mirrett P. Early repair and breast-feeding for infants with cleft lip. Plast Reconstr Surg 79:879, 1987.
8. Matthew OP. Nipple units for newborn infants: A functional comparison. Pediatrics 81:688, 1988.
9. Vandenberg KA. Nippling management of the sick neonate in the NICU: the disorganized feeder. Neonatal Network 9:9, 1990.
10. Porterfield HW. Feeding infants with cleft lip, cleft palate, or both. Cleft Palate J 25:80, 1988.
11. Lee J, Nunn J, Wright C, Height and weight achievement in cleft lip and palate. Arch Dis Child 76(1):70, 1997.
12. Klein MD. Feeding Techniques for Children who have Cleft Lip and Palate. Tucson: Therapy Skill Builders, 1988.
13. American Cleft Palate Educational Foundation, University of Pittsburgh.
14. Danner SC, Cerutti ER. Nursing your Baby with a Cleft Palate or Cleft Lip. Rochester, N.Y.: Childbirth Graphics, 1990.
15. Cudmore RE. Oesophageal atresia and tracheo-oesophageal fistula. In: Lister J, Irving I, eds. Neonatal Surgery. 3d ed. London: Butterworth, 1990; 231.
16. Howard ER. Paediatric abdominal surgery. In: O'Higgins NJ, Chisholm GD, Williamson RCN, eds. Surgical Management. 2d ed. Oxford: Butterworth, Heinemann, 1991; 636.

17. Rideout DT, Hayashi AH, Gillis DA, et al. The absence of clinically significant tracheomalacia in patients having esophageal atresia without tracheoesophageal fistula. J Pediatr Surg 26:1303, 1991.
18. Bar-Maor JA, Shoshany G, Sweed Y. Wide gap esophageal atresia: a new method to elongate the upper pouch. J Pediatr Surg 24:882, 1989.
19. Schmittenbecher PP, Mantel K, Hofmann U, et al. Treatment of congenital tracheoesophageal fistula by endoscopic laser coagulation: Preliminary report of three cases. J Pediatr Surg 27:26, 1992.
20. Ohkawa H, Ochi G, Yomazaki Y, et al. Clinical experience with a sucking sump-catheter in the treatment of esophageal atresia. J Pediatr Surg 24:333, 1989.
21. Beasley S, Myers NA, Auldist AW. Management of the premature infant with esophageal atresia and hyaline membrane disease. J Pediatr Surg 27:23, 1992.
22. Heird WC, Kashyap S, Gomez M. Parenteral alimentation of the neonate. Semin Perinatol 15:493, 1991.
23. Chittmittrapap S, Spitz L, Kiely EM, et al. Anastomotic leakage following surgery for esophageal atresia. J Pediatr Surg 27:29, 1992.
24. Fonkalsrud EW, Foglia RP, Ament ME, et al. Operative treatment for the gastroesophageal reflux syndrome in children. J Pediatr Surg 24:525, 1989.
25. Lindahl H, Rintala R, Louhimo I. Failure of the Nissen fundoplication to control gastroesophageal reflux in esophageal atresia patients. J Pediatr Surg 24:985, 1989.
26. Rowe MJ, O'Neill JA, Grosfeld JL, et al. Hypertrophic pyloric stenosis. In: Essentials of Pediatric Surgery. St. Louis: Mosby; 481, 1995.
27. Quinn D, Shannon LF. Congenital anomalies of the gastrointestinal tract. Pt 1. The stomach. Neonatal Network 14(8):63, 1995.
28. Janik JS, Wayne ER. Pyloric stenosis in premature infants. Arch Pediatr Adolesc Med 150(2):223, 1996.
29. Raffensperger JG. Omphalocele and gastroschisis. In: Raffensperger JG, ed. Swenson's Pediatric Surgery. 5th ed. New York: Appleton and Lange, 1990; 782.
30. Bruce J, Afshani E, Korp MP, et al. Omphalocele with pyloroduodenal obstruction by extrinsic hepatic compression: a case report. J Pediatr Surg 23:1018, 1988.
31. Howard ER. Paediatric abdominal surgery. In: O'Higgins NJ, Chisholm GD, Williamson RCN, eds. Surgical Management. 2nd ed. Oxford: Butterworth, Heinemann, 1991; 628.
32. Irving IM. Umbilical abnormalities. In: Irving IM, Lister J, eds. Neonatal Surgery. 3d ed. London: Butterworth, 1990; 376.
33. Moore TC, Nur K. An international survey of gastroschisis and omphalocele (490 cases). III. Factors influencing outcome of surgical management. Pediatr Surg Int 2:27, 1987.
34. DeLorimier AA, Adzick NS, Harrison MR. Amnion inversion in the treatment of giant omphalocele. J Pediatr Surg 26:804, 1991.
35. Ein SH, Bernstein A. A 24-year follow-up of a large omphalocele: From silon pouch to pregnancy. J Pediatr Surg 25:1190, 1990.
36. Swift RI, Singh MP, Ziderman DA, et al. A new regime in the management of gastroschisis. J Pediatr Surg 27:61, 1992.
37. Shah R, Woolley MM. Gastroschisis and intestinal atresia. J Pediatr Surg 26:788, 1991.

38. Langer JC, Bell JG, Castillo RO, et al. Etiology of intestinal damage in gastroschisis. II. Timing and reversibility of histological changes, mucosal function, and contractility. J Pediatr Surg 25:1122, 1990.
39. Zivkovic SM. Repair of gastroschisis using umbilical cord as a patch. J Pediatr Surg 26:1179, 1991.
40. Bealer JF, Graf J, Bruch SW, et al. Gastroschisis increases small bowel nitric oxide synthase activity. J Pediatr Surg 31(8):1043, 1996.
41. Walker J, Taylor CJ. Fluid and electrolyte management and nutritional support. In: Irving IM, Lister J, eds. Neonatal Surgery. 3d ed. London: Butterworth, 1990; 37-50.
42. Couper RTL, Durie PR, Stafford SE, et al. Late gastrointestinal bleeding and protein loss after distal small-bowel resection in infancy. J Pediatr Gastroenterol Nutr 9:454, 1989.
43. Reynolds M. Diaphragmatic anomalies. In: Raffensperger JG, ed. Swenson's Pediatric Surgery. 5th ed. New York: Appleton and Lange, 1990; 721.
44. Johnston PW, Bashner B, Liberman R, et al. Clinical use of extracorporeal membrane oxygenation in the treatment of persistent pulmonary hypertension following surgical repair of congenital diaphragmatic hernia. J Pediatr Surg 23:908, 1988.
45. Atkinson JB, Ford EG, Humphries B, et al. The impact of extracorporeal membrane support in the treatment of congenital diaphragmatic hernia. J Pediatr Surg 26:791, 1991.
46. Michalevicz D, Chaimoff CH. Use of a Silastic sheet for widening the abdominal cavity in the surgical treatment of diaphragmatic hernia. J Pediatr Surg 24:265, 1989.
47. Bartlett RH, Cassaniga AB, Tomasian J, et al. Extracorporeal membrane oxygenation (ECMO) in neonatal respiratory failure, 100 cases. Ann Surg 204:236, 1986.
48. Wilson JM, Lund DP, Lillehai C, et al. Delayed repair and preoperative ECMO does not improve survival in high-risk congenital diaphragmatic hernia. J Pediatr Surg 27:368, 1992.
49. Perlman M, Kirpalani H. Nutrition. In: Residents' Handbook of Neonatology. St Louis: Mosby Year Book, 1992; 61.
50. Spigland N, Yazbeck S. Complications associated with surgical treatment of congenital intrinsic duodenal obstruction. J Pediatr Surg 25:1127, 1990.
51. Hancock BJ, Wiseman NE. Congenital duodenal obstruction: The impact of an antenatal diagnosis. J Pediatr Surg 247:1027, 1989.
52. Kern IB, Leece A, Bohane T. Congenital short gut, malrotation, and dysmotility of the small bowel. J Pediatr Gastroenterol Nutr 11:411, 1990.
53. Usmani SS, Kenigsberg K. Intrauterine volvulus without malrotation. J Pediatr Surg 26:1409, 1991.
54. Boutlon JE, Ein SH, Reilly BJ, et al. Necrotizing enterocolitis and volvulus in the premature neonate. J Pediatr Surg 24:901, 1989.
55. Miller V. Growth and development of endodermal structures. In: Dobbing J, Davis J, eds. Scientific Foundations of Pediatrics. 2d ed. Baltimore: University Park Press, 1981; 460.
56. Tumock RR, Brereton RJ, Spitz L, et al. Primary anastomosis in apple-peel bowel syndrome. J Pediatr Surg 26:718, 1991.
57. Sullivan PB. Hirschsprung's disease. Arch Dis Child 74(1):5, 1996.

58. Ryan ET, Ecker JL, Christakis NA, et al. Hirschsprung's disease: Associated abnormalities and demography. J Pediatr Surg 27:76, 1992.
59. Hirobe S, Doody DP, Ryan DP, et al. Ectopic class II major histocompatability antigens in Hirschsprung's disease and neuronal intestinal dysplasia. J Pediatr Surg 27:357, 1992.
60. Larsson LT, Malmfors G, Ekblad E, et al. NPY hyperinnervation in Hirschsprung's disease: Both adrenergic and nonadrenergic fibers contribute. J Pediatr Surg 26:1207, 1991.
61. Torig GM, Brereton RJ, Wright VM. Complications of endorectal pullthrough for Hirschsprung's disease. J Pediatr Surg 26:1202, 1991.
62. Levy M, Reynolds M. Morbidity associated with total colon Hirschsprung's disease. J Pediatr Surg 27:364, 1992.
63. Swenson O, Raffensperger JG. Hirschsprung's disease. In: Raffensperger, JG, ed. Swenson's Pediatric Surgery. 5th ed. New York: Appleton and Lange, 1990; 555.
64. Marty TL, Seo T, Matlak ME, et al. Gastrointestinal function after surgical correction of Hirschsprung's disease: Long term follow-up in 135 patients. J Pediatr Surg 30(5):655, 1995.
65. Meconium ileus, meconium peritonitis, and the meconium plug syndrome. In: Raffensperger JG, ed. Swenson's Pediatric Surgery. 5th ed. New York: Appleton and Lange, 1990; 537-38.
66. Howard ER. Paediatric abdominal surgery. In: O'Higgins NJ, Chisolm GP, Williamson RCN, eds. Surgical Management. 2d ed. Oxford: Butterworth, Heinemann, 1991; 640.
67. Ein S, Shandling B, Reilly BJ, et al. Bowel perforation with non-operative treatment of meconium ileus. J Pediatr Surg 22:146, 1987.
68. Fitzgerald R, Conlon K. Use of the appendix stump in the treatment of meconium ileus. J Pediatr Surg 24:899, 1989.
69. Coran AG, Drongowski RA. Body fluid compartment changes following neonatal surgery. J Pediatr Surg 24:829, 1989.
70. Somppi E, Tammela O, Ruuska T, et al. Outcome of patients operated on for esophageal atresia: 30 years' experience. J Pediatr Surg 33:1341, 1998.
71. Ure BM, Slany E, Eypasch EP, et al. Quality of life more than 20 years after repair of esophageal atresia. J Pediatr Surg 33:511, 1998.
72. Kavvadia V, Greenough A, Davenport M, et al. Chylothorax after repair of congenital diaphragmatic hernia—risk factors and morbidity. J Pediatr Surg 33:500, 1998.

Nutritional Care for High-Risk Newborns (Rev. 3d. Ed.)
S. Groh-Wargo, M. Thompson, J. Cox, editors
© 2000, Precept Press, Inc., Chicago

27

GASTROESOPHAGEAL REFLUX

Melody Thompson, MS, RD, LD

Gastroesophageal reflux (GER) is the return of gastric contents into the esophagus.[1] Reflux can either be occult ("asymptomatic," i.e., remaining in the esophagus with no clinical symptoms) or regurgitant ("symptomatic," manifested as spitting up with little or no effort.) Reflux is a common physiological event occurring with varying degrees of frequency in most healthy individuals, but it is particularly common in infancy.[2-4] GER in infants appears to be caused by transient spontaneous relaxations of the lower esophageal sphincter (LES) and/or transient increases in intra-abdominal pressure rather than lower baseline LES tone, as was previously thought.[5-7] The availability of gastric contents is important in the pathogenesis of GER.[8] Pathologic reflux is manifested by three main categories of symptoms: regurgitation-malnutrition symptoms (including emesis, failure to thrive), symptoms indicative of esophagitis (including epigastric pain, irritability, feeding problems, anemia), and respiratory symptoms (including aspiration pneumonia, bronchospasm, apnea).[9] Frequent regurgitation is the symptom most strongly correlated with pathologic GER.[10,11] Although some infants with GER demonstrate slow gastric emptying, most have normal gastric emptying times.[12-16]

The incidence of GER (in a particular infant or a total population) depends on a variety of factors, including gestational age, chronologic age, state (awake, asleep, crying), position, feeding, care-giving activities, and additional medical problems. GER is more common in preterm infants than in term infants or older children.[17,18] In asymptomatic infants, GER incidence increases significantly between two and four months and decreases after one year.[19] Most infants have more GER when awake (especially postcibal), followed by active sleep and movement.[20-22] Asymptomatic infants have less GER during quiet sleep, whereas symptomatic infants have more GER when sleeping.[22,23] Crying appears to decrease reflux frequency and duration as compared to the state of wakefulness without crying.[24] Prone positioning and small, frequent feedings are associated with a decreased incidence of reflux.[25,26] Sucking on a pacifier has no effect on the total duration of esophageal acid exposure. This nonnutritive sucking decreases reflux frequency only when the infant is in a seated position (e.g., in a car seat).[27] Certain care-giving activities (e.g., suctioning, diaper change) are associated with an increased incidence of reflux.[17] Other care-giving activities are associated with a decreased incidence of reflux. For example, infants have less GER when tube-fed than when fed orally;[28] and use of mechanical ventilation is associated with less reflux than that seen in infants with no assisted ventilation.[29] GER is frequently seen in infants with neurodevelopmental disabilities,[30] with cystic fibrosis,[31] and following repair of congenital diaphragmatic hernia[32] esophageal atresia/tracheoesophageal fistula,[33] and surgical gastrointestinal anomalies.[92,93] Cow's milk protein allergy may also be associated with reflux in up to one-third of infants with GER.[34-36,94]

Clinically, the diagnosis of GER is often presumed, based on symptoms and systematic elimination of other possible diagnoses. Clinical symptoms are not a reliable indicator of GER in preterm infants.[95] A careful workup is important, therefore, in confirming the diagnosis of pathologic GER.[9] The accuracy of diagnosis may be improved by using at least two of the following tests:[37]

- Esophageal pH monitoring (documents esophageal acidification)[38]
- Barium esophogram (demonstrates anatomic abnormalities)[39]
- Endoscopy with biopsy (allows assessment of esophagitis)[39,40]
- GE Scintiscan (can demonstrate evidence of aspiration pneumonia)[41]

Twenty-four-hour esophageal pH monitoring has long been considered the "gold standard" in diagnosing GER.[42] Normal ranges have been published for healthy term and preterm infants.[17,19] Most investigators quantify reflux index (percent of time with pH < 4), number of episodes > 5 minutes, duration of longest episode, and total number of episodes in 24 hours. Short-term pH studies are not reliable in infants < 1 year of age.[43] Some researchers are now proposing the use of ultrasound in the diagnosis of GER.[44] The presence of lipid-laden alveolar macrophages or lactose in bronchial fluid has been proposed as a marker for GER, although neither test is capable of differentiating aspiration directly from feedings or from refluxed gastric contents.[45,46]

Studies linking GER to other clinical occurrences have been inconclusive.[47,48] Generally, *causal* relationships cannot be proven between GER and apnea,[49-51] bradycardia,[52] apparent life-threatening events,[53] feeding hypoxemia,[54] bronchopulmonary dysplasia,[55] and other respiratory symptoms.[96]

Chronic untreated GER can advance to severe esophagitis, esophageal obstruction due to strictures, aspiration pneumonitis, or failure to thrive. Sandifer's syndrome (esophagitis, abnormal posturing, anemia) is also associated with chronic GER.[9]

The occurrence of mild GER is normal and cannot be prevented; however, pathologic GER and its complications may be prevented by employing the treatment methods below. Preterm infants with pathologic GER consume more hospital resources than do preterm infants without GER,[97,98] but the developmental outcome in both of these groups appears to be similar.[98]

Treatment Nutrition

For healthy, growing babies, GER is a benign condition without clinical consequences. Parents of "spitters" can be reassured that GER is common and will be outgrown. They may wish to carefully feed and burp the baby and avoid overfeeding.

Parental reassurance has recently been promoted as the first-line (and, in many cases, only) "treatment" of physiologic GER.[56,57] Taking a feeding history and observing a feeding may give the best diagnostic clues. Psychosocial factors in the pathogenesis of the infant's symptoms may need to be considered.[58] Sound (although quickly dispensed) medical advice (e.g., to burp frequently) if enacted aggressively, can exacerbate the problem and escalate the treatment. (An enlightening case study has been published.[59])

For pathologic GER, a variety of treatment modalities have been investigated, including:

Altering the size and frequency of feedings. Small, frequent feedings are recommended for the treatment of GER. Larger feeding volumes are associated with a significant increase in both the total amount of GER and the maximum continuous episode of GER during postcibal esophageal pH monitoring.[26] Continuous tube feedings (the epitome of increased frequency, low-volume feedings) have been shown to resolve GER-related emesis and failure to thrive in infants without other medical problems.[60] Fortunately, continuous, or small, frequent feedings are typically used in the neonatal intensive care unit (NICU), so this would not represent a change in practice.

Altering the formula. GER is seen in both breast-fed and formula-fed infants. Healthy breast-fed infants demonstrated episodes of shorter duration (compared with infants fed whey dominant formulas) only in active sleep.[61] No differences were seen between the two groups in quiet or indeterminate sleep or awake states. In general, changing formula has not been proven to affect the incidence of GER in formula-fed infants. Term infants demonstrate the same amount of reflux on milk-based, soy-based, or whey hydrolysate formulas.[62] No difference in reflux was found in infants fed different whey-to-casein ratios.[63] In infants with GER and cow's milk protein allergy, however, a diet free from cow's milk protein (casein-hydrolysate formula) was associated with a significant improvement in reflux symptoms.[34] Similarly, infants and children with eosinophilic esophagitis and GER had dramatic improvement of their reflux when treated with an amino-acid-based formula and avoidance of intact proteins.[64] Thus, for a subset of infants, GER may be a manifestation of a hypersensitivity reaction that is treatable by dietary manipulation.

Preterm infants demonstrated the same amount of GER on formula enriched with medium-chain triglycerides (3.7 g fat/100 ml, 87.6% MCT by weight) as on standard formula.[65] A low-fat, high-carbohydrate formula did not improve reflux measurements in preterm infants.[66]

Increasing the osmolality of the feeding may result in increased GER.[67] Increasing formula concentration (e.g., from 20 to 24 cal/oz) will slightly increase osmolality. Concentrated formulas, however, can improve caloric intake in reduced formula volume with the goal of reducing GER.

Thickening the feedings. The practice of thickening formula in the treatment of GER is common but controversial. Thickening feedings (in the United States, usually with dry rice cereal) has not been shown to reduce objective measurements (by esophageal pH monitoring and gastroesophageal scintigraphy) of GER in infants.[68-71] In fact, the use of thickened formula is associated with an increase in duration of the longest reflux episodes. Thus, thickened feedings could lead to occult reflux of long duration, possibly increasing the risk for esophagitis and respiratory dysfunction.[69]

Clinically, episodes of emesis may be fewer with thickened feedings in many infants.[68,69] Some infants, however, regurgitate more often while on thickened feedings.[68] It is impossible to predict whether thickening feedings will improve or worsen reflux in an individual infant. Coughing is observed more often in infants who receive thickened feedings compared to unthickened feedings.[72] Because the etiology and implications of this increased coughing are unknown, the investigators recommend avoiding thickened feedings for infants with nonregurgitant reflux.

The use of thickened feedings in the NICU is associated with technical difficulties, undesirable side effects, and social/educational dilemmas. Thickened feedings may be too thick to flow through a feeding tube or require too much effort for a baby to take by nipple. Constipation may occur in babies whose feedings are thickened with rice cereal.[9]

Pumped human milk may not thicken with cereal (presumably due to the amylase content of human milk.) Direct breast-feeding is not possible when attempting to thicken human milk. This may be frustrating and undesirable for both the mother and the infant.

The implicit feeding messages imparted to parents of infants whose feedings are thickened are counter to accepted data. Parents may perceive that starting solid foods early and giving food in a bottle rather than by spoon constitute optimal and current infant feeding practices. Thickening formula with cereal may result in a high-carbohydrate, low-nutrient intake, especially if the infant takes a reduced volume of thickened formula.

A European panel has recently recommended thickened feedings as a first phase intervention in infantile regurgitant reflux if parental reassurance alone has failed.[73] Recognizing that thickening the feedings does not have a beneficial effect on GER, this group recommends thickened formula to decrease the amount and severity of regurgitation. Prethickened infant formulas are now commercially available (in the United States as Enfamil AR, Mead Johnson Nutritionals, Evansville, Ind.). There are no published safety or efficacy studies of these formulas.[73] The nutrient profile of prethickened formulas (intended for term infants) is not appropriate for the preterm baby.

Nonnutrition Treatment

Positioning. Ironically, the "chalasia chair" (infant seat formerly used for supine propping of infants with GER) increased rather than decreased the incidence of GER. Horizontal prone[25,74] or 30° elevated prone positioning[75,76] has been associated with fewer and briefer episodes of GER than supine or 30° elevated supine positioning. Elevated prone positioning is difficult to maintain. Horizontal prone positioning has been shown to be as effective as the elevated prone position in treating reflux.[74,77] Recent studies show that left-lateral positioning is comparable to prone in reducing reflux index and the duration of prolonged episodes.[77,99]

Infant position while sleeping has recently been studied in relation to the incidence of Sudden Infant Death syndrome (SIDS). The supine position confers the lowest risk for SIDS and is recommended by the American Academy of Pediatrics (AAP) for all healthy infants.[78-80] However, preterm[81] and term[82] babies may be noted to have improved respiratory function when lying prone. The prone position is also associated with decreased crying time in term infants[83] and with decreased energy expenditure in preterm infants.[84] Certainly, positions are varied in the NICU, where infants are electronically and visually monitored.

The AAP recommends that healthy preterm infants (as well as term infants) after hospital discharge be placed supine to sleep. The infant's bed should be free of soft surfaces and gas-trapping objects. The AAP notes, however, that symptomatic GER may be an indication for a prone sleeping position.[79,80]

Medications. Studies of the use of metaclopramide, domperidone, and cisapride in treating GER in infancy have recently been extensively reviewed.[4] Cisapride, a prokinetic drug, has been used in treating GER and esophagitis in infancy, although its use may be associated with cardiac arrhythmias, especially if the infant is receiving certain antibiotics or other QT-prolonging medications concurrently.[85,86] Cisapride was recently taken off the market.[100] Acid-reducing agents (including antisecretory and acid-neutralizing drugs) also may be used in infancy (see Appendix E).[1]

Surgery. Pediatric surgical treatment of GER is usually the Nissen fundoplication. This procedure involves wrapping the gastric fundus 360° around the distal esophagus, which is pulled below the diaphragm. Surgical treatment is usually reserved for severe cases that are refractory to long-term medical management or in which complications of GER are life-threatening (such as recurrent aspiration pneumonia, failure to thrive, and/or anemia due to blood loss from esophagitis). The most frequent complications of antireflux surgery are recurrent reflux due to wrap disruption (7.1%), respiratory problems (4.4%), gas bloat (3.6%), and intestinal obstruction (2.6%).[87] Neurologically impaired patients who need a long-term feeding tube may not require an antireflux procedure with the placement of a percutaneous endoscopic gastrostomy.[88,89] Performing a 24-hour pH probe study before surgery may assist in this determination.[89]

Care-giving activities. GER in infants has been shown to be most severe after a diaper change (due to increase in intra-abdominal pressure).[47,90] The reflux index also may be increased after nursing care (chest physiotherapy, oropharyngeal or endotracheal suction) to a much greater degree than the postcibal increase.[17] At this writing, one study investigating the impact of altering these care-giving practices on the incidence of GER has been published. In this study, modifying the technique of performing physiotherapy on infants with cystic fibrosis improved measurements of GER compared with standard physiotherapy.[91]

Case Study

JS was born at 30 weeks' gestation weighing 1,200 g. He was admitted to the NICU with diagnoses of prematurity and respiratory distress. Within the first two weeks he was weaned from the ventilator and parenteral nutrition. At three weeks, when his feedings were advanced to 180 ml/kg/day of 20 kcal/oz premature formula, he began having frequent regurgitation. His abdominal X-ray and exam were benign. He continued to have one or two stools per day that were negative for occult blood and reducing substances. With a presumptive diagnosis of GER, his feeding volume was decreased to 150 ml/kg/day and formula was concentrated to 24 kcal/oz. He was placed in a prone position for one-half hour after each feeding. His continued frequent emeses prompted the intern to gradually restrict feeding volumes to 110 ml/kg/day. JS began losing weight and suffered an episode of aspiration pneumonia. Management was changed to include continuous nasogastric tube feedings and positioning prone or left lateral around the clock. Volume was advanced over three days to 160 ml/kg/day (128 kcal/kg/day), and JS began gaining weight at 20 g/day. Emesis diminished and resolved after four days of continuous feeding, which was continued for another week. Nipple-feedings were then introduced, and JS was weaned quickly from continuous to bolus feedings. Shortly thereafter (at 7 weeks of age, weighing 1,560 g), JS began regurgitating again after feedings. Again, his exams were benign. Feedings were changed from 45 ml every four hours to 34 ml every three hours. Regurgitation continued despite prone positioning and smaller, more frequent feedings. His formula was thickened with rice cereal, which reduced the frequency of regurgitation, but JS became irritable and fed poorly. Rice cereal was discontinued. Continuous night feedings were instituted with small-volume nipple-feedings (every two to three hours, on modified-demand schedule) during the day. Within 10 days, JS was weaned from continuous night feedings and was taking 35-50 ml every two and a half to three and a half hours with one or two "wet burps" daily. He was discharged weighing 1,840 g on frequent demand feedings of Similac NeoSure concentrated to 24 kcal/oz with instructions about careful burping and guidelines to avoid overfeeding.

References

1. Orenstein SR. Gastroesophageal reflux. Pediatr Rev 13:174, 1992.
2. Orenstein SR. Infantile reflux: different from adult reflux. Am J Med 103:114S, 1997.
3. Marcon MA. Advances in the diagnosis and treatment of gastroesophageal reflux disease. Curr Opin Pediatr 9:490, 1997.
4. Vandenplas Y, Belli C, Benhamou P, et al. A critical appraisal of current management practices for infant regurgitation—recommendations of a working party. Eur J Pediatr 156:343, 1997.
5. Omari TI, Barnett C, Snel A, et al. Mechanisms of gastroesophageal reflux in healthy premature infants. J Pediatr 133:650, 1998.
6. Omari TI, Barnett C, Snel A, et al. Mechanisms of gastroesophageal reflux in premature infants with chronic lung disease. J Pediatr Surg 34:1795, 1999.
7. Sondheimer JM. Gastroesophageal reflux: Update on pathogenesis and diagnosis. Pediatr Clin North Am 35:103, 1988.
8. Vargas JH. Gastroesophageal reflux: Mechanisms in infants. J Pediatr Gastroenterol Nutr 21:479, 1995.

9. Orenstein SR. Controversies in pediatric gastroesophageal reflux. J Pediatr Gastroenterol Nutr 14:338, 1992.
10. Orenstein SR. Gastroesophageal reflux. Pediatr Rev 20:24, 1999.
11. Heine RG, Jaquiery A, Lubitz L, et al. Role of gastro-oesophageal reflux in infant irritability. Arch Dis Child 73:121, 1995.
12. Hillemeier AC, Lange R, McCallum R, et al. Delayed gastric emptying in infants with gastroesophageal reflux. J Pediatr 98:190, 1981.
13. Hillemeier AC. Reflux and esophagitis. In: Walker WA, Durie PR, Hamilton JR, et al., eds. Pediatric Gastrointestinal Disease. Philadelphia: Decker, 1991; 420.
14. Rosen PR, Treves S. The relationship of gastroesophageal reflux and gastric emptying in infants and children: Concise communication. J Nucl Med 25:571, 1984.
15. Billeaud C, Guillet J, Sandler B. Gastric emptying in infants with or without gastro-oesophageal reflux according to the type of milk. Eur J Clin Nutr 44:577, 1990.
16. Ewer AK, Durbin GM, Morgan ME, et al. Gastric emptying and gastro-oesophageal reflux in preterm infants. Arch Dis Child Fetal Neonatal Ed 75:F117, 1996.
17. Newell SJ, Booth IW, Morgan MEI, et al. Gastro-oesophageal reflux in preterm infants. Arch Dis Child 64:780, 1989.
18. Marino AJ, Assing E, Carbone MT, et al. The incidence of gastro-sophageal reflux in preterm infants. J Perinatol 15:369, 1995.
19. Vandenplas Y, Sacre-Smits, L. Continuous 24-hour esophageal pH monitoring in 285 asymptomatic infants 0-15 months old. J Pediatr Gastroenterol Nutr 6:220, 1987.
20. Jeffery HE, Heacock HJ. Impact of sleep and movement on gastro-sophageal reflux in healthy, newborn infants. Arch Dis Child 66:1136, 1991.
21. De Ajuriaguerra M, Radvanyi-Bouvet MF, Huon C, et al. Gastroesophageal reflux and apnea in prematurely born infants during wakefulness and sleep. Am J Dis Child 145:1132, 1991.
22. Vandenplas Y, De Wolf D, Deneyer M, et al. Incidence of gastro-sophageal reflux in sleep, awake, fasted, and postcibal periods in asymptomatic and symptomatic infants. J Pediatr Gastroenterol Nutr 7:177, 1988.
23. Dreizzen E, Escourrou P, Odievre M, et al. Esophageal reflux in symptomatic and asymptomatic infants: Postprandial and circadian variations. J Pediatr Gastroenterol Nutr 10:316, 1990.
24. Orenstein SR. Crying does not exacerbate gastroesophageal reflux in infants. J Pediatr Gastroenterol Nutr 14:34, 1992.
25. Orenstein SR, Whitington PF, Orenstein DM. The infant seat as treatment for gastroesophageal reflux. New Engl J Med 309:760, 1983.
26. Sutphen JL, Dillard VL. Effect of feeding volume on early postcibal gastroesophageal reflux in infants. J Pediatr Gastroenterol Nutr 7:185, 1988.
27. Orenstein SR. Effect of nonnutritive sucking on infant gastro-sophageal reflux. Pediatr Res 24:36, 1988.
28. Abe T, Hata Y, Sasaki F, et al. The effect of tube feeding on postprandial gastroesophageal reflux. J Pediatr Surg 28:56, 1993.
29. Newell SJ, Morgan MEI, Durbin GM, et al. Does mechanical ventilation precipitate gastro-oesophageal reflux during enteral feeding? Arch Dis Child 64:1352, 1989.

30. Roberts K. Gastroesophageal reflux in infants and children who have neurodevelopmental disabilities. Pediatr Rev 17:211, 1996.

31. Heine RG, Button BM, Olinsky A, et al. Gastro-oesophageal reflux in infants under 6 months with cystic fibrosis. Arch Dis Child 78:44, 1998.

32. Kieffer J, Sapin E, Berg A, et al. Gastroesophageal reflux after repair of congenital diaphragmatic hernia. J Pediatr Surg 30:1330, 1995.

33. Biller JA, Allen JL, Schuster SR, et al. Long-term evaluation of esophageal and pulmonary function in patients with repaired esophageal atresia and tracheoesophageal fistula. Dig Dis Sci 32:985, 1987.

34. Cavataio F, Iacono G, Montalto G, et al. Clinical and pH-metric characteristics of gastro-oesophageal reflux secondary to cow's milk protein allergy. Arch Dis Child 75:51, 1996.

35. Iacono G, Carroccio A, Cavataio F, et al. Gastroesophageal reflux and cow's milk allergy in infants: A prospective study. J Allergy Clin Immunol 97:822, 1996.

36. Staiano A, Troncone R, Simeone D, et al. Differentiation of cows' milk intolerance and gastro-oesophageal reflux. Arch Dis Child 73:439, 1995.

37. Meyers WF, Roberts CC, Johnson DG, et al. Value of tests for evaluation of gastroesophageal reflux in children. J Pediatr Surg 20:515, 1985.

38. Vandenplas Y, Derde MP, Piepsz A. Evaluation of reflux episodes during simultaneous esophageal pH monitoring and gastroesophageal reflux scintigraphy in children. J Pediatr Gastroenterol Nutr 14:256, 1992.

39. Hillemeier AC. Gastroesophageal reflux. Diagnostic and therapeutic approaches. Pediatr Clin No Am 43:197, 1996.

40. Friesen CA, Zwick DL, Streed CJ, et al. Grasp biopsy, suction biopsy, and clinical history in the evaluation of esophagitis in infants 1-6 months of age. J Pediatr Gastroenterol Nutr 20:300, 1995.

41. McVeagh P, Howman-Giles R, Kemp A, et al. Pulmonary aspiration studied by radionuclide milk scanning and barium swallow roentgenography. Am J Dis Child 141:917, 1987.

42. Dalt LD, Mazzoleni S, Montini G, et al. Diagnostic accuracy of pH monitoring in gastro-oesophageal reflux. Arch Dis Child 64:1421, 1989.

43. Barabino A, Costantini M, Ciccone MO, et al. Reliability of short-term esophageal pH monitoring versus 24-hour study. J Pediatr Gastroenterol Nutr 21:87, 1995.

44. Westra SJ, Derkx HHF, Taminiau JAJM. Symptomatic gastroesophageal reflux: Diagnosis with ultrasound. J Pediatr Gastroenterol Nutr 19:58, 1994.

45. Nussbaum E, Maggi JC, Mathis R, et al. Association of lipid-laden alveolar macrophages and gastroesophageal reflux in children. J Pediatr 110:190, 1987.

46. Hopper AO, Kwong LK, Stevenson DK, et al. Detection of gastric contents in tracheal fluid of infants by lactose assay. J Pediatr 102:415, 1983.

47. Byrne WJ. Reflux and related phenomenon. J Pediatr Gastroenterol Nutr 8:283, 1989.

48. Novak DA. Gastroesophageal reflux in the preterm infant. Clin Perinatol 23:305, 1996.

49. Kahn A, Rebuffat E, Sottiaux M, et al. Lack of temporal relation between acid reflux in the proximal esophagus and cardiorespiratory events in sleeping infants. Eur J Pediatr 151:208, 1992.

50. Sacre L, Vandenplas Y. Gastroesophageal reflux associated with respiratory abnormalities during sleep. J Pediatr Gastroenterol Nutr 9:28, 1989.

51. Paton JY, Nanayakkara CS, et al. Observations of gastroesophageal reflux, central apnoea and heart rate in infants. Eur J Pediatr 149:608, 1990.

52. Suys B, De Wolf D, Hauser B, et al. Bradycardia and gastroesophageal reflux in term and preterm infants: Is there any relation? J Pediatr Gastroenterol Nutr 19:187, 1994.

53. Newman LJ, Russe J, Glassman MS, et al. Patterns of gastroesophageal reflux (GER) in patients with apparent life-threatening events. J Pediatr Gastroenterol Nutr 8:157, 1989.

54. Rosen CL, Glaze DG, Frost JD Jr. Hypoxemia associated with feeding in the preterm infant and full-term neonate. Am J Dis Child 138:623, 1984.

55. Sindel BD, Maisels MJ, Ballantine TVN. Gastroesophageal reflux to the proximal esophagus in infants with bronchopulmonary dysplasia. Am J Dis Child 143:1103, 1989.

56. Vandenplas Y, Belli D, Cadranel S, et al. Dietary treatment for regurgitation—recommendations from a working party. Acta Paediatr 87:462, 1998.

57. Vandenplas Y, Belli D, Benhamou P-H, et al. Current concepts and issues in the management of regurgitation of infants: A reappraisal. Acta Paediatr 85:531, 1996.

58. Fleisher DR. Functional vomiting disorders in infancy: Innocent vomiting, nervous vomiting, and infant rumination syndrome. J Pediatr 125:S84, 1994.

59. Satter E. How to Get Your Kid to Eat....But not too Much. Palo Alto: Bull Publishing, 1987; 127-130.

60. Ferry GD, Selby M, Pietro TJ. Clinical response to short-term nasogastric feeding in infants with gastroesophageal reflux and growth failure. J Pediatr Gastroenterol Nutr 2:57, 1983.

61. Heacock HJ, Jeffery HE, Baker JL, et al. Influence of breast versus formula milk on physiological gastroesophageal reflux in healthy, newborn infants. J Pediatr Gastroenterol Nutr 14:41, 1992.

62. Tolia V, Lin C-H, Kuhns LR. Gastric emptying using three different formulas in infants with gastroesophageal reflux. J Pediatr Gastroenterol Nutr 15:297, 1992.

63. Khoshoo V, Zembo M, King A, et al. Incidence of gastroesophageal reflux with whey- and casein-based formulas in infants and in children with severe neurological impairment. J Pediatr Gastroenterol Nutr 22:48, 1996.

64. Kelly KJ, Lazenby AJ, Rowe PC, et al. Eosinophilic esophagitis attributed to gastroesophageal reflux: Improvement with an amino acid-based formula. Gastroenterology 109:1503, 1995.

65. Sutphen JL, Dillard VL. Medium chain triglyceride in the therapy of gastroesophageal reflux. J Pediatr Gastroenterol Nutr 14:38, 1992.

66. Vandenplas Y, Sacre L, Loeb H. Effects of formula feeding on gastric acidity time and oesophageal pH monitoring data. Eur J Pediatr 148:152, 1988.

67. Sutphen JL, Dillard VL. Dietary caloric density and osmolality influence gastroesophageal reflux in infants. Gastroenterology 97:601, 1989.

68. Orenstein SR, Magill HL, Brooks P. Thickening of infant feedings for therapy of gastroesophageal reflux. J Pediatr 110:181, 1987.

69. Vandenplas Y, Sacre L. Milk-thickening agents as a treatment for gastroesophageal reflux. Clin Pediatr 26:66, 1987.

70. Bailey DJ, Andres JM, Danek GD, et al. Lack of efficacy of thickened feeding as treatment for gastroesophageal reflux. J Pediatr 110:187, 1987.

71. Vandenplas Y, Hachimi-Idrissi S, Caseels A, et al. A clinical trial with anti-regurgitation formula. Eur J Pediatr 153:419, 1994.

72. Orenstein SR, Shalaby TM, Putnam PE. Thickened feedings as a cause of increased coughing when used as therapy for gastroesophageal reflux in infants. J Pediatr 121:913, 1992.

73. Vandenplas Y, Lifshitz JZ, Orenstein S, et al. Nutritional management of regurgitation in infants. J Am Coll Nutr 17:308, 1998.

74. Oenstein SR. Prone positioning in infant gastroesophageal reflux: Is elevation of the head worth the trouble? J Pediatr 117:184, 1990.

75. Orenstein SR, Whitington PF. Positioning for prevention of infant gastroesophageal reflux. J Pediatr 103:534, 1983.

76. Meyers WF, Herbst JJ. Effectiveness of positioning therapy for gastroesophageal reflux. Pediatrics 69:768, 1982.

77. Tobin JM, McCloud P, Cameron DJS. Posture and gastro-oesophageal reflux: A case for left lateral positioning. Arch Dis Child 76:254, 1997.

78. American Academy of Pediatrics Task Force on Infant Positioning and SIDS. Positioning and SIDS. Pediatrics 89:1120, 1992.

79. American Academy of Pediatrics Task Force on Infant Positioning and SIDS. Infant sleep position and sudden infant death syndrome (SIDS) in the United States: Joint commentary from the American Academy of Pediatrics and selected agencies of the federal government. Pediatrics 93:820, 1994.

80. American Academy of Pediatrics Task Force on Infant Positioning and SIDS. Positioning and Sudden Infant Death Syndrome (SIDS): Update. Pediatrics 98:1216, 1996.

81. Martin RJ, DiFiore JM, Korenke CB, et al. Vulnerability of respiratory control in healthy preterm infants placed supine. J Pediatr 127:609, 1995.

82. Adams JA, Zabaleta IA, Sackner MA. Comparison of supine and prone noninvasive measurements of breathing patterns in fullterm newborns. Pediatr Pulmonol 18:8, 1994.

83. Orenstein SR. Effects on behavior state of prone vs. seated positioning for infants with gastroesophageal reflux. Pediatrics 85:765, 1990.

84. Masterson J, Zucker C, Schulze K. Prone and supine positioning effects on energy expenditure and behavior of low birth weight neonates. Pediatrics 80:689, 1987.

85. Scott RB, Ferreira C, Smith L, et al. Cisapride in pediatric gastroesophageal reflux. J Pediatr Gastroenterol Nutr 25:499, 1997.

86. Hill SL, Evangelista JK, Pizzi AM, et al. Proarrhythmia associated with cisapride in children. Pediatrics 101:1053, 1998.

87. Fonkalsrud EW, Ashcraft KW, Coran AG, et al. Surgical treatment of gastroesophageal reflux in children: A combined hospital study of 7467 patients. Pediatrics 101:419, 1998.

88. Borowitz SM, Sutphen JL, Hutcheson RL. Percutaneous endoscopic gastrostomy without an antireflux procedure in neurologically disabled children. Clin Pediatr 36:25, 1997.

89. Sulaeman E, Udall JN Jr, Brown RF, et al. Gastroesophageal reflux and nissen fundoplication following percutaneous endoscopic gastrostomy in children. J Pediatr Gastroenterol Nutr 26:269, 1998.

90. Spitzer AR, Boyle, JT, Tuchman DN, et al. Awake apnea associated with gastroesophageal reflux: A specific clinical syndrome. J Pediatr 104:200, 1984.

91. Button BM, Heine RG, Catto-Smith AG, et al. Postural drainage and gastro-oesophageal reflux in infants with cystic fibrosis. Arch Dis Child 76:148, 1997.

92. Koivusalo A, Rintala R, Lindahl H. Gastroesophageal reflux in children with a congenital abdominal wall defect. J Pediatr Surg 34:1127, 1999.

93. Jolley SG, Lorenz ML, Hendrickson M, et al. Esophageal pH monitoring abnormalities and gastroesophageal reflux disease in infants with intestinal malrotation. Arch Surg 134:747, 1999.

94. Cavataio F, Carroccio A, Iacono G. Milk-induced reflux in infants less than one year of age. J Pediatr Gastroenterol Nutr 30:S36, 2000.

95. Snel A, Barnett CP, Cresp TL, et al. Behavior and gastroesophageal reflux in the premature neonate. J Pediatr Gastroenterol Nutr 30:18, 2000.

96. Vijayaratnam V, Lin CH, Simpson P, et al. Lack of significant proximal esophageal acid reflux in infants presenting with respiratory symptoms. Pediatr Pulmonol 27:231, 1999.

97. Frakaloss G, Burke G, Sanders MR. Impact of gastroesophageal reflux on growth and hospital stay in premature infants. J Pediatr Gastroenterol Nutr 26:146, 1998.

98. Ferlauto JJ, Walker MW, Martin MS. Clinically significant gastroesophageal reflux in the at-risk premature neonate: relation to cognitive scores, days in the NICU, and total hospital charges. J Perinatol 18:455, 1998.

99. Ewer AK, James ME, Tobin JM. Prone and left lateral positioning reduce gastro-oesophageal reflux in preterm infants. Arch Dis Child Fetal Neonatal Ed 81:F201, 1999.

100. Office of Public Affairs, US Food and Drug Administration. Janssen pharmaceutica stops marketing cisapride in the US. http://www.fda.gov/bbs, April. 2000.

Bibliography

Borowitz SM. Gastroesophageal reflux in babies: Impact on growth and development. Inf Young Children 10:14, 1997.

Nelson SP, Chen EH, Syniar GM, et al. Prevalence of symptoms of gastroesophageal reflux during infancy. A pediatric practice-based survey. Arch Pediatr Adolesc Med 151:569, 1997.

Nelson SP, Chen EH, Syniar GM, et al. One-year follow-up of symptoms of gastroesophageal reflux during infancy. Pediatrics 102:e67, 1998.

Orenstein SR, Cohn JF, Shalaby TM, et al. Reliability and validity of an infant gastroesophageal reflux questionnaire. Clin Pediatr 32:472, 1993.

Orenstein SR, Shalaby TM, Cohn JF. Reflux symptoms in 100 normal infants: Diagnostic validity of the infant gastroesophageal reflux questionnaire. Clin Pediatr 35:607, 1996.

Nutritional Care for High-Risk Newborns (Rev. 3d. Ed.)
S. Groh-Wargo, M. Thompson, J. Cox, editors
© 2000, Precept Press, Inc., Chicago

28

SHORT BOWEL SYNDROME

Jacqueline Jones Wessel, MEd, RD, LD, CNSD

SHORT BOWEL SYNDROME (SBS) in the neonate has been defined as the anatomic or functional absence of more than 50% of expected small intestine.[1] This is a good working definition, because SBS cannot strictly be defined anatomically; absorption of nutrients may not correlate with the length of the remaining intestine if this bowel is damaged. Functionally, an infant may behave as having SBS with only a modest resection of bowel.[2,3] In animal studies, surgical intestinal ligation and re-anastomosis without resection has a significant effect on gut growth and maturation with decreased disaccharidase activity, especially lactase and sucrase.[4]

The injury and loss of intestine may be a result of necrotizing enterocolitis (NEC), intestinal atresias, volvulus, gastroschisis, or vascular infarct.[1] The basic defect in SBS is that of a smaller surface area of intestine for absorption, coupled with a more rapid transit time.[1,2] The resulting diarrhea and malabsorption of nutrients varies with the extent and site of intestinal resection and the functional adaptation of the remaining intestine (see Table 28.1).[5]

Normal small bowel length in the term neonate has been estimated to be 240 cm, or about five times the crown-heel length.[6,7] The length of the colon is about 40 cm. Intestinal length in the preterm infant has been measured and nomograms developed.[8] Total bowel length, including both small and large intestine, is 142 ± 22 cm in preterm infants 19-27 weeks and 304 + 44 cm in infants 35 weeks and older.[8] The doubling in length of jejunum, ileum, and colon in the latter part of pregnancy gives the preterm infant a better outlook in terms of gut growth potential. This growth has been documented by studying the same infant over time.[9]

Good outcome, defined as the ability to ultimately be able to sustain growth on enteral nutrition (EN), has been reported with remaining intestine of 15 cm of jejunum-ileum with an ileocecal valve and 40 cm without the valve.[10] Reports describe survival with normal growth and eventual transition from total parenteral nutrition (TPN) to EN with as little as 11 cm jejunum-ileum with an ileocecal valve and 25 cm without the valve.[11-14] Mortality for infants with surgically treated NEC is increasing as sicker and smaller infants are being treated.[14] Late deaths due to sepsis, stricture, and hepatic failure, have been seen in many centers.[14] A review of seven patient with very short bowel syndrome suggests that infants with < 6 cm of small bowel beyond the ligament of Treitz will inevitably die of their disease or of treatment complications.[15] The definitions of outcome based on bowel length assume that remaining gut is functional. It is important that the surgeon note not only the length of remaining bowel but also the estimate of its integrity at the time of resection. The effect of the ileocecal valve (ICV) on growth, time to independence from parenteral nutrition, and overall survival has been discussed.[10,14,16,17] There is a trend for infants without an ICV to require a longer interval on parenteral nutrition than those with an ICV.[14,16,17]

Growth data of infants receiving prolonged TPN have been found to be adequate in two studies, with developmental outcome positive for the majority.[18,19] One long-term study of EN-fed SBS infants showed that growth was dependent on the length of remaining bowel. Those with resection of < 50 cm of small intestine had normal or near-normal growth; those with > 50 cm resected had below-normal weight gain and malabsorption of fat, bile acids, vitamin D, iron, and zinc.[20]

In healthy infants, absorption of fluids and nutrients occurs throughout the small intestine. Half of the total mucosal surface area is contained within the proximal one-fourth of the small intestine.[2] The duodenum and jejunum are the main sites of digestion and absorption of carbohydrates, proteins, and fats as well as the absorptive sites of most minerals, including iron and calcium.[21] Fat- and water-soluble vitamins are also primarily absorbed in the proximal bowel, with the exception of vitamin B_{12}, which is absorbed in the distal ileum. The ileum can compensate for the loss of the jejunum, but because of the specific roles of the ileum, such as bile salt resorption, the reverse is not true.[22] Bile salt resorption is necessary for enterohepatic circulation. A decrease in the bile acid pool impairs micelle formation, resulting in decreased fat absorption and steatorrhea. This also affects the absorption of fat-soluble vitamins (see Figure 28.1 and Table 28.1 and Chapter 14).

The role of the ileocecal valve in slowing transit time and acting as physiological barrier to bacteria from the colon is extremely important. Bacterial colonization of the small intestine can reduce absorption of vitamin B_{12}, deconjugate bile salts, reduce bile salt resorption, and impair gut function.[1,2]

The colon is important for water and mineral absorption. This role can be impaired by the direct dumping of irritants such as dihydroxy

Table 28.1.   Possible Implications of Intestinal Resections

Proximal small bowel	Distal small bowel/colon	
Duodenum-jejunum	*Ileum*	*Ileocecal valve*
⇩ Secretin	⇩ ⇩ Vitamin B12 absorption	⇩ Transit time
⇩ Cholecystikinin	⇩ Bile salt reabsorption	⇧ Malabsorption
⇩ Pancreatic secretions	⇩ Enterohepatic circulation	⇧ Bacterial overgrowth
⇩ Bilary secretions	Resulting in:	⇩ Vitamin B_{12} absorption
⇩ Fat digestion, absorption	⇩ Bile acid pool	⇩ Folate absorption
⇩ Fat-soluble vitamin absorption	⇩ Micelle formation	
⇩ Protein digestion, absorption	⇩ Long-chain fat absorption	
⇧ Mineral losses: Ca, Fe, Mg, Cu, Cr, Mn	⇩ Fat-soluble vitamin absorption	*Colon*
⇧ Losses of water-soluble vitamins	⇧ Steatorrhea	⇩ Water absorption
⇩ Surface area for absorption	⇧ Potential for cholelithiasis	⇩ Sodium absorption
⇩ Disaccharidase	⇧ Dihydroxy bile salts	⇩ Risk of renal oxalate stones
⇩ ⇩ Lactase	⇧ Trace element losses	
⇩ Sucrase	⇩ Colonic fluid absorption	
⇧ Substrate for bacterial overgrowth	⇧ Bile diarrhea	
⇧ Osmotic diarrhea	⇧ Risk of renal oxalate stones	

bile acids, which are produced by unabsorbed conjugated bile salts.[1,2] Carbohydrate malabsorbed by the small intestine is fermented by colonic bacteria to short-chain fatty acids. The colon has a potential role in salvaging malabsorbed carbohydrate by absorbing short-chain fatty acids. Studies using pectin, which is completely fermented in the colon by intestinal bacteria to short-chain fatty acids, have shown a beneficial effect upon intestinal adaptation in animals.[23,24] Short-chain fatty acids have been shown to be trophic to the large bowel and important in maintaining the integrity of the colonic epithelium.[25] They have been shown to enhance mucosal hyperplasia in the large intestine.[24] The absorption of SCFAs from the colon enhances the absorption of sodium and water from the lumen of the colon.[26,27] A recent study suggests that the fecal SCFA profile may predict gastrointestinal disease in preterm infants.[28] One human case report in a three-year-old child has shown increased nitrogen absorption and prolonged transit time with a pectin-supplemented diet.[29] In research studies, addition of short-chain fatty acids to TPN has been shown to decrease the bowel atrophy commonly seen with TPN therapy without enteral feedings.[30,31]

One infant formula (Isomil DF; Ross Products Division, Abbott Laboratories, Columbus, Ohio) and several pediatric formulas are available with added fiber (see Appendix K). The soy polysaccharide fiber used is considered to be a mix of insoluble and soluble fiber, but appears to act as if it has a higher percentage of soluble fiber. This may be due to the manufacturing process. In studies, soy polysaccharide fiber has been comparable to pectin, which is considered a soluble fiber.[32] The degradation and fermentation process that produces short-chain fatty acids typically occurs in the large bowel, but when there is no large bowel, it occurs in the small intestine. Studies have shown that the addition of fiber, soy polysaccharide,[33] and pectin[24] enhances small intestine adaptation. In the animal study by Michail et al., animals fed Isomil DF showed significantly higher sucrase and lactase levels in the proximal bowel after a small-bowel resection than those fed Isomil.[33] Clinically, some have used the commercially available liquid preparation of pectin (example: Certo brand) in a 1-3% concentration (ie 1-3 cc to 100 cc formula). More studies are needed to confirm effects of fiber on intestinal adaptation in infants.

Dietary fiber can inhibit mineral absorption through the chelating effect of fiber; the effect is dependent on the type and amount of fiber in the diet.[34] The soluble fibers are currently thought to decrease mineral absorption more than the insoluble fibers, and increasing the amount of fiber lowers mineral retention.[34]

Glutamine is considered to be the primary gut fuel. After an exploratory laparotomy, gut consumption of glutamine is increased.[35-37] Glutamine supplementation in TPN may prevent the intestinal atrophy seen in the use of TPN without EN.[38] Supplemental glutamine may also decrease bacterial translocation-the emigration of G.I. bacteria in damaged gut through the intestinal mucosa into the mesenteric lymph nodes and the bloodstream.[35] It is thought that supplemental glutamine might support gut metabolism in an infant with intestinal immaturity.[35] Glutamine is absent in commercially available TPN solutions at this time.[36] Glutamine with growth hormone and a modified diet has been used in adults in a pharmacologic bowel compensation program.[39-41] However, animal studies have not shown that the combination of glutamine and growth hormone enhances intestinal adaptation.[42]

Gastric acid hypersecretion can be a problem after a large bowel resection, with reports varying in frequency from 17% to 50%.[5,43] Hypersecretion of gastric acid appears to be associated with the extent of the resection (more common with greater resection), and the initiation of enteral feedings.[43] Digestion and absorption of nutrients may be affected by excess gastric acid entering the small bowel. This may also lead to peptic ulcer disease and breakdown at the anastomosis site. Intravenous ranitidine has been shown to be effective in inhibiting acid secretion, and cimetidine is also used for this purpose.[2,44] Because the hypersecretion is usually transitory, caution is advised in the long-term use of H_2 antagonists such as ranitidine and cimetidine. These agents may decrease intrinsic factor secretion,

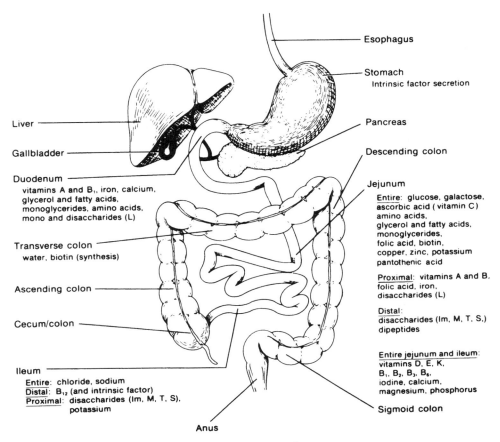

Figure 28.1. Sites of nutrient absorption.

The exact sites for absorption of manganese, cobalt, selenium, molybdenum, and cadmium are unknown. L = lactose; IM = isomaltose; M = maltose; T = trehalose; S = sucrose.

(Reprinted from Caldwell MD, Kennedy-Caldwell C. Surg Clin North Am 61:491 1981, with permission from WB Saunders.)

which may alter vitamin B_{12} absorption as well as increase the potential for bacterial contamination of the small bowel.[2]

Renal oxalate stone formation may be a problem in SBS. Normally, dietary oxalate is bound to calcium in the intestine, forming calcium oxalate, which is nonabsorbable and is excreted in the feces. After an ileal resection, bile salt resorption may be sufficiently decreased to impair micelle formation and fatty acid absorption. These fats bind calcium, leaving oxalate in an absorbable form.[2,5] Oxalate can be absorbed in large amounts in infants with a functional colon and then must be excreted by the kidneys. Hyperoxaluria may result and may lead to nephrolithiasis.[2,5]

Previously, infants with an ileostomy were felt to be less likely to form urinary oxalate stones.[5,45] Recent reports, however, indicate excessive oxalate excretion in the urine of patients with and without an ileostomy.[46] Extra calcium in the diet may decrease the problem with renal calculi.[22] Because ascorbic acid can be metabolized to oxalate, excessive doses of vitamin C should be avoided.[5]

When foods are consumed, a mild oxalate restriction may be beneficial, but inasmuch as most of these foods are not appropriate for the infant, oxalate restriction generally is not a matter for concern. Sources include spinach, rhubarb, citrus fruits, chocolate, cola drinks, and tea.[5]

Preventive Nutrition

With the possible exception of NEC, conditions leading to SBS are not prevented by nutrition therapy (see Chapter 25).

Treatment Nutrition

Parenteral Therapy

The initial nutrition therapy is parenteral (see Table 28.2). Because of the possible long-term nature of TPN support, central venous access is preferred.[1] Providing sufficient calories to sustain growth necessitates the use of > 10% dextrose solutions, as well as optimal fat and amino acid intake. TPN should be monitored carefully and advanced as tolerated, taking any other conditions such as prematurity into account (see Chapters 10 and 11). Because of the long-term nature of TPN support, a pediatric amino acid solution may help. The addition of cysteine HCL to solutions formulated with a pediatric amino acid product will increase plasma taurine concentrations to within the normal reference range.[47]

TPN-associated liver disease is a leading cause of death in TPN-dependent SBS, with hepatic failure occurring in 3-19% of children with SBS acquired as a neonate.[3,9,48-51] Cholestasis occurs in 30-60% of infants with SBS.[9,49-51] Although the exact mechanism of TPN-induced liver disease is not known, theories include excess administration of nutrients and inadequate secretion of certain G.I. hormones needed for normal hepatic function.[52,53] Sepsis that occurs early in life when the liver may be more vulnerable to insults may also play an important role in the development of cholestasis and liver disease in infants with SBS.[48,108] When fat malabsorption occurs with cholestasis

Table 28.2.   Progression of Nutritional Management

I.V. fluids (usually only one day):

Stabilize fluids (dextrose and electrolytes)

Total parenteral nutrition:

Offer replacement fluids as needed
Increase substrate gradually to allow for expected growth
Initiate nonnutritive oral motor program

Combined parenteral and enteral nutrition:

Initiate continuous NG or GT enteral 24-hr infusion
Wean gradually from parenteral nutrition
Begin small bolus feeding(s) by mouth to retain swallow
Introduce small amount of solids if developmentally appropriate

Enteral nutrition:

Wean from continuous infusion to all-bolus feedings
Continue developmental feeding skill progression
Manage macronutrient malabsorption
Look for possible micronutrient deficiencies
Monitor growth closely

additional supplemental fat soluble vitamins are suggested in the following doses:[109]

Vitamin A	3,000-10,000 IU/day
Vitamin D (25 OH)	400-4000 IU/day
Vitamin E	25 IU/kg/day
Vitamin K	2.5-5.0 mg/d

Monitoring of vitamin nutritional status is required.

Careful calculation of nutrient needs for growth should be ongoing in order to avoid unneeded amounts of macronutrients. Early introduction of enteral feedings, even if at a gut-priming rate of 1 cc/hour, may have a protective effect.[52] If cholestasis occurs, the amounts of copper and manganese should be decreased, due to their biliary excretion.[1,54,108]

The benefit from cycling TPN in an attempt to decrease the incidence of cholestasis is debated. Georgeson et al. use cycling with an aggressive surgical program to combat cholestasis.[55] Others have used cycling in an effort to prevent cholestasis;[56,57] still others feel cycling offers no benefits.[54] From a practical perspective, it is help-ful to give the long-term TPN infant a "window" or time off TPN for greater freedom of movement. When doing this, the infusion rate should be gradually decreased when coming off infusion and slowly moved up when restarting TPN in order to avoid swings in blood glu-cose.[52] A commonly used taper is to cut the rate in half one hour before and one hour after full infusion times.

Zinc losses increase as stool output increases. Zinc losses from ileostomy fluid may be 12 mg/L and 17 mg/L from diarrhea.[58] The reported deficiency symptoms include suboptimal growth, diarrhea, perineal and perioral skin rash, impaired wound healing, and alope-cia.[59-63] Zinc balance studies suggest that stool zinc losses are highest during periods of negative zinc balance. After repletion, stool con-centration of zinc is significantly reduced.[59]

Sodium (Na) needs may be markedly increased. Patients with fis-tulas, ostomies, or abnormal losses need appropriate electrolyte replacement (see Table 28.3). Using a replacement solution such as 5% dextrose with ½ normal saline and 15 mEq/L of K to replace gas-tric drainage may prove to be easier to manage than to make up for these losses through TPN. The use of urine as well as serum elec-trolytes is helpful in determining needs. Urine electrolytes are more helpful in determining total body sodium status than are serum elec-trolytes. When depleted, the body retains sodium, and urinary sodi-um decreases. This change will occur before any change is noted in serum sodium. Sodium-depleted infants will not grow well.[67-70] To supplement sodium, an average output can be determined and an estimate of sodium loss can be determined. Sodium supplementation can be added to parenteral or enteral nutrition and urine electrolytes used to titrate the amount of supplementation needed. A thorough discussion of neonatal postoperative fluid and electrolyte manage-ment is beyond the scope of this chapter; however, several excellent references have been published.[65,66,71,72]

Enteral Management

Because the small bowel mucosa has been shown to undergo atro-phy with long-term TPN therapy, it is important to begin gradual EN feedings once the patient is stable and G.I. motility has returned.[73-77] Early EN feedings appear to decrease the incidence of TPN-associ-ated cholestasis.[52,73] Intestinal adaptation, characterized by cellular hyperplasia, villous hypertrophy, intestinal lengthening, motility improvement, and hormonal changes (such as elevated gastrin lev-els), increases absorptive capacity.[74] This response frequently takes more than a year; a 1989 study reported that calcium absorption con-tinued to improve for more than two years.[5,74,76]

Table 28.3   Pediatric GI Losses[64-66]

	Sodium (mEq/L)	Potassium (mEq/L)	Chloride (mEq/L)	Bicarbonate (mEq/L)
Gastric	140	15	155	-
Ileostomy	80-140	15	115	40
Colon	50-80	10-30	40	20-25
Diarrhea	10-90	10-80	10-110	30
Normal Stool	5 mEq/d	10 mEq/d	10 mEq/d	0

Much research activity continues to examine factors trophic for gut regrowth, including glutamine, long chain polyunsaturated fatty acids such as decosahexaenoic acid (DHA) and arachidonic acid (AA), enteroglucagon, ornithine decarboxylase, diamine oxidase, putrescine, spermidine, and spermine, as well as short-chain fatty acids specifically for the colon.[23,30,31,78,79] The adaptation process appears to result in the increased expression of the sodium glucose cotransporter gene (SGLT1) which leads to an increase in nutrient transport.[80] Epidermal growth factor and its receptor appear to be necessary for intestinal adaptation to occur.[81]

Components of an ideal formula for infants with SBS remain controversial (see Table 28.4).[82-84] Practically speaking, Alimentum (Ross) and Pregestimil (Mead Johnson Nutritionals, Evansville, Ind.) are most often used, with transition to a premature infant formula possible in some patients.[2,5,21] An amino-acid-based complete infant formula such as Neocate (Scientific Hospital Supplies North America, Gaithersburg, MD) may result in greater feeding tolerance in some patients.[83] The use of commercial products with fiber, or supplemental fiber may have specific benefits. (see discussion earlier in chapter) Adult formulas are not recommended because they will not meet the infant's unique nutritional needs without supplementation.

Human milk may have potential benefits. Colostrum-induced mucosal growth has been documented in animals.[3,78] Human milk's bile-salt stimulated lipase as well as lymphocytes, macrophages, short-chain peptides, and free amino acids seem to be absorbed well.[85]

Enteral feedings are often started with a continuous infusion into the stomach through either a nasogastric tube or a gastrostomy.[52,74] Continuous feedings are used to maximize absorption[77,86] (see Chapter 18). Jejunal feedings are usually contraindicated, for the reason that they bypass needed intestine for optimal digestion and absorption. An oral motor stimulation program should be initiated, starting with nonnutritive sucking, progressing to small-volume bottle feedings as tolerated. Patients with SBS have difficulty learning feeding skills, often needing intense intervention (see Chapter 19).[87] Infants with smaller resections may do well on small bolus tube feedings or may progress to bottle feedings after achieving full continuous enteral feedings. Nippling is often started during a window or time-off period from the continuous infusion. Ideally, the amount given should equal the hourly continuous feeding rate. This should be viewed as an enteral change; no other increases should be made that day in order to monitor the effect of a bolus feeding.

The length of time to achieve full enteral feedings depends on the length, absorptive surface area, and condition of the remaining intestine, as well as the nutrient needs of the infant. Infants with concomitant disorders such as bronchopulmonary dysplasia (BPD) have increased caloric needs that increase the enteral goals and lengthen the time for the progression to full EN feedings.

Feedings are generally advanced gradually and TPN reduced to equal the appropriate fluids for the infant. As EN feedings replace PN fluids, caloric intake may decrease. The PN solution, if infused through a central venous catheter, may be higher in calories per unit volume than the EN product. Factoring in the effects of malabsorption unique to each case may mean that the needed calories per kilogram for appropriate growth will greatly increase as the percentage of enteral feedings increases. To counter the problem of increased calorie needs as PN is decreasing, the PN solution may need to be more calorically dense or total fluid volume may need increasing. Also, continuous EN feedings may not deliver all the calories and nutrients contained in the product, especially if it is human milk (see Chapter 18).

Feedings are generally advanced until stool output increases to about 40 cc/kg and/or significant malabsorption occurs. A higher volume of accepted stool output has been used in one study.[88] This method is feasible, but astute fluid and electrolyte management is essential as dehydration can occur rapidly. Stool pH of < 5.5 and the presence of reducing substances can be used as indicators of carbohydrate malabsorption.[89-92] Fecal reducing substance tests such as Clinitest (Ames Division, Miles Laboratories, Elkhart, Ind.) are used, but may underestimate the degree of malabsorption of carbohydrate. Because sucrose is not a reducing sugar, sucrose malabsorption is not identified by this test unless acid hydrolysis is done prior to the test.[90] The Harriet Lane Handbook includes this procedure.[91]

Breath hydrogen has been used to indicate carbohydrate malabsorption, but it is not practical for daily assessments.[93] Fecal fat tests can be helpful in determining fat losses (see Chapter 3).[90] As a research tool, bomb calorimetry has been used to determine the caloric equivalent in the stool.[94]

The literature is sparse on progression of strained baby foods for the infant with SBS. In theory and in practice, most infant cereals

Table 28.4. Characteristics of Components Desired in a Formula Designed for Infants with Short Bowel Syndrome

Protein

Better tolerated than fats or carbohydrates[20]
Free amino acids may be helpful[83]
Casein hydrolysates tolerated well; casein not superior to casein hydrolysates[82]

Carbohydrates

May not be tolerated well
Each unit of lactase available for digestion matched by 2 units of sucrase and 6-8 units of maltase[19]
Lactose-containing formulas may increase diarrhea
Lactase preparations would seem to be beneficial, but have not been studied In this population
Preemie formulas (1/2 lactose) often tolerated after initial trial of protein hydrolysate formula
Glucose polymers tolerated well, have a lower osmolality than glucose, can be hydrolyzed by maltase[1,2,20,22]

Fat

May be poorly absorbed
Decreased micelle formation hinders long-chain triglyceride (LCT) fat absorption
Medium-chain triglyceride (MCT) fats better absorbed than LCT fats, but not as effective in stimulating mucosal hyperplasia[84]
Combination MCT / LCT fats tolerated well
Essential fatty acids required, but not supplied by MCT fats

Vitamins

Need for additional fat-soluble vitamins when on all-enteral feedings if cholestasis or steatorrhea present
If premature, increased needs

Minerals

Need for additional sodium and zinc if jejunostomy or ileostomy is present (increased losses)
Need for additional calcium due to malabsorption
If loss or damage to duodenum, consider iron malabsorption
If premature, increased needs

and starches are tolerated well, as are meats. Vegetables and fruits are generally tolerated, although in practice not as well as cereals. Because simple sugars and lactose-containing foods may increase stool output, they should be introduced carefully into the diet.

D-lactic acidosis has been reported to result from excessive D-lactate production by intestinal bacteria from malabsorbed carbohydrate in young children with SBS who are on a mixed diet. This acidosis causes drowsiness and mental confusion.[95-97]

Bacterial overgrowth may occur as a result of poor motility and dilated bowel. Stasis of intestinal contents leads to bacterial overgrowth, which can alter absorption and cause increased stooling.[98] The 13C-xylose breath test has been used for diagnosis of overgrowth.[99] For infants prone to overgrowth, routine scheduled antibiotic treatment may be useful.

Follow-up Issues

The potential for nutritional deficiencies and altered growth in infants with SBS is great. A multidisciplinary team approach, including a nutritionist, is appropriate. Because of the possibility of altered feeding development, the resources of occupational therapy and/or speech pathology are beneficial. The inclusion of a social worker on the team would seem essential in view of the financial and emotional cost of this chronic condition.

Surgical reassessment plays a role in follow-up, especially when gut adaptation does not seem to be working after one year.[12,49] Some infants go home with ostomies, and others have the bowel reconnected during the initial hospitalization. Creative surgical techniques such as colon interposition, reversal of small areas of intestine, and the creation of intestinal valves have been developed to decrease transit time.[8] For infants with dilated bowel, intestinal tapering and lengthening (the Bianchi procedure) have been successful.[9,49,100-105]

Intestinal transplantation can be considered only when all other treatment options have been exhausted.[50,51,106] This is an area of intensive research. The two major problems preventing successful outcome appear to be the classic graft rejection and graft-versus-host disease, as well as disturbed function of the graft by transplantation.[107]

Infants with SBS present a complex picture to the practitioner. Less than 30 years ago, death was inevitable for infants with this diagnosis.[49] Much has been learned regarding treatment, especially PN therapy. More research needs to be done, specifically in the area of enhanced adaptation and gut growth.

Case Study

Infant A was a 32 weeks' gestation, 1,500 g premature infant who developed NEC on the seventh day of life. Exploratory laparotomy showed necrotic distal ileum, ascending, and transverse colon. A resection of ileum, ileocecal valve and colon was performed, leaving 38 cm of proximal bowel. An ostomy was made and a gastrostomy tube (G-tube) inserted. The remainiing intestine appeared to the surgeons to be healthy. The descending colon was intact but not connected.

TPN was started on postoperative day 2 and a central venous catheter was inserted on day 4. TPN was gradually increased to 3 g/kg/day protein, using a pediatric amino acid solution, and 3 g/kg/day fat, with 20% dextrose solution providing 105 kcal/kg/day. An oral motor stimulation plan was started on day 5.

EN feedings were started on day 10 at 1 cc/hour continuous feeds through the G-tube. A protein hydrolysate formula was used. (Mother did not wish to breast-feed.) Feedings were advanced by 1 cc/hour/day as long as stool output was < 30 cc/kg/day and Clinitests were not > 1%. When feedings reached 5 cc/hour, a one-hour window off the enteral drip was created and a 5 cc bottle of formula was given for oral stimulation. Feedings were gradually increased, with two more bottles added to the feeding plan.

An attempt was made to change the infant to a premature infant formula, starting at ¼ protein hydrolysate to premature formula, then ½ to ½, etc. Stool output increased with each increase in amount of premature formula to > 30 cc/kg/day but decreased after the third day. The transition to premature formula was integrated with other enteral increases. Change to full premature formula was not successful, and the infant was kept on a formula consisting of 3/4 premature formula and ¼ protein hydrolysate formula. Growth averaged 25 g/day during this time.

When EN feedings had reached 50% of the projected goal of 120 kcal/kg/day, the decision was made to discharge the infant on home TPN 14 hours/day and enteral drip feedings 21 hours/day, with three bottles taken by mouth during the time off continuous feedings.

Cereal was added by spoon at 6 months corrected age, followed by starchy vegetables, meats, then other vegetables and fruits. Teething biscuits and crackers were added when interest developed at 7 months corrected age. The infant was kept on a lactose and mild oxalate-restricted diet. Foods high in sucrose also were limited.

Continued progress was made, and at 8 months corrected age TPN was discontinued. Additional sodium bicarbonate and chloride were added to the formula. The transition to all-oral feedings occurred over the next 18 months, with the last year spent weaning off of nocturnal continuous feedings of a pediatric tube-feeding formula. The toddler was at this time at the 50th percentile for weight, height, and head circumference. The surgical plan for reconnection of the remaining colon was to be set after toilet training occurred, due to expected problems with frequent stooling. Vitamin B_{12} status was evaluated, and the toddler was to start monthly B_{12} injections at 3 years of age.

References

1. Ziegler MM. Short bowel syndrome in infancy: Etiology and management. Clin Perinatol 13:167, 1986.
2. Taylor SF, Sokol RJ. Infants with short bowel syndrome. In: Hay WW, ed. Neonatal nutrition and metabolism. St. Louis: Mosby Year Book, 1991; 437.
3. Cooper A, Floyd TF, Ross AJ, et al. Morbidity and mortality of short bowel syndrome acquired in infancy: An update. J Pediatr Surg 18:711, 1984.
4. Stringel G, Uauy R, Guertin L. The effect of intestinal anastomosis on gut growth and maturation. J Pediatr Surg 24:1086, 1989.
5. Biller JA. Short small bowel syndrome. In: Grand RJ, Sutphen JL, Dietz WH, eds. Pediatric nutrition. Boston: Butterworths, 1987; 481.
6. Reiquam CW, Allen RP, Akers DR. Normal and abnormal small bowel lengths. Am J Dis Child 134:593, 1980.
7. Siebert JR. Small intestine length in infants and children. Am J Dis Child 18:593, 1980.
8. Touloukian RJ, Smith GJ. Normal intestinal length in preterm infants. J Pediatr Surg 18:720, 1983.
9. Caniano DA, Starr J, Ginn-Pease ME. Extensive short bowel syndrome in neonates: Outcome in the 1980's. Surgery 105:119, 1989.
10. Wilmore DW. Factors correlating with a successful outcome following extensive intestinal resection in newborn infants. J Pediatr 80:88, 1972.
11. Dorney SF, Ament ME, Berquist WE, et al. Improved survival in very short small bowel of infancy with use of long-term parenteral nutrition. J Pediatr 107:521, 1985.
12. Iacono G, Carrioco A, Montalto G, et al. Extreme short bowel syndrome: A case for reviewing the guidelines for predicting survival. J Pediatr Gastroenterol Nutr 16:216, 1993.
13. Grosfeld JL, Cheu H, Schlatter M, et al. Changing trends in necrotizing enterocolitis: Experience with 302 cases in two decades. Ann Surg 214:300, 1991.
14. Ladd AP, Rescoria FR, West KW, et al Long term follow-up after bowel resection for necrotizing enterocolitis: Factors affecting outcome. J Pediatr Surg 33:967, 1998.
15. Hancock BJ, Wiseman NE. Lethal short bowel syndrome. J Pediatr Surg 25:1131, 1990.
16. Georgeson KE, Breaux Jr CW. Outcome and intestinal adaptation in neonatal short-bowel syndrome. J Pediatr Surg 27:344, 1992.
17. Goulet OJ, Revillon Y, Jan D, et al. Neonatal short bowel syndrome. J Pediatr 119:18, 1991.

18. Ralston CW, O'Connor MJ, Ament ME, et al. Somatic growth and developmental functioning in children receiving prolonged home total parenteral nutrition. J Pediatr 105:842, 1984.

19. Lin CH, Rossi TM, Herlinger LA. Nutritional assessment of children with short bowel syndrome receiving home parenteral nutrition. Am J Dis Child 141:1093, 1987.

20. Ohkochi V, Igarashi Y, Tazawa Y, et al. Evaluation of the nutritional condition and absorptive capacity of nine infants with short bowel syndrome. J Pediatr Gastroenterol Nutr 5:198, 1986.

21. Conrad, M. Iron absorption. In: Johnson LR, ed. Physiology of the gastrointestinal tract. New York: Raven Press, 1987; 1437.

22. Klish WJ. The short gut. In: Walker WA, Watkins JB, eds. Nutrition in pediatrics. Boston: Little, Brown, 1985; 561.

23. Sakata T, Yajima T. Influence of short chain fatty acids in the epithelial cell division of the GI tract. Q J Exp Physiol 69:639, 1984.

24. Koruda MJ, Rolandelli RH, Settle RG, et al. The effect of pectin supplemented elemental diet on intestinal adaptation to massive small bowel resection. J Parenter Enter Nutr 10:343, 1986.

25. Roediger WEW. Bacterial short chain fatty acids and mucosal diseases of the colon. Br J Surg 75:346, 1988.

26. Ruppin H, Bar-Meir S, Soergel K, et al. Absorption of short chain fatty acids by the colon. Gastroenterology 78:1500, 1980.

27. Roediger WEW, Moore A. The effect of short chain fatty acids on sodium absorption in the isolated human colon perfused through the vascular bed. Am J Dig Dis 26:100, 1981.

28. Szylit O, Maurage C, Gasqui P, et al. Fecal short chain fatty acids predict digestive disorders in premature infants. JPEN 22:136, 1998.

29. Finkel Y, Brown G, Smith HL, et al. The effects of a pectin supplemented elemental diet in a boy with short gut syndrome. Acta Paediatr Scand 79:983, 1990.

30. Koruda MJ, Rolandelli RH, Settle RG, et al. Effect of parenteral nutrition supplemented with short chain fatty acids on adaptation to massive small bowel resection. Gastroenterology 95:715, 1988.

31. Lo CW, Walker WA. Changes in the gastrointestinal tract during enteral or parenteral feeding. Nutr Rev 47:193, 1989.

32. McIntyre A, Young GP, Taranto T, et al. Different fibers have different regional effects on luminal contents of rat colon. Gastroenterology 101:1274, 1991.

33. Michail S, Mohammadpour M, Park JHY, Vanderhoof JA. Soy polysaccharide-supplemented soy formula enhances mucosal disaccharidase levels following massive small intestinal resection in rats. J Pediatr Gastroenterol Nutr 24:140, 1997.

34. Wang Y, Funk MA, Garleb KA, Chevreau N. The effect of fiber source in enteral products on fecal weight, mineral balance, and growth rate in rats. JPEN 18:340, 1994.

35. Souba WW, Klimberg VS, Plumley DA, et al. The role of glutamine in maintaining a healthy gut and supporting the metabolic response to injury and infection. J Surg Res 48:383, 1990.

36. Souba WW, Smith RJ, Wilmore DW. Glutamine metabolism by the intestinal tract. J Parenter Enter Nutr 9:608, 1985.

37. Klimberg VS, Souba WW, Salloum RM, et al. Intestinal metabolism after massive small bowel resection. Gastroenterology 95:715, 1988.

38. Hwang TL, O'Dwyer ST, Smith RJ, et al. Preservation of small bowel mucosa using glutamine enriched parenteral nutrition. Surg Forum 38:56, 1987.
39. Wilmore DW, Lacey JL, Soultanakis R, et al. Factors predicting a successful outcome after pharmacologic bowel compensation. Ann Surg 226:288, 1997.
40. Byrne TA, Morrisey TB, Nattakom TV, et al. Growth hormone, glutamine, and a modified diet enhance nutrient absorption in patients with severe short bowel syndrome. JPEN 19:296, 1995.
41. Byrne TA, Persinger RL, Young LS, et al. A new treatment for patients with short bowel syndrome: Growth hormone, glutamine, and a modified diet. Ann Surg 222:242, 1995.
42. Vanderhoof JA, Kollman KA, Griffin S, et al. Growth hormone and glutamine do not stimulate intestinal adaptation following massive small bowel resection in the rat. J Pediatr Gastroenterol Nutr 25:327, 1997.
43. Hyman PE, Everett SL, Harada T. Gastric acid hypersecretion in short bowel syndrome in infants: Association with extent of resection and enteral feeding. J Pediatr Gastroenterol Nutr 5:191, 1987.
44. Hyman PE, Garvey TQ, Abrams CE. Tolerance to intravenous ranitidine. J Pediatr 110:794, 1987.
45. Modigliani R, Labayle D, Aymes C, Denvil R. Evidence for excessive absorption of oxalate by the colon in enteral hyperoxaluria. Scand J Gastroenterol 13:187, 1978.
46. Buchman AL, Moukarzel aa, Ament ME. Excessive urinary oxalate excretion occurs in long-term TPN patients both with and without ileostomies. J Am Coll Nutr. 14:24, 1995.
47. Helms RA, Storm MC, Christensen ML, et al. Cysteine supplementation results in normalization of plasma taurine concentrations in children receiving home parenteral nutrition. J Pediatr 134:358, 1999.
48. Sondheimer JM, Asturias E, Cadnapaphornchai M. Infection and cholestasis in neonates with intestinal resection and long-term parenteral nutrition. J Pediatr Gastroenterol Nutr 27:131, 1998.
49. Galea MH, Holliday H, Carachi R, et al. Short bowel syndrome: A collective review. J Pediatr Surg 27:592, 1992.
50. Simmons MG, Georgeson KE, Figueroa R, Mock DL. Liver failure in parenteral nutrition dependent children with short bowel syndrome. Transplant Proc 28:2701, 1996.
51. Teitelbaum H, Drongowski R, Spivak D. Rapid development of hyperbilirubinemia in infants with short bowel syndrome as a correlate to mortality: Possible indications for early small bowel transplant. Transplant Proc 28:2699, 1996.
52. Vanderhoof JA. Clinical management of the short bowel syndrome. In: Balistreri WF, Vanderhoof JA, eds. Pediatric gastroenterology and nutrition. London: Chapman and Hall Medical, 1990; 24.
53. Vileisis RA, Inwood RJ, Hunt CE. Prospective controlled study of parenteral nutrition-associated cholestatic jaundice: Effect of protein intake. J Pediatr 96:893, 1980.
54. Warner BW. Parenteral nutrition in the pediatric patient. In: Fischer JE, ed. Parenteral nutrition. Boston: Little, Brown, 1991; 299.
55. Georgeson KE, Halpin D, Figeroa R, et al. Sequential intestinal lengthening procedures for refractory short bowel syndrome. J Pediatr Surg 29:316, 1994.

56. Meehan JJ, Georgeson KE. Prevention of liver failure in parenteral nutrition-dependent children with short bowel syndrome. J Pediatr Surg 32:473, 1997.
57. Collier S, Crough J, Hendricks K, Caballero B. Use of cyclic parenteral nutrition in infants less than 6 months of age. Nutr Clin Prac 9:65, 1994.
58. Shulman RJ. Zinc and copper balance studies in infants receiving TPN. Am J Clin Nutr 49:879, 1989.
59. Latimer JS, McClain CJ, Sharp HL. Clinical zinc deficiency during zinc supplemented parenteral nutrition. J Pediatr 97:434, 1980.
60. Weber TR, Sears N, Dacies B, et al. Clinical spectrum of zinc deficiency in pediatric patients receiving total parenteral nutrition. J Pediatr Surg 16:236, 1981.
61. Friel JK, Gibson RS, Peliowski A, et al. Serum zinc, copper, and selenium concentrations in preterm infants receiving parenteral nutrition supplemented with zinc and copper. J Pediatr 104:736, 1984.
62. Zlotkin SH, Buchanan BE. Meeting zinc and copper intake requirements in the parenterally fed preterm and full term infant. J Pediatr 103:441, 1983.
63. Greene HL, Hambridge KM, Schanler R, et al. Guidelines for the use of vitamins, trace elements, calcium, magnesium, and phosphorus in infants and children receiving total parenteral nutrition: Report of the Subcommittee on Pediatric Parenteral Nutrient Requirements from the Committee on Clinical Practice Issues, American Society for Clinical Nutrition. Am J Clin Nutr 48:1334, 1988.
64. Baker RD, Baker SS, Davis AM. Pediatric Enteral Nutrition. New York: Chapman & Hall, 1997; 430.
65. Heird WC, Winters RW Fluid therapy for the pediatric surgical patient. In: Winters RW, ed. Principles of pediatric fluid therapy. Boston: Little, Brown, 1982; 595.
66. Winters RW, Heird WC. Special problems of the pediatric surgical patient. In: Winters RW, ed. Principles of pediatric fluid therapy. Boston: Little, Brown, 1982; 612.
67. Mews CF. Topics in neonatal nutrition: Early ileostomy closure to prevent chronic salt and water losses in infants. J Perinatol 12:297, 1992.
68. Sacher P, Hirsig J, Gresser J, Spitz L. The importance of oral sodium replacement in ileostomy patients. Prog Pediatr Surg 24:226, 1989.
69. Bower TR Pringle KC, Soper RT. Sodium deficit causing decreased weight gain and metabolic acidosis in infants with ileostomy. J Pediatr Surg 23:567, 1988.
70. Schwarz KB, Ternberg JL, Bell MJ, Keating JP. Sodium needs of infants and children with ileostomy. J Pediatr 102:509, 1983.
71. John E, Kladianou M, Vidyasagar D. Electrolyte problems in neonatal surgical patients. Clin Perinatol 16:219, 1989.
72. Ichikawa I, ed. Pediatric textbook of fluids and electrolytes. Baltimore: Williams and Wilkins, 1990.
73. Feldman EJ, Dowling RH, McNaughton J, et al. Effects of oral versus intravenous nutrition on intestinal adaptation after small bowel resection in the dog. Gastroenterology 70:712, 1976.
74. Purdum PP, Kirby DE Short bowel syndrome: A review of the role of nutrition support. J Parenter Enter Nutr 15:93, 1990.
75. Vanderhoof JA, Langnas AN, Pinch IW, et al. Short bowel syndrome. J Pediatr Gastroenterol Nutr 14:359, 1992.

76. Giuttebel MC, Saint Aubert B, Colette C, et al. Intestinal adaptation in patients with short bowel syndrome: Measurement by calcium absorption. Dig Dis Sci 34:709, 1989.

77. Buts JP, Morin CL, Ling V. Influence of dietary components on intestinal adaptation after small bowel resection in rats. Clin Invest Med 2:59, 1979.

78. Heird WC, Schwartz SM, Hansen IH. Colostrum induced enteric mucosal growth in beagle puppies. Pediatr Res 18:512A, 1984.

79. Kollman KA, Lien EL, Vanderhoof JA. Dietary lipids influence intestinal adaptation after massive bowel resection. J Pediatr Gastroenterol Nutr 28:41, 1999.

80. Sigalet DL, Martin, GR. Mechanisms underlying intestinal adaptation after massive intestinal resection in the rat. J Pediatr Surg 33:889, 1998.

81. Helmrath MA, Shin CE, Erwin CR, et al. Intestinal adaptation is enhanced by epidermal growth factor independent of increased ileal epidermal growth factor receptor expression. J Pediatr Surg 33:980, 1998.

82. Vanderhoof JA, Grandjean CJ, Burkley KT, et al. Effect of casein versus casein hydrolysate on mucosal adaptation following small bowel resection in infant rats. J Pediatr Gastroenterol Nutr 3:262, 1984.

83. Bines J, Francis D, Hill D. Reducing parenteral requirement in children with short bowel syndrome: Impact of an amino acid-based complete infant formula. J Pediatr Gastroenterol Nutr 26:123, 1998.

84. Vanderhoof JA, Grandjean CJ, Burkley KT, et al. Effect of high percentage medium chain triglyceride diet in mucosal adaptation following small bowel resection in rats. J Parenter Enter Nutr 8:685, 1984.

85. Lawrence RA. Breastfeeding: A guide for the medical profession. 5th Ed. St. Louis: Mosby, 1999.

86. Parker P, Stroop S, Greene H. A controlled comparison of continuous versus intermittent feeding in the treatment of infants with intestinal disease. J Pediatr 99:360, 1987.

87. Linscheid TR, Tarnowski KJ, Rasnake LK, et al. Behavioral treatment of food refusal in a child with short gut syndrome. J Pediatr Psych 12:451, 1987.

88. Alkalay AL, Fleisher DR, Pomerance JJ, Rosenthal P. Management of premature infants with extensive bowel resection with high volume enteral infusates. Isr J Med Sci 31:298, 1995.

89. Ameen VZ, Powell GK, Jones LA. Quantitation of fecal carbohydrate excretion in patients with short bowel syndrome. Gastroenterology 92:493, 1987.

90. Merritt RJ, Hack, S. Infant feeding and enteral nutrition. Nutr Clin Pract 3:47, 1988.

91. Siberry GK, Iannone R, eds. Harriet Lane handbook. 15th Ed. St. Louis: Mosby, 2000; 262.

92. Kerry KR, Anderson CM. A ward test for sugar in feces. Lancet 1:981, 1964.

93. Shermeta DW, Ruaz E, Fink BB, et al. Respiratory hydrogen secretion: A simple test of bowel adaptation in infants with short gut syndrome. J Pediatr Surg 16:271, 1981.

94. Mezoff A, Heubi J, Cornett L, et al. Enteral feeding tolerance in short bowel syndrome. Unpublished data. Children's Hospital Medical Center, Cincinnati.

95. Perlmutter DH, Boyle JT, Campos JM, et al. D-lactic acidosis in children: An unusual metabolic complication of small bowel resection. J Pediatr 102:234, 1983.

96. Gurevitch J, Sela B, Jonas A, et al. D-lactic acidosis: A treatable encephalopathy in pediatric patients. Acta Paediatrica 82:11, 1993.

97. Bongaerts G, Tolboom J, Naber T, et al. D-lactic acidemia and aciduria in pediatric and adult patients with short bowel syndrome. Clin Chem 41:107, 1995.

98. Kaufman SS, Loseke CA, Lupo JV, et al. Influence of bacterial overgrowth and intestinal inflammation on duration of parenteral nutrition in children with short bowel syndrome. J Pediatr 131:356, 1997

99. Dellert SF, Nowicki MJ, Farrell MK, et al. The 13C-xylose breath test for the diagnosis of small bowel bacterial overgrowth in children. J Pediatr Gastroenterol Nutr 25:153, 1997.

100. Bianchi A. Intestinal lengthening: An experimental and clinical review. J R Soc Med 77:35, 1984.

101. Thompson JS, Vanderhoof JA, Antonson DI. Intestinal tapering and lengthening for the short bowel syndrome. J Pediatr Gastroenterol Nutr 4:495, 1985.

102. Figueroa-Colon R, Harris PR, Birdsong E, et al. Impact of intestinal lengthening on the nutritional outcome for children with short bowel syndrome. J Pediatr Surg 31:912,1996.

103. Saday C, Mir E. A surgical model to increase the intestinal absorptive surface: Intestinal lengthening and growing neomucosa in the same approach. J Surg Res 62:184, 1996.

104. Chaet MS, Farrell MK, Ziegler MM, Warner BW. Intensive nutritional support and remedial surgical intervention for extreme short bowel syndrome. J Pediatr Gastroenterol Nutr 19:295, 1994.

105. Warner BW, Chaet MS. Non transplant surgical options for management of the short bowel syndrome. J Pediatr Gastroenterol Nutr 17:1, 1993.

106. Wood RFM. International symposium on small bowel transplantation. Transplant Proc 22:2423, 1990.

107. Watson AJM, Lear PA. Current status of intestinal transplantation. Gut 30:1771, 1989.

108. Suita S, Masumoto K, Yamanouchi T, et al. Complications in neonates with short bowel syndrome and long-term parenteral nutrition. JPEN 23:S106, 1999.

109. Molleston JP. Acute and chronic liver disease. IN Walker WA and Watkins JB, eds. Nutrition in Pediatrics. Hamilton: BC Decker Inc, 1997; 568-569.

Nutritional Care for High-Risk Newborns (Rev. 3d. Ed.)
S. Groh-Wargo, M. Thompson, J. Cox, editors
© 2000, Precept Press, Inc., Chicago

29

OSTEOPENIA
OF
PREMATURITY

Susan K. Krug, MS, RD, LD

Introduction

Preterm infants frequently have decreased bone mass or osteopenia when compared with an intrauterine model.[1-3] This osteopenia of prematurity develops when supplies of mineral substrate are inadequate to maintain the normal remodeling, mineralization, and growth of bone.[4-7] The severity of osteopenia among preterm infants varies from mild demineralization to overt rickets and nontraumatic fractures.

Reports of severe osteopenia (rickets) of prematurity increased as survival of infants with birth weights of < 1,500 g improved. Several studies reported the presence of rickets in > 30% of very low birth weight (VLBW) infants surveyed.[8-11] Milder forms of osteopenia were present in an even greater number of VLBW infants.[9,10] These surveys were completed in nurseries using unfortified human milk, soy formula, or standard cow's milk-based formula as the routine feeding. Although controlled clinical trials using mineral-fortified feedings demonstrate improved bone mineralization,[12,13] no systematic surveys are available that evaluate the incidence of osteopenia among VLBW infants managed using parenteral and enteral feedings that optimize calcium and phosphorus intake.

Risk Factors

Fetal accretion rates for calcium (Ca) and phosphorus (P) increase throughout pregnancy, with maximal rates of Ca (120-150 mg/kg/day) and P (75-85 mg/kg/day) being achieved during the third trimester.[14-16] Preterm birth interrupts the maternal-fetal transfer of minerals, placing the infant at risk for osteopenia unless an adequate, alternate mineral supply is provided and maintained. The development and severity of osteopenia is influenced by the infant's mineral stores at birth, the mineral intake after birth, and alterations in mineral excretion associated with diet or medications.[3,8,11,17-25] Risk factors associated with the disorder are given in Table 29.1.

Clinical Findings

Osteopenia of prematurity is clinically silent. Many infants with mild osteopenia are not identified, and the condition spontaneously resolves over a period of several months with nutrition management.[11,26] Those with severe osteopenia often go undetected until nontraumatic fractures or rachitic respiratory distress develop.[27-29] Diagnosis of rickets usually occurs between 2 to 4 months chronological age. On clinical examination, craniotabes and frontal bossing are commonly found. Nontraumatic fractures of ribs or extremities may be present. Other rachitic features that have been reported include thickening of wrists and ankles, palpable enlargement of the costochondral junctions (rachitic rosary) and late onset respiratory distress associated with softening of the ribs with poor chest wall compliance.[7,11,17,21,27-29]

Impaired rates of linear growth have been reported among preterm infants with suspected osteopenia based on elevated peak plasma alkaline phosphatase values.[30,31] On follow-up at 9 and 18 months corrected age, this group of infants continued to have shorter lengths than a control group of preterm infants.[30]

Enamel hypoplasia has also been associated with osteopenia of prematurity. These changes, however, do not become apparent until the affected teeth erupt.[32]

Biochemical Findings

Infants with osteopenia of prematurity typically have low-normal or low serum P values.[5,8,22-24,33,34] Serum Ca levels may be low, normal, or high.[5,34-36] Concurrently, urinary P is low and urinary Ca is elevated.[5,22,23,33,36] Renal tubular reabsorption of P (TRP) increases to > 95%.[37] Although low levels of serum 25-hydroxyvitamin D (25-OH D) have been reported, values usually are within normal limits if infants are given daily doses of 160-400 IU vitamin D enterally or at least 25

Table 29.1. Risk Factors Associated with Osteopenia of Prematurity

< 34 wk gestation at birth*[2,11,17]
< 1,500 g birth weight*[11,17]

Delayed establishment of full enteral feedings
    Complicated neonatal course[8,11]
    Prolonged parenteral nutrition[11,18,20]

Use of enteral feedings with low mineral content/bioavailability
    Unsupplemented human milk[8,22,23]
    Soy-based infant formulas[8,24]
    Standard term milk-based formulas[12]

Chronic use of medications that increase mineral excretion
    Diuretics[11,21]
    Dexamethasone[25]
    Sodium bicarbonate[21]

Cholestatic jaundice[18,19,20]

* Risk for osteopenia increases with decreasing gestational age and/or birth weight.

IU/dl parenterally.[35,38-42] Serum 1,25-dihydroxyvitamin D (1,25-[OH]$_2$ D) levels are high or high-normal.[35,37,42-44] These laboratory findings indicate that preterm infants can absorb and hydroxylate enough vitamin D to maintain a normal status. Impaired bone mineralization results primarily from inadequate Ca and P intake. Low serum and urinary P with hypercalciuria suggest P to be the limiting nutrient. Reference values for biochemical measurements commonly used in evaluating infants for osteopenia are listed in Tables 29.2 and 29.3.

Serial measurement of serum or plasma alkaline phosphatase (AP) has been recommended for screening for osteopenia of prematurity.[48,52,53] AP values rise during periods of increased bone turnover and may reflect either growth or demineralization. In preterm infants, AP values up to five times the adult reference range are considered normal. Infants free of liver disease who have AP values greater than five times the adult reference range may have osteopenia and merit further evaluation.[48,52-55] However, normal or even low AP values may be present when rickets or fractures are diagnosed radiographically.[10,56] These seemingly contradictory findings may reflect the sequence of events. The rise in AP identifies the period in which remodeling of bone occurs; the X-ray measures the resulting structural changes when the AP level may have dropped.[5] Laboratory methods are now available to measure bone isoforms of alkaline phosphatase (BAP). The relationships between BAP and bone mineral content are similar to those reported for AP.[57,58]

The recent identification of markers for bone formation and resorption has renewed interest in finding biochemical indexes that will detect the presence of metabolic bone disease prior to the development of radiographic changes. Two commonly reported serum markers for bone formation include osteocalcin and carboxy-terminal propeptide of type I collagen (PICP),[57-59] and two markers for bone resorption include serum pyridinoline cross-linked telopeptide of type I collagen (ICTP) and urinary pyridinium (Pyd) cross-links.[59-60] Limited reference data for bone markers in preterm and term infants are currently available.[57,59] The reported confidence intervals for reference ranges in healthy subjects are broad, indicating a limited use in screening individuals. However, these markers will provide valuable information in longitudinal studies and have potential for identifying early response to treatment of metabolic bone disease.[57-61]

Radiographic Studies

Radiographs of the wrist or ankle, including the distal portion of the associated long bone, are used to verify the presence of rickets or fractures.[10,11,17,56] Milder forms of osteopenia can be detected through radiographs; several methods for scoring its severity based on radiographic changes have been described.[9,17,56] Radiographic evidence of impaired bone mineralization is often present by the end of the first month of life. In a retrospective review of 25 infants with birth weights of < 1,000 g, early radiographic changes representing demineralization in the metaphyses of long bones and in the margins of other bones were noted within the first 2 months of life (mean age: 24 days) of all infants studied. General demineralization was present in 67% of the infants by 2½ months (mean age: 40 days), and active rickets was identified in 44% by 3½ months (mean age: 83 days). Healing of rickets was noted to be present by 4 to 4½ months.[9] This progression of radiographic findings is consistent with a prospective follow-up study that reported resolution of rickets among affected infants between six months and one year chronological age.[11]

Bone mineral content (BMC) and bone mineral density (BMD) can be measured at specific sites using single photon absorptiometry (SPA) or dual energy x-ray absorptiometry (DXA).[3,62-64] DXA also is used to measure total body BMC and BMD, and equipment adapted for pediatric scans has been validated in infants as small as 2,000 g.[65-69] BMC and BMD measurements provide more sensitive assessments of bone mineral status than radiographic scoring.[12,13,70-74] Until recently, SPA and DXA have been used primarily for research. However, equipment for bone mineral assessment is becoming available for clinical care and can be useful in monitoring the progress of

Table 29.2.   Serum Laboratory Reference Values

Substance	Gestational age	Reference range
Calcium	Preterm[*]	8.3-10.5 mg/dl
	Term[†]	8.7-10.8 mg/dl
Phosphorus	Preterm[*]	4.7-8.5 mg/dl
	Term[†]	5.6-8.4 mg/dl
25-OH D[‡]		18-90 ng/ml
1,25-[OH]$_2$ D[‡]		13-117 pg/ml
Alkaline phosphatase[§]		< 5 times upper adult reference standard[ʃ]

[*]   Data for healthy, growing preterm infants ages 10-55 days[45]
[†]   Data for healthy term infants < 6 mo (mean ± 2 S.D.)[46]
[‡]   Data for healthy term infants < 6 mo (mean ± 2 S.D.)[47]
[§]   Standard for preterm infants[48]
[ʃ]   Reference values vary depending on methodology used. The adult reference standard for the colorimetric assay used at the University of Cincinnati Medical Center is 35-95 U/L.

infants with osteopenia. Data on small populations of term and preterm infants are now available for BMC and BMD measurements.[69,75-76]

When an estimate of bone mineral status is desired and these techniques are not available, the measurement of the cortical area of the humerus has been recommended as a simple, practical alternative.[9,77] This measurement provides more objective data than radiographic scoring and can be completed on a routine chest radiograph that includes the humerus.

Preventive Nutrition

The goal for health care providers is to prevent osteopenia of prematurity. Theoretically, this could be achieved by giving feedings that contain Ca and P at levels equivalent to in utero accretion rates within the first few days of life. However, neonatal complications and feeding intolerance frequently delay the provision of an adequate mineral intake.

Preterm infants often require total or partial parenteral nutrition (PN) during the first few days or weeks of life. The amount of Ca and P given parenterally is limited by the solubility of Ca and P salts.[78,79] Problems with precipitation result in Ca and P intakes below fetal accretion rates during PN feeding. The use of PN solutions containing up to 15 mM/L each of Ca and P (60 mg Ca/dl and 46.5 mg P/dl) has been shown to improve mineral status in preterm infants when compared to standard PN solutions containing 5 mM/L or less of Ca

Table 29.3. Urine Laboratory Reference Values

Substance	Feeding method	Reference values
Phosphorus*		Median (90% range)
	Breast	0.91 (0.03-4.00)mM/L
		0.094 (0.003-0.258) mM/kg/d
	Formula	8.01 (6.03-11.8) mM/L
		0.84 (0.62-1.35)mM/kg/d
Calcium*	Breast	1.45 (0.32-4.84) mM/L
		0.145 (0.040-0.342) mM/kg/d
	Formula	0.50 (0.20-2.10) mM/L
		0.062 (0.037-0.105) mM/kg/d
Urine calcium/creatinine ratio[†]		Median (95%ile)
< 7 mo		0.29 mg/mg (0.86 mg/mg)
7-18 mo		0.21 mg/mg (0.60 mg/mg)
Tubular reabsorption of phosphate (TRP)‡		85-90%

* Data for healthy term, male infants ages 1-6 mo.[45] Daily excretion rates are based on 72-hr balance studies.
† Data for healthy term infants based on spot urine collections.[49]
‡ Values > 95% are consistent with inadequate P intake.[50] Calculation for TRP (%)[51]: [1 – (urine P x plasma creatinine) / (urine creatinine x plasma P)] x 100

and P.[15,80-82] Therefore, the goal of PN for preterm infants should be to optimize Ca and P intake while avoiding precipitation of mineral salts (see Chapters 11 and 12 for additional information on Ca and P in PN).

Enteral nutrition (EN) provides the safest and most effective route for meeting Ca and P requirements. Human milk fortified with Ca and P and preterm infant formula have been shown to improve mineral retention and bone mineral status in VLBW infants.[12,70,83-89] A variety of methods and feedings are used to initiate EN in preterm infants, but once feeding tolerance has been demonstrated, fortified human milk or a preterm formula should be given.[90] Prolonged use of low-mineral formulas, including unfortified human milk and term infant formulas, increases the risk for osteopenia of prematurity.

Soy-based infant formulas are not recommended for preterm infants because of low bioavailability of Ca and P.[24] Ca and P supplementation of soy-based infant formula does improve mineral retention, but weight gain, serum protein and albumin, and energy efficiency remain higher among infants fed preterm formulas.[91] For preterm infants with lactose intolerance, adding a lactase preparation to preterm formula may provide an alternative to soy-based infant formula.[92]

Nutrient priming is an EN technique that introduces very small quantities of human milk or formula to even critically ill neonates within the first few days of life. Systematic, gradual advances in volume have been successful in promoting earlier tolerance of full EN without adverse consequences.[93-95] The early establishment of feedings provided by this technique has the potential to improve mineral intake among infants at highest risk for osteopenia.

The length of time preterm infants should be fed fortified human milk or preterm formula remains unresolved.[70,96-100] After hospital discharge, the rate of bone mineralization continues to be related to the mineral content of the milk or formula fed.[99-100] The transition to unsupplemented breast-feeding or standard infant formula at discharge may result in lower BMCs during the first year of life and is of particular concern among preterm infants discharged at weights < 1,800 grams. The recent introduction of preterm discharge formulas now enables clinicians to provide preterm infants a mineral-enriched feeding at home. A comparable study formula used until 9 months adjusted age promoted greater growth and bone mineralization than a standard infant formula.[100] For preterm infants with complex medical problems and prolonged hospitalizations, a prudent approach is to continue fortified human milk or preterm formula until a term weight of 3.0-3.5 kg is reached.[101] At that time, a preterm discharge formula or lower level of human milk fortification may be recommended.

Providing 160-400 IU vitamin D/day is adequate to maintain a normal vitamin D status among preterm infants.[35,38,40,119] Supplementing up to 2,000 IU/day has not been effective in reducing the incidence of osteopenia.[41,56]

Studies evaluating long-term bone mineralization outcomes in preterm infants are positive. By age 2 years, the BMCs of former preterm infants fed unsupplemented human milk after hospital discharge were comparable to those of infants fed standard infant formula posthospitalization.[102] Former preterm infants evaluated at ages 3 and older had BMCs similar to those of age-matched controls.[103-104] Higher intakes of human milk have been associated with higher BMCs at age 5 years.[105] Further investigation of this latter unexpected outcome is in progress.

Treatment Nutrition

Even with a well-designed preventive program, cases of severe osteopenia may still occur.[34,106] Screening for osteopenia can be incor-

Table 29.4.   Monitoring During Treatment of Nutritional Rickets in Very Low Birth Weight Infants

Test	Frequency
Serum	
Ca, P, Na, K, creatinine	One or twice/wk
Urine	
Ca, P, creatinine	Once or twice/wk
Acid/base status	Weekly
Serum	
25-OH D	Monthly
1,25-[OH]2 D	Once every 1-3 mo
X-ray films	
Wrists or knees	Once every 1-3 mo
Other sites	Upon clinical indication

Reprinted with permission from Koo and Tsang and Mosby Year Book.[107]

porated into routine neonatal care through biweekly measurement of serum Ca, P, and AP and bimonthly forearm X-rays.[106] Screening is particularly important for infants with three or more risk factors (Table 29.1) associated with osteopenia of prematurity. When screening identifies an infant to be at risk for osteopenia, measurement of urinary mineral excretion, serum 25-OH D and 1,25-[OH]$_2$ D, and bone mineral content, if available, should be considered. Infants requiring treatment need regular monitoring to determine effectiveness and duration of therapy. Monitoring guidelines are outlined in Table 29.4.

Infants with severe osteopenia who weigh < 3.5 kg are treated by advancing to or continuing feedings of fortified human milk or preterm formula.[34,106] When these feedings are not available, tolerated, or desired for other medical or nutritional reasons, daily supplementation with 100 mg/kg Ca and 50 mg/kg P in divided doses should be sufficient to promote improved mineralization.[107,108] Intakes of 400 IU vitamin D are adequate for infants with normal levels of serum 25-OH D.

Calcium additives commonly used for supplementation include calcium gluconate, calcium lactate, calcium gluceptate, and calcium glubionate. Phosphorus is given in the form of mono- or dibasic salts of potassium phosphate or sodium phosphate.[107,109] The supplements selected may vary depending on availability, osmolality, solubility, and fluid limitations. The use of Ca and P supplements is not without risk. Serum mineral or electrolyte status can be altered, and intestinal obstruction has been associated with Ca supplementation of enteral feedings.[110-111] Acidosis has occurred in response to phosphate supplementation.[107,109] To minimize problems, incremental advancement of supplements, beginning at 50% of the target dose, is recommended. Infants should be carefully monitored for acid/base, serum mineral and electrolyte status as well as G.I. tolerance. Supplementation should be based on each infant's response to therapy.

For the PN-fed infant with osteopenia, the Ca and P content of the PN solution should be at maximum. EN should be introduced as soon as medically safe, with advancement to mineral-fortified feedings made as tolerated. Evaluation for aluminum toxicity should be considered in infants with osteopenia who have been on long-term PN (see Chapter 11).[112,113]

Caution should be used when supplementing Ca and P in infants receiving chronic diuretic therapy. Furosemide, as well as spironolactone and chlorothiazides, has been associated with increased urinary calcium excretion.[114,115] High urinary Ca places infants at risk for developing nephrocalcinosis.[114,116-118] Periodic renal ultrasonography and monitoring of urinary excretion of Ca are suggested.

Treatment for osteopenia of prematurity continues until biochemical indexes are normal and radiographic evidence of healing is present. At that time, infants are changed to a standard infant diet for age; a preterm discharge formula may be recommended. Follow-up evaluation of mineral status is recommended to ensure that therapy has been adequate.

Case Study

JM was a 750 g girl born at 26 weeks' gestation by dates and clinical examination. She required mechanical ventilation for the first 20 days of life; supplemental oxygen by nasal cannula was required until 60 days. Furosemide was given at a dose of 1 mg/kg on six occasions.

PN was started on day of life (DOL) 2 and continued until DOL 25. PN solutions containing Ca and P each at 5 mM/L provided an average volume of 160 ml/kg/day prior to initiation of enteral feeding. Feedings of human milk were started on DOL 15. Feeding volume was gradually advanced to 100 ml/kg/day by DOL 25 and maintained between 160-180 ml/kg/day after DOL 35. A multivitamin containing 400 IU vitamin D was started on DOL 25. At age 75 days, JM was noted to have pain and swelling in her left arm. On X-ray she was found to have a fractured left radius. Wrist X-rays were diagnostic for rickets. Laboratory studies were consistent with osteopenia of prematurity: Ca = 9.4 mg/dl, P = 3.2 mg/dl, AP = 680 U/L (nl: < 480 U/L), 25-OH D = 48 ng/ml, 1,25-[OH]2 D = 98 pg/ml, urine Ca = 5.0 mM/L, urine P = 0.02 mM/L. Her weight at diagnosis was 1,935 g.

Treatment consisted of splinting her left arm and fortifying her human milk feedings with Similac Natural Care (Ross Products Division, Abbott Laboratories, Columbus, Ohio) at the standard ratio of 50:50. Feeding volume was adjusted as needed to maintain an intake of 150-170 ml/kg/day providing about 155-175 mg Ca/kg/day and 80-90 mg P/kg/day. Vitamin D supplementation was given as 0.5 ml/day Vidaylin ADC Vitamins + iron to provide a total intake of about 400 IU/day. After two weeks of therapy, JM was discharged home. At this time, her growth measurements were: weight, 2,500 g; length, 44 cm; and head circumference, 33 cm. Laboratory values were Ca = 9.7 mg/dl, P = 5.6 mg/dl, AP = 430 U/L, urine Ca = 1.9 mM/L, P = 0.7 mM/L. Her diet consisted of breast-feeding on demand, with 200 ml Similac Natural Care given daily by using a nursing supplementer/training device. Dietary therapy continued until JM was six months old (adjusted age). At that time, radiographs showed complete healing of her fracture and rickets, and all laboratory indexes were within the normal range for age.

References

1. Steichen JJ, Gratton TL, Tsang RC. Osteopenia of prematurity: The cause and possible treatment. J Pediatr 96:528, 1980.
2. Greer FR, McCormick A. Bone growth with low bone mineral content in very low birth weight premature infants. Pediatr Res 20:925, 1986.
3. Lyon AJ, Hawkes DJ, Doran M, et al. Bone mineralization in preterm infants measured by dual energy radiographic densitometry. Arch Dis Child 64:919, 1989.
4. Koo WWK, Steichen JJ. Osteopenia and rickets of prematurity. In: Polin SA, Fox WW, eds. Fetal and Neonatal Physiology. Philadelphia: Saunders, 1998; 2335.
5. Bishop N. Bone disease in preterm infants. Arch Dis Child 64:1403, 1989.
6. Bishop NJ. Nutritional management of bone mineralization and metabolic bone disease. Semin Neonatol 1:11, 1996.
7. Mayne, PD, Kovar IZ. Calcium and phosphorus metabolism in the premature infant. Ann Clin Biochem 28:131, 1991.
8. Callenbach JC, Sheehan MB, Abramson SJ, et al. Etiologic factors in rickets of very low birthweight infants. J. Pediatr 98:800, 1981.
9. Masel JP, Tudehope D, Cartwright D, et al. Osteopenia and rickets in the extremely low-birth-weight infant—a survey of the incidence and a radiological classification. Australas Radiol 26:83, 1982.
10. Lyon AJ, McIntosh N, Wheeler K, et al. Radiological rickets in extremely low birthweight infants. Pediatr Radiol 17:56, 1987.

11. Koo WWK, Sherman R, Succop P, et al. Fractures and rickets in very low birthweight infants: Conservative management and outcome. J Pediatr Orthop 9:326, 1989.
12. Greer FR, Steichen JJ, Tsang RC. Effect of increased calcium, phosphorus and vitamin D intake on bone mineralization in very low birth weight infants fed formula with Polycose and medium-chain triglycerides. J Pediatr 100:951, 1982.
13. Horsman A, Ryan SW, Congdon PJ, et al. Bone mineral accretion rate and calcium intake in preterm infants. Arch Dis Child 64:910, 1989.
14. Ziegler E, O'Donnel A, Nelson S, et al. Body composition of the reference fetus. Growth 40:329, 1976.
15. Forbes G. Calcium accumulation by the human fetus. Pediatrics 57:976, 1976.
16. Shaw JCL. Parenteral nutrition in the management of sick low birthweight infants. Pediatr Clin North Am 20:333, 1973.
17. Koo WWK, Gupta JM, Nayanar VV, et al. Skeletal changes in preterm infants. Arch Dis Child 57:447, 1982.
18. Amir J, Katz K, Grunebaum M, et al. Fractures in premature infants. J Pediatr Orthop 8:41, 1988.
19. Thomas PS, Glasgow JFT. Bone disease in infants with prolonged obstructive jaundice. Pediatr Radiol 2:125, 1974.
20. Toomey F, Hoag R, Batton D, et al. Rickets associated with cholestasis and parenteral nutrition in premature infants. Radiology 142:85, 1982.
21. Chudley AE, Brown DR, Holzman IR, et al. Nutritional rickets in 2 very low birthweight infants with chronic lung disease. Arch Dis Child 55:687, 1980.
22. Sagy M, Birenbaum E, Balin A, et al. Phosphate-depletion syndrome in a premature infant fed human milk. J Pediatr 96:683, 1980.
23. Rowe J, Rowe D, Horak E, et al. Hypophosphatemia and hypercalciuria in small premature infants fed human milk: evidence for inadequate dietary phosphorus. J Pediatr 104:112, 1984.
24. Shenai JP, Jhaveri BM, Reynolds JW, et al. Nutrition balance studies in very low birthweight infants: role of soy formula. Pediatrics 67:631, 1981.
25. Weiler HA, Wang Z, Atkinson SA. Dexamethasone treatment impairs calcium regulation and reduces bone mineralization in infant pigs. Am J Clin Nutr 61:805, 1995.
26. Congdon PJ, Horsman A, Ryan SW, et al. Spontaneous resolution of bone mineral depletion in preterm infants. Arch Dis Child 65:1038, 1990.
27. Geggel RL, Pereira GR, Spackman TJ. Fractured ribs, unusual presentation of rickets in premature infants. J Pediatr 93:680, 1978.
28. Gefter WB, Epstein DM, Anday EK, et al. Rickets presenting as multiple fractures in premature infants on hyperalimentation. Radiology 142:371, 1982.
29. Glasgow JFT, Thomas PS. Rachitic respiratory distress in small preterm infants. Arch Dis Child 52:268, 1977.
30. Lucas A, Brooke OG, Baker BA, et al. High alkaline phosphatase activity and growth in preterm neonates. Arch Dis Child 64:902, 1989.
31. James JA, Mayne PD, Barnes IC, et al. Growth velocity and plasma alkaline phosphatase activity in the preterm infant. Early Hum Dev 11:27, 1985.

32. Seow WK, Masel JP, Weir C, et al. Mineral deficiency in the pathogenesis of enamel hypoplasia in prematurely born, very low birthweight children. Pediatric Dent 11:297, 1989.

33. Lyon AJ, McIntosh N. Calcium and phosphorus balance in extremely low birthweight infants in the first six weeks of life. Arch Dis Child 59:1145, 1984.

34. Cooke RJ. Rickets in a very low birth weight infant. J Pediatr Gastroenterol Nutr 9:397, 1989.

35. Koo WWK, Sherman R, Succop P, et al. Serum vitamin D metabolites in very low birthweight infants with and without rickets and fractures. J Pediatr 114:1017, 1989.

36. Lyon AJ, McIntosh N, Wheeler K, et al. Hypercalcaemia in extremely low birthweight infants. Arch Dis Child 59:1141, 1984.

37. Koo WWK, Tsang RC, Succop P, et al. Minimal vitamin D and high calcium and phosphorus needs of preterm infants receiving parenteral nutrition. J Pediatr Gastroenterol Nutr 8:225, 1989.

38. Koo WWK, Krug-Wispe S, Neylan M, et al. Effect of three levels of vitamin D intake in preterm infants receiving high mineral-containing milk. J Pediatr Gastroenterol Nutr 21:182, 1995.

39. Hillman LS, Hoff N, Salmons S, et al. Mineral homeostasis in very premature infants: Serial evaluation of serum 25-hydroxyvitamin D, serum minerals, and bone mineralization. J Pediatr 106:970, 1985.

40. Cooke R, Hollis B, Conner C, et al. Vitamin D and mineral metabolism in the very low birth weight infant receiving 400 IU of vitamin D. J Pediatr 116:423, 1990.

41. Robinson MJ, Merrett AL, Tetlow VA, et al. Plasma 25-hydroxyvitamin D concentrations in preterm infants receiving oral vitamin D supplements. Arch Dis Child 56:144, 1981.

42. Huston RK, Reynolds JW, Jensen C, et al. Nutrient and mineral retention and vitamin D absorption in low-birth-weight infants: Effect of medium-chain triglycerides. Pediatrics 72:44, 1983.

43. Steichen JJ, Tsang RC, Greer FR, et al. Elevated serum 1,25 dihydroxyvitamin D concentrations in rickets of very low-birth-weight infants. J Pediatr 99:293, 1981.

44. Markestad T, Aksnes L, Finne PH, et al. Plasma concentrations of vitamin D metabolites in premature infants. Pediatr Res 18:269, 1984.

45. Meites S, ed. Pediatric clinical chemistry reference (normal) values, 3d ed. Washington, D.C.: American Association for Clinical Chemistry Press, 1989; 85-86, 219-20.

46. Specker BL, Lichtenstein P, Mimouni F, et al. Calcium-regulating hormones and minerals from birth to 18 months of age: A cross-sectional study. II. Effects of sex, race, age, season and diet on serum minerals, parathyroid hormone and calcitonin. Pediatrics 77:891, 1986.

47. Lichtenstein P, Specker BL, Tsang RC, et al. Calcium-regulating hormones and minerals from birth to 18 months of age: A cross-sectional study. I. Effects of sex, race, age, season and diet on vitamin D status. Pediatrics 77:883, 1986.

48. Kovar I, Mayne P, Barltrop D. Plasma alkaline phosphatase activity: A screening test for rickets in preterm neonates. Lancet 1:308, 1982.

49. Sargent JD, Stukel TA, Kresel J, et al. Normal values for random urinary calcium to creatinine ratios in infancy. J Pediatr 123:393, 1993.

50. Koo WWK, Tsang RC. Calcium, magnesium and phosphorus. In: Tsang RC, ed. Nutrition in Infancy. Philadelphia: Hanley and Belfus, 1988; 175.
51. Dalton RN, Haycock GB. Laboratory investigation. In: Holliday MA, Barratt TM, Avner ED, eds. Pediatric Nephrology. 3rd ed. Baltimore: Williams & Wilkins, 1994; 414.
52. Walters EG, Murphy JF, Henry P, et al. Plasma alkaline phosphatase activity and its relation to rickets in pre-term infants. Ann Clin Biochem 23:652, 1986.
53. Crofton PM, Hume R. Alkaline phosphatase isoenzymes in the plasma of preterm and term infants: Serial measurements and clinical correlation. Clin Chem 33:1783, 1987.
54. Koo WWK, Succop P, Hambidge M. Serum alkaline phosphatase and serum zinc concentrations in preterm infants with rickets and fractures. Am J Dis Child 143:1342, 1989.
55. Ryan SW, Truscott J, Simpson M, et al. Phosphate, alkaline phosphatase and bone mineralization in preterm neonates. Acta Paediatr 82:518, 1993.
56. Evans JR, Allen AC, Stinson DA, et al. Effect of high-dose vitamin D supplementation on radiographically detectable bone disease of very low birth weight infants. J Pediatr 115:779, 1989.
57. Pittard WB, Geddes KM, Hulsey TC, et al. Osteocalcin, skeletal alkaline phosphatase, and bone mineral content in very low birth weight infants: A longitudinal assessment. Pediatr Res 31:181, 1992.
58. Panteghini M, Pagani F. Biological variation in bone-derived biochemical markers in serum. Scand J Clin Lab Invest 55:609, 1995.
59. Lieuw-a-Fa M, Sierra RL, Specker BL. Carboxy-terminal propeptide of human type I collagen and pyridinium cross-links as markers of bone growth in infants 1 to 18 months of age. J Bone Miner Res 10:849, 1995.
60. Eriksen EF, Charles P, Melsen F, et al. Serum markers of type I collagen formation and degradation in metabolic bone disease: correlation and bone histomorphometry. J Bone Miner Res 8:127, 1993.
61. Demers LM. Clinical usefulness of markers of bone degradation and formation. Scand J Clin Lab Invest 57 (suppl 227):12, 1997.
62. Minton SD, Steichen JJ, Tsang RC. Bone mineral content in term and preterm appropriate-for-gestational-age infants. J Pediatr 95:1037, 1979.
63. Greer FR, Lane J, Weiner S, et al. An accurate and reproducible absorptiometric technique for determining bone mineral content in newborn infants. Pediatr Res 17:259, 1983.
64. Mimouni F, Tsang RC. Bone mineral content: Data analysis. J Pediatr 113:178, 1988.
65. Chan GM. Performance of dual-energy x-ray absorptiometry in evaluating bone, lean body mass, and fat in pediatric subjects. J Bone Miner Res 7:369, 1992.
66. Brunton JA, Bayley HS, Atkinson SA. Validation and application of dual-energy x-ray absorptiometry to measure bone mass and body composition in small infants. Am J Clin Nutr 58:839, 1993.
67. Koo WWK, Walter J, Bush AJ. Technical considerations of dual-energy x-ray absorptiometry-based bone mineral measurement for pediatric studies. J Bone Miner Res 10:1998, 1995.

68. Koo WWK, Massom LR, Walters J. Validation of accuracy and precision of dual energy x-ray absorptiometry for infants. J Bone Miner Res 10:1111, 1995.

69. Picaud JC, Rigo J, Nyamugabo K, et al. Evaluation of dual-energy x-ray absorptiometry for body-composition assessment in piglets and term human neonates. Am J Clin Nutr 63:157, 1996.

70. Abrams SA, Schanler RJ, Garza C. Bone mineralization in former very low birthweight infants fed either human milk or commercial formula. J Pediatr 112:956, 1988.

71. Pettifor JM, Rajah R, Venter A, et al. Bone mineralization and mineral homeostasis in very low-birth-weight infants fed either human milk or fortified human milk. J Pediatr Gastroenterol Nutr 8:217, 1989.

72. Schanler RJ, Abrams S, Sheng H. Mineral status in preterm infants as measured by single photon absorptiometry. In: Yasumura S, ed. Advances in in vivo Body Composition Studies. New York: Plenum Press, 1990; 39.

73. Koo WWK, Sherman R, Succop P, et al. Sequential bone mineral content in small preterm infants with and without fractures and rickets. J Bone Miner Res 3:193, 1988.

74. James JR, Congdon PJ, Truscott J, et al. Osteopenia of prematurity. Arch Dis Child 61:871, 1986.

75. Lapillonne AA, Glorieux FH, Salle BL, et al. Mineral balance and whole body bone mineral content in very low-birth-weight infants. Acta Paediatr Suppl 405:117, 1994.

76. Koo WWK, Bush AJ, Walters J, et al. Postnatal development of bone mineral status during infancy. J Am Coll Nutr 17:65, 1998.

77. Poznanski AK, Kuhns LR, Guire KE. New standards of cortical mass in the humerus of neonates: A means of evaluating bone loss in the premature infant. Pediatr Radiol 134:639, 1980.

78. Eggert LD, Rusho WJ, MacKay MW. Calcium and phosphorus compatibility in parenteral nutrition solutions for neonates. Am J Hosp Pharm 39:49, 1982.

79. Dunham B, Marcuard S, Khazanie PG, et al. The solubility of calcium and phosphorus in neonatal total parenteral nutrition solutions. J Parenter Enter Nutr 15:608, 1991.

80. Koo WWK, Hollis BW, Horn J, et al. Stability of vitamin D2, calcium, magnesium, and phosphorus in parenteral nutrition solution: Effect of in-line filter. J Pediatr 108:478, 1986.

81. MacMahon P, Blair ME, Treweeke P, et al. Association of mineral composition of neonatal intravenous feeding solutions and metabolic bone disease of prematurity. Arch Dis Child 64:489, 1989.

82. Prestidge LL, Schanler RJ, Shulman RJ, et al. Effect of parenteral calcium and phosphorus therapy on mineral retention and bone mineral content in very low birth weight infants. J Pediatr 122:761, 1993.

83. Shenai JP, Reynolds JW, Babson SG. Nutritional balance studies in very-low-birth-weight infants: Enhanced nutrient retention rates by an experimental formula. Pediatrics 66:233, 1980.

84. Rowe JC, Goetz CA, Carey DE, et al. Achievement of in utero retention of calcium and phosphorus accompanied by high calcium excretion in very low birth weight infants fed a fortified formula. J Pediatr 110:581, 1987.

85. Raschko PK, Hiller JL, Benda GI, et al. Nutritional balance studies of VLBW infants fed their mothers' milk fortified with a liquid human milk fortifier. J Pediatr Gastroenterol Nutr 9:212, 1989.

86. Moyer-Mileur L, Chan GM, Gill G. Evaluation of liquid or powdered fortification of human milk on growth and bone mineralization status of preterm infants. J Pediatr Gastroenterol Nutr 15:370, 1992.

87. Itabashi K, Hayashi T, Tsugoshi T, et al. Fortified preterm human milk for very low birth weight infants. Early Hum Dev 29:339, 1992.

88. Schanler RJ, Abrams SA. Postnatal attainment of intrauterine macromineral accretion rates in low birth weight infants fed fortified human milk. J Pediatr 126:441, 1995.

89. Pohlandt F. Prevention of postnatal bone demineralization in very low-birth-weight infants by individually monitored supplementation with calcium and phosphorus. Pediatr Res 35:125, 1994.

90. Churella HR, Bachhuber WL, MacLean WC. Survey: Methods of feeding low-birth-weight infants. Pediatrics 76:243, 1985.

91. Hall RT, Callenbach JC, Sheehan MB, et al. Comparison of calcium- and phosphorus-supplemented soy isolate formula with whey-predominant premature formula in very low birth weight infants. J Pediatr Gastroenterol Nutr 3:571, 1984.

92. Carlson SJ, Rogers RR, Lombard KA. Effect of a lactase preparation on lactose content and osmolality of preterm and term infant formulas. J Parenter Enter Nutr 15:564, 1991.

93. Dunn L, Hulman S, Weiner J, et al. Beneficial effects of early hypocaloric enteral feeding on neonatal gastrointestinal function: Preliminary report of a randomized trial. J Pediatr 112:622, 1988.

94. Slagle TA, Gross SJ. Effect of early low-volume enteral substrate on subsequent feeding tolerance in very low birth weight infants. J Pediatr 113:526, 1988.

95. Meetze WH, Valentine C, McGuigan JE, et al. Gastrointestinal priming prior to full enteral nutrition in very low birth weight infants. J Pediatr Gastroenterol Nutr 15:163, 1992.

96. Raupp P, von Kries R, Schmiedlau D, et al. Biochemical evidence for the need of long-term mineral supplementation in an extremely low birth weight infant fed own mother's milk exclusively during the first 6 months of life. Eur J Pediatr 149:806, 1990.

97. Hall RT, Wheeler RE, Montalto MB, et al. Hypophosphatemia in breast-fed low-birth-weight infants following initial hospital discharge. Am J Dis Child 143:1191, 1989.

98. Abrams SA, Schanler RJ, Tsang RC, et al. Bone mineralization in former very low birth weight infants fed either human milk or commercial formula: One year follow-up observation. J Pediatr 114:1041, 1989.

99. Chan, GM. Growth and bone mineral status of discharged very low birth weight infants fed different formulas or human milk. J Pediatr 123:439, 1993.

100. Bishop NJ, King FJ, Lucas A. Increased bone mineral content of preterm infant fed with a nutrient enriched formula after discharge from hospital. Arch Dis Child 68:573, 1993.

101. Koo WWK, Tsang RC. Mineral requirements of low-birth-weight infants. J Am Coll Nutr 10:474, 1991.

102. Schanler RJ, Burns PA, Abrams SA, et al. Bone mineralization outcomes in human milk-fed preterm infants. Pediatr Res 31:583, 1992.

103. Hori C, Tsukahara H, Fujii Y, et al. Bone mineral status in preterm-born children: assessment by dual-energy x-ray absorptiometry. Biol Neonate 68:254, 1995.

104. Rubinacci A, Sirtori P, Moro G, et al. Is there an impact of birth weight and early life nutrition on bone mineral content in preterm born infants and children? Acta Paediatr 82:711, 1993.

105. Bishop NJ, Dahlenburg SL, Fewtrell MS, et al. Early diet of preterm infants and bone mineralization at age five years. Acta Paediatr 85:230, 1996.

106. Koo WWK, Oestreich A, Sherman R, et al. Failure of high calcium and phosphorus supplementation in the prevention of rickets of prematurity. Am J Dis Child 140:857, 1986.

107. Koo WWK, Tsang RC. Rickets in infants. In: Nelson NM, ed. Current Therapy in Neonatal-Perinatal Medicine. vol. 2. Philadelphia: B. C. Decker, 1990; 353.

108. Greer FR, Steichen JJ, Tsang RC. Calcium and phosphate supplements in breast milk-related rickets: Results in a very-low-birth-weight infant. Am J Dis Child 136:581, 1982.

109. Atkinson SA. Calcium, phosphorus and vitamin D needs of low birth-weight infants on various feedings. Acta Paediatr Scand (suppl) 351:104, 1989.

110. Cleghorn GJ, Tudehope DI. Neonatal intestinal obstruction associated with oral calcium supplementation. Aust Paediatr J 17:298, 1981.

111. Koletzko B, Tangemann R, von Kries R, et al. Intestinal milk-bolus obstruction in formula fed premature infants given high doses of calcium. J Pediatr Gastroenterol Nutr 7:548, 1988.

112. Sedman AB, Klein GL, Merritt RJ, et al. Evidence of aluminum loading in infants receiving intravenous therapy. New Engl J Med 312:1337, 1985.

113. Koo WWK, Kaplan LA, Krug-Wispe SK, et al. Response of preterm infants to aluminum in parenteral nutrition. J Parenter Enter Nutr 13:516, 1989.

114. Hufnagle KG, Khan SN, Penn D, et al. Renal calcifications: A complication of long-term furosemide therapy in preterm infants. Pediatrics 70:360, 1982.

115. Atkinson SA, Shah JK, McGee C, et al. Mineral excretion in premature infants receiving various diuretic therapies. J Pediatr 113:540, 1988.

116. Jacinto JS, Modanlou HD, Crade M, et al. Renal calcification incidence in very low birth weight infants. Pediatrics 81:31, 1988.

117. Ezzedeen F, Adelman RD, Ahlfors CE. Renal calcification in preterm infants: Pathophysiology and long-term sequelae. J Pediatr 113:532, 1988.

118. Rowe JC, Carey DE, Goetz CA, et al. Effect of high calcium and phosphorus intake on mineral retention in very low birth weight infants chronically treated with furosemide. J Pediatr Gastroenterol Nutr 9:206, 1989.

119. Backstrom MC, Maki R, Kuusela A-L, et al. Randomised controlled trial of vitamin D supplementation on bone density and biochemical indices in preterm infants. Arch Dis Child Fetal Neonatal Ed. 80:F161, 1999.

Bibliography

American Academy of Pediatrics Committee on Nutrition. Calcium requirements of infants, children, and adolescents. Pediatr 104:1152, 1999.

Feark J, Petersen S, Peitersen B, et al. Diet and bone mineral content at term in premature infants. Pediatr Res 47:148, 2000.

Fewtrell MS, Prentice A, Cole TJ, et al. Effects of growth during infancy and childhood on bone mineralization and turnover in preterm children aged 8-12 years. Acta Paediatr 89:148, 2000.

Kurl S, Heinonen K, Lansimies E, et al. Determinants of bone mineral density in prematurely born children aged 6-7 years. Acta Paediatr 87:650, 1998.

Narbona E, Maldonade J, Ocete E, et al. Bone mineralization status measured by dual energy radiographic densitometry in preterm infants fed commercial formulas. Early Hum Develop 53:S173, 1998.

Nutritional Care for High-Risk Newborns (Rev. 3d. Ed.)
S. Groh-Wargo, M. Thompson, J. Cox, editors
© 2000, Precept Press, Inc., Chicago

30

RENAL DYSFUNCTION

Nancy S. Spinozzi, RD

RENAL DYSMATURITY, CONGENITAL RENAL anomalies, and postnatally acquired renal dysfunction resulting in both acute and chronic renal insufficiency are encountered in the neonatal population. Fluid, electrolyte, and nutritional consequences of these disorders require specific nutritional therapy.

Renal Dysmaturity

Decreased glomerular filtration and tubular resorption and a decreased glucose threshold are associated with prematurity.[1] These alterations in renal function result in increased renal losses of water and nutrients, including sodium, bicarbonate, and glucose. Frequently, the ability to excrete nitrogenous waste and potassium is decreased. Preterm infants are therefore at risk for dehydration and its metabolic sequelae-hyponatremia, metabolic acidosis, mild azotemia, hyperkalemia, and renal wasting of nutrients. These acute complications may require treatment initially, but resolve as renal function improves with increasing postnatal and gestational age. Very low birth weight (VLBW) infants may be at greater risk of developing "late hyponatremia" or hyponatremia that develops beyond the first two weeks of life due to immature renal function and low sodium intake.[2] VLBW infants who are fed human milk, even when fortifier is added, receive 30 to 45% less sodium than those fed

---

The contributions of Jean B. Crouch, MPh, RD, CNSD to this chapter in the previous edition are gratefully acknowledged.

premature infant formula, and may require additional sodium supplementation.[2]

The most common method to assess glomerular filtration rate (GFR) in the newborn is by calculation of creatinine clearance. The formula for making this calculation is as follows:

$$CrCl\ (ml/min/1.73m^2) = K \times Length\ (cm)/P_{Cr}$$

[CrCl = cratinin clearance; K =0.34 in premature infants $\leq$ 34 weeks' gestation and 0.44 in infants 35 weeks to term; P_{Cr} = plasma creatinine (mg/dl).]

GFR doubles from birth to two weeks of age, increases to more than half the adult level by two months of age, and reaches maturity by about 2 years of age.[3]

Acute Renal Insufficiency

Acute renal insufficiency is characterized by renal tubular damage and/or a severe decrease in glomerular filtration rate (GFR).[4] Acute impairment of renal function in this patient population is most commonly related to asphyxia, sepsis, advanced dehydration, renal vein/artery thrombosis, and medication-induced injury (including indomethacin, gentamicin, and amphotericin).[5] Typical symptomatology includes oliguria or anuria, azotemia, hyperkalemia, hyperphosphatemia, edema, hypertension, and altered sodium, chloride, and acid/base balance. Urine output, < 1ml/kg/hour over 12 hours occurring after the first 24 hours of life may indicate the presence of oliguria. Nonoliguric renal failure is usually detected by a rapid rise in serum creatinine, which fails to decline below maternal levels or a serum creatinine > 1.5 mg/dl.[6]

Chronic Renal Insufficiency

The incidence of chronic renal insufficiency (CRI) in children is equally divided between congenital and acquired etiologies.[7] In neonates, the predominant diagnoses include renal hypoplasia, renal dysplasia, and obstructive uropathy. CRI may be acquired as the result of asphyxia, vascular accidents, or hypotension.

The usual consequences of CRI are similar to those of acute renal insufficiency but also include anemia, renal osteodystrophy, anorexia resulting in undernutrition, and growth failure. Most of these abnormalities adversely affect growth; it is essential that they be identified early and managed aggressively.[8-10] Growth delay is evident in > 50% of children when CRI is first noted, especially if renal impairment began prior to the first birthday.[11]

Other Renal Disorders

Hypertension and nephrocalcinosis are two additional renal disorders that may arise in the neonate. Hypertension in young infants may be the result of renal vascular disorders, coarctation of the aorta, bronchopulmonary dysplasia, extracorporeal membrane oxygenation, or endocrine or seizure disorders. Hypertension may also result from methylxanthine, steroid, or pancuronium use.[12] Irritability, tachypnea, diarrhea, and vomiting have been associated with infantile hypertension. Although these associated symptoms may have some nutritional consequences, hypertension is generally treated with antihypertensive medication, not dietary modification.[5]

Hypercalciuria is common in very low birth weight (VLBW) infants.[13-15] The reported incidence of nephrocalcinosis (calcium deposits within the renal parenchyma) in VLBW infants varies widely.[14] Although hypercalciuria does not always lead to nephrocalcinosis, several factors may increase the occurrence of both of these findings in sick, VLBW infants. These factors include immature renal function, decreased GFR, low citrate excretion, increased urine alkalinity, hypervitaminosis D, phosphorus deficiency, and acid/base disturbances. Furosemide, xanthines, and glucocorticoids have been shown to increase calcium excretion in this population and may significantly increase the risk of stone formation.[15] Acute complications of nephrocalcinosis may include hematuria, urinary tract infections, and pain. Although nephrocalcinosis may resolve spontaneously over time, calcifications may persist beyond infancy. Irreversible renal compromise, including hypertension and tubular dysfunction, has been reported.[13,15]

Preventive Nutrition

Although renal insufficiency is generally a result of factors unrelated to nutrition, it may arise as a consequence of severe dehydration. There is wide individual variation in renal function and fluid losses in the first one to two weeks of life, particularly in extreme prematurity. Close monitoring is central to nutrition management. Important parameters in monitoring fluid, electrolyte, and renal function include daily weight change, serum and urine electrolytes, and fluid intake and output. Monitoring can be simplified as renal function and metabolic stability improve with increasing age.

A weight loss of > 2-5% over 24 hours suggests a fluid deficit, as does hypernatremia in the face of negative fluid and sodium balance.[16] The estimated insensible fluid losses shown in Table 30.1 and urine output are subtracted from fluid intake to determine fluid balance. Sodium balance is determined by comparing sodium intake to urine sodium loss. These determinations are also useful in assessing hyponatremia and sodium deficit or overload, as well as fluid overload, which is characterized by congestive heart failure, pulmonary edema, hypertension, and weight gain. The newborn's water compartment, through which sodium is distributed, represents about 80% of body weight and is used as a factor in calculating the total body sodium deficit (0.8 x weight). In older infants and children, this compartment drops to 60-70% of body weight (0.6-0.7 x weight). The total body sodium (Na^+) deficit can be estimated using the equation: Na^+ deficit (mEq) = 0.8 x wt (kg) x [desired serum Na^+ (mEq/dl) – actual serum Na^+ (mEq/dl)].[6,16] To avoid rapid osmotic and hemodynamic shifts, the deficit should be replaced gradually.

Nutrition management is one important factor in minimizing the potential for nephrocalcinosis. As skeletal growth correlates with linear growth, so do calcium and phosphorus intake. Prevention of nephrocalcinosis includes enhancement of growth and determination and provision of appropriate intakes of calcium and phosphorus. Vitamin D excess, which may induce hypercalemia and hypercalciuria, must be avoided. Electrolyte and acid/base balance must be maintained. Monitoring the urine calcium–creatinine ratio in patients at increased risk for nephrocalcinosis may provide early detection of individual infants who may need dietary manipulation. Infants with urine calcium–creatinine ratios of > 0.2-0.35 mg/mg may require attention to renal solute load and adequate fluid intake, acid/base balance, and electrolyte homeostasis.[14,18,19] Also, an alteration in diuretic therapy may be indicated.[14,19] Restriction of mineral intake may not be effective in reducing calcium excretion and may increase the risk of developing metabolic bone disease.[14]

Treatment Nutrition

Management of renal insufficiency includes treatment of the underlying disorder concurrent with supportive nutritional therapy. Nutrition management is critical in minimizing morbidity and offsetting the need for advanced therapy. Fluid, electrolyte, calorie, and nutrient needs vary with the amount of residual renal function and the medical or surgical treatment.

In high output renal failure, fluid intakes of 150-200 cc/kg/day are sometimes required to maximize remaining renal function. Supplementation with 5 mEq/kg/day or more of sodium and/or bicarbonate may be needed to replace excess losses of these electrolytes.[20-22]

In oliguria and anuria, fluid balance is generally managed by restricting intake to equal urine output plus insensible losses until urine output is normalized.[6] It is often necessary to restrict fluid intake to < 100 cc/kg/day. Sodium, potassium, phosphorus, and protein intake must also be adjusted to maintain homeostasis. When impaired renal function persists and limited fluid intake must continue, nutrition becomes a primary focus of medical management.

Nutrition management of conditions associated with renal insufficiency are summarized in Table 30.2. Whether the infant is able to feed by mouth or nasogastric (NG) tube or requires parenteral nutrition (PN) support, the principles of management are similar.[26] In a recent study, 26 infants with CRI not receiving dialytic support were found to achieve at least normal growth rates when caloric intake was maintained between 8-12 cal/cm/day (around 115-170 kcal/kg/day), with a protein intake of ≤ 0.15 g/cm/day (about 2.2 g/kg/day, but not less than Recommended Dietary Allowances for height-age).[23] Length is preferred over weight in determining nutrient intake because it can be accurately assessed and is independent of fluctuations in total body water. Length or height has been shown to provide a more reliable index of creatinine production and lean body mass.[27,28]

Enteral nutrition is preferred over PN whenever possible, but particularly in the neonate with renal insufficiency. Even with central venous access, it is difficult to optimize PN support within the confines of any significant fluid restriction. The effect of uremia combined with renal immaturity on amino acid requirements remains unclear. Parenteral essential amino acid solutions have not been shown to be superior over standard solutions in this patient population (see Chapters 8-12.)[29]

When a formula is designed to meet the specific needs of an infant whose renal function is compromised, many factors must be simultaneously considered. The nutritional needs of the rapidly growing infant, including energy, protein, minerals and vitamins must be met in spite of limited fluid, protein, and electrolyte tolerance. Restriction of fluid intake along with protein and mineral needs determine the specific concentration of the formula base. Energy needs, above that provided by the formula base, determine use of additional carbohydrate and fat.

For example, if fluid tolerance is only 100 ml/kg/day, and protein needs are the equivalent of 2.2 g/kg/day, 28 kcal/oz Similac PM 60:40 (Ross Products Division, Abbott Laboratories, Columbus, Ohio) is needed to provide adequate protein needs. This concentration alone does not provide adequate energy intake. Energy intake is important, not only to support normal growth and development, but to prevent catabolism, which provides an endogenous source of urea, potassium, and phosphorus. Carbohydrate and fat are added to the formula

Table 30.1. Insensible Water Loss During
the First Week of Life

Birth weight (g)	Insensible water loss* (ml/kg/24 hr)
750-1,000	82
1,001-1,250	56
1,251-1,500	46
> 1,501	26

Adapted with permission from Cloherty and Stark[17]
* Insensible water loss is influenced by phototherapy (⇧ ≈ 40%), radiant warmers
 (⇧ ≈ 50%), fever, and humidification of environment and gas (⇩),
 postnatal age (⇩).

to increase caloric density up to 45 cal/oz or more without increasing protein, phosphorus, and electrolyte concentration.[23,30] But if fluid tolerance is at least 180 cc/kg/day, as in high-output renal failure, standard-strength formula may be used, with additions of carbohydrate and fat to supply adequate calories as needed to support growth.

Glucose polymers are an ideal source of carbohydrate, since osmolality increases only moderately even at high concentrations. Glucose polymers are usually well tolerated, do not significantly alter flavor, and do not increase renal solute load. Adding vegetable oil to increase caloric density of formula is inexpensive and does not increase osmolality. If feedings are given slowly or by continuous infusion pump, and fat tends to separate from the feeding solution, an emulsified oil may be used (see Appendix K). Fat may delay gastric emptying, which may not be a problem unless gastroesophageal reflux is present. To ensure tolerance, the caloric density of formula is usually increased gradually, by 2 cal/oz every 12-24 hours, until energy intake is within the normal range and/or weight gain occurs. Carbohydrate should comprise 35-65%, and fat should comprise 30-55% of total energy intake. Protein supplements may be needed, particularly with peritoneal dialysis, if protein requirements exceed the infant's tolerance of phosphorus or potassium in the base formula.

Breast milk is often desirable, in that protein quality is high, but the amount of protein is low; it is also low in phosphorus and electrolytes. However, iron and vitamin D content is also low, and these nutrients must be supplemented. If nutritional needs are greater than what can be met at breast or if quantification of intake is necessary for optimal management, breast milk may be pumped and formula powder, carbohydrate or fat may be added. Feedings may then be given by tube, bottle or nursing supplementer.[22,30]

Table 30.2. Major Nutritional Considerations for Infants with Chronic Renal Insufficiency (CRI)

Nutrient	Indication	Modification	Reference
Energy	CRI without dialysis	8-12 kcal/cm/d or ≥ RDA to promote anabolism	20,23
	Peritoneal dialysis	≥ RDA, depending on dialysate dextrose absorption	
	Hemodialysis	≥ RDA or ≈ 10-12 kcal/cm/d	
Protein	CRI without dialysis	≤ 0.15 g/cm/d or 2.2 g/kg/d 0-6 mo; 1.6 g/kg/d 6-12 mo	23, 25
	Peritoneal dialysis	≥ RDA to maintain normal serum albumin or 2.4-4.0 g/kg/d	
	Hemodialysis	≤ 0.3 g/cm/d or 3.3 g/kg/d 0-6 mo; 2.4 g/kg/d 6-12 mo	
Phosphorus (P)	CRI	200 mg/d age 0-2 mo 400 mg/d age 2-6 mo	24
	Hyperphosphatemia	Similac PM 60/40* (low P content); use Ca carbonate or Ca acetate for P binding effects; avoid P binding agents containing aluminum; if parenterally fed, reduce phosphorus by 1/3 to 1/2	20, 24, 25
	Hypophosphatemia (due to anabolic state)	Standard infant formula	
Calcium (Ca)	CRI	400 mg/d age 0-2 mo 500 mg/d age 2-6 mo	20, 24
	Hypocalcemia (secondary to ⇩ rate of conversion to active vitamin D and ⇩ Ca absorption)	Vitamin D analogs (DHT† or Rocaltrol‡) and Ca carbonate or Ca acetate to maintain nl serum Ca levels; avoid Ca gluconate due to aluminum contamination	
	Nephrocalcinosis (due to hypercalciuria)	Ensure adequate phosphorus and fluid intake; avoid excess vitamin D intake	15
Sodium (Na)	Hypertension; fluid retention	Adjust Na intake if excessive (usually 1-3 mEq/kg/d); adjust fluid intake (may need ≤ 100 ml/kg/d)	20, 24
	Hyponatremia or losses to peritoneal dialysate	Up to 5-10 mEq/kg/d in divided doses to achieve nl serum Na levels	

Table 30.2. Major Nutritional Considerations for Infants with Chronic Renal Insufficiency (CRI) (continued)

Nutrient	Indication	Modification	Reference
Potassium (K)	Hyperkalemia	Decrease intake to maintain nl serum K levels	24
	Hypokalemia (secondary to dialysate losses, diarrhea, or diuretic therapy)	Increase intake to maintain nl serum K levels	
Iron	Anemia (secondary to ⇩ production of erythropoetin)	Standard iron administration if stores are adequate; iron as needed (2-6 g/kg/day) if stores are low; erythropoetin intramuscular injections	25
Vitamins	CRI	Standard dose of infant multivitamins (1 ml/d)	25
	Dialysis (secondary to losses of water-soluble vitamins into dialysate)	Standard dose of infant multivitamins (1 ml/d) Folic acid, 1 mg/d	

* Similac PM 60/40, Ross Products Division, Abbott Laboratories, Columbus, Ohio
† DHT (dihydrotachysterol), Roxane Laboratories, Columbus, Ohio
‡ Rocaltrol (calcitriol), Roche Laboratories, Nutley, N.J.

For formula fed infants, Similac PM 60:40 is usually preferred particularly during the initial advancement of feedings because it contains a moderate amount of high-quality protein, and is low in sodium, potassium, and phosphorus.[31] Infants experiencing formula intolerance should be given the formula best tolerated, regardless of its protein, mineral, and electrolyte content. Dilutional strategies and caloric replacement can be implemented to alter electrolyte and/or protein excess.

Once anabolism is achieved, Similac PM 64/40 may provide inadequate quantities of electrolytes and minerals, especially phosphorus; standard formulas such as Enfamil with iron (Mead Johnson, Evanston Ill.), Similac, or even soy formulas may then be used. Carnation Good Start (Carnation, Glendale, Calif) contains a moderate amount of phosphorus and is lower in sodium and potassium than other standard formulas.[22]

Experience using products such as AminAid (McGaw Laboratories, Irvine, Calif.), Travasorb Renal (Baxter-Clintec, Deerfield, Ill.), and Nepro and Suplena (Ross), has been reported only in adults and older children. These products do not contain appropriate or adequate amounts of minerals, electrolytes, or vitamins for infants. For these reasons, general use of these products for infants is not recommended.

Protein-free infant formula bases such as Protein-Free Diet Powder (Mead Johnson) and Pro-Phree (Ross) require added protein and perhaps other nutrients as determined on an individual basis. These products are used less often than more standard formulas because of cost and the complexity of supplementation required.

Detailed instructions given to parents prior to their infant's discharge regarding formula preparation and supplementation are necessary to avoid confusion and potential preparation errors. This is particularly true when using formulas such as protein-free formula bases, although standard formulas often require multiple supplements as well. Errors in formula preparation could significantly compromise medical management. It is often helpful for parents to actually do formula preparation and supplement dosing before the infant is discharged.

A standard dose of a routine liquid multivitamin supplement should be given daily. Supplementation with vitamin D as dihydrotachysterol or calcitriol and often calcium (as carbonate or acetate) is routinely prescribed for infants with CRI. Such supplementation is needed because of the infant's decreased rate of conversion to the active form of vitamin D and depressed G.I. absorption of Ca.[32-34] Serum Ca and P levels are routinely monitored during calcitriol therapy to avoid hypercalcemia and soft-tissue calcification. The serum Ca (mg/dl) x serum P (mg/dl) product should not exceed 70.[6] Chronic acidosis can contribute to bone demineralization and hypercalciuria. Acidosis may be treated with sodium citrate or sodium bicarbonate, initially at 2-3 mEq/kg/day in divided doses, then adjusted as necessary.

Consistent and adequate nutritional intake is essential in these infants. This is not only to promote optimal growth, but also to prevent the catabolism that would result in rising blood urea nitrogen (BUN) levels, hyperkalemia, and hyperphosphatemia. Yiu et al. found that feedings by NG tube were necessary in > 50% of 26 infants studied in order to achieve intake compliance.[23] Anorexia associated with chronic renal disease is known to interfere with adequate nutritional intake, potentially leading to malnutrition and ultimately to growth failure.[31] It may be unrealistic to expect a sick infant to spontaneously and regularly take adequate amounts of formula, especially if the formula contains supplemental calories due to restricted volume.

Dialysis becomes necessary once kidney function deteriorates to the point that conservative management (diet/medication) can no longer maintain normal fluid, electrolyte and acid-base balance or prevent accumulation of endogenous or exogenous toxins. Dialysis is a technically difficult procedure to perform in the newborn; therefore, every attempt should be made to exhaust conservative treatment regimens prior to beginning dialysis. Although continuous hemofiltration (with or without dialysate) may be used in the NICU, peritoneal dialysis or hemodialysis is required if renal failure becomes chronic.[30,35] In infants, peritoneal dialysis is preferred over hemodialysis.[36] Nutrition management of patients continues to be critical in achieving optimal growth and effectiveness of dialytic therapy. Urea kinetic modeling (UKM) uses measurements of urea in blood and dialysate to assess the adequacy of nutritional intake and to determine the optimal dialysis prescription. Although the principles of UKM are similar for infants and adults, interpretation of these calculations may be quite different and are reviewed elsewhere.[37,38]

Modifications in nutrient intake for infants on peritoneal dialysis and hemodialysis are shown in Table 30.2.[15,20-25] Numerous studies have shown that there is dextrose absorption from and protein loss to peritoneal dialysate. The extent to which the infant experiences these processes varies from one infant to another as well as at any point during a single infant's treatments. Regular monitoring of standard laboratory indexes (BUN, sodium (Na), potassium (K), Ca, P, albumin, pH, and total CO_2) and assessment of growth (length, weight, and head circumference) are most often preferred and are usually sufficient indicators of nutritional adequacy and metabolic stability.

The ultimate goal of treatment for children with chronic renal failure remains transplantation. Transplantation in the infant or child < 2 years of age poses more technical and management issues than in the older child. It is generally recommended that transplantation in the infant be done at a pediatric center where staff is experienced at performing transplants in this age group.

In summary, nutrition management is paramount to attenuating the morbidity associated with neonatal renal dysfunction. Nutrition intervention usually involves restricting the intakes of fluid, protein, and electrolytes while providing supplemental sources of energy. Nutrient needs vary with the infant's age and growth rate as well as the specific renal disorder and treatment. Regardless of the route, adequate intake must be ensured to promote optimal growth and to prevent the adverse metabolic effects of catabolism.

Case Study

MD was a 39 weeks' gestation female infant. At birth, weight was 3,200 g (50th-75th percentile for gestational age on Lubchenco growth chart), length was 50 cm (75th percentile), and head circumference was 33.5 cm (50th percentile). She was admitted in no acute distress, but was noted to be oliguric from birth. Serum chemistries at 2 days of age were remarkable for a creatinine of 3.2 mg/dl, BUN 30 mg/dl, P 7.6 mg/dl, Ca 8 mg/dl, and K 4.8 mEq/dl. An abdominal ultrasound test revealed bilateral dysplastic/hypoplastic kidneys.

At 3 days of age, enteral feedings were initiated with Similac PM 60/40. Insensible fluid loss was estimated using Table 30.1: 26 ml/kg/day x 3.2 kg = 83 ml/day. Urine output measured 257 ml/day. Thus, fluids were restricted to 340 ml/day (110 cc/kg/day), in order to maintain fluid balance.

Nutrition goals were established that included 10 kcal/cm/day and < 0.15 g protein/cm/day. To achieve these goals within the fluid restriction, formula was supplemented to 44 kcal/oz. Advancement of calories to 40 kcal/oz was accomplished by increasing formula caloric density 2 kcal/oz/12-24 hours by adding glucose polymers and vegetable oil. The base formula was concentrated at this point to 22 and then to 24 kcal/oz in order to provide adequate protein. MD tolerated advancement well, without vomiting or diarrhea and with minimal spitting. This intake provided 160 kcal/kg/day with a protein intake of 2.2 g/kg/day.

MD gained ≥ 20 g/day and her weight and length consistently followed the 50th percentiles for age. However, MD's renal function continued to deteriorate. At discharge, serum creatinine was 6.8 mg/dl. Other blood laboratory values were within normal limits, indicating appropriate nutrition and medication management: BUN 12 mg/dl, Ca 10.6 mg/dl, P 6.0 mg/dl, Na 140 mEq/L, K 4.5 mEq/L, and albumin 4.1 g/dl. Note: Serum Ca 10.6 mg/dl x serum P 6.0 mg/dl product was 63.6, which is < 70, thus requiring no further manipulation of mineral intake at that time.

MD was discharged home on Similac PM 60/40 24 kcal/oz increased to 44 kcal/oz by Polycose (Ross Laboratories) and corn oil. Although she was able to take most of her total daily intake by mouth, supplemental continuous nighttime NG feedings were necessary to ensure adequate and consistent intake. Supplements included a standard pediatric multivitamin (1 cc/day) and iron (2 mg/kg/day).

References

1. Costarino AT, Baumgart S. Controversies in fluid and electrolyte therapy for the premature infant. Clin Perinatol 15:863, 1988.
2. Kloiber LL, Winn NJ, Shaffer SG, et al. Late hyponatremia in very-low-birth-weight infants. Incidence and associated risk factors. J Am Diet Assoc 96:880. 1996.
3. Corey HE, Spitzer A. Renal blood flow and glomerular filtration rate during development. In: Edelmann CM, ed. Pediatric kidney disease. 2d ed. Boston: Little, Brown, 1992; 57.
4. Siegel NJ. Acute renal failure. In: Tune BM, Mendoza SA, eds. Pediatric nephrology. New York: Churchill Livingstone, 1984; 304.
5. Arant BS. Renal disorders of the newborn infant. In: Tune BM, Mendoza SA, eds. Pediatric nephrology. New York: Churchill Livingstone, 1984; 111.
6. Karlowicz MG, Adelman RD. Acute renal failure in the neonate. Clin Perinatol 19:139, 1992.
7. Fine RN. Growth in children with renal insufficiency. In: Nessenson A, Fine RN, Gentile D, eds. Clinical dialysis. New York: Appleton-Century-Crofts, 1984; 661.
8. Broyer M. Growth in children with renal insufficiency. Pediatr Clin North Am 29:991, 1982.
9. Rizzoni G, Broyer M, Guest G, et al. Growth retardation in children with chronic renal disease: Scope of the problem. Am J Kidney Dis 7:256, 1986.
10. Rizzoni G, Basso T, Setari M. Growth in children with chronic renal failure on conservative treatment. Kidney Int 26:52, 1984.
11. Foreman JW, Chan JCM. Chronic renal failure in infants and children. J Pediatr 113:793, 1988.
12. Rasoulpour M, Marinelli KA. Systemic hypertension. Clin Perinatol 19:121, 1992.
13. Ezzedeen F, Adelman RD, Ahlfors CE. Renal calcification in preterm infants: Pathophysiology and long-term sequelae. J Pediatr 113:532, 1992.
14. Adams ND, Rowe JC. Nephrocalcinosis. Clin Perinatol 19:179, 1992.
15. Karlowicz MG, Adelman RD. Renal classification in the first year of life. Pediatr Clin No Am 42:1397, 1995.
16. Simmons CF. Fluid and electrolyte management of the newborn. In: Cloherty JP, Stark AR, eds. Manual of neonatal care. 3d ed. Boston: Little, Brown, 1991; 460.
17. Cloherty JP, Stark AR, eds. Manual of neonatal care. Boston: Little, Brown, 1998.
18. Jones CA, King S, Shaw NJ et al. Renal calcification in preterm infants: follow-up at 4-5 years. Arch Dis Child 76:F185, 1997.
19. Sargent JD, Studel TA, Kresel J, et al. Normal values for random urinary calcium to creatinine ratios in infancy. J Pediatr 123:393, 1993.
20. Weiss RA. Dietary and pharmacologic treatment of chronic renal failure. In: Edelmann CM, ed. Pediatric kidney disease. 2d ed. Boston: Little, Brown, 1992; 57.

21. Rodriquez-Soriano J, Arant BS, Brodehi J, et al. Fluid and electrolyte imbalances in children with chronic renal failure. Am J Kidney Dis 7:268, 1986.

22. Brizee L. Nutrition for children with chronic renal failure. Nutr Focus 10:4, 1995.

23. Yiu VW, Harmon WE, Spinozzi n et al. High-calorie nutrition for infants with chronic renal disease. J Renal Nutr 6:203, 1996.

24. Hendricks KM, Walker WA. Manual of pediatric nutrition, 2d ed. Philadelphia: Decker, 1990; 266.

25. Stover J, Nelson P. Nutritional recommendations for infants, children and adolescents with ESRD. In: Gillit D, Stover J, Spinozzi NS, eds. A clinical guide to nutritional care in ESRD. Chicago: American Dietetic Association, 1987; 71.

26. Brewer ED. Supplemental enteral tube feeding in infants undergoing dialysis—indications and outcome. Semin Dialysis 7:429, 1994.

27. Grayston JE. Creatinine excretion during growth. In: Cheer DB, ed. Human growth. Philadelphia: Lea and Febiger, 1968; 182.

28. Viteri FE, Alvarado J. The creatinine height index: Its use in the estimation of the degree of protein depletion and repletion in protein calorie malnourished children. Pediatrics 46:696, 1970.

29. Grupe WE. Nutritional considerations in the management of infants and children with renal disease. In: Lebenthal E, ed. Textbook of gastroenterology and nutrition in infancy, 2d ed. New York: Raven Press, 1989; 630.

30. Spinozzi NS, Nelson P. Nutrition support in the newborn intensive care unit. J Renal Nutr 6:188, 1996.

31. Wassner SJ, Abitbol C, Alexander S, et al. Nutritional requirements for infants with renal failure. Am J Kidney Dis 7:300, 1986.

32. Mehls O, Salusky IB. Recent advances and controversies in childhood renal osteodystrophy. Pediatr Nephrol 1:212, 1987.

33. Tamanaha K, Mak RH, Rigden SP, et al. Long-term suppression of hyperparathyroidism by phosphate binders in uremic children. Pediatr Nephrol 1:145, 1987.

34. Schiller LR, Santa Ana CA, Sheikh MS, et al. Effect of the time of administration of calcium acetate on phosphorus binding. n Engl J Med 320:1110, 1989.

35. Coulthard MG, Vernon B. Managing acute renal failure in very low birthweight infants. Arch Dis Child 73:F187, 1995.

36. Kohaut EC, Whelchel J, Iraldo FB, et al. Aggressive therapy for infants with renal failure. Pediatr Nephrol 1:150, 1987.

37. Harmon WE. Kinetic modeling of hemodialysis in children. Semin Dialysis 7:392, 1994.

38. Schleifer CR, Teehan BP, Brown JM, et al. The application of urea kinetic modeling to peritoneal dialysis: a review of methodology and outcome. J Renal Nutr 3:2, 1996.

39. Salusky IB, Kopple JD, Fine RN. Continuous ambulatory peritoneal dialysis—a 20 months' experience. Kidney Int 23(S15):S101, 1983.

40. Grupe WE, Harmon WE, Spinozzi NS. Protein and energy requirements in children receiving chronic hemodialysis. Kidney Int 24:S6, 1983.

Bibliography

Bailie MD. Renal function and disease. Clin Perinatol 19:1-273, 1992.

Edelman CM Jr, ed. Pediatric kidney disease, 2d ed. vols. 1 and 2. Boston: Little, Brown, 1992.

Nutritional Care for High-Risk Newborns (Rev. 3d. Ed.)
S. Groh-Wargo, M. Thompson, J. Cox, editors
© 2000, Precept Press, Inc., Chicago

31

NEUROLOGICAL IMPAIRMENT

Nancy L. Nevin-Folino, MEd, RD, LD, CSP, FADA

T HE EFFECTS OF GENETIC abnormalities, congenital anomalies, or perinatal trauma on the central nervous system (CNS) often have an impact on nutrition. Growth patterns may be affected, and the metabolism of some nutrients may be altered by the disease itself or by drugs used in its treatment. Feeding behaviors and digestive patterns may require alternative feeding methods. The extent of the impact on nutrition, not always evident at birth, becomes apparent as the infant grows or fails to grow and acquires or fails to acquire feeding skills.

The initial signs and symptoms of neurological impairment may be subtle. An infant who has slow feeding skills or sucking or swallowing difficulties that cannot be attributed to gestational immaturity or physical or medical compromise may be neurologically impaired. Neurologic and metabolic screening should be considered to identify underlying conditions.[1,2] Sick or premature infants should have newborn metabolic screening samples taken by at least seven days of life even if feedings have been slow or delayed, because catabolism will lead to elevated blood amino acids in affected babies.[1] In many states, regulations require routine screening for phenylketonuria, galactosemia, and maple sugar urine disease, because these are the most common metabolic diseases that may cause neurological compromise if nutritional management is not started early in infancy. Additional screening for errors in metabolism may be indicated.[3]

Common diagnoses of the neonatal period that have neurologic implications that may involve nutrition problems are listed in Table 31.1. The medical diagnosis clarifies the cause of the neurological

The thoughtful guidance of David N. Franz, MD, assistant professor of neurology and pediatrics, Wright State University School of Medicine, is gratefully acknowledged.

insult, but may or may not provide direction for nutrition assessment and care.

Preventive Nutrition

Neurometabolic diagnoses or inborn errors of metabolism are definitive for nutrition intervention. Table 31.2 outlines inborn errors of metabolism that present in the neonatal period; Table 31.3 profiles clinical manifestations. Nutrition intervention in these cases may prevent, reduce severity, or delay the onset of neurological compromise. If a woman has an inborn error of metabolism, preventive nutrition begins ideally with dietary control before conception and throughout the pregnancy. The fetus of a woman with phenylketonuria is at risk for intrauterine growth retardation, mental retardation, microcephaly, and cardiac anomalies. This risk increases if maternal dietary management or compliance is inadequate.

The dietary management of inborn errors of metabolism may require that a specific nutrient or nutrients be restricted, eliminated, or supplemented. Indepth descriptions of nutrition intervention for inborn errors of metabolism are reviewed elsewhere.[2,4,5] As with other restricted or defined diets, nutrient intake should be analyzed routinely to ensure adequate intake of all nutrients, including energy, essential amino acids, essential fatty acids, vitamins, minerals, and trace elements.

Maternal abuse of alcohol, cigarettes, and illicit drugs may affect neurological outcome. Newborns with fetal alcohol syndrome (FAS) may have slow fetal and postnatal growth and may exhibit CNS dysfunction, including mild-to-moderate mental retardation, microcephaly, hypotonia, poor motor coordination, irritability during infancy, and hyperactivity during childhood. Prevention of FAS is well documented.[7] Other intrauterine drug exposures can cause neuroanatomic damage or alterations in the neurotransmitter systems that control state regulation, muscle tone, and responsivity. Cocaine exposure is associated with shorter gestation, increased risk of intraventricular hemorrhage, and higher incidence of both cognitive and motor developmental delay.[12,13] In addition, the psychosocial environment and lifestyle of a mother who has abused substances, particularly multiple drugs, during her pregnancy may also be predictive factors of poor function and neurobehavioral outcome for her infant.[14,15]

Prevention of neural tube defects (NTD) with folic acid supplementation before conception and during pregnancy has been clearly established.[16] Although nutritionists often meet the mother after NTD have been diagnosed in her infant, the mother should be counseled to begin folic acid supplementation and continue supplementation throughout her child-bearing years. Other neurological diseases

Table 31.1. Common Neonatal Diagnoses with Neurologic Implications that May Involve Nutrition Problems[4,6-11]

Genetic

Chromosomal abnormalities
— Fragile X
— Trisomy 13
— Trisomy 18
— Trisomy 21
Neurometabolic disorders
Neuromuscular dystrophies
Spina bifida

Congenital

Drug exposure
Fetal alcohol syndrome
Hydrocephalus
Intrauterine growth retardation
Intrauterine infections
— Cytomegalovirus
— Herpes simplex virus
— Syphilis
Small for gestational age
Uncontrolled maternal neurometabolic disorder during pregnancy

Perinatal or birth trauma

Asphyxia
Intraventricular hemorrhage
Meconium aspiration
Sepsis

may present during the neonatal period in which nutrition plays no preventive role. However, timely nutrition assessment may prevent, modify, or compensate for nutrition problems that may occur in this population.

Treatment Nutrition

Although neurological diseases in infancy (other than neurometabolic diseases) do not require specific nutrition therapy or treatment, a variety of conditions that affect nutrition may be associated with neurological disease.[8,9] Table 31.4 lists some of the conditions that may be present in the infant who is neurologically impaired and gives information on their nutrition implications. Feeding intolerance associated with birth asphyxia may be caused by altered motor patterns, including intestinal motor activity. Manometric studies have identified altered intestinal motility in infants with birth asphyxia and altered motor activity. Feeding intolerance may resolve as intestinal motility and motor patterns become more normal.[17]

Nutrition Assessment

Standard growth charts are used to plot serial measurements, except when disease-specific growth charts are available such as those for children with Down syndrome, Turner syndrome, cerebral palsy, Williams syndrome, and Prader-Willi syndrome[18]. Growth in infants with neurological or developmental handicaps may vary from normal (Table 31.4); such variations must be taken into consideration when using anthropometric progress to assess the adequacy of nutrition. Evaluation of anthropometric measurements requires the judgment of someone who is familiar with growth expectations for infants with the neurologically impairing condition.[22,23]

Head circumference measurements should be compared to those of the normal population as defined on the National Center for Health Statistics (NCHS) growth charts, and there should be no abrupt deviations. Microcephaly, or poor head growth, is associated with poor neurodevelopmental outcome.[10,24-26] Unless they are extremely ill, premature infants experience an accelerated rate of head growth, usually during the first eight weeks of postnatal life, representing expected "catch-up" growth.[27-29] Such growth must be distinguished from accelerated head growth due to pathologic conditions such as hydrocephalus, subdural collections, intracranial hemorrhage, intracranial cysts and tumors, or other disorders causing brain swelling or encephalopathy.[11]

Length should be measured and plotted frequently to identify variations from the norm. It is important, although often difficult to determine, if lagging linear growth is the result of inadequate nutrition or a symptom of a disease or condition. Some genetic and congenital disorders may include short stature or slow linear growth.[25,26] Brain injury involving the pituitary gland may also affect growth. A significant delay in linear growth may affect calorie needs. In these cases, linear growth rather than age may determine ideal weight. When determining calorie needs, height age and ideal weight for height (or length) are usually considered in addition to actual weight and age.[25]

Weight must be assessed in relationship to age, length, and average daily increments. (See Appendix D.) Average weight for length or height (50th percentile ranking) may be a more appropriate determination of ideal weight than weight for age. If the infant is over- or

Table 31.2.   Inborn Errors of Metabolism with Presentation in the Neonatal Period

Disorders of carbohydrate metabolism

1. Galactosemia
2. Hereditary fructose intolerance
3. Fructose–1,6–diphosphatase deficiency
4. Glycogen storage disease, type I
5. Glycogen storage disease, type II
6. Glycogen storage disease, type III
7. Glycogen storage disease, type IV
8. Pyruvate dehydrogenase deficiency
9. Pyruvate carboxylase deficiency
10. Phosphoenolpyruvate carbokinase deficiency

Disorders of amino acid metabolism

11. Maple syrup urine disease
12. Hypervalinemia
13. Periodic hyperlysinemia
14. Hyper-β-alaninemia
15. Nonketotic hyperglycinemia
16. Phenylketonuria
17. Hereditary tyrosinemia
18. Pyroglutamic aciduria
19. Hyperornithinemia-hyperammonemia-homocitrullinuria syndrome
20. Lysinuric protein intolerance
21. Methylene tetrahydrofolate reductase deficiency
22. Sulfite oxidase deficiency

Organic acidemias

23. Methylmalonic acidemia
24. Propionic acidemia
25. Isovaleric acidemia
26. 3–methyl crotonyl CoA carboxylase deficiency
27. Multiple carboxylase deficiency
28. Glucaric acidemia, type II
29. Ethylmalonic–adipic aciduria
30. Hydroxymethylglutaryl CoA lyase deficiency
31. 2–methyl–3hydroxyutyric acidemia
32. D–glyceric acidemia

Urea cycle defects

33. Carbamyl phosphate sythetase deficiency
34. Ornithine transcarbamylase deficiency
35. Cutrullinemia
36. Argininosuccinic aciduria
37. Arginase deficiency

Lysosomal storage disorders

38. GM_1 gangliosidosis type I
39. Gaucher's disease, infantile form (glucocerebrosidase deficiency)
40. Niemann-Pick disease, types A and B (sphinomyelinase deficiency)
41. Wolam disease (acid lipase deficiency)
42. Farber disease (ceramidase deficiency)
43. Mucopolysaccharidosis type VII (β-glucronidase deficiency)
44. Fucosidosis
45. I-cell disease (mucolipidosis, type II)
46. Sialidosis type II (neuraminidase deficiency)

Other disorders

47. Congenital adrenal hyperplasia
48. Lysosomal acid phosphatase deficiency
49. Menke kinky hair syndrome
50. Hereditary orotic aciduria
51. Cystic fibrosis
52. Hypophosphatasia
53. Crigler-Najjar syndrome
54. $α_1$-antitrypsin deficiency
55. Fatty acyl CoA dehydrogenase deficiency
57. Zellweger syndrome
58. Neonatal adrenoleukodystrophy

Reprinted with permission[1]

Table 31.3.   Major Clinical Manifestations of the Inborn Errors
of Metabolism in the Neonatal Period

Clinical findings	Associated disorders (Numbers refer to those listed in table 31.2)
Failure to thrive, poor feeding	Essentially all
Vomiting	1-3, 11-13, 16-20, 23-31, 41, 42, 47, 48
Diarrhea	1-4, 17, 20, 41, 51
Lethargy or coma	3, 11-15, 18-20, 23-27, 49, 50, 55, 56
Hypotonicity or hypertonicity	1, 3-12, 14, 15, 18, 22-27, 30, 32-37, 39, 40, 42, 43, 49, 50, 57, 58
Seizures	1-4, 6, 9-11, 13-15, 19-25, 27, 28, 30-36, 42, 44, 47, 49, 52, 55-58
Respiratory distress and/or apnea	3-6, 8-11, 15, 21-25, 30, 33-38, 55
Jaundice	1, 2, 7, 17, 40, 41, 49, 53, 54
Hepatomegaly	1-7, 19, 20, 23, 30, 34, 36-41, 43-46, 54, 56, 57
Coarse facial features	38, 43-46
Abnormal odor	11, 16, 17, 25-28
Dysmorphic features (multiple minor anomalies)	28, 49, 57, 58
Abnormal eye findings (cataract, retinopathy, other)	1, 22, 38, 40, 42, 43, 45, 46, 49, 57, 58
Abnormal hair	20, 36, 49
Macroglossia	5, 38, 42

Reprinted with permission[1]

underweight, measurements of lean body mass and muscle mass may be helpful in determining ideal weight.[30]

No definitive method has been devised to accurately assess the weight contribution of excess spinal fluid when it is present, but approximations can be obtained using computerized tomography (CT) scans or magnetic resonance imaging (MRI).[31]

Feeding assessment may reveal oral, pharyngeal, or esophageal dysfunction.[32] Choking may occur frequently and may signal increased risk of aspiration. Frequent aspiration and respiratory tract infections may prevent adequate nutrient intake or increase metabolic needs. The incidence of gastroesophageal reflux, which is higher in infants with neurodevelopmental disabilities, may require medical or surgical intervention to prevent respiratory compromise and to allow adequate nutrition and growth.[33] Feedings that take longer than 30 minutes may tire the infant, frustrate the care-giver, and prevent adequate intake of nutrients. Alternative feeding methods may need to be considered (see Chapter 18). When swallowing disorders are suspected, videofluoroscopy is recommended to identify the specific problem and design a plan of treatment (see Chapters 18 and 19). When dealing with the sometimes complex feeding problems of a neurologically-impaired infant, involvement of an interdisciplinary team is helpful in developing a comprehensive treatment plan.[34]

Nutrition Intervention

Neurometabolic disease are treated by limiting the specific amino acid, carbohydrate, or fat that cannot be normally metabolized. Carnitine deficiency may be caused by inadequate intake in very prematurely born infants, or by a primary defect in metabolism, decreased uptake by cells, or increased renal excretion. Normal doses for premature infants is 5-10 mg/kg/day. Doses for infants with metabolic errors in carnitine metabolism may be in the range of 50-100 mg/kg/d.[5,35-37]

Beyond the Recommended Dietary Allowances (RDA), no specific guidelines are available for nutrition of the neurologically-impaired infant. Infants who develop nutrition problems or exhibit factors that may contribute to increased risk for the development of nutrition problems must be treated individually (Table 31.4). The most frequent nutrition problem encountered is an alteration in the amount of calories an infant requires. Congenital hypotonia, or inactivity due to disability or delayed development, may decrease expected caloric needs. Hypertonia, or spasticity, may increase expected caloric needs. Serial assessment of intake and anthropometric measurements determines the specific calorie needs of an individual infant and how well these needs are met. If calorie needs are < 75% of the RDA, supplementation of vitamins and minerals may be necessary. When growth is less than expected, concentrated formula, supplements, or alternative feeding methods may be needed. If cereal or other complex carbohydrate sources are used to thicken formula or other liquids to facilitate swallowing, nutrient intake imbalances may occur.

At discharge, families and care-givers may need education and specific instruction in special formula preparation, nutrient supplements, or tube-feeding. If the infant does not give clear hunger and satiety cues, the family and care-givers may also need guidelines for expected weight gain and amounts of formula or food to give. Feeding should not be the single focus of care and interaction with the infant. Infants with decreased metabolic needs or decreased mobility may be placed at increased risk of obesity if feedings are used to replace the usual bonding and activities that take place with

Table 31.4. Frequently Reported Nutrition-Related Problems in Infants with Neurologic Impairment

Condition	Altered growth needs	Altered energy needs	Altered nutrient	Formula intolerance	Feeding problems	Constipation/ diarrhea	Other
Cerebral palsy	X	X	X		X	X	Poor appetite
Neuromuscular dysfunction		X			X	X	
Spina bifida	X	X	X			X	
Chromosonal abnormalities	X	X	Possible		X	X	Gum disease
Neurometabolic disease		X	X	X	X		May need specialized nutrients
Neurologic damage due to sepsis		X		X	X		
Drug exposure/fetal alcohol syndrome	X			X	X	X	
Birth asphyxia	X			X	X	X	
Neonatal seizures			X	X	Possible	X	Drug/nutrient interactions
Neurologic impairment of unknown cause	X	X			X	X	Drug/nutrient interactions

Adapted from Byler and Lucas,[19] with additional data from Briggs et al,[7] Fanaroff and Martin,[9] Berman et al,[20] and reference 21.

unaffected infants.[22] Infants with increased metabolic demands need time and energy to "work" on other aspects of their development.

Follow-up Guidelines

Infants with neurometabolic disorders are usually followed by specialists familiar with these disorders. Follow-up is often complex and, at least initially, may be needed weekly to monitor serum levels of specific metabolites and to adjust dietary intake. Many states have regional clinics with a complete team of experienced health professionals to follow these patients.

If a baby requires any special formula or has nutritional needs that vary from the normal, this information should be communicated to the primary health care provider. It is helpful to give a complete report, including intake recommendations, for all nutrients that are different from normal infant guidelines. Suggestions for monitoring, diet advancement, and expected growth should be included.

When establishing a schedule for follow-up nutrition assessment, the following factors should be considered:[23,24]

- Extent to which intake recommendations vary from the norm
- Complexity of formula preparation or other aspects of the nutritional care plan
- Feeding modality
- Number of nutrients that require monitoring
- Growth and dietary history
- Other professional involvement
- Capabilities and resources of the caregivers

Case Study

TH, born at 33 weeks' gestation, weighed 1,250 g. He was 37 cm long and his head circumference was 27.5 cm. His Apgar scores were 1 at one minute of age and 6 at five minutes of age. Diagnoses included premature birth, intrauterine growth retardation, intrauterine asphyxia, and gastroesophageal reflux. Neurologic sequelae included dysphagia, generalized hypotonia, and increased irritability with stimulation. A gastrostomy and fundoplication were performed at 2 months of age.

Parenteral nutrition was required for the first 7 days of age. Enteral nutrition (human milk) began at 5 days of age. At 2 weeks of age, enteral feedings included human milk combined with equal portions of Similac Natural Care (Ross Products Division, Abbott

Laboratories, Columbus, Ohio). Head circumference progressed from below 2 standard deviations (SD) below the mean to 2 SD below the mean at 4 weeks of age. Length and weight progressed likewise by 7 weeks of age (term date). Subsequent growth continued at 2 SD below the mean, with normal rates of gain on 125 cal/kg/day on human milk without formula supplement. Poly Vi-Flor (Mead Johnson, Evansville, Ind.) 1.0 ml/day and Fer-In-Sol (Mead Johnson) 0.3 ml/day were given to ensure adequate vitamin and mineral intake. It was assumed that at least initially, TH would continue growth at 2 SD below the mean.

Because TH was fed solely by gastrostomy tube at discharge and because his hunger and satiety cues were not clear due to his irritability, the parents were given guidelines for expected growth and intake needs during the first few weeks after discharge (see chart below). Instructions were also given to help parents read hunger and satiety cues and to appropriately respond to these as much as possible for feedings. In an effort to help TH establish his own body rhythms and work toward longer sleep periods at night, parents were given expected total feeding volumes for 24 hours. Dividing this into 24 individual hours, the parents could then calculate how much milk he would need based on how many hours it had been since his last feeding. For example, if his last feeding began at 8 a.m. and it was now 11 a.m., he would need three hours' worth of milk (or 3 oz initially, using the table below) at his 11 a.m. feeding. Parents could also give six feedings a day during the day of the required volume and allow TH to sleep through the night. This plan allowed flexibility and parental involvement, yet ensured adequate nutritional intake. The parents would also know how to judge subsequent weight gain.

Date	Expected weight	Expected needs for milk intake over 24 hours	Expected needs for milk intake per hour
12/11	8 lb 11 oz to 8 lb 13 oz	24 oz, or 4 oz every 4 hr	30 cc for every hour
12/25	9 lb 7 oz to 9 lb 14 oz	26-27 oz, or 4½ oz every 4 hr	33 cc for every hour
1/25	11 lb to 12 lb	30-33 oz, or 5 to 5½ oz every 4 hr	40 cc for every hour

Follow-up was arranged to determine subsequent growth expectations and nutritional needs. Referral to a rehabilitation service was made to provide oral-motor and physical therapy.

References

1. Burton B. Inborn errors of metabolism: The clinical diagnosis in early infancy. Pediatrics 79:359, 1987.
2. Burton BK. Inborn errors of metabolism in infancy: A guide to diagnosis. Pediatrics 102:e69, 1998.
3. Acosta PB, Yannicelli S. A practitioner's guide to selected inborn errors of metabolism. Columbus, Ohio: Ross Laboratories, 1992.
4. Chen H. Medical genetics handbook. St. Louis: Warren H. Green, 1988.
5. Acosta PB. The Ross metabolic formula system nutrition support protocols. Columbus, Ohio: Ross Laboratories, 1997.
6. Hendricks KM, Walker WA. Manual of pediatric nutrition. Philadelphia: Decker, 1990.
7. American Academy of Pediatrics Committee on Substance Abuse and Committee on Children with Disabilities. Fetal alcohol syndrome and fetal alcohol effects. Pediatrics 91:1004, 1993.
8. Fenichel GM. Neonatal neurology, 2d ed. New York: Churchill Livingstone, 1990.
9. Fanaroff AA, Martin RJ: Neonatal-perinatal medicine: Diseases of the fetus and infant. St. Louis: Mosby Year Book, 1997.
10. Lipper EG, Lee KS, Gartner LM, et al. Determinants of neurobehavioral outcome in low-birth-weight infants. Pediatrics 67:502-505, 1981.
11. Milhorat TH. Neurosurgery of the newborn. In: Avery GB, ed. Neonatology: Pathophysiology and management of the newborn, 3d ed. Philadelphia: J Lippincott, 1994.
12. Tronick EZ, Frank DA, Cabral H, et al. Late dose–response effects of prenatal cocaine exposure on newborn neurobehavioral performance. Pediatr 98:76-83, 1996.
13. Singer T, Yamashita TS, Hawkins S, et al. Increased incidence of intraventricular hemorrhage and developmental delay in cocaine-exposed, very low birth weight infants. J Pediatr 124:765-71, 1994.
14. Napiorkowski B, Lester BM, Freier C, et al. Effects of in utero substance exposure on infant neurobehavior. Pediatr 98:71-75, 1996.
15. Jacobson JL, Jacobson SW, Sokol RJ, et al. Effects of alcohol use, smoking, and illicit drug use on fetal growth in black infants. J Pediatr 124:757-64. 1994.
16. Daly LE, Kirke PN, Molloy A, et al. Folate levels and neural tube defects: implications for prevention. JAMA 272:1698-1702, 1995.
17. Berseth CL, McCoy HH. Birth asphyxia alters neonatal intestinal motility in term neonates. Pediatrics 90:669, 1992.
18. Bonnema S. Neurological compromise. In: Cox JH (ed). Nutrition manual for at-risk infants and toddlers. Chicago: Precept Press, 1997, pg 113.
19. Position of the American Dietetic Association: Nutrition in comprehensive program planning for persons with developmental disabilities. J Am Diet Assoc 92:613-615, 1992.
20. Behrman RE, Kliegman RM, Nelson WE, et al. Nelson textbook of pediatrics. Philadelphia: Saunders, 1996.
21. Manual of Pediatric Nutrition. St. Paul: Twin Cities District Dietetic Association, 1990.

22. Cronk C, Crocker AC, Pueschel SM, et al. Growth charts for children with Down syndrome: 1 month to 18 years of age. Pediatrics 81:102, 1988.

23. Shaddix TE. Nutrition implications in children with cerebral palsy. Nutr Focus 6:1, 1991.

24. Gross SJ, Oehler JM, Echerman CO. Head growth and developmental outcome in very low-birth-weight infants. Pediatrics 71:70, 1983.

25. Ross G, Lipper EG, Auld PAM. Growth achievement of very low birth-weight premature children at school age. J Pediatr 117:307, 1990.

26. Hack M, Breslau N, Weissman B, et al. Effect of very low birthweight and subnormal head size on cognitive abilities at school age. N Engl J Med 325:231, 1991.

27. Altigani M, Murphy JF, Newcombe RG, et al. Catch up growth in preterm infants. Acta Paediatr Scand (suppl) 357:3, 1989.

28. Fitzhardinge PM. Follow-up studies of the high-risk newborn. In: Avery GB, ed. Neonatology: Pathophysiology and management of the newborn, 3d ed. Philadelphia: Lippincott, 1994.

29. Rickard K, Brady MS, Gresham EL. Nutrition management of the chronically ill child. Pediatr Clin North Am 24:157, 1977.

30. Wordarski LA. An interdisciplinary nutrition assessment and intervention protocol for children with disabilities. J Am Diet Assoc 90:1563, 1990.

31. Condon B, Wyper D, Grant R, et al. Use of magnetic resonance imaging to measure intracranial cerebrospinal fluid volume. Lancet 1:1355-57, 1986.

32. Reilly S, Skuse D, Poblete X. Prevalence of feeding problems and oral motor dysfunction in children with cerebral palsy: A community survey. J Pediatr 129:76-83, 1996.

33. Roberts KB. Gastroesophageal reflux in infants and children who have neurodevelopmental disabilities. Pediatr Rev 17:211-212, 1996.

34. Wordaski LA, Bundschuh E, Forbus WR. Interdisciplinary case management: A model for intervention. J Am Diet Assoc 88:332, 1988.

35. Tao RC, Yoshimura NN. Carnitine metabolism and its application in parenteral nutrition. J Parenter Enter Nutr 4:469, 1980.

36. Innis SM. Fat. In: Tsang RC, Lucas A, Uauy R, et al. (eds). Nutritional needs of the preterm infant: Scientific basis and practical guidelines. Baltimore: Williams and Wilkins, 1993, 65-87.

37. Pons R, DeVivo DC. Primary and secondary carnitine deficiency syndromes. J Child Neurol 10(Suppl):2S8-2S24, 1995.

Bibliography

Pipes PL, Glass RP. Nutrition and feeding of children with developmental disability and related problems. In: Pipes PL, ed. Nutrition in infancy and childhood, 4th ed. St. Louis: Times Mirror/Mosby, 1997.

Ekvall SW, ed. Pediatric nutrition in chronic diseases and development disorders: Prevention, assessment, and treatment. New York: Oxford University Press, 1993.

Issacs JS, Cialone J, Horsley JW, et al. Children with special health care needs: A community nutrition pocket guide. Columbus: Ross Product

Division of Abbott Laboratories. Order through University of Alabama Sparks Clinics 1-205-934-5471.

Nutritional Care for High-Risk Newborns (Rev. 3d. Ed.)
S. Groh-Wargo, M. Thompson, J. Cox, editors
© 2000, Precept Press, Inc., Chicago

32

INFANTS
OF
DIABETIC MOTHERS

Susan K. Hooy, RD, and
Karen Amorde-Spalding, MS, RD, CSP

INFANTS OF DIABETIC MOTHERS (IDMs) experience alterations in the delivery and utilization of metabolic fuels during gestation. These alterations can cause multiple neonatal complications (see Table 32.1). The severity of maternal disease influences the neonatal course. According to the system detailed in Table 32.2,[1] classification of maternal diabetes is based on onset and duration of the disease and presence of vascular disease. Recent advancements in obstetrical management of diabetes have greatly reduced the incidence of complications in IDMs. The mechanisms responsible for the complications seen in the IDM have yet to be fully elucidated. Maternal hyperglycemia results in an altered milieu of metabolic fuels that produce teratogenic effects in the fetus in addition to fetal hyperinsulinemia.[2,3] Those complications of nutritional interest in the IDM are discussed in this chapter.

Hypoglycemia is a common metabolic problem in the IDM during the neonatal period. Hypoglycemia may be defined as serum glucose levels < 40 mg/dl in infants.[4] The incidence of hypoglycemia is greater in infants of mothers with pregestational diabetes (50-75%) than those of mothers with gestational diabetes (25%).[5,6] Hypoglycemia is also more likely in macrosomic IDMs (47%) than in those IDMs born < 4 kg (20%).[7]

Maternal hyperglycemia results in elevation of fetal serum glucose levels, which in turn causes fetal pancreatic islet cell hypertrophy with beta cell hyperplasia. The result is fetal hyperinsulinemia.[8] Hypoglycemia may then result because of the sudden cessation of maternal glucose delivery to the infant immediately after birth while elevated insulin levels persist. Although this condition usually subsides within the first three days of life, hypoglycemia in the IDM occasionally persists longer. In those cases, other possible etiologies should be investigated.[9]

Also common in the IDM is neonatal hypocalcemia. As many as 50% of infants born to mothers with insulin-dependent diabetes develop hypocalcemia (< 7 mg/dl) within the first three days of life.[7,8] In contrast, the incidence of hypocalcemia in infants of mothers with gestational diabetes is similar to infants born to mothers without diabetes.[8] The incidence of hypocalcemia is also related to severity of maternal disease, birth asphyxia, and prematurity.[10]

The etiology of hypocalcemia is not well understood. Normally, fetal parathyroid hormone (PTH) levels are suppressed by relatively high serum calcium levels delivered to the fetus. Serum PTH levels rise in response to decreasing serum calcium levels after birth. IDMs exhibit a delay in PTH response compared to other infants.[11,12] Hyperphosphatemia, common in both the normal newborn and in the IDM, and low magnesium levels seen in some IDMs may play a role in depressing PTH secretion.[8,11] Hypocalcemia typically resolves within the first three days of life.

Hypomagnesemia (< 1.5 mg/dl) is seen in ≤ 33% of IDMs.[8] Like hypocalcemia, the incidence and severity depend on maternal disease; the disorder resolves within the first three days of life.[11]

The incidence of macrosomia, weight > 90% for age, or large for gestational age (LGA), is 20-30% in IDMs, compared to 10% in normal pregnancies.[5,13,14] Insulin functions as a growth hormone in fetal development.[8] Fetal hyperinsulinemia results in increased organ size, particularly the heart and liver, but not kidney or brain.[2,15] Persistently elevated insulin and glucose levels lead to enhanced deposition of fat in the third trimester.[8]

Large infants are more susceptible to birth injury and asphyxia, with related neurologic sequelae.[2] To prevent these complications, large infants may be delivered prior to term. IDMs are also at risk for premature birth as a result of maternal complications such as preeclampsia. The incidence of premature birth in one series of insulin-dependent diabetes pregnancies was 26%, compared to 10% of nondiabetes pregnancies.[16]

In contrast to the increased risk of macrosomia, some IDMs are small for gestational age (SGA) as a consequence of either maternal low blood sugar[17] and/or maternal vascular disease.[14] In one series, the incidence of intrauterine growth retardation (IUGR) was 20% in infants born to mothers with class F diabetes.[18]

An estimated 10-20% of IDMs have cardiomegaly.[19] Cardiomyopathy may also be present, although it is often asymptomatic.[20] Cardiorespiratory symptoms, if present, typically resolve within 1-2 weeks of age, whereas radiographic signs of cardiomyopathy may

Table 32.1. Complications Associated with Infants
of Diabetic Mothers

Hypoglycemia	Respiratory distress
Hypocalcemia	Respiratory distress syndrome
Hypomagnesemia	Congenital anomalies
Macrosomia	Hyperbilirubinemia
Birth injury	Polycythemia
Asphyxia	Neurologic impairment
Cardiomyopathy	

persist for weeks to months.[19-21] Typically, treatment is not necessary. When pharmicotherapy is required, propranolol is used.[20]

IDMs have lower bone mineral content than normal infants. The etiology for this condition is not well understood, but may be related to elevated vitamin D_3 in IDMs.[22] The consequence of lower bone mineral content in IDMs has not been determined.

Respiratory distress is frequently seen in IDMs secondary to cardiac or respiratory compromise.[2] Respiratory distress syndrome (RDS) may result from delayed production of mature surfactant secondary to hyperinsulinemia.[23,24] High insulin levels may inhibit cortisol activity in lecithin synthesis.[24] Recent studies indicate that RDS may more often be a consequence of premature delivery, independent of fetal insulin levels.[25,26]

IDMs may also have mild neurologic impairment independent of perinatal complications such as birth injury, asphyxia or hypoglycemia.[6,27] The etiology of the neurologic impairment remains uncertain. Macrosomic IDMs also have abnormal iron indexes, with iron deficiency of the liver, heart, and brain.[28] Iron deficiency may play a role in neonatal muscle tone and neurodevelopment and may explain the difficulty some infants have with nipple-feeding during the early neonatal period.[28,29]

Maternal hyperglycemia in the first trimester is associated with specific congenital anomalies in the IDM.[30-32] Malformations of the ears, and in the skeletal, renal, gastrointestinal, cardiovascular, and central nervous systems are listed in Table 32.3.

Preventive Nutrition

Preventing disorders of growth and congenital anomalies depends upon strict maternal metabolic control beginning prior to concep-

Table 32.2. The White System for Classification of Diabetes in Pregnancy (revised)[1]

Gestational diabetes	Abnormal GTT, diet management alone, or insulin required with diet management
Class A	Diet alone, any duration or onset age
Class B	Onset age 20 yr or older and duration < 10 yr
Class C	Onset age 10-19 yr or duration 10-19 yr
Class D	Onset age < 10 yr, duration > 20 yr, background retinopathy, or hypertension (not preeclampsia)
Class R	Proliferative retinopathy or vitreous hemorrhage
Class F	Nephropathy with > 500 mg/d proteinuria
Class RF	Criteria for both classes R and F coexist
Class H	Arteriosclerotic heart disease clinically evident
Class T	Prior renal transplantation

tion.[3] Neonatal hypoglycemia and other transient metabolic complications are prevented with strict control of maternal blood glucose in the third trimester and perinatal period.[32]

When the infant is born, early enteral nutrition (EN) may maintain normal blood glucose levels in an infant with mildly depressed blood glucose levels.[32] If enteral feedings are not possible, glucose is given parenterally until adequate EN feedings are established.

Treatment Nutrition

During the neonatal period, IDMs are at risk for metabolic derangements requiring immediate medical treatment. Glucose supplementation should be given to infants with blood glucose levels < 40 mg/dl. The route of glucose supplementation is dependent on the presence or absence of symptoms.[33-35] Ideally, enteral feedings are used to accomplish the overall goal of maintaining serum glucose in the normal range. If I.V. support is required, glucose is administered at an initial rate of 6-8 mg/kg/min, with subsequent advances of 10-15% increments until the plasma glucose level stabilizes or a glucose infusion rate of 15-20 mg/kg /min is reached.[36] Bolus infusion is indicated if continuous infusion fails to normalize blood glucose or if the blood glucose is very low. As a result of the neonate's underlying hyperinsulinemia, rebound hypoglycemia may follow a bolus infusion. A continuous infusion of dextrose follows a bolus infusion in order to maintain normal blood glucose levels.[34-35] I.V. support can be slowly reduced as enteral bolus feedings are advanced.[32] Figure 32.1

outlines a stepwise protocol to manage hypoglycemia used by one hospital. The addition of glucose polymers to formula may raise prefeeding glucose levels but does not permit less frequent feedings.[37] Hypocalcemia and hypomagnesemia may also require I.V. supplementation and are generally managed by the medical team.[5,38]

Although the full-term, appropriate-for-gestational-age (AGA) IDM appears to have the same nutrient needs as the normal full-term infant, IDMs who are SGA or have cardiac or other anomalies may require an altered nutrient intake specific to their condition. IDMS who are LGA may be at risk for obesity later in life.[39] Current evidence suggests that macrosomic IDMs appear similar to the general population at 1 year, so that their nutrient needs in the first year of life are no different from those of the healthy term infant.[40] Because macrosomic IDMs have abnormal iron indexes, supplemental iron in the newborn period has been suggested, but no specific dose recommendations have been made.[28,53]

For several reasons, IDMs often take oral feedings poorly and may require tube-feeding.[34] The etiology may be multifactorial. Frequently, IDMs are delivered prematurely; therefore, even though they may be LGA, they are developmentally unable to successfully nipple-feed in the early neonatal period. In addition, IDMs may suffer from other complications, such as congenital heart disease or respiratory distress, that may affect their ability to nipple-feed.[2] Independent of these complications, some IDMs are hypotonic and do not nipple-feed well in the early neonatal period.[27,34] This is most often seen in macrosomic infants. Experienced nurses, lactation specialists, and occupational therapists play a pivotal role in supporting development of feeding behaviors.

There are no contraindications to breast-feeding the IDM. Successful lactation is most likely to occur with careful diet management to avoid maternal hypoglycemia and early intervention for breast-feeding–related problems.[41] Expressed human milk may be tube-fed in the early neonatal period if the infant nipple-feeds poorly or requires early feeding to correct hypoglycemia. Precise measurements of volume and energy intakes are not necessary as long as euglycemia can be maintained. When detailed intake data are important, pre- and postfeeding weights may be reliable.[42] Breast-feeding may be especially beneficial for the LGA infant, because breast-fed babies tend to be leaner after the first 6 months of life, and they tend to be less obese later in life.[43,54]

IDMs given nothing by mouth for more than five days should be considered for parenteral nutrition (PN) support even if they are LGA, and especially if they are premature. The addition of amino acids increases the potential net glucose load; consequently, continuous close monitoring of blood glucose levels will be necessary to avoid unexpected hypoglycemia secondary to the IDMs underlying hyperinsulinemia.[44]

Table 32.3. Congenital Anomalies in Infants of Diabetic Mothers

Skeletal and central nervous system

    Caudal regression syndrome
    Neural tube defects, excluding anencephaly
    Anencephaly with or without herniation of neural elements
    Microcephaly

Cardiac

    Transposition of the great vessels with or without ventricular septal defect
    Ventricular septal defects
    Coarctation of the aorta with or without ventricular septal defect or patent ductus arteriosus
    Atrial septal defects
    Cardiomegaly

Renal Anomalies

    Hydronephrosis
    Renal agenesis
    Ureteral duplication

Gastrointestinal

    Duodenal atresia
    Anorectal atresia
    Small left colon syndrome

Other

    Single umbilical artery

Source: Reece EA, Hobbins JC: Diabetic embryopathy: Pathogenesis, prenatal diagnosis and prevention. Obstet Gynecol Survey 41:325-335, 1986; with permission.

Using galactose as an enteral carbohydrate source to maintain normal blood glucose levels is also of theoretical interest. Galactose clearance does not require insulin and does not stimulate insulin secretion.[32] Galactose or a metabolite of galactose may be involved in the regulation of hepatic glucose metabolism, resulting in either hepatic glycogen synthesis or hepatic glucose production.[45,46] Using

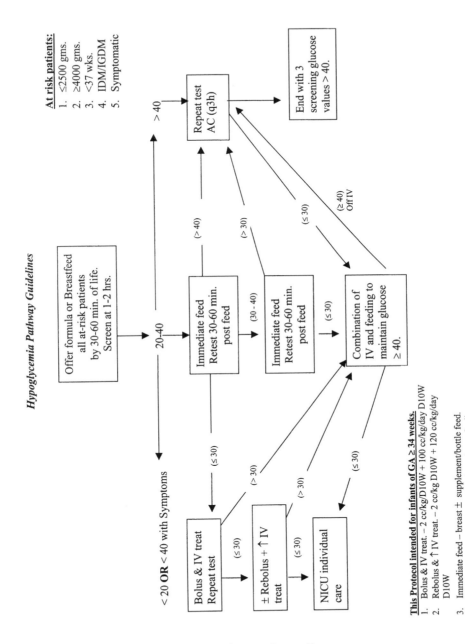

Figure 32.1. Neonatal hypoglycemia pathway.

Source: MetroHealth Medical Center, Cleveland, Ohio; with permission.

lactose-containing human milk or cow's milk-based formulas rather than soy or hydrolyzed formulas may help to attentuate plasma insulin concentrations in IDMs and maintain normal blood glucose levels.[46]

Follow-up Issues

Elevated amniotic fluid insulin concentrations during weeks 32-38 of gestation are correlated with macrosomia at birth and with obesity during childhood.[47] IDMs who are macrosomic at birth appear similar to the general population with respect to their heights and weights at one year of life. However, infants who had elevated amniotic fluid insulin tend to become obese at about 6 years of age whether or not they were macrosomic at birth.[47] Because of the IDM's potential for childhood obesity, regular height and weight measurements should be followed and weight control counseling provided if weight gain becomes accelerated.

The altered maternal metabolism seen in pregnant diabetics may cause IDMs to become obese, score lower on newborn behavioral tests, and score lower on standard I.Q. tests during early childhood.[40] Lower newborn behavioral scores and lower early childhood I.Q. scores are correlated with poor second and third trimester glycemic regulation and maternal lipid metabolism (serum free fatty acids and β-hydroxybutyrate), respectively.[48] These altered maternal metabolic fuels may be only a marker for and not the etiology of the lower developmental and I.Q. scores.[49] These findings provide additional motivation for close maternal metabolic control, but do not respond to nutritional intervention during infancy or childhood.

IDMs are at a greater risk for insulin-dependent diabetes mellitus later in life than the general population.[50] They are at increased risk because of genetic factors and possibly because of the altered glucose availability during intrauterine life, which by itself appears to increase the risk of diabetes.[50]

The relationship between feeding infants intact cow's milk or soy protein in the first year of life and the increasing incidence of diabetes in the general population has been the focus of considerable attention. This complicated relationship has not been fully analyzed. However, until the results of prospective, randomized trials are available the American Academy of Pediatrics recommends the following. In families with a strong history of diabetes, breast-feeding and avoidance of cow's milk/products containing cow's milk protein are strongly encouraged during the first year of life. Since the antigenicity of infant formulas and cow's milk may be different, commercial formulas based on cow's milk protein remain the appropriate alternative to human milk.[51]

To summarize, IDMs are at risk for several neonatal complications as a result of alterations in the delivery and utilization of metabolic fuels. Metabolic complications include hypoglycemia, hypocalcemia, and hypomagnesemia. Other complications include macrosomia, respiratory and cardiac disease, neurologic sequelae, and congenital anomalies.

Immediate medical treatment is required for the metabolic complications seen in the neonatal period. With modern management, fewer morbidities are expected in IDMs.[52] Although long-term complications remain a concern, the only one that may respond to nutritional intervention is obesity.

Case Study

Baby girl S was a 4.2 kg birth weight LGA infant delivered by repeat cesarean section for failure to progress after a trial of labor at 38-39 weeks' gestation to a 24-year-old woman with gestational diabetes controlled by diet. The mother received sporadic prenatal care and her hemoglobin A_{1c} was 9.8% at the time of delivery. Apgar scores of the baby were 8 at one minute and 9 at five minutes.

The initial blood sugar concentration was 25 mg/dl at 30 minutes of life. The physical examination was unremarkable and the baby was asymptomatic. A 30-cc formula feeding was given, but the repeat blood sugar 30 minutes later was still low at 28 mg/dl. A peripheral I.V. line was placed, and a CBC and blood culture sent. A bolus of dextrose 10% (2 cc/kg) was given followed by a continuous infusion of 100 cc/kg/day (6.9 mg/kg/min), along with every 2° ad lib formula feedings. Serum blood sugar rose to 54 mg/dl by 3 hours of age. The I.V. rate was then tapered over the next 12 hours, with the infant feeding well from the bottle and taking about 45-60 ml every three hours.

The infant was noted to have a heart murmur on the second day of life (DOL). A chest x-ray from the first DOL had revealed mild cardiomegaly. An echocardiogram showed septum and ventricular thickening consistent with mild hypertrophic cardiomyopathy of the IDM. No medical therapy was required.

The infant was discharged weighing 3.8 kg after a three-day hospitalization. The baby was taking ad lib bottle feedings well every three to four hours. A follow-up appointment was made with the primary care physician.

References

1. Hare JW, White P. Gestational diabetes and the White Classification. Diab Care 3(2):394, 1980.
2. Cowett RM, Shulman DI, Root AW, et al. Endocrine diseases. In: Sweet AY, Brown EG, eds. Fetal neonatal effects of maternal disease. St. Louis: Mosby Year Book, 1991; 302.
3. Goto MP, Goldman AS. Diabetic embryopathy. Curr Opin Pediatr 6:486, 1994.
4. American Academy of Pediatrics Committee on Nutrition. Hypoglycemia. Kleinman RE, ed. Pediatric nutrition handbook. 4th ed. Elk Grove Village, Ill.: American Academy of Pediatrics, 1998; 387.
5. Otaga ES. The infant of the diabetic mother. In: Rudolph AM, Hoffman JIE, Rudolph CD, ed. Rudolph's pediatrics. 19th ed. Norwalk, Conn.: Appleton and Lange, 1991; 202.
6. Rizzo TA, Ogata ES, Dooley SL, et al. Perinatal complications and cognitive development in 2- to 5-year-old children of diabetic mothers. Am J Obstet Glynecol 171:706, 1994.
7. Cordero L, Landon MB. Infant of the diabetic mother. Clin Perinatol 20(3):635, 1993.
8. Cowett RM. The infant of the diabetic mother. In: Cowett RM, ed. Principles of perinatal-neonatal metabolism. New York: Springer-Verlag, 1991; 678.
9. Polk DH. Disorders of carbohydrate metabolism. In: Taeusen HW, Ballard RA, Avery ME, eds. Schaffer and Avery's diseases of the newborn. 6th ed. Philadelphia: Saunders, 1991; 970.
10. Tsang RC, Chen IW, Friedman MA, et al. Parathyroid function in infants of diabetic mothers. J Pediatr 86:399, 1975.
11. Noguchi A, Eren M, Tsang RC. Parathyroid hormone in hypocalcemic and normocalcemic infants of diabetic mothers. J Pediatr 97:112, 1980.
12. Tsang RC, Kleinman LI, Sutherland JM, et al. Hypocalcemia in infants of diabetic mothers. J Pediatr 80:384, 1972.
13. Lubchenco LO. The infant who is large for gestational age. In: Schaffer AJ, Markowicz M, eds. The high risk infant. (vol. 14 in major problems in clinical pediatrics) Philadelphia: Saunders, 1976; 165.
14. Small M, Cameron A, Lunan B, et al. Macrosomia in pregnancy complicated by insulin-dependent diabetes mellitus. Diab Care 10(5):534, 1987.
15. Breitweser JA, Meyer RA, Sperling MA, et al. Cardiac septal hypertrophy in hyperinsulinemic infants. J Pediatr 96:535, 1980.
16. Greene MF, Hare JW, Krauhe J, et al. Prematurity among insulin requiring diabetic gravid women. Am J Obstet Gynecol 161:106, 1989.
17. Langer O, Levy J, Brustman L, et al. Glycemic control in gestational diabetes mellitus—how tight is tight enough: Small for gestational age versus large for gestational age? Am J Obstet Glynecol 161(3):646, 1989.
18. Kitzmiller JL, Brown ER, Phillipe M, et al. Diabetic nephropathy and perinatal outcome. Am J Obstet Gynecol 141:741, 1981.
19. Way GL, Wolfe RR, Eshaghpour E, et al. The natural history of hypertrophic cardiomyopathy in infants of diabetic mothers. J Pediatr 95:1020, 1979.

20. Walther FJ, Siassi B, King J, et al. Cardiac output in infants of insulin-dependent diabetic mothers. J Pediatr 107(1):109, 1985.

21. Gutgesell HP, Mullins CE, Gillette PC, et al. Transient hypertrophic subaortic stenosis in infants of diabetic mothers. J Pediatr 89:120, 1976.

22. Demarini S, Specker BL, Sierra RI, et al. Evidence of increased intrauterine bone resorption in term infants of mothers with insulin-dependent diabetes. J Pediatr 126:796, 1995.

23. Kitzmiller JL, Cloherty JP, Younger MD, et al. Diabetic pregnancy and perinatal morbidity. Am J Obstet Gynecol 131:560, 1978.

24. Robert MF, Neff RR, Hubbell JP, et al. Association between maternal diabetes and the respiratory-distress syndrome in the newborn. N Engl J Med 294(7):357, 1976.

25. Kjos SL, Walther FJ, Montoro M, et al. Prevalence and etiology of respiratory distress in infants of diabetic mothers: Predictive value of fetal lung maturation tests. Am J Obstet Gynecol 163:898, 1990.

26. Ferroni KM, Gross TL, Sokol RJ, et al. What affects fetal pulmonary maturation during diabetic pregnancy? Am J Obstet Gynecol 150:270, 1984.

27. Robinson R. Neurological development in infants of diabetic mothers. Dev Med Child Neurol 12:227, 1970.

28. Petry CD, Eaton MA, Wobken JD, et al. Iron deficiency of liver, heart and brain in newborn infants of diabetic mothers. J Pediatr 121:109, 1992.

29. Lukens JN. Iron metabolism and iron deficiency anemia. In: Miller DR, Baehner RL, McMillan CW, eds. Blood diseases of infancy and childhood, 5th ed. St. Louis: Mosby, 1984; 115.

30. Reece EA, Homko CJ, Wu YK, et al. Metabolic fuel mixtures and diabetic embryopathy. Clin Perinatol 20(3):517, 1993.

31. Adashi EY, Pinto H, Tyson JE. Impact in diabetic pregnancy. Am J Obstet Gynecol 133:268, 1979.

32. Pildes RS. Infants of diabetic mothers. In: Avery GB, ed. Neonatology, pathophysiology and management of the newborn. 3d ed. Philadelphia: Lippincott, 1987; 339.

33. Cowett RM. The infant of the diabetic mother. In: Hay WW Jr, ed. Neonatal nutrition and metabolism. St. Louis: Mosby Year Book, 1991; 419.

34. Kliegman RM, Behrman RE. The fetus and the neonatal infant. In: Behrman RE, Kliegman RM, Nelson WE, Vaughan VC, eds. Nelson textbook of pediatrics. 14th ed. Philadelphia: Saunders, 1992; 492.

35. Lillien LD, Pildes RS, Srinivasan G, et al. Treatment of neonatal hypoglycemia with minibolus and intravenous glucose infusion. J Pediatr 97:295, 1980.

36. American Academy of Pediatrics. Pediatric Nutrition Handbook, 4th ed. Elk Grove Village, Ill.: American Academy of Pediatrics, 1998; 391.

37. Costalos C, Russell G, Al Rahim Q, et al. Effects of plasma glucose concentration of light-for-date infants and infants of diabetic mothers of feeds supplemented with a glucose polymer. Acta Paediatr Scand 74:382, 1985.

38. Robson AM. General considerations in the care of sick children. In: Behrman RE, Kliegman RM, Nelson WE, Vaughan VC, eds. Nelson textbook of pediatrics. 14th ed. Philadelphia: Saunders, 1992; 212.

39. Vohr BR, Lewis PL, Oh W. Somatic growth of children of diabetic mothers with reference to birth size. J Pediatr 97:196, 1980.
40. Silverman BL, Rizzo T, Green DC, et al. Long-term prospective evaluation of offspring of diabetic mothers. Diabetes 40 (suppl. 2):121, 1991.
41. Ferris AM, Dalidowitz CK, Ingardia FD, et al. Lactation outcome in insulin-dependent diabetic women. J Am Diet Assoc 88:137, 1988.
42. McCoy R, Kadowaki C, Wilks S, et al. Nursing management of breast feeding for preterm infants. J Perinat Neonat Nurs 2:42, 1988.
43. Dewey KG, Heinig JM, Nommsen LA, et al. Growth of breast-fed and formula-fed infants from 0-18 months: The DARLING study. Pediatrics 89:1035, 1992.
44. Freedland RA, Briggs S. A biochemical approach to nutrition. London: Chapman and Hall, 1977; 40.
45. Kliegman RM, Sparks JW. Perinatal galactose metabolism. J Pediatr 107:831, 1985.
46. Kliegman RM, Morton S. Galactose assimilation in pups of diabetic canine mothers. Diabetes 36:1280, 1987.
47. Metzger BE, Silverman BL, Freinkel N, et al. Amniotic fluid insulin concentration as a predictor of obesity. Arch Dis Child 65:1050, 1990.
48. Rizzo T, Freinkel N, Metzger BE, et al. Correlations between antepartum maternal metabolism and newborn behavior. Am J Obstet Gynecol 163:1458, 1990.
49. Rizzo T, Metzger BE, Burns WJ, et al. Correlations between antepartum maternal metabolism and intelligence of offspring. N Engl J Med 325:911, 1991.
50. Warram JH, Krolewski AS, Gottlieb MS, et al. Differences in risk of insulin-dependent diabetes in offspring of diabetic mothers and diabetic fathers. N Engl J Med 311:149, 1984.
51. American Academy of Pediatrics, Work group on cow's milk protein and diabetes mellitus. Infant feeding practices and their possible relationship to the etiology of diabetes mellitus. Pediatrics 94:752, 1994.
52. Cordero L, Trever SH, Landon MC, Gabbe SG. Management of infants of diabetic mothers. Arch Pediatr Adolesc Med 152:249, 1998.
53. American Academy of Pediatrics, Committee on Nutrition. Iron fortification of infant formulas. Pediatrics 104:119, 1999.
54. Agostoni C. Breast feeding and childhood obesity. Pediatr Res 47:3, 2000.

SECTION V

DISCHARGE
AND
FOLLOW-UP

Nutritional Care for High-Risk Newborns (Rev. 3d. Ed.)
S. Groh-Wargo, M. Thompson, J. Cox, editors
© 2000, Precept Press, Inc., Chicago

33

NUTRITIONAL CONCERNS AT TRANSFER OR DISCHARGE

Janice Hovasi Cox, MS, RD, and Denise Doorlag, OTR

AS NEONATAL MEDICAL AND surgical care have become more sophisticated, smaller and sicker infants are now surviving. Regardless of whether these infants continue to have complex medical problems beyond the neonatal period, discharge planning is an essential aspect of comprehensive medical care that provides a smooth transition from the neonatal intensive care unit (NICU) to the hospital providing primary care and/or to the home. The purpose of this chapter is to briefly describe nutrition issues that arise during this transition.

Criteria for Transfer or Discharge

Earliest possible NICU discharge is desired for high-risk infants to (1) decrease the period of separation from parents and reduce the adverse effects of separation on parenting, (2) reduce the risk of hospital acquired morbidity, (3) focus NICU resources on infants who require intensive medical care rather than routine care, and (4) reduce medical care costs.[1,2] However, higher rates of hospital readmission and death during the first year of life among low-birth-weight (LBW) infants who require neonatal intensive care indicate that family and community health care providers must be sufficiently prepared to assume the responsibility for the infant's care when NICU discharge occurs. Causes for hospital readmission commonly include failure to thrive and feeding problems. Medical treatments or equipment needed, referring hospital staff, equipment availability and capability, the infant's physiologic maturity, and parental readiness must be considered.[3] Depending upon the infant's condition and needs, many persons may be involved in planning for transfer or discharge, including the neonatologist, primary care physician, nurse, social worker, occupational or physical therapist, dietitian, community support services, and the infant's family.

Proposed guidelines for hospital discharge of high-risk neonates include several aspects that may be applied to nutrition (Table 33.1). Physiologic maturity, ability to nipple-feed and sustain an acceptable pattern of weight gain, and parental readiness are most often cited as the criteria for discharge.[1-7] Parameters of physiologic maturity related to nutrition include the ability to maintain adequate body temperature and growth in an open bed with appropriate clothing and adequate hemoglobin and hematocrit levels (or evidence of adequate reticulocyte activity).[3,4] Metabolic screening is completed within the guidelines of individual states with additional follow-up or appropriate referral provided for infants with abnormal results.

A consistant pattern of sufficient weight gain is often used as a criterion for discharge, although the definitions of "consistent" and "sufficient" vary, based on maturity and individual growth patterns.[1,2,7,8] Previous guidelines for NICU discharge have included achieving a minimum weight of 1,800 to 2,000 g.[2,7,9] A specific achieved weight is not always useful as a predictor of readiness for discharge because progression toward physiological maturity, weight gain patterns, and suckling ability are affected by many factors. Infants who are small for gestational age at birth are more physiologically mature relative to their weight at birth, and these infants may be ready for discharge at 1,300 g.[2] Infants who experience respiratory, gastrointestinal, or neurologic dysfunction regardless of birthweight or gestational age at birth may not be ready for hospital discharge until they are byond 40 weeks' postmenstrual age and have achieved a weight beyond 2,000 g.[9] A "consistent pattern of sufficient weight gain" may be interpreted as that which maintains or improves the infant's weight status compared with potmenstrual-age-matched peers using standardized growth tables or charts, or at least 15-20 g/day for a period of three days[3] (see Table 34.1, Table 34.3, and Appendix D).

Most infants progress toward physiological maturity in tandem with their suckling ability so they are able to nipple-feed adequate amounts of breast milk or formula by the time they are able to maintain cardiopulmonary stability and are ready for hospital discharge. Intake may be considered adequate if it supports growth that is within normal limits. (See "Feeding Recommendations" below.) Before transfer to a less acute medical setting, infants are usually weaned from parenteral nutrition. Enteral nutrition usually has progressed to bolus nasogastric or orogastric tube feedings, but if the need for alternative feeding methods extends beyond the need for other technical support, infants may be transferred to a less intensive medical care setting. If neurologic or alimentary tract dysfunction precludes oral feeding for an extended period of time, infants may be discharged to their home with parenteral nutrition and/or tube feedings, provided that nutrition and feeding assessments are completed before discharge with treatment plans clearly identified, including appropriate follow-up.[3] Caring for an infant who is difficult to feed can be frustrating, causing parental feelings of failure or inadequacy. Multidisciplinary follow-up may be needed to provide ongoing assessment and recommendations as well as emotional support.

Parents should be able to demonstrate the ability to feed their infant, whether by breast, bottle, or feeding tube. They may need help reading their infant's hunger and satiety cues, especially if the infant is < 40 weeks' gestation at discharge, requires some or all of the feedings given by tube, or has sustained neurological damage (see Chapters 18, 19, and 31). Parents should be able to demonstrate or describe formula preparation and/or dosing of nutrient supplements. When needed, special recipes, feeding instructions, or counseling should be provided to meet the individual infant's nutritional needs within the framework of the family's learning styles, abilities, and functional level of literacy and understanding.

Communication

A written summary of nutrition issues is an integral part of a discharge plan to facilitate a smooth transition from the intensive medical care setting to the home or local hospital.[2] Parameters of nutrition assessment and nutrition care plans that may be important to include in discharge summaries are given in Table 33.4. Each professional involved in nutrition follow-up of the infant should receive a discharge summary; this group includes the primary care physician, nutritionist, public health dietitian or nurse, visiting nurse, and/or early intervention program personnel. Computer-generated discharge summaries may be helpful for this purpose (see Chapter 6).

Table 33.1.   Guidelines for Establishing Readiness for Discharge Applied to Nutrition[1-7]

Infant

• Adequate weight gain is sustained
• Normal body temperature is maintained
• Cardiopulmonary stability is achieved
• Feeding skills to support normal growth are consistently demonstrated
• Metabolic screening is performed
• Hematologic status is assessed and treatment is established (if needed)
• Nutritional risks/problems are identified and treatment is established
   (if needed)

Family

• Ability to adequately feed infant, whether by breast, bottle, or alternative
   feeding method, including accurate assessment of feeding cues, is
   demonstrated
• Ability to procure, safely handle, and accurately prepare formula
   (if needed) is demonstrated
• Ability to accurately administer nutrient supplements (if needed) is
   demonstrated

Community

• Primary medical care providers are identified and accept responsibility for
   care of infant after hospital discharge
• Follow-up nutrition care providers are identified (if needed), appropriate
   referrals made
• Information regarding growth expectations and nutrition care plan has
   been given to the primary medical care provider and nutrition care
   provider when indicated

Feeding Recommendations

Breast-feeding

Human milk is the optimal food for infants regardless of gestational maturity at birth. Smaller, less mature infants may require fortification of human milk with protein, minerals, and vitamins for a time to provide adequate amounts of nutrients that support rapid growth.[17] At the same time that infants develop proficiency nursing at the breast, their need for nutrient supplements likely diminishes

Table 33.2.   Causes of Delayed and Dysfunctional Feeding
Problems

Delayed progress in feedings skills	Dysfunctional feeding skills
Premature birth	Physical or structural deficits
Frequent or prolonged illness	Neurological deficits
Decreased exposure to more advanced feeding techniques	
Parental misperceptions or lack of information	

if the breast milk supply is adequate. It is not clear whether human milk fortifiers continue to provide benefit in supporting growth beyond hospital discharge, although if the breast milk supply is not adequate, supplementation with premature infant formula or enriched formula is usually recommended.[18] (See Table 33.5 for specific discharge feeding recommendations.)

The need for neonatal intensive medical/surgical care can present many challenges to successful breast feeding (see Chapter 17). At discharge, issues of adequate milk supply and the infant's breast-feeding ability require individualized assessment and strategies to support breastfeeding success. Table 33.6 contains guidelines for establishing successful breast-feeding. Several professional and parent breast-feeding education resources are available. [19-22]

Formula

If human milk is not available, formula is prescribed at hospital discharge based on individual needs. Premature infant formulas are generally indicated for infants up to 1,850 to 2,000 g body weight.[7,18,23] Infants with increased mineral needs may continue to receive these formulas up to 3,500 grams body weight,[24] but intake of premature infant formula in amounts > 500 ml per day may provide excessive vitamin A and D intake.[25] Enriched formulas (NeoSure, Ross Products Division, Abbott Laboratories, Columbus, Ohio; and EnfaCare, Mead Johnson Nutritionals, Evansville, Ind.) provide energy, protein, vitamins, and minerals in amounts greater than standard infant formulas, but less than premature infant formulas to support rapid growth and prevent nutrient depletion without providing excess nutrients[24-31] (see Appendix K).

Volumes given should support at least 20 g/day weight gain. Unlike their term counterparts who may have experienced their most rapid gain of 30-35 g/day during 32-36 weeks' gestation in utero, preterm infants may show similar rates of gain during 38-48 weeks postconceptual age.[32-35] This catch-up growth seems to depend most upon nutrient intake and absence of continuing medical compromise.

Table 33.3.   Feeding Concerns for High-Risk Newborns at Discharge[11-16]

Feeding problem	Symptoms/characteristics	Recommendations
State/Physiological Stability	State stability: • Sleepy baby or quickly becomes sleepy • Poor waking cues or may sleep poorly • Cries frequently • Fussy with feedings • Difficulty achieving quiet alert state • Difficulty initiating sucking • Difficulty focusing on feeding Physiological stability: • Color changes • Stress signs • Sweating • Apnea/bradycardia • Shuts down • Hiccoughs	Calming techniques: • Provide pacifier • Swaddle/contain • Watch for subtle/early hunger cues • Begin feeding during quiet alert state • Provide slow rhythmic movement • Speak in quiet, modulated voice or no auditory stimulation at all • Look closely at environment for sources of excessive stimulation Alerting techniques: • Vary pitch of voice • Change diaper • Frequent burping • Keep unswaddled • Wipe face with a cool cloth
Endurance	• Sleepy baby, does not wake for feedings • Does not wake often enough for feedings • Slow, "pokey" eater • Feeding lasts longer than 30-45 minutes before finishing feeding • Increased liquid loss as feeding progresses • Sucking becomes disorganized as feeding progresses • Baby takes long pauses to breathe • Baby has very short sucking bursts • Indicates satiety or falls asleep	• Consider a faster flow nipple if coordination is not an issue • Offer chin and cheek support • Limit feeding to 20-30 minutes; discontinue feeding when infant is fatigued • Consider feeding supplements/concentrated feedings • Look closely at environment for sources of excessive stimulation • Support flexed position, head aligned with body
Suck/swallow/breathe coordination	• Gulping • Coughing/choking • Excessive liquid loss • Gasping for breath • Takes 1-2 sucks then pulls away • Oxygen desaturation • Apnea with or without bradycardia • Periodic breathing	• Adjust flow of milk from nipple (slow flow nipple) • Begin nursing after initial let down/ejection reflex • Reduce distractions in environment • Swaddle or contain baby in flexed position, head aligned with body • Help baby pace feeding by allowing breaks for breathing • Baby may need a feeding evaluation*

Table 33.3. Feeding Concerns for High-Risk Newborns at Discharge (continued)[11-16]

Feeding problem	Symptoms/characteristics	Recommendations
Swallowing mechanism	• Takes pacifier but not breast/bottle • Holds liquid in mouth before swallowing • Excessive liquid loss • Audible hard swallows • *Frequent* coughing/choking • Recurrent aspiration pneumonia	• Adjust flow of milk from nipple (e.g. use slow flow nipple) • Feeding evaluation* and/or videofluorscopic swallow study to rule out delayed or dysfunctional swallow
Oral motor control/coordination	• Weak suck or noisy sucking • Tongue retraction or abnormal movement • Arching backward, altered trunk tone • Inconsistent success with various nipples • Nipple biting/munching instead of sucking • Excessive liquid loss even with reduced milk flow • Frequent coughing/choking even with reduced milk flow • Lack of feeding skill progression at appropriate age intervals • *Frequent* gagging • Aversive or defensive behaviors • Abnormal anatomy • Hypertonia—or hypotonia • Recurrent aspiration pneumonia	• Feeding evaluation* • Nutrition evaluation by a registered dietitian to assess nutrition intake and provide recommendations to optimize nutrient intake and support the achievement growth and development potential

* These assessments are best performed by a feeding therapist (Occupational Therapist, Speech Pathologist, or Physical Therapist) or a developmental therapist who is trained/experienced in feeding newborns.

Average daily nutrient needs and intake to support catch-up growth may exceed that of the normal term newborn.[36] The European Society for Pediatric Gastroenterology and Nutrition (ESPAN) recommends 165 kcal/kg/day.[37] Various sources indicate average daily intakes of 137-165 kcal/kg/day.[26,29,32] Average intakes of > 200 kcal/kg/day may be consumed by a significant number of infants.[26,29] The rate of weight gain beyond this time period closely mimics that of term-born post-conceptual age matched peers, indicating only gradual or no catch-up growth beyond this initial period for even as late as eight years.[32,38,39] At least some degree of catch-up growth may occur at any time when a growth limiting condition such as congenital cyanotic heart disease, bronchopulmonary dysplasia, or psychosocial neglect is resolved.[40]

Infants who cannot tolerate these larger volumes of milk or formula due to impaired pulmonary, cardiac, hepatic, renal, alimentary tract, or neurological function may require feedings of higher caloric density or supplemental tube-feedings. Standard concentrated liquid or powdered infant formulas may be prepared at greater caloric density as long as the potential renal solute load is within the limits of renal function. Recipes for formula concentrations of 24, 27, and 30 kcal/oz are given in Appendix I.

If the volume of milk or formula intake is adequate to meet vitamin and mineral needs but growth is insufficient, modular components of carbohydrate, fat, and/or protein may be added to meet a specific infant's needs. Care must be taken to provide an appropriate balance of these macronutrients, with protein providing 7-16%, fat 30-55%, and carbohydrate 30-60% of total calories.[40] One must also consider availability, cost, and ease of preparation when designing special preparations of formulas to be used at home.

Vitamins

Recommendations for oral intake of vitamins by premature LBW infants who have reached 1,800-2,000 g of weight is similar to that for full-term infants (see Chapter 15). Infants who receive human milk fortifier, premature infant formula, or enriched formula after discharge as recommended in Table 33.6 generally do not need additional vitamin supplements if daily milk or formula intake is meeting energy needs. Vitamin D intake with enriched formulas are at least 150 IU/day. Although intake of standard infant formula or human milk may be higher per unit of body weight than full-term infants, total volume of intake may not be adequate to provide recommended amounts of vitamins. A daily dose of 0.5-1.0 ml of a standard multivitamin supplement is recommended until standard infant formula or human milk intake reaches 750 ml/day (or until body weight is 3.5-4.0 kg). Infants fed human milk should continue to receive supplement of 200-400 IU of vitamin D until other dietary sources are added.[18,41]

Table 33.4. Nutrition Information for Inclusion in Discharge Summaries

Anthropometry (actual measurements and percentile ranking)

Birth weight, length, and head circumference
Discharge weight, length, and head circumference
Rate of weight gain to be expected during first few weeks after discharge

Laboratory

Metabolic screening results
Hemoglobin and hematocrit
Other pertinent laboratory values that require follow-up such as elevated serum
    alkaline phosphatase or bilirubin, low serum phosphorus, protein, prealbumin,
    or other nutrient level

Intake

Length of time infant received parenteral nutrition
Enteral feedings used during hospitalization
Formula intolerances, if any
Feeding regimen recommended at discharge, including:
— Breast-feeding (progress toward full feedings at breast)
— Formula (kind, strength, amount, frequency of feeding)
— Formula recipe (if nonstandard)
— Supplements (kind and dose)
— Changes in intake expected during first few weeks after discharge
— Oral motor treatment plan (if needed)
— Handling/positioning techniques (if needed)

Other

Infants discharged while receiving parenteral nutrition need specific nutrient
prescription and recommended schedule for laboratory monitoring

Guidelines for progression to full oral feedings may be needed for infants who still
require tube feedings at discharge

Other special considerations may include use of specific nipples or bottles (as with
cleft palate), oxygen delivery during feedings, oral-motor treatment regimens, and
recommendations for introduction of solid foods

Referrals

— NICU follow-up clinic
— Special Supplemental Food Program for Women, Infants, and Children
— Children's Rehabilitative Services for feeding therapist/specialist follow-up
— Services for Children with Special Health Care Needs (Crippled Children's
    Services)

Minerals

Iron (Fe) supplementation is needed for LBW infants beyond 1 to 2 months of age receiving human milk or low-iron infant formulas. The recommended dose is 2-4 mg/kg/day, given orally as ferrous sulfate.[40] Standard and premature formulas fortified with Fe provide 2 mg/kg/day at intakes of 120 kcal/kg/day.

The calcium (Ca) and phosphorus (P) content of human milk and standard infant formulas and the zinc content of standard formulas may not be sufficient during the rapid growth phase of the premature infant from 38-48 weeks postconceptual age to support normal mineral accretion rates.[28] Continued use of human milk fortifier, premature formula, or enriched formula should be considered during this phase, particularly if osteopenia of prematurity has been identified (see Chapter 29). If these products are unavailable or impractical, Ca and P supplements may be considered.[42] When Ca supplements are given to infants who are also receiving calciuretic medications, care should be taken to avoid hypercalciuria, and monitoring urine Ca–creatinine ratios should be considered. Ca and P supplements may be absorbed better if administered separately, because simultaneous addition of these minerals may result in precipitation (see Chapters 15 and 16 and Appendix L for doses and product information).

Food and Milk

Recommendations for starting foods other than human milk or infant formula are the same as for term-born infants of same postconceptual age. (These are described in detail in Chapter 34, Table 34.4.) Whole cow's milk should not replace human milk or Fe-fortified infant formula until one year beyond term to ensure adequate intake of Fe, vitamins B_6, C, and essential fatty acids.

NICU follow-up Programs

Follow-up programs that have been developed in conjunction with many NICUs vary in purpose, structure, staff, and site, depending on the characteristics and needs of the population and the resources of the institution and the community.

Purpose

The developmental outcome and diagnosis of developmental problems and referral for early intervention are often the primary focus of NICU follow-up for the benefit of the patient as well as to establish efficacy of neonatal care.[4] Programs may also include general

Table 33.5. Discharge Feeding Guidelines for Infants < 37 Weeks' Gestational Age and ≤ 1850 g at Birth*

Infants with Highest Nutrient Needs	Infants with High Nutrient Needs
1. Birth weight < 1,000 g or 2. Birth weight ≥ 1,000 g and Discharge weight < 1,850 g or 3. Serum prealbumin < 10 mg/dL or 4. Growth < -2 SD/5th percentile[†] or 5. Bronchopulmonary dysplasia[§] or 6. Osteopenia[‡]	1. Birthweight ≥ 1,000 g and 2. Discharge weight > 1,850 g and 3. Growth ≥ -2 SD or 5th percentile[†]
Breast-fed: 1. See table 33.6. 2. Provide high-protein, high-mineral supplement such as human milk fortifier or enriched formula until nutrient deficiency is corrected; explore alternative feeding techniques (i.e. cup, syringe, etc.) with family to minimize exposure to artificial nipple 3. Supplement with 1 dose/d multivitamin drops until 5 kg (11#) and iron 2-4 mg/kg/d	**Breast-fed:** 1. See table 33.6. 2. If breast milk supply is insufficient, supplement with enriched or standard formula (see below) 3. Supplement with 1 dose of multivitamin drops daily until weight is 5 kg (11#) 4. Supplement with 2-4 mg iron/kg/d
Formula-fed: 1. 24 kcal/oz premature infant formula with iron until 1,850 g/4 lb (or at most 3,500 g/7 lb 11 oz) 2. 22 kcal/oz enriched formula with iron from 1,850 g (or 3,500 g) until catch-up growth complete or until 9 mo to 1 yr corrected age 3. Standard 20 kcal/oz formula may be considered once growth parameters achieve expected genetic potential for corrected age; continue until 1 yr corrected age 4. Either formula provides 2 mg/kg/day iron; may need additional iron for a total of 4 mg/kg/d	**Formula-fed:** 1. Enriched 22 kcal/oz with iron formula until catch-up growth is completed, then standard 20 kcal/oz with iron formula up to 1 yr corrected age 2. If already following genetic growth channel, standard 20 kcal/oz with iron formula up to 1 yr corrected age 3. Supplement with 1/2 to 1 dose of multivitamin drops daily if standard formula is used until intake is regularly ≥ 32 oz/d 4. Formula provides 2 mg/kg/d iron; may need additional iron for a total of 4 mg/kg/d

Reassess growth and intake at 2 wk follow-up visit, every 4-6 wk thereafter until 6 m corrected age, then every 2 mo. Spoon feedings are started based on oral motor development/readiness, usually around 4-6 mo corrected age.

* These are general guidelines; discharge instructions must be individualized to accommodate specific needs. Infants > 37 weeks' gestational age or > 1,850 g birth weight without chronic disease or condition may be discharged on standard nutrition regimen for normal term infants.

† Growth is evaluated in standard deviations from the mean on the Oregon Growth Chart and in percentile rank on the National Center for Health Statistics (NCHS) Charts or the Gairdner/Pearson growth charts; growth parameters that plot below the 25th percentile on the VLBW Infant Health and Development Program (IHDP) growth charts are roughly equivalent to the 5th percentile on the NCHS or Gairdner/Pearson charts or at -2 SD on the Oregon chart.

§ If bronchopulmonary dysplasia is significant at discharge and requires treatment with supplemental oxygen, diuretics and/or steroid therapy, nutritional needs may be altered.

‡ Osteopenia: serum phosphorus < 4 mg/dl, serum alkaline phosphatase > 600 IU/L, or bone demineralization noted on x-ray.

Adapted from Groh-Wargo S, Cox JH. Prematurely born infants. In: Nutrition manual for at-risk infants and toddlers. Chicago: Precept Press, 1997: 91.

pediatric care during the early months of transition from the NICU to home.[2,8,43,44] The most significant concerns at this time are monitoring growth, development, and nutrition; managing residual health problems or concerns; identifying and treating new health problems; immunization schedules; and parental education and reassurance.[7,44] It is also an opportune time to confirm that issues identified prior to discharge have been addressed and that the parents are receiving the support they need. Although generally not the primary focus of follow-up, clinical research concerning the outcome of specific groups of infants is paramount in providing perspective and direction for care during the neonatal period and beyond. Follow-up programs also provide an opportunity for education of therapists or educators specializing in infant development, primary care physicians, pediatric residents, nursing staff, and dietitians.

Structure

Identification of infants to be followed and the frequency and duration of follow-up are determined based on program purpose. Eligibility criteria usually include birth-weight or gestational age at birth; perinatal or neonatal complications associated with long-term risk for adverse outcome; or identified medical, social, or developmental problems.[4,46] Risk factors that may be associated with nutritional problems after hospital discharge are given in Table 33.7. Many of these factors may be included as criteria for eligibility in NICU follow-up programs. Infants who may be at risk for developing nutritional problems but who are not eligible for comprehensive NICU follow-up may be eligible for other avenues of nutrition follow-up through the federal Food Supplemental Program for Women, Infants, and Children, early intervention programs that provide services identified by Public Law 102-119 (previously 99-457, Part H)[47] public health agencies, or home health care providers.

The schedule of visits may include a visit within a few weeks of discharge from the unit to access initial adaptation to the home environment. Nutrition assessment may play an integral part of early follow-up.[2,3,6,7,44] (Guidelines for growth and nutrition assessment are given in Chapter 34, Tables 34.1 and 34.3). Subsequent follow-up usually is based on ages that coincide with developmental milestones, normally at 4, 8 and/or 12, 18 or 24, and 36 or 48 months.[1,48] Age is "corrected for prematurity;" for example, an infant born at 32 weeks' gestation who is now 12 weeks old has a "corrected age" of one month, or the infant is one month beyond the term date. Infants at highest risk for nutritional problems after discharge may benefit from nutrition assessment and intervention throughout this follow-up period (see Table 33.7).

Table 33.6. Establishing Successful Breast-feeding in the Premature Infant

- Create ideal mealtime environment: minimal amounts of bright light, noise, or other distracting stimulation, and appropriate room temperature

- Observe infant's cues for stress, relaxation, and early hunger cues; infant is calm but alert when feedings are started; feeding is stopped if stress signals are observed

- Feed infant at breast on demand every 1 1/2 to 3 hrs, or at least 8-12 times/d, with no more than one period of prolonged sleep of up to 5 hrs

- Generous use of pillows may be needed to support comfortable position for infant and mother; infant's head and body are in alignment; infant's body is flexed, chin tucked, shoulders and arms forward; infant's mouth is positioned directly at mother's nipple. Position breast using C-cup hold so infant can fully and easily grasp nipple; mother's thumb and index finger can come forward to support jaw or cheeks if necessary

- Initiate let-down and express some milk before infant is placed at breast to better encourage latching-on

- Infant is able to establish a pattern of sucking bursts with pauses for swallowing and breathing; stopping occasionally for burping or to rest may be needed; infant is able to empty breast with at least 10 min of active nursing—however, overemphasis on time elapsed rather than quality of nursing may interfere with breast-feeding success; feeding sessions that last longer than 30 min may tire both infant and mother and may also limit breast-feeding success

- Empty breasts by pumping after feedings if needed for the first 2-3 wk at home to ensure that breasts are being emptied and to further stimulate adequate milk supply; use cup, syringe, or bottle-feeding of this hind milk to ensure adequate caloric intake. If milk supply is greater than infant's needs, encourage feeding pattern that allows infant to empty at least one breast per feeding to ensure that the infant receives hind milk

- Adequacy of intake may be assessed by weighing infant before and after feedings using a scale specifically designed for accurate measurement of minute weight increments—most premature born infants newly discharged from NICU weigh 4-5 lb (1,800-2,250 g), so that intake at individual feedings is generally around 11/2 to 2 oz (45 to 60 ml)

- Weighing infant within 24 hr after hospital discharge and again within 48-72 hr provides a timely assessment of intake and fluid balance during initial discharge period and provides reassurance to parents regarding breast-feeding success. Adequacy of intake may be assessed by weighing infant regularly; average daily weight gain is generally at least 20-25 g/d (or 5-6 oz/wk) during first few weeks after discharge

- Supplement using recommendations in Table 33.6; supplements are generally decreased or eliminated as soon as possible after discharge based on weight gain and other nutrient needs, though iron supplementation may be required throughout the first year

- Use of supplemental nursing device may be helpful for mother who has not yet achieved adequate milk supply or for infant able to nurse at breast but needs nutrient supplements or extra calories

Adapted from Groh-Wargo S, Cox JH. Prematurely born infants. In: Nutrition manual for at-risk infants and toddlers. Chicago: Precept Press, 1997; 89.

Staff and Site

Personnel involved in follow-up varies with program purpose and institution resources. The physician involved is often a neonatologist

Table 33.7.   Infants at Highest Risk for Nutritional Problems
After Discharge from Neonatal ICU

Very low birth weight infants (< 1,500 g birth weight)
Extremely low birth weight infants (< 1,000 g birth weight)
Small-for-gestational-age infants
Breast-fed infants
Infants on special formulas
Infants on parenteral nutrition > 4 wk during hospitalization
Infants on parenteral nutrition after hospital discharge
Infants with a diagnosis of any of the following*
 Bronchopulmonary dysplasia
 Chronic renal insufficiency
 Congenital alimentary tract anomalies
 Cyanotic congenital heart disease
 Inborn errors of metabolism
 Malabsorption
 Osteopenia of prematurity
 Poverty or low socioeconomic status
 Severe neurological impairment
 Short bowel syndrome
Infants with gastrostomies or tracheostomies
Infants who require tube feedings at home
Infants who fail to gain at least 20 g/d prior to discharge

* For full discussion of diseases listed, see various chapters of section IV of this book.

or a pediatrician with special training in infant development. Nurses and social workers provide assessment of health, parenting, social, and financial needs and are often the liaison between the NICU and various community or home health agencies. Developmental testing may be performed by any of several professionals trained in developmental follow-up. These professionals may be skilled in occupational or physical therapy or psychology. Nutritionists may be available on a routine or consultative basis, although evidence suggests that if a registered dietitian provides routine assessment and intervention during the first year after discharge, catch-up growth in weight, length, and head circumference is enhanced.[43] Other consultants may include representatives from audiology, ophthalmology, and speech pathology.

Follow-up visits are often conducted within the institution that is affiliated with the NICU. If regions serviced by the NICU are large and distance is a significant barrier to follow-up, additional sites may be used. Some institutions are able to provide home visits, at least for initial follow-up. Regardless of the specific agency, personnel, or site, communication among all who are involved in the health and welfare of these patients is paramount if comprehensive care and a smooth transition from NICU to home is the goal.

The time surrounding transfer or discharge from the NICU is a time of transition in the nutritional care of the high-risk infant. Growth patterns may be changing, beginning catch-up growth, or settling into genetic patterns. The method of feeding may be changing from tube to bottle or breast. Enriched feedings are replaced with standard infant formulas or unsupplemented breast milk. Parents become fully responsible for the feeding of their infant and may be unsure of themselves or their infant's feeding cues and abilities. Parent education must be individualized to meet the specific needs of the infant and the parents' level of understanding, especially if the infant has feeding problems.[49] Planning for the infant's transfer or discharge from the NICU involves assessment of the infant's nutritional status and projecting the infant's nutritional needs and growth expectations. This nutrition information must then be effectively communicated to the parents and the health care providers who will be responsible for the infant after transfer or discharge from the NICU.

References

1. American Academy of Pediatrics Committee on Fetus and Newborn. Hospital discharge of the high-risk neonate—proposed guidelines. Pediatr 102:411, 1998.
2. Cruz H, Guzman N, Rosales M, et al. Early hospital discharge of preterm very low birth weight infants. J Perinatol 17:29-32, 1997.
3. Raddish M, Merritt TA. Early discharge of premature infants: a critical analysis. Clin Perinatol 25:449, 1998.
4. Joint Committee on High-Risk Infant Environment, Intervention and follow-up. Discharge planning and neonatal follow-up. American Public Health Association, Maternal and Child Health Section, 1991.
5. Hurt H. Continuing care of the high-risk infant. Clin Perinatol 11:3, 1984.
6. Gershan LA, Kliegman RM. Early discharge of low birth weight infants: An opportunity to evolve and to create partnerships. J Pediatr 127:272, 1995.
7. American Academy of Pediatrics and American College of Obstetrics and Gynecology. Guidelines for perinatal care. 3rd ed. Elk Grove Village, Ill: American Academy of Pediatrics; and Washington, D.C.: American College of Obstetricians and Gynecologists, 1992.
8. Kotagal UR, Perlstein PH, Gamblian V, et al. Description and evaluation of a program for the early discharge of infants from a neonatal intensive care unit. J Pediatr 127:285, 1995.
9. Rawlings JS, Scott JS. Postconceptional age of surviving preterm low-birth-weight infants at hospital discharge. Arch Pediatr Adolesc Med 150:260, 1996.

10. Lau C, Schanler RJ. Oral motor function in the neonate. Clin Perinatol 23:161, 1996.

11. Als H et al. Manual for assessment of preterm infant behavior (APIB). In: Fitzgerald HE, Lester BM, Yogman MW, eds. Theory and research in behavioral pediatrics, vol 1. New York: Plenum Press, 1982; 65-132.

12. Arvedson JC, Brodsky L. Pediatric swallowing and feeding: Assessment and management. San Diego: Singular Publishing Group Inc, 1993.

13. Shriver-Shaker C. Nipple feeding premature infants: a different perspective. Neonatal Network, 8:9, 1990.

14. VandenBerg K. Nippling management of the sick neonate in the NICU: The disorganized feeder. Neonatal Network 9:9, 1990.

15. Wolf LS, Glass RP. Feeding and swallowing disorders in infancy: Assessment and management. Tucson, Ariz.: Therapy Skill Builders, 1992.

16. Gray K, King W. Feeding assessment. In: Cox JH, ed. Nutrition manual for at-risk infants and toddlers. Chicago:Precept Press, 1997; 33-42.

17. Bier JAB, Ferguson AE, Morales Y, et al. Breastfeeding infants who were extremely low birth weight. Pediatrics 1997;100(6). URL: http://www.pediatrics.org/cgi/content/full/6/e3

18. Groh-Wargo S, Cox JH. Prematurely born infants. In: Nutrition manual for at-risk infants and toddlers. Chicago: Precept Press, 1997, 81-96.

19. O'Leary M. You can breast-feed your preterm infant (video and pamphlets, 1989). Health Sciences Center for Educational Resources, SB-56, University of Washington, Seattle 98195, 206/545/1186.

20. Danner S, Cerutti E. Nursing your premature baby (pamphlet, 1990). Childbirth Graphics L&D, Box 20540, Rochester, NY 14602-0540, 716/272-0300.

21. LeLeche League International. Breast-feeding your premature baby (pamphlet, 1990). LeLeche League International, Box 1209, Franklin Park, IL 60131, 847/455-7730.

22. Meier P. Professional guide to breastfeeding premature infants. Columbus, Ohio: Ross Products Division, Abbott Laboratories, 1997.

23. Ziegler EE. Infants of low birth weight special needs and problems. Am J Clin Nutr 41:440, 1985.

24. Wheeler RE and Hall RT. Feeding of premature infant formula after hospital discharge of infants weighing less than 1800 grams at birth. J Perinatol 16:111, 1996.

25. Nako Y, Fukushima N, Tomomasa T, et al. Hypervitaminosis D after prolonged feeding with a premature formula. Pediatrics 92:862, 1993.

26. Lucas A, Bishop NJ, King FJ, et al. Randomised trial of nutrition for preterm infants after discharge. Arch Dis Child 67:324, 1992.

27. Lucas A, King F, Bishop NB. Postdischarge formula consumption in infants born preterm. Arch Dis Child 67:691, 1992.

28. Friel JK, Andrews WL, Matthew JD, et al. Improved growth of very low birth weight infants. Nutr Res 13:611, 1993.

29. Bishop NJ, King FJ, Lucas A. Increased bone mineral content of preterm infants fed with a nutrient enriched formula after discharge from hospital. Arch Dis Child 68:573, 1993.

30. Bhatia J, Rassin DK. Feeding the premature infant after hospital discharge: Growth and biochemical responses. J Pediatr 118:515, 1991.

31. Altigani M, Murphy JF, Gray OP. Plasma zinc concentration and catch-up growth in preterm infants. Acta Paediatr Scand (suppl) 357:20, 1989.

32. Brandt I. Growth dynamics of low-birth-weight infants with emphasis on the perinatal period. In: Falkner F, Tanner J, eds. Human growth: vol. 2 Postnatal growth. New York: Plenum Press, 1978; 572.
33. Manser JJ. Growth in the high-risk infant. Clin Perinatol 11:19, 1984.
34. Altigani M, Murphy JF, Newcombe RG, et al. Catch-up growth in preterm infants. Acta Paediatr Scand (suppl) 357:3, 1989.
35. Ernst JA, Bull MJ, Rickard KA, et al. Growth outcome and feeding practices of the very low birth weight infant (less than 1500 grams) within the first year of life. Pediatrics 117:S156, 1990.
36. Reichman B, Chessex P, Putet G, et al. Partition of energy metabolism and energy cost of growth in the very low-birth-weight infant. Pediatrics 69:446, 1982.
37. European Society of Paediatric Gastroenterology and Nutrition (ESPGAN), Committee on Nutrition of the Preterm Infant. Nutrition and feeding of preterm infants. Acta Paediatr Scand (suppl) 336:3, 1987.
38. Casey PH, Kraemer HC, Bernbaum J, et al. Growth status and growth rates of a varied sample of low birth weight preterm infants: A longitudinal cohort from birth to three years of age. J Pediatr 119:599, 1991.
39. Kitchen WH, Doyle LW, Ford GW, et al. Very low birth weight and growth to age 8 years. Am J Dis Child 146:40, 1992.
40. Fomon SJ. Nutrition of normal infants. St. Louis:Mosby, 1993.
41. American Academy of Pediatrics Committee on Nutrition. Nutritional needs of low-birth-weight infants. Pediatrics 75:976, 1985.
42. Hall RT, Wheeler RE, Rippetot LE. Calcium and phosphorus supplementation after initial hospital discharge in breast-fed infants of less than 1800 grams birthweight. J Perinatol 13:272, 1993.
43. Bryson SR, Theriot L, Ryan NJ, et al. Primary follow-up care in a multidisciplinary setting enhances catch-up growth of very-low-birth-weight infants. J Am Diet Assoc 97:386, 1997.
44. Bernstein S, Heimler R, Sasidharan P. Approaching the management of the neonatal intensive care unit graduate through history and physical assessment. Pediatr Clin North Am 45:79, 1998.
45. Joint Committee on High-Risk Infant Environment, Intervention and follow-up. Discharge planning and neonatal follow-up. Maternal and Child Health Bureau, U.S. Department of Health and Human Services, Roll Laboratories and College of Public Health, University of South Florida, 1991.
46. Kelleher KJ, Casey PH, Bradley RH, et al. Risk factors and outcomes for failure to thrive in low birth weight preterm infants. Pediatrics 91:941, 1993.
47. Department of Education. Early intervention program for infants and toddlers with handicaps. Federal Register 54:26305, 1989.
48. Perinatal Association of Michigan. Report of task force on developmental assessment of neonatal intensive care unit graduate, 1984.
49. Costello A, Bracht M, Van Camp K, et al. Parent information binder: individualizing education for parents of preterm infants. Neonatal Network 15:43, 1996.

Nutritional Care for High-Risk Newborns (Rev. 3d. Ed.)
S. Groh-Wargo, M. Thompson, J. Cox, editors
© 2000, Precept Press, Inc., Chicago

34

ROUTINE NUTRITION CARE DURING FOLLOW-UP

Lea Theriot, MS, LDN, RD

THE PURPOSE OF PROVIDING consistent nutrition follow-up for infants after discharge from the neonatal intensive care unit (NICU) is to support optimal growth, development, and nutrition status and to identify infants requiring referral for further evaluation or nutrition intervention. Nutrition follow-up may be provided by physicians, nurses, nurse practitioners, or registered dietitians. These professionals may encounter infants receiving care in physicians' offices, NICU follow-up clinics, emergency rooms, public health departments, or in homes. This chapter provides a literature review of growth and feeding practices after NICU discharge and suggestions for nutrition assessment and intervention during infancy.

Growth After Discharge

Optimal growth for this population has yet to be definitely established. Many factors may affect growth including birth weight; gestational age; intrauterine growth retardation; maternal drug use during pregnancy; nutrition; early growth delay; presence of a nurturing environment; and the severity, duration, and kinds of neonatal illness. Reports, although numerous, seem to lack agreement at first glance, most likely due to the varied methods of reporting.[1-21] Some investigators use chronologic age, which is age in months from date of birth. Others use corrected or adjusted age, which is age in months from estimated term date. Infants whose growth is appropriate for

The contributions of Janice Stice, MPH, ERD, to this chpater in the previous edition are gratefully acknowledged.

gestational age (AGA) may not be reported separately from those born small for gestational age (SGA). The definition or interpretation of catch-up growth may vary. A weight that plots above the fifth percentile may be considered adequate catch-up growth, or catch-up growth may be reported only if the mean weight of a group of infants coincides with the mean weight on a standard growth chart. Growth charts used for comparison are not the same for all studies.

Although a review of the literature may seem contradictory and confusing, several observations recur or are in close agreement.

- Better postnatal growth occurs in infants who also have good developmental outcome. This group of infants also tends to have a shorter, more benign neonatal course, lower incidence of chronic disease, and lower incidence of rehospitalization.[1-4, 22, 23]
- Between term and four months beyond term, the heaviest group of low-birth-weight (LBW) infants (2,000 to 2,500 g birth weight) may exhibit faster growth and equal or greater percentile ranking for weight, length, and head circumference than term-born peers (see the Infant Health Development Program (IHDP) growth charts in Appendix D). This may also be true for many infants of lower birth weight.[5-8,71]
- Mean values for weight and length for children with birth weights of < 1,500 g approach but do not achieve the mean for postmenstrual age-matched children up to 8 years of age.[5,6,8-13] Individual children with weight and height below the 10th percentile at 2 years of age are more likely to remain below the 10th percentile at 5 and 8 years of age.[8,11]
- Regardless of whether early catch-up growth has occurred, the rate of gain beyond four months' post-term for weight and length of infants born prematurely is not strikingly different from that of term infants of similar postmenstrual age.[8,9,14,16]
- Catch-up growth may occur later during the first year in infants whose growth-limiting condition resolves during that time. Rates of daily weight gain have been reported and are given in Table 34.1 and Chapter 2. Rates of monthly linear and head circumference growth are given in Table 34.1.
- Head growth, as measured by the occipitofrontal circumference shows the least difference between low-birth-weight preterm infants and normal term infants. Catch-up growth measured by increasing head circumference (reflecting brain growth) is usually better and earlier than catch-up weight gain or linear growth.[5,6,7,8,9,17,18] This must be differentiated from excessive growth due to intracranial hemorrhage, infection, or hydrocephaly.[24,26,27] Head circumference growth that has not achieved normal percentile ranking by 8 months postterm date has been associated with poor cognitive function, academic achievement, and behavior at 8 years of age.[25,71] However, normal development at 18 months of age has been reported in extremely low birth weight

infants (< 1,000 g birth weight) in spite of head growth that did not catch up with that of larger premature infants or term infants.[20]

- SGA infants, whether symmetrically or asymmetrically growth retarded, demonstrate catch-up growth. At least two-thirds are likely to achieve growth that plots within normal percentiles, although most do not achieve the mean. Growth deficits may persist into early childhood when compared with normal term infanmts or AGA low-birth-weight infants.[19,28-33] Zinc supplementation may improve weight gain.[29]

Observations of large groups of prematurely born infants can guide our expectations, but may not determine ideal or abnormal growth for an individual infant. The Intrauterine and Postnatal Growth Chart published by by Babson and Benda,[34] the National Center for Health Statistics (NCHS) Physical Growth Percentiles,[35] and the Infant Health and Development Program (IHDP) Growth Percentiles[36] are the charts most often used to assess growth (see Appendix D). Additional information regarding the use and comparison of these growth charts is given in Table 34.2. The infant's age used for plotting growth should be calculated from term date rather than birth date. This is often referred to as the infant's corrected age or "adjusted age." The literature reports use of corrected or adjusted age until 18 months for evaluation of head circumference, until 24 months for evaluation of weight, and until 42 months for length.[8] In practice, corrected or adjusted age is often used at least until 18 months or until 36 months for assessment of all parameters of growth. Weight-for-length grids may also be used to provide a means of assessment independent of age.[35-37] Because some infants do not catch-up to normal percentiles, several guidelines are provided to identify infants who are at increased nutritional risk and require further evaluation. (See Table 34.3 for guidelines.)

The growth of breast-fed infants often differs from that of formula-fed infants. Term breast-fed infants gain weight faster than formula-fed infants during the first two months, then less rapidly from 2-12 months of age. Linear growth is only slightly lower, so that weight for length is also lower. Accelerated head growth is frequently reported, with the mean of breast-fed infants just slightly below the NCHS 75th percentile.[38,39] The growth of premature infants who are breast-fed beyond term has not been extensively reported. Although weight gain, linear growth, and head growth up to 3 months corrected age is lower in infants fed human milk after initial hospitalization than in those fed enriched formula, differences at 3 years do not appear significant.[40]

Table 34.1.   Growth velocity of preterm infants from term
to 24 months*

Age from term (mo)	Weight (g/day)	Length (cm/mo)	Head circumference (cm/mo)
1	26-40	3.0-4.5	1.6-2.5
4	15-25	2.3-3.6	0.8-1.4
8	12-17	1.0-2.0	0.3-0.8
12	9-12	0.8-1.5	0.2-0.4
18	4-10	0.7-1.3	0.1-0.4

*   range includes ± 1 SD

References: 8, 9, 14

Feeding Practices

Although many factors may affect the growth outcome of these infants, reports suggest that feeding practices in the premature infant population may further limit the potential for catch-up growth.[6,41,42] The impact of nutrition separate from other factors may be difficult to differentiate in this population, although malnutrition during infancy is clearly related to poorer physical and developmental outcome.[43,44]

Use of nutrient-enriched formulas (see Appendix K) shows significant advantage for the preterm infant after hospital discharge. Greater weight gain and greater mean length and head circumference are seen in infants receiving nutrient-enriched formulas, with additional improvements in plasma zinc concentrations, net mineral retention, and bone mineral content.[40,45-47] Nutrient-enriched formulas contain higher amounts of protein, electrolytes, and most minerals and vitamins than standard formulas per unit of volume and per unit of energy, but lower amounts of these nutrients contained in premature infant formulas.

Breast-feeding mothers may have concerns about adequate milk production, milk composition, and the infant's ability to nurse adequately, particularly if feeding skills are not fully mature. Some infants may require supplemental vitamins, minerals or all nutrients depending upon the mother's milk supply and the infant's clinical condition[48] (see Table 33.5). After the infant's hospital discharge, breast-feeding support may be lacking and expectations for growth unrealistic, prompting inappropriate supplementation and early weaning. Maternal education is one of the key determinants of successful breast-feeding.[49] (See Table 33.6 for suggestions to establish successful breast-feeding in premature infants.)

Table 34.2. Growth Charts Commonly Used To Monitor Premature Infants

GROWTH CHART	DATA CHARACTERISTICS	ADVANTAGES	DISADVANTAGES
National Center for Health Statistics (NCHS)[35]	• Small sample size • Large intervals between data • Term to 36 mo (length) • 2 to 18 yr (height) • Includes weight for length (height) • Separate charts for males, females	• Widely available • Allows comparison with post-menstrual age-matched term infants for "ideal" growth • Includes weight for length/BMI	• Requires correcting/ adjusting age for preterm infants • Difficult to interpret when catch-up growth has not occurred • Does not include < 40 wk gestation
Intrauterine and Postnatal Growth Chart (Oregon)[34]	• 26-40 wk gestation are crossectional data • Data from term to 12 mo are from 4,000 term infants • Male and female data combined	• Growth from premature birth through one year corrected age plotted on same chart • Weight, length, and head circumference on one chart	• Requires correcting/ adjusting age for preterm infants • Males and females combined • Does not go beyond 12 mo corrected age • Does not include weight for length • Difficult to interpret when catch-up growth has not occurred • Uses logarithmic scale
Growth and Developmental Records (Gairdner/Pearson)[70]	• 24-40 wk gestation are crossectional data • Data from term to 2 yr are from term infants • Separate charts for males, females • Data similar to NCHS charts	• Growth from premature birth through 2-yr corrected age plotted on same chart • Weight, length, and head circumference on one chart	• Requires correcting/ adjusting age for preterm infants • Does not include weight for length • Difficult to obtain/costly • Uses logarithmic scale
Infant Health and Development Program (IHDP) Growth Percentiles[36]	• Data from LBW* and VLBW* infants from 40 wk gestation to 36 mo corrected age • Separate charts for males, females • Data collected before enriched formulas were available	• Growth may be assessed against infants of similar birth weight • Includes weight for length	• Requires correcting/ adjusting age for preterm infants • Does not include data < term • Does not determine "normal" or abnormal growth • Infants who fall < 50th %ile may need further nutrition evaluation (< 5th %ile on other charts)

* BMI = body mass index; LBW = low birth weight or 1,500 to 2,500 g birth weight;
VLBW = very low birth weight or < 1,500 g birth weight

Feeding practices that are inconsistent with the present American Academy of Pediatric guidelines for infant feeding are commonly encountered (see Table 34.4 for feeding recommendations during the first year).[6,50,51] Introduction of solid foods before developmental readiness may result in "forced" feedings of solids and may decrease formula or human milk consumption, often reducing protein and mineral intake. Use of cow's milk in place of iron-fortified infant formula may not only decrease total iron intake, but may cause a significant loss of iron through the G.I. tract.[52] Whole cow's milk may also provide an excess intake of protein and a higher potential renal solute load while providing inadequate amounts of copper, linoleic acid, and vitamins C and E.[53-55] Feeding cow's milk with reduced fat content may decrease overall energy intake and further compromise essential fatty acid intake.[6,54]

Feeding problems are frequently encountered during follow-up of high-risk neonates. A delay in feeding skills may be related to frequent or prolonged illness, decreased exposure to more advanced feeding techniques, or parents' misperceptions or lack of information. Infants with neurological or anatomical abnormalities may have poor suck-swallow coordination, excessive tongue thrust, problems with gag reflex, or gastroesophageal reflux. Respiratory or cardiac compromise may increase the work of breathing and compromise an infant's ability to eat by decreasing feeding endurance or interest.[56] (See chapters in Section IV for nutrition recommendations specific to diagnoses.)

Feeding methods may also affect nutrient intake and development of feeding skills. Hunger and satiety cues must be accurately interpreted and appropriate actions taken. Guidelines and client instruction materials regarding recognition of feeding cues and appropriate feeding methods have been published.[42,57-60]

Nutrition Assessment and Intervention

Infants who require intensive medical care as neonates may continue to have increased medical, nutritional, developmental, emotional, and financial needs after hospital discharge. Timely identification of problems and intervention to treat or resolve these problems by knowledgeable health care providers can have a significant impact on the progression of disability in this population.[56] There are data to support the efficiency of a multidisciplinary approach in following high-risk infants, especially the very-low-birth-weight infants.[61]

Most NICUs have established programs for follow-up, but the schedule, availability of health care providers, and focus may vary significantly. If there is an early hospital discharge program, or if the NICU staff continues to provide medical management, follow-up

Table 34.3. Criteria for Referral to Registered Dietitian During Follow-up

Anthropometric 'red flags'	Clinical 'red flags'	Feeding/Diet 'red flags'
Weight for age or weight for length at or below 5th percentile (or below 50th percentile on IHDP growth charts)	**Vomiting**—chronic vomiting, particularly if accompanied by other signs and symptoms such as: diarrhea or dehydration; growth faltering, pain or obvious discomfort or frequent respiratory tract infections; diarrhea, atopic dermatitis or wheezing; forceful vomiting, or vomitus which contains bile (green) or blood (red or "coffee ground" appearance)	Low iron formula, Similac Special Care, Enfamil Premature Formula, goat's milk, or a product other than an infant formula for infants
Weight for age or weight for length at or above 95th percentile		Adding more or less water than can directions call for; supplements added to formula
Weight loss or significant decline in percentile ranking, particularly if weight precedes length in decline	**Diarrhea**—frequent/chronic loose, watery, large, bulky or unusually foul smelling stools, particularly if accompanied by other signs and symptoms such as vomiting or dehydration, gas and bloating, skin breakdown in diaper area; grey, white or pale colored stools.	Cow's milk as the main source of nutrition during the first year instead of formula or breast milk; Low-fat milk (especially skim milk) < 2 yr of age
Poor rate of weight gain for age (corrected age in infants and toddlers up to 24 mo):	Note: Stools of breast-fed babies may be quite frequent (often occur with every feeding) during the first few weeks of life.	< 24 oz formula/day for infants; < 16 oz milk/day for toddlers and no other significant source of dairy products in diet; > 32 oz cow's milk/d for toddlers (over 1 yr of age)
< 20 g/d (< 5 oz/wk) term-3 mo	**Constipation**—hard, dry, infrequent stools that are difficult to pass.	Use of infant feeders, tube feedings or parenteral nutrition (TPN or "hyperal")
< 15 g/d (< 3 1/2 oz/wk) 3-6 mo		Infants > 6 mo corrected age not yet starting spoon feedings or toddlers > 12 mo of age not yet taking finger foods; daily food intake regularly excludes one or more basic food groups > 12 mo of age
< 10 g/d (< 2 oz/wk) 6-9 mo	**Chronic illness or medical conditions such as:** AIDS/HIV+, multiple allergy/food intolerance, bronchopulmonary dysplasia, cyanotic cardiac anomalies, cerebral palsy, cystic fibrosis, Down syndrome, failure to thrive, fetal alcohol syndrome or other intrauterine drug exposure, gastrointestinal disease, kidney or liver disease, seizure disorder, spina bifida	Feeding duration > 30 min for infants or > 45 min for toddlers (excluding breaks for diapering, playing, etc.); < 5 feedings/d for infants; < 4 feedings/d for toddlers
< 7 g/d (< 1 1/2 oz/wk) 9-12 mo		Parents have difficulty interpreting or responding appropriately to feeding cues
< 1 kg (2 lb)/6 mo 1-2 yr	**Chronic use** of medications such as antibiotics, anticholinergics, anticonvulsants, antidiuretics, laxatives, or others that may affect nutritional status	Fussy or distressed during feeding; has trouble breathing during feeding; difficult to wake for feedings, tires easily or has difficulty finishing feedings; frequently gags, coughs or chokes during feedings; refuses to eat, is difficult to feed, or arches backward when feeding; mealtimes are frustrating to parent or infant/child
< 0.7 kg (1 1/2 lb)/6 mo 2-5 yr		Parents have nutrition questions or concerns not addressed in standard nutrition education materials
Disproportional head growth		

Reprinted with permission from Cox JH, ed. Nutrition manual for at-risk infants and toddlers. Chicago, Ill.: Precept Press, 1997; 186.

visits may be scheduled within five to seven days of hospital discharge, then weekly or monthly until the local health care provider assumes complete responsibility for medical management.[62] If the primary focus of follow-up is developmental outcome, visits may be scheduled less regularly, corresponding to ages when developmental milestones are likely to be achieved at 6, 12, 18, and 36 months of age. Programs that focus on screening for neurodevelopmental abnormalities generally do not provide primary care and do not address early medical-, growth- or nutrition-related problems.

The potential for subsequent growth and feeding difficulties is higher in infants who require extensive mediacal care as neonates. (See Table 33.7 for a list of those at risk.) A strong relationship exists between growth and developmental outcome, indicating the need for early, periodic and frequent follow-up that includes nutrition screening and a mechanism for intervention/referral to address nutrition problems. Evidence suggests that if a registered dietitian provides the assessment and intervention during the first year after discharge, catch-up growth in weight, length and head circumference is enhanced.[61] The last is of considerable interest, as head growth is a refelction of brain growth, and 80% of the adult head size is normally achieved by the first year of age.

Use of a nutrition screening tool (see Figure 34.1) facilitates history taking and organizes data for quick and accurate identification of problems and need for further assessment. The nutrition screen is designed to identify adequacy of growth and nutrient intake, the appropriateness of feeding, and the presence of clinical conditions that may interfere with adequate nutrition. Guidelines for identification of infants who may require further evaluation of growth and feeding are given in Table 34.3.

Nutrition assessment includes anthropometric measurements of weight, length, and head circumference. Growth achievement and growth velocity may be compared to norms. (See Table 13.1 and Appendix D.) Records of laboratory assessments and dietary intake are reviewed when available. Direct observation of a feeding helps to assess behaviors and skills to determine whether a simple intervention or referral to a feeding therapist may be needed. (See Appendices N and O.) A sample reporting form for nutrition assessment is given in Figure 34.2. Once nutrition assessment is complete, intervention may include: 1) a review of the infant's growth and goals for future growth, 2) recommendations for formula/dietary changes, 3) nutrition counseling for caregivers regarding formula preparation, introduction of solids, supplement doses, and feeding methods, and/or 4) referrals to other team professionals or community agencies.

Infants can be referred to a variety of federal, state, and local programs for additional nutrition intervention. The federal Special Supplemental Food Program for Women, Infants, and Children provides food and nutrition counseling. The infant's length, weight, and

Table 34.4.   Suggested Infant Feeding Schedule

Age*	Daily food intake	Rationale/comments
Birth to 4 mo	Breast-feeding 8-12 times/day initially, 6-10 times/day after 6-8 wk; infant formula 6-8 times/day initially, 5-7 times/day after 6-8 wk Human milk or iron fortified infant formula 18-32 oz/day	Sucking and rooting reflexes allow milk/formula intake; prominent extrusion reflex and lack of mature head and trunk control preclude use of spoon feedings; water not routinely recommended
4 to 6 mo	Human milk or iron-fortified infant formula 5-6 times/day for a total intake of 27-45 oz/day	Water may be given as additional source of fluid only, not a substitute for formula
	Iron-fortified infant cereal 1-6 tblsp per day; begin with rice, then individually add barley, oats, and wheat after 6 mo of age	Decreased extrusion reflex allows transfer of solid foods from spoon to back of mouth for swallowing. Increased head and trunk control allow head to remain erect/steady and sitting with minimal support throughout feeding of solid foods
6 to 8 mo	Human milk or iron-fortified infant formula 3-5 times/day for a total intake of 24-32 oz/day Cup may be offered in addition to breast or bottle Daily food intake gradually increases to include: Iron-fortified infant cereal 4-6 tblsp Vegetables 3-4 tblsp Fruits 3-4 tblsp Meats 1-2 tblsp Unsweetened fruit juice 2-4 oz (citrus juices started after 7 mo of age) Crackers, toast, dry unsweetened cereal	Dietary source of iron is needed when foods are added to diet of breast-fed infant, as food may interfere with absorption of breast milk iron Ability to remove food from spoon with lips, bite soft foods, and control liquids offered from cup increases. Foods become a significant source of vitamins A, C, and B complex, also iron and protein Offer in spouted or child size cup May provide some relief during teething
9 to 10 mo	Human milk or iron-fortified infant formula 2-4 times/day for a total intake of 24-32 oz/day Daily food intake gradually increases to include: Iron-fortified infant cereal 4-6 tblsp Vegetables 6-8 tblsp Fruits 6-8 tblsp Meats, fish, poultry, eggs, yogurt, cottage cheese, or cheese 3-4 tblsp Crackers, toast, dry unsweetened cereal, soft cooked noodles or rice 3-4 tblsp Unsweetened fruit juice 4 oz Soft, chopped or ground table foods gradually replace strained or mashed foods.	Chewing and biting skills begin to mature As human milk or formula intake decreases, introduce other food sources of calcium, B complex vitamins and protein

Table 34.4. Suggested Infant Feeding Schedule (continued)

Age*	Daily food intake	Rationale/comments
11 to 12 mo	Human milk or iron-fortified infant formula 2-4 times/day for a total intake of 24-32 oz/day; amount gradually decreases to around 20-24 oz/day as intake of solid foods increases	Rotary chewing motion develops, allowing a gradual increase in food textures. Encourage self-feeding with finger foods and child-sized spoon to enhance development of fine motor skills
	Soft, chopped or ground table foods continue to replace strained or mashed foods as above	As human milk or infant formula decreases, select a variety of foods to meet nutritional needs

* If infant is prematurely born, use corrected age. See text. See Table 33.5 for low-birth-weight infant recommendations prior to term age.

Adapted with permission from: American Dietetic Association. Pediatric manual of clinical dietetics. Chicago: The ADA, 1996; 59-62.

head circumference, hemoglobin and hematocrit are monitored every six months at recertification appointments. All LBW and VLBW infants qualify for the program in their first year of life if the family meets income eligibility standards. A registered dietitian provides nutrition assessment and is available to provide further nutrition consultation, intervention, or dietary recommendations when needed.

Federal Public Law 102-119 (previously 99457, Part H) mandates early intervention for infants and risk for developmental delay, including nutrition assessment and intervention, as part of case management and the individual family service plan.[63-65] Children's Rehabilitative Services or Children's Special Health Care Services (CHSCS) may provide additional support services or funding for special formula or feeding equipment. These programs commonly have income eligibility guidelines but may supplement private medical insurance reimbursement.

Local health departments or nursing agencies often can provide such nutrition services as growth assessment and parent education. Programs may include visits by health care providers directly in the infant's home, particularly when the infant's care is complicated, the infant's health is fragile, or the family's transportation is limited. Home visits also allow assessment of the infant in his/her own physical and psychosocial environment.

In summary, as the survival of high risk infants increases, more health care professionals will encounter these infants in a variety of settings. Assessment of growth, feeding practices, and nutrient intake may identify infants who are at increased nutritional risk.

Figure 34.1. Nutrition Screening Form[67-69]

Name _____DOB_____ Corrected age_____

Fill in the information requested and answer each question by marking
YES or NO as appropriate.

				YES	NO
Weight_____;	_____%ile	Below the 5th%ile?*		❑	❑
Length_____;	_____%ile	Below the 5th%ile?*		❑	❑
Head circumference_____;	_____%ile	Below the 5th%ile?*		❑	❑
Weight/length_____%ile	Below the 5th%ile or above the 95th%ile?*			❑	❑

Previous weight/date_____   (Hospital discharge weight or last clinic visit.)

Rate of weight gain_____
< 20 gm/day (5 oz/wk) term-3 months*   ❑   ❑
< 15 gm/day (31/2 oz/wk) 3-6 months*
< 10 gm/day (2 oz/wk) 6-9 months*
< 7 gm/day (11/2 oz/wk) 9-12 months*
< 1 kg (2 lb)/6 months from 1-2 years*
*using corrected age   < 0.7 kg (11/2 lb)/6 months from 2-5 years

Hemoglobin: 11 gm/dl or LESS   ❑   ❑

Hematocrit: 34% or LESS   ❑   ❑

Diagnoses: Does your child have any of these diagnoses
or chronic conditions?   ❑   ❑

___ Anemia	___ Heart Disease	___ Fetal Alcohol Syndrome
___ Cerebral Palsy	___ Cystic Fibrosis	___ Lung Disease
___ Kidney Disease	___ Liver Disease	___ Gastrointestinal Disease
___ Spina Bifida	___ Down Syndrome	___ Neuromuscular Disease
___ Seizure Disorder	___ Failure to Thrive	___ Poor Growth

Other _____

Does your child frequently experience any of the following?   ❑   ❑

___ Diarrhea   ___ Constipation   ___ Vomiting or reflux

Does your child take medications regularly (excluding vitamins, iron or fluoride)?   ❑   ❑

If yes, please list: _____

Does your child need special formula or nutrient supplements
(including vitamins, iron, fluoride?)   ❑   ❑

If yes, please list: _____

Do you use a recipe for formula preparation other than the one
on the printed label?   ❑   ❑

___ More water   ___ Less water   ___ Other ingredients added

Does your child use a feeding tube or other special feeding equipment?   ❑   ❑

Does your child have any food allergies?   ❑   ❑
If yes, please list:_____

Figure 34.1. Nutrition Screening Form (continued)

	YES	NO
If your child is less than 12 months of age, does he/she do any of the following?	❑	❑

____ If formula fed, drink less than 24 ounces a day
____ If formula fed, take the bottle to bed
____ If breast fed, take less than 5 breast feedings a day
____ Take solid foods from the bottle
____ Drink more than 4 oz of cow's milk a day

If your child is over 12 months of age, does he/she do any of the following? ❑ ❑

____ Drink more than 32 oz of cow's milk per day
____ Take less than 16 oz of cow's milk or 2 slices of cheese per day
____ Refuse to eat any vegetables, fruits or juices
____ Refuse to eat any meat, beans, peanut butter or eggs
____ Take the bottle to bed

Does your child experience any of the following? ❑ ❑

____ 7 months of age or older and has not started spoon feedings
____ 10 months of age or older and consistently refuses lumpy or textured foods
____ 12 months of age or older and drinks liquids primarily from bottle
____ 15 months of age or older and does not finger feed
____ 18 months of age or older and does not use a spoon yet

Does your child frequently experience any of the following? ❑ ❑

____ Happy at beginning of feeding, then often gets fussy or distressed
during feedings
____ Frequently has trouble breathing while eating
____ Tires easily with feedings, *or* frequently has difficulty finishing feedings
____ Eats slowly, usually takes more than 30 minutes (infant)/45 minutes (toddler) to eat
____ Usually has difficulty sucking, swallowing, or chewing
____ Frequently gags, coughs, *or* chokes during feedings
____ Fussy for most of feeding, arches backward, *or* doesn't seem to enjoy eating
____ Refuses to eat or is difficult to feed
____ Picky eater, eats very little, not interested in food or eating, *or* has poor appetite

Do you ever find that you are almost out of food at the end of the month? ❑ ❑

Do you have any questions or concerns about your child's nutrition? ❑ ❑
If yes, please list: _____

If you are breastfeeding, do you have any questions or concerns
about breastfeeding? ❑ ❑
If yes, please list: _____

A **YES** response indicates that nutrition intervention and/or a referral to a registered dietitian is needed; nutritional risk may be present.

A **NO** response indicates no nutritional risk in that particular area.

If all items are checked **NO**, no nutrition intervention or referral to a registered dietitian is needed at this time.

Is referral/intervention indicated? ❑ ❑

Signature of screener _____ Date _____

Figure 34.2. Nutrition Consultation Report

PATIENT'S NAME _____ DOB_____ DATE_____

SUBJ: (DIET HISTORY)

OBJ: (ANTHROPOMETRIES/LAB)   AGE: _____   CORRECTED AGE: _____

WEIGHT:

_____; _____%ile   _____ gm/day; _____ lb/wk

LENGTH/HEIGHT:

_____; _____%ile   _____ cm/mo; _____ in/mo

HEAD:

_____; _____%ile   _____ cm/mo; _____ cm/mo

WEIGHT FOR LENGTH/HEIGHT:

_____%ile   IDEAL WEIGHT FOR LENGTH/HEIGHT: _____

LABS:

ASSESS:

 GROWTH:

 INTAKE:

 FEEDING SKILLS/DEVELOPMENT:

PLAN:

 NUTRITION RECOMMENDATIONS:

 REFERRALS:

 FOLLOW-UP:

 Signed: _____

Infants and their families can then be referred to appropriate health care providers, programs, or agencies for additional nutrition intervention to support optimal growth, development, and nutritional status.

References

1. Hack M, Merkatz IR, McGrath SK, et al. catch-up growth in very-low-birth-weight infants. Am J Dis Child 138:370, 1984.
2. Ross G, Krauss AN, Auld AM. Growth achievement in low-birth-weight premature infants: Relation to neurobehavorial outcome at one year. J Pediatr 103:105, 1983.
3. Hack M, Merkatz IR, Gordon D, et al. The prognostic significance of postnatalgrowth in very low birth weight infants. Am J Obstet Gynecol 143:693, 1982.
4. Saigal S, Rosenbaum P, Stoskopf B, et al. follow-up of infants 501-1,500 gm birth weight delivered to residents of a geographically defined region with perinatal intensive care facilities. J Pediatr 100:606, 1982.
5. Casey PH, Kraemer HC, Bernbaum J, et al. Growth patterns of low birth weight preterm infants: A longitudinal analysis of a large, varied sample. J Pediatr 117:298, 1990.
6. Ernst JA, Bull MJ, Rickard KA, et al. Growth outcome and feeding practices of the very low birth weight infant (less than 1,500 grams) within the first year of life. J Pediatr 117:S156, 1990.
7. Altigani M, Murphy JF, Newcombe RG, et al. catch-up growth in preterm infants. Acta Paediatr Scand (suppl) 357:3, 1989.
8. Brandt I. Growth dynamics of low-birth-weight infants with emphasis on the perinatal period. In: Falkner F, Tanner JM, eds. Human growth. vol. 2. Postnatal growth. New York: Plenum Press, 1978; 557-617.
9. Casey PH, Kraemer HC, Bernbaum J, et al. Growth status and growth rates of a varied sample of low birth weight preterm infants: A longitudinal cohort from birth to three years of age. J Pediatr 119:599, 1991.
10. Kitchen WH, Ford GW, Doyle LW. Growth and very low birth weight. Arch Dis Child 64:379, 1989.
11. Kitchen WH, Doyle LW, Ford GW, et al. Very low birth weight and growth to age 8 years. Am J Dis Child 146:40, 1992.
12. Scottish Low Birth Weight Study Group. The Scottish low birthweight study. I. Survival, growth, neuromotor and sensory impairment. Arch Dis Child 67:675, 1992.
13. Barros FC, Huttly SRA, Victora CG, et al. Comparison of the causes and consequences of prematurity and intrauterine growth retardation: A longitudinal study in southern Brazil. Pediatrics 90:238, 1992.
14. Fomon SJ. Nutrition of normal infants. St. Louis:Mosby, 1993.
15. Fomon SJ, Haschke F, Ziegler EE, et al. Body composition of reference children from birth to 10 years. Am J Clin Nutr 35:1169, 1982.
16. Baumgartner RN, Roche AF, Himes JH. Incremental growth tables: Supplementary to previously published charts. Am J Clin Nutr 43:711, 1986.
17. Wright CM, Waterston A, Aynsley-Green A. Effect of deprivation on weight gain in infancy. Acta Paediatr 83:357, 1994.

18. Eriksson M, Jonsson B, Steneroth G, et al. Cross-sectional growth of children whose mothers abused amphetamines during pregnancy. Acta Paediatr 83:612-17, 1994.

19. Hack M, Weissman B, Borawski-Clark E. catch-up growth during childhood among very-low-birth-weight children. Arch Pediatr Adolesc Med 150:1122, 1996.

20. Sheth RD, Mullett MD, Bodensteiner JB, et al. Longitudinal head growth in developmentally normal preterm infants. Arch Pediatr Adolesc Med 149:1358, 1995.

21. Saigal S, Rosenbaum P, Stoskopf B, et al. Comprehensive assessment of the health status of extremely bow birth weight children at eight years of age: Comparison with a reference group. J Pediatr 125:411, 1994.

22. Robertson C, Hrynchyshun B. Population-based study of the incidence, complexity, and severity of neurologic disability among survivors weighing 500-1,200 gms at birth: A comparison of two birth cohorts. Pediatrics 90:750, 1992.

23. Vaughn VD. On the utility of growth curves. JAMA 267:975, 1992.

24. Manser JJ. Growth in the high-risk infant. Clin Perinatol 11:19, 1984.

25. Hack M, Breslau N, Weissman B, et al. Effect of very low birth weight and subnormal head size on cognitive abilities at school age. N Engl J Med 325:231, 1991.

26. Sher PK, Brown SB. A longitudinal study of head growth in pre-term infants. II: Differentiation between 'catch-up' head growth and early infantile hydrocephalus. Dev Med Child Neurol 17:711, 1975.

27. Löppönen T et al. Growth in patients with shunted hydrocephalus. Pediatrics 95:917, 1995.

28. Albertsson-Wikland K, Wennergren M, et al. Longitudinal follow-up of growth in children born small for gestational age. Acta Paediatr 82:438, 1993.

29. Castillo-Dur·n C, Rodriquez A, Venegas G, et al. Zinc supplementation and growth of infants born small for gestational age. J Pediatr 127:206, 1995.

30. Hokken-Koelega ACS, de Ridder MAJ, Lemmen RJ, et al. Children born small for gestational age: do they catch up? Pediatr Res 38:267, 1995.

31. Strauss RS, Dietz WH. Effects of intrauterine growth retardation in premature infants on early childhood growth. J Pediatr 131:95, 1997.

32. Sung I-K, Vohr B, and Oh W. Growth and neurodevelopmental outcome of very low birth weight infants with intrauterine growth retardation: Comparison with control subjects matched by birth weight and gestational age. J Pediatr 123:618, 1993.

33. Williams SP, Durbin GM, Morgan MEI, et al. catch-up growth and pancreatic function in growth retarded neonates. Arch Dis Child 73:F158, 1995.

34. Babson SG, Benda GI. Growth graphs for the clinical assessment of infants of varying gestational age. J Pediatr 89:814, 1976.

35. Hamill PVV, Drizd FA, Johnson CL, et al. Physical growth: National Center for Health Statistics percentiles. Am J Clin Nutr 32:607, 1979.

36. Guo SS, Roche AF, Chumlea WC, et al. Growth in weight, recumbent length, and head circumference for preterm low-birth-weight infants during the first three years of life using gestation-adjusted ages. Early Hum Dev 47:305, 1997.

37. Guo SS, Wholihan K, Roche AF, et al. Weight-for-length reference data for preterm, low-birth-weight infants. Arch Pediatr Adolesc Med 150:964, 1996.
38. Heineig MJ, Nommsen LA, Peerson JM, et al. Energy and protein intakes of breast-fed and formula-fed infants during the first year of life and their association with growth velocity: the DARLING study. Am J Clin Nutr 58:152-161, 1993.
39. Dewey KG, Peerson JM, Brown KH, et al. Growth of breast-fed infants deviates from current reference data: a pooled analysis of US, Canadian, and European data sets. Pediatrics 96:495, 1995.
40. Wheeler RE and Hall RT. Feeding of premature infant formula after hospital discharge of infants weighing less than 1800 grams at birth. J Perinatol 16:111, 1996.
41. Ernst J, Bull M, Rickard K, et al. Feeding practices of the very-low-birth-weight infant within the first year. J Am Diet Assoc 82:158, 1983.
42. Gardner S, Hagedorn M. Physiologic sequelae of prematurity: The nurse practitioner's role. IV. Feeding difficulties and growth failure. J Pediatr Health Care 5:306, 1991.
43. Chase, HP, Martin, HP. Undernutrition and child development. N Engl J Med 282:933, 1970.
44. Walter T, De Andraca 1, Chadud P, et al. Iron deficiency anemia: Adverse effects of infant psychomotor development. Pediatrics 84:7, 1989.
45. Lucas A, King F, Bishop NB, King FJ, et al. Randomised trial of nutrition for preterm infants after discharge. Arch Dis Child 67:324, 1992.
46. Friel JK, Andrews WL, Matthew JD, et al. Improved growth of very low birth weight infants. Nutr Res 13:611, 1993.
47. Rajaram S, Carlson SE, Koo WK, et al. Plasma mineral concentrations in preterm infants fed a nutrient-enriched formula after hospital discharge. J Pediatr 126:791, 1995.
48. Kavanaugh K, Mead L, Meier P, et al. Getting enough: Mothers' concerns about breastfeeding a preterm infant after discharge. JOGNN 24:23, 1995.
49. Michaelsen KF, Larsen PS, Thomsen BL, et al. The Copenhagen cohort study on infant nutrition and growth: duration of breast feeding and influencing factors. Acta Paediatr 83:565, 1994.
50. American Academy of Pediatrics Committee on Nutrition. The use of whole cow's milk in infancy. Pediatrics 89:1105, 1992.
51. American Academy of Pediatrics Committee on Nutrition. On the feeding of supplemental foods to infants. Pediatrics 65:1178, 1980.
52. Ziegler EE, Fomon SJ, Nelson SE, et al. Cow milk feeding in infancy: Further observations on blood loss from the gastrointestinal tract. J Pediatr 116:11, 1990.
53. Ziegler EE. Milk and formulas for older infants. J Pediatr 117:576, 1990.
54. Martinez GA, Ryan AS, Malec DJ. Nutrient intakes of American infants and children fed cow's milk or infant formula. Am J Dis Child 139:1010, 1985.
55. Shank JS, Dorsey JL, Cooper WT, et al. The vitamin E status of infants receiving cow's milk or milk based formula (abstr). Fed Proc 46:1194, 1987.

56. Bernstein S, Heimler R, Sasidharan P. Approaching the management of the neonatal intensive care unit graduate through history and physical assessment. Pediatr Clin North Amer 45:79, 1998.

57. Finney J. Preventing common feeding problems in infants and young children. Pediatr Clin North Am 33:775, 1986.

58. Pridham K. Feeding behavior of 6-12 month infants: Assessment and sources of parental information. J Pediatr 117:2, 1990.

59. Satter E. Child of mine: Feeding with love and good sense. Palo Alto, Calif.: Bull Publishing, 1986.

60. Satter E. The feeding relationship. J Am Diet Assoc 86:35, 1986.

61. Bryson SR, Theriot L, Ryan NJ, et al. Primary follow-up care in a multidisciplinary setting enhances catch-up growth of very-low-birth-weight infants. J Am Diet Assoc 97:386, 1997.

62. Cruz H, Guzman N, Rosales M, et al. Early hospital discharge of preterm very low birth weight infants. J Perinatol 17:29-32, 1997.

63. Department of Education. Early intervention program for infants and toddlers with handicaps. Federal Register 54:26305, 1989.

64. Hine RJ, Cloud HH, Carithers T, et al. Early nutrition intervention services for children with special health care needs. J Am Diet Assoc 89:1636, 1989.

65. Holland M. Early intervention. In: Cox JH, ed. Nutrition manual for at-risk infants and toddlers. Chicago: Precept Press, 1997.

66. American Dietetic Association. Pediatric manual of clinical dietetics. Chicago:The ADA, 1996; 59-62.

67. Bayerl CT and Ries JD. Early start: Nutrition services in early intervention in Massachusetts. Zero to three 12:29-31, 1992.

68. Campbell MK, Kelsey KS. The Peach survey: a nutrition screening tool for use in early intervention programs. J Am Diet Assoc 94:1156-58, 1994.

69. Cox JH. Nutrition screening form and referral criteria. In: Nutrition manual for at-risk infants and toddlers. Chicago:Precept Press, 1997; 184-186.

70. Gairdner D, Peterson J. Growth and development record: Preterm—2 years, length/weight/head circumference. Welwyn Garden City, Hertfordshire, England: Castelmead Press, 1988. (Table 34.2 Growth charts commonly used to monitor premature infants)

71. Kennedy TS, Oakland MJ, Shaw RD. Growth patterns and nutritional factors associated with increased head circumference at 18 months in normally developing, low-birth-weight infants. J Amer Dietet Assoc 99:1522, 1999.

Appendix A

Perspectives on the Neonatal Nutritionist's Role

Melody Thompson, MS, RD, LD

The National Research Council (NRC), the American Academy of Pediatrics (AAP), the American College of Obstetricians and Gynecologists (ACOG), the American Dietetic Association (ADA), the American Society for Parenteral and Enteral Nutrition (ASPEN), and the Joint Commission on Accreditation of Health Care Organizations (JCAHO), all endorse the involvement of registered dietitians in the care of high-risk infants.[1-5] These organizations recognize that nutrition support plays a fundamental role in the recovery of vulnerable infants and that registered dietitians (RDs) are the appropriate health care professionals to provide, oversee, and/or coordinate this medical nutrition therapy.

Historical Perspective

In 1975, Karyl Rickard, RD, PhD, and Edwin Gresham, MD, published a paper on nutritional considerations for the newborn requiring intensive care in which they described the contribution of the dietitian.[6] One of their stated objectives was to encourage nutritionists and dietitians to collaborate with neonatologists and other team members to establish nutrition programs as part of the comprehensive medical care for high-risk neonates. Dr. Rickard, along with Mary Sue Brady, RD, DMSc, and Judith Ernst, RD, DMSc, have been pioneers in establishing and developing the neonatal nutritionist's role and training, as well as in devising protocols for nutritional management of low-birth-weight infants.[7]

In 1977, the Ohio Department of Health provided grant funding for six neonatal nutritionist positions in level III neonatal intensive care units (NICUs) in Ohio. The current Ohio Neonatal Nutritionists (ONN) group evolved from the support and encouragement that these original nutritionists provided to one another. The objectives of ONN are to (1) provide members a network of professional support, (2) promote the role of the neonatal nutritionist, and (3) share and disseminate state-of-the-art neonatal nutrition information. The ONN group publishes a newsletter, has prepared educational materials for parents of high-risk infants, and has completed a national survey of nutrition services in NICUs in the United States.[8,9] A similar survey has recently been completed in Canada.[46]

Current Status

Neonatal nutritionists are advanced-level clinical dietitians who provide medical nutrition therapy to high-risk infants. They are registered dietitians with prior pediatric or neonatal experience. About half of currently employed neonatal nutritionists or neonatal RDs hold a master's degree.[8] (The terms neonatal nutritionist and neonatal RD will be used interchangeably in this discussion.)

Most neonatal RDs are employed in NICUs that provide care for the most critically ill infants. These units may be referral centers affiliated with medical schools. Teaching and research, as well as patient care, may be part of the mission, and a multidisciplinary staff is employed. Usually, the neonatal RD position is budgeted in the department of dietetics/nutrition services.[8] Some neonatal RD positions are budgeted in neonatology/pediatrics (or other hospital departments) or are funded by grants.

Some nurseries only provide care for moderately ill infants—those needing further hospitalization but not requiring transport to a referral center. The degree of sophistication of practice in these NICUs or "special care nurseries" varies considerably. Some small units transport all but the most stable babies. Others provide ventilator management and parenteral nutrition but not surgical or medical subspecialty services. Depending on the size, activity, and needs of the unit, an RD's services may be utilized.

As for staffing depth in these specialized nurseries, Mayfield et al. have recommended that one neonatal RD should be provided for each 30 inpatients.[10] Similarly, if the recommendation for RD staffing is the same as that for social workers according to the AAP and ACOG, there should be one full-time registered dietitian for every 30 beds.[2] The Ohio Neonatal Nutritionists' survey showed that the amount of time devoted by the neonatal RD to the NICU was direct-

Table A.1.   Model Job Description for a Neonatal Nutritionist

The neonatal nutritionist functions within a multidisciplinary team to provide nutritional care for all infants in the Neonatal Intensive Care Unit. This includes nutrition assessment and intervention, education of staff and families, development of policies and procedures, participation in research projects, and serving as a consultant to the entire health care team.

I. Responsibilities:

A.   Participates in direct patient care by providing medical nutrition therapy that includes
   1.   Coordinates nutrition screening for all new patients to determine nutritional risk
   2.   Assesses nutrition status and develops a nutrition care plan based upon individual need. This includes:
      - Collection of pertinent medical, biochemical, anthropometric, social, and nutritional data
      - Identification of current, past, or potential nutritional problems
      - Calculation of individualized nutrient requirements
      - Recommendations for type, amount, and route of nutrition support
      - Documentation in medical record
   3.   Evaluates and modifies nutrition care plan on an ongoing basis
   4.   Promotes and supports initiation and maintenance of lactation
   5.   Participates in neonatal teaching rounds and attends interdisciplinary patient care conferences
   6.   Instructs patients' families regarding special nutrition care plans either during the hospitalization and/or at discharge. Develops teaching materials as needed
   7.   Identifies community resources and makes referrals for continuity of nutrition care after discharge
   8.   Participates in neonatal follow-up clinic and/or provides outpatient counseling as needed.
   9.   Acts as a resource person to families, medical staff and community health professionals
B.   Develops and conducts professional education for physicians, nurses, neonatal nurse practitioners, registered dietitians, dietetic interns and students, and other health care professionals involved in the care of the high-risk newborn
C.   Develops and implements standards of care for the neonatal unit to ensure the provision of optimal nutrition care
D.   Pursues new knowledge in neonatal nutrition by reviewing and evaluating current literature, attending and/or presenting at conferences, and participating in practice groups in order to maintain a high level of expertise
E.   Participates in nutrition-related research projects

II. Background and education requirements:

A.   Registered/licensed dietitian
B.   Master's degree preferred
C.   2-5 years related clinical experience or traineeship/fellowship in neonatal nutrition

ly related to the number of NICU beds.[8] In units with 30 or more beds, neonatal RDs are more likely to devote 40 or more hours weekly to NICU-related activities, but in smaller units they may work part-time in the NICU and cover other areas as well (most frequently, other pediatric units or maternity/obstetric units).

Role of the Neonatal Nutritionist

In most settings, neonatal nutritionists have multifaceted roles. They are usually involved in patient care (clinical), including physician consultation (formal consultation and medical rounds), education (inservice, outreach), research, and administrative responsibilities. Most of their time is spent in direct patient care and medical rounds with physicians.[8] Because the members of ONN have been frequently asked to provide information about the neonatal RD's role, they have developed a model job description that can be adapted to the individual setting (Table A.1).

Patient Care and Physician Consultation Rounds

Neonatal RDs are responsible for medical nutrition therapy that includes nutrition screening and assessment and the development of nutrition care plans in the inpatient and/or outpatient setting.[5] They provide recommendations to physicians and other health care professionals when participating in medical rounds, in informal consultation, and/or in the medical record.[11] They provide nutrition information to the professional staff and families. They promote breastfeeding and maintenance of lactation.[12,13] They identify and communicate with institutional and community providers of continuing nutrition care after the baby's discharge from the hospital, furnishing information on medical history, nutritional status, and nutritional goals.

Neonatal nutritionists usually work autonomously, organizing daily activities around regularly scheduled clinics, rounds, or team meetings. They have their own record-keeping systems, which may include a visible card file or notebook, worksheets, and/or computer-generated records (see Figures A.1, 4.1, and 4.2).

Education and Research

As recommended by the American Dietetic Association, neonatal RDs develop and conduct inservice programs on neonatal nutrition topics for physicians, nurses, dietetic interns/students, and other team members in their own hospitals.[14,15] In states with regionalized perinatal care, the neonatal RD in a referral center may provide pro-

Figure A.1.   RD's patient record

(Used by permission of Michelle Moser Johnson, RD, LD, Neonatal Nutritionist, St. Christopher's Hospital for Children, Philadelphia, PA)

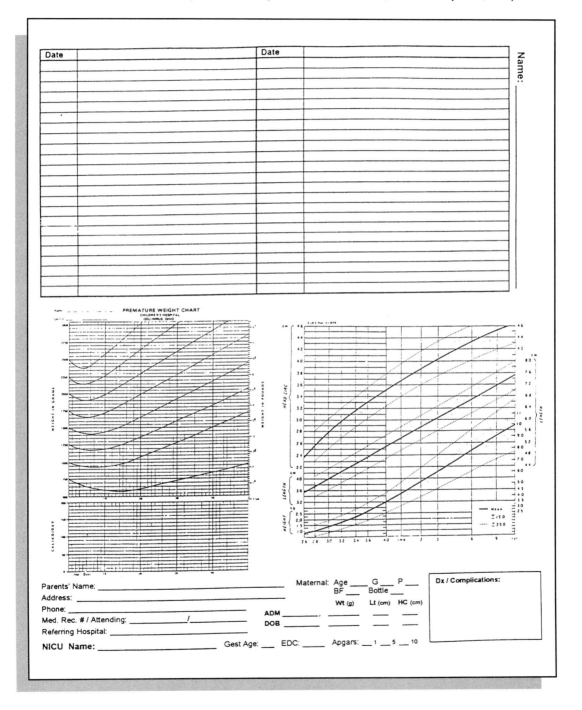

Figure A.1.   RD's patient record (continued)

DATE							
Wt a/c (g)	/	/	/	/	/	/	/
ENTERAL							
kcal/kg/d							
cc/kg/d							
pro g/kg/d							
Fe mg/kg/d							
PARENTERAL							
tpn							
lipids							
kcal/kg/d							
cc/kg/d							
pro g/kg/d							
lipids g/kg/d							
dextrose g/kg/d							
Tot. kcal/kg/d							
Tot. cc/kg/d							
Tot. pro g/kg/d							
Wt change g/d							
uop cc/kg/hr							
Stool Ct.							
Stool cc/kg/d							
Gastric op cc/d							

Date		Date	

grams and consultation for health professionals in the perinatal region served.

Continuing education is a priority for neonatal RDs through reading medical literature, attending hospital lectures, and traveling to neonatal nutrition conferences. Some enroll in college courses and obtain advanced degrees.

Neonatal nutritionists may also teach at the college level. Indeed, the ONN survey found that 41.8% of neonatal RDs have teaching affiliations with a university or college,[8] a surprising statistic in view of the fact that others found that less than 10% of advanced-level RDs have faculty appointments.[16]

Neonatal RDs may contribute to team research efforts or may develop their own research projects.[17] Finding time for research may be a problem unless research time is included in the job description.

A few RDs are employed in nontraditional neonatal nutritionist positions. Instead of being focused on direct patient care, their job responsibilities are more heavily weighted in other aspects of the neonatal RD's role, notably in education and research. One RD who carries the title of perinatal nutrition educator devotes her time entirely to disseminating information on perinatal education topics to health professionals in a wide area of her state. The assignment includes educational site visits, conducting inservice programs, preparing a quarterly newsletter devoted to perinatal nutrition, and serving as an advisor to a number of perinatal organizations. Another RD, a neonatal research nutritionist, spends the majority of her time developing and conducting nutrition research projects, then analyzing and reporting study results. Still another research nutritionist reports that results from clinical research, her primary responsibility, have an important influence on nutrition policy in the institution with which she is affiliated.

Administration and Other Aspects

Administrative responsibilities in which neonatal RDs are involved include development of policies, procedures, protocols, standards of care, and quality assurance.[18] Examples of these include feeding protocols, policies and procedures for the use of human milk in the NICU, standards of nutrition care for babies with various diagnoses, and quality assurance monitors for Formula Room procedures. Neonatal nutritionists may also supervise dietetic technicians or Formula Room personnel.

It is not unusual for the roles of health professionals to overlap. Role overlap for the neonatal RD most frequently occurs with the pharmacist and/or nurse. Some flexibility is needed among team members to adapt their specific roles to the individual job setting. Maintaining the unique aspects of one's own contribution may require assertiveness balanced with a respect for the unique contributions of other team members.

Although most neonatal nutritionists provide nutrition assessments, calculations, consultations, and counseling, fewer than 20% charge for these services.[8] Because lack of funding for a neonatal RD position is perceived as a barrier to the generation of the position, hospital decision-makers may be influenced by the knowledge that the position could generate income.[19] Although managed care may be changing this orientation in many locations, published resources are available to assist in setting up a fee-for-service program.[20]

Cost-Effectiveness and Outcome Studies

In the current health care environment, consumers (and payers) are seeking economical yet high-quality care. They expect that this care will lead to positive health outcomes. A new emphasis is being placed on interventions that lead to consistent, measurable outcomes. Specific interventions are being scrutinized to find evidence that they are cost effective.

Variability in medical practice in neonatal intensive care units is now being identified.[21-24] General nutrition policies vary among NICUs even in the same city.[25] Infants grow differently in different NICUs.[26,47] Are some practices associated with improved outcomes? Does the intervention of a registered dietitian in the NICU have an impact on the patients' outcomes? If so, what is that impact, and can it be measured? What do we know so far?

Valentine and Schanler compared nutritional milestones in 533 low-birth-weight infants before and after the addition of a registered dietitian to the NICU team.[27] Similar nutrition protocols were used in the two years evaluated. Before the RD started, 273 infants started total parenteral nutrition (TPN) 3.6 ± 0.2 days after birth and were continued on it for 19 ± 1 days. With an RD in the nursery, 260 infants began TPN 2.7 ± 0.1 days after birth and were on it 16 ± 1 days. The initiation (9 ± 1 vs 12 ± 1 days) and complete attainment (19 ± 1 vs 23 ± 1 days) of tube feedings and complete attainment of oral feedings (40 ± 2 vs 48 ± 2 days) occurred sooner with an RD in the nursery (P < 0.02) than before. Thus, the interventions of a neonatal nutritionist resulted in earlier initiation of feedings and achievement of complete enteral and oral nutrition, along with less reliance on TPN. A cost savings of 16% (due to less TPN use) was realized.

Lair et al. compared routine intervention (twice weekly evaluations and recommendations by a Neonatal Nutrition Support Team [NNST]) with intervention on consultation only for 341 infants <1,250 g at birth.[28] The NNST consisted of a full-time dietitian assisted by a pharmacist and a neonatologist. The 168 infants receiving routine intervention regained birth weight earlier and made the transition from intensive care one week earlier than did the 173 infants who were seen on consultation only. This result is even more remarkable considering that educational and program effects of the NNST may have influenced all of the NICU patients—not just those in the intervention group.

In an outpatient setting, Bryson et al. observed the growth outcomes of 75 former very-low-birth-weight (VLBW) infants.[29] Forty-two infants received follow-up care on an as-needed basis in a general pediatric follow-up clinic. (In this clinic, referral to a registered dietitian was based on perceived patient need by a physician.) Another 33 infants received routine nutrition intervention from a registered dietitian as part of a multidisciplinary comprehensive care clinic. The two groups differed significantly in the number of infants exhibiting catch-up growth for length and head circumference. By 12 months corrected age, 12 (57%) of the general pediatric clinic infants and 26 (87%) of the comprehensive care clinic infants were at the fifth percentile or greater for length ($p < 0.05$); 11 (52%) of the general pediatric clinic infants and 27 (90%) of the comprehensive care clinic infants were at the fifth percentile or greater for head circumference ($p < 0.05$). The authors conclude that multidisciplinary primary care that includes the services of a registered dietitian who participates in the assessment and care of each patient can enhance the catch-up growth of VLBW infants through 12 months corrected age.

Dietitians in NICUs have implemented a variety of interventions, including global nutrition screening, frequent nutrition assessment, neonatal nutrition education for NICU team members, monitored feeding protocols, standards of nutrition care, weekly nutrition rounds, written and verbal recommendations, and policy revisions. These interventions by registered dietitians have resulted in improved infant weight gain,[30,31] improved overall growth,[29,32,33] and a lower incidence of growth failure.[29,34] Infants regain birth weight sooner when a dietitian intervenes.[28,35,36] Additionally, nutrient intakes have improved due to dietitians' interventions, including higher calorie intakes,[30,32,36,37,48] more rapid attainment of higher calories,[35,38] higher protein intakes,[30-32,48] higher calcium, phosphorus, and magnesium intakes,[30] and higher intakes of vitamins A and D.[36] The surveillance and recommendations of dietitians reduces errors in TPN orders.[30] Infants can be taken off TPN sooner[27,38,48] and initiate feedings earlier[27,35,48] when dietitians are actively involved in their care. Infants may even be discharged from the hospital sooner when dietitians provide intensive nutrition care.[31,39]

The ADA has developed standards of professional practice for dietetics professionals.[40] According to standard 5, the registered dietitian systematically evaluates the quality and effectiveness of practice and revises practice as needed to incorporate the results of evaluation. Eck[41] and Naglak[42] encourage dietitians to incorporate outcomes research into routine clinical practice. Since dietitians often report lack of resources or financial support as obstacles to

Figure A.2.   Sample RD case study[43]

REGISTERED DIETITIAN/ NUTRITIONIST CASE 15

Site:	Home infusion agency
Client:	11-week-old female
Diagnosis or Condition:	Congestive heart failure, cardiac hypertrophy, malnutrition (weight < 5th%ile). Post-surgery complications. Baby discharged with NG tube feeds
Intervention:	Mother trained to place NG tubes so baby could receive specialized concentrated infant formula not nippled from bottle. Increased formula volume to match weight gain and promote catch-up growth. RD updated insurance case managers on progress and conducted a weekly weight check. Contacts: nine home visits, three telephone conversations over three months
Outcomes:	Successful transition from 50% NG feeds/50% oral to 100% oral feeds in three months. Steady weight gain
Interventions Avoided:	Total = $6,930 (Surgery for permanent G-tube, $5,700; further malnutrition, complications with worsening cardiac condition, rehospitalizations, tube-feeding equipment/formula for approximately three months, $1,230; noncompliance by caregiver since weekly weight gain was shown)
Intervention Costs:	Total = $4,392 (Of this total, approximately $520 for RD services; the remainder is RN services and daily charges for supplies, pump, bags, etc.)
Cost savings of Intervention:	Saved $2,538 over three months

incorporating research into clinical practice,[41] perhaps documenting a few case studies would be a good starting point. An example[43] is shown in Figure A.2. Eventually, the neonatal RD may want to become more involved in outcomes research and writing. If she has no prior experience, she may be able to collaborate with academic or research-oriented dietitians.[41] Other resources[44,45] are available for dietitians who are interested in outcomes research. More outcome studies published in peer-reviewed journals are needed.

References

1. Committee on Nutrition Status during Pregnancy and Lactation, Food and Nutrition Board. Nutrition Services in Perinatal Care. 2nd ed. Washington, D.C.: National Academy Press, 1992.
2. American Academy of Pediatrics and The American College of Obstetricians and Gynecologists. Guidelines for Perinatal Care. 4th ed. Elk Grove Village, IL: AAP, 1997.
3. ASPEN Board of Directors. Standards for hospitalized pediatric patients. Nutr Clin Pract 11:217, 1996.
4. The Joint Commission on Accreditation of Health Care Organizations. Comprehensive accreditation manual for hospitals, 1996. Oakbrook Terrace, IL: JCAHO, 1996.
5. American Dietetic Association. Position of The American Dietetic Association: The role of registered dietitians in enteral and parenteral nutrition support. J Am Diet Assoc 97:302, 1997.
6. Rickard K, Gresham E. Nutritional considerations for the newborn requiring intensive care. J Am Diet Assoc 66:592, 1975.
7. Rickard KA, Ernst JA, Brady MS, et al. Nutritional outcome of 207 very low-birth-weight infants in an intensive care unit. J Am Diet Assoc 81:674, 1982.
8. Ohio Neonatal Nutritionists. Nutrition services in neonatal intensive care: A national survey (conducted in April 1990).
9. Thompson M, Price P, Stahle DA. Nutrition services in neonatal intensive care: A national survey. J Am Diet Assoc 94:440, 1994.
10. Mayfield SR, Albrecht J, Roberts L, et al. The role of the nutritional support team in neonatal intensive care. Semin Perinatol 13:88, 1989.
11. Mueller CM, Colaizzo-Anas T, Shronts EP, et al. Order writing for parenteral nutrition by registered dietitians. J Am Diet Assoc 96:764, 1996.
12. American Dietetic Association. Position of The American Dietetic Association: Promotion of breast-feeding. J Am Diet Assoc 97:662, 1997.
13. Helm A, Windham CT, Wyse B. Dietitians in breastfeeding management: An untapped resource in the hospital. J Hum Lact 13:221, 1997.
14. American Dietetic Association. Position of The American Dietetic Association: Nutrition education for health care professionals. J Am Diet Assoc 98:343, 1998.
15. Booth MB. Teaching and learning in a neonatal intensive care unit. Arch Dis Child 78:275, 1998.
16. Kane MT, Estes CA, Colton DA, et al. Role delineation for dietetic practitioners: Empirical results. J Am Diet Assoc 90:1124, 1990.
17. Dwyer JT. Scientific underpinnings for the profession: Dietitians in research. J Am Diet Assoc 97:593, 1997.
18. American Dietetic Association Pediatric Nutrition Practice Group. Quality assurance criteria for pediatric nutrition conditions: a model. Chicago: ADA, 1990.

19. Smith AE, Smith PE. Reimbursement for clinical nutrition services: a 10-year experience. J Am Diet Assoc 92:1385, 1992.

20. American Dietetic Association. Nutrition Entrepreneur's Guide to Reimbursement Success. Chicago: American Dietetic Association, 1995.

21. Richardson DK, Shah BL, Frantz ID, et al. Perinatal risk and severity of illness in newborns at 6 neonatal intensive care units. Am J Public Health 89:511, 1999.

22. Ringer SA, Richardson DK, Sacher RA, et al. Variations in transfusion practice in neonatal intensive care. Pediatrics 101:194, 1998.

23. Kahn DJ, Richardson DK, Gray JE, et al. Variation among neonatal intensive care units in narcotic administration. Arch Pediatr Adolesc Med 152:844, 1998.

24. Perlstein PH, Atherton HD, Donovan EF, et al. Physician variations and the ancillary costs of neonatal intensive care. Health Serv Res 32:299, 1997.

25. Olsen I, Awnetwant E, Cardi G, et al. Variations in nutrition personnel and practice among 7 neonatal intensive care units. J Am Diet Assoc 97:A-30, 1997.

26. Rubin LP, Richardson DK, Bednarek FJ, et al. Longitudinal growth in hospitalized VLBW infants: Identification of patient characteristics and inter-NICU differences. Pediatr Res 41:239A, 1997.

27. Valentine C, Schanler RJ. Neonatal nutritionist intervention improves nutritional support and promotes cost containment in the management of low birth weight (LBW) infants. ASPEN 17th Clinical Congress nutrition practice poster 46, Feb 14-17, 1993.

28. Lair C, Albrecht J, Kennedy KA. Randomized controlled trial of neonatal nutrition support team (NNST) services. Pediatr Res 43:177A, 1998.

29. Bryson SR, Theriot L, Ryan NJ, et al. Primary follow-up care in a multidisciplinary setting enhances catch-up growth of very-low-birthweight infants. J Am Diet Assoc 97:386, 1997.

30. Elsaesser KR. Dietitian intervention in neonatal intensive care reduces errors and improves clinical outcomes. J Am Diet Assoc 98:A-22, 1998.

31. LaBarre DJ, Maher MM, Raye JR, et al. The effect of a monitored feeding protocol on very, very low birth weight infants. J Am Diet Assoc 87:A-58, 1987.

32. Carlson SJ, Redlin J. Use of nutrition outcome monitors in intensive care nurseries. J Am Diet Assoc 97:A-102, 1997.

33. Henry B, Smith S, Naber M, et al. Nutrition screening with home care services connects pediatric patients for dietitian intervention. ASPEN 23rd Clinical Congress nutrition practice poster 76, Jan 31-Feb 3, 1999.

34. Smith S, Henry B, Sajous C. Development and efficacy of nutritional screening criteria for neonatal ICU patients. ASPEN 23rd Clinical Congress nutrition practice poster 28, Jan 31-Feb 3, 1999.

35. Urrutia JG, Gupta U, Kuzma-O'Reilly B. Fifteen year comparison of nutritional support for very low birth weight neonates. Pediatr Res 41:183A, 1997.

36. Price P, Carde KA, Flammang AM, et al. Identifying priorities for a nutrition support team (NST) in a neonatal intensive care unit (NICU). ASPEN 14th Clinical Congress nutrition practice poster 81, Jan 28-31, 1990.

37. Ford A, Lalla S, Korones S. Implementation of clinical nutrition protocols in a neonatal intensive care unit (NICU). ASPEN 15th Clinical Congress nutrition practice poster 47, Jan 27-30, 1991.

38. Han-Markey T, August D, Schumacher R. Impact of the nutrition support team (NST) on neonatal nutrition care. ASPEN 18th Clinical Congress Nutrition Practice Poster 43, Jan 30-Feb 2, 1994.

39. Stave VS, Robbins S, Fletcher AB. A comparison of growth rates of premature infants prior to and after close nutritional monitoring. Clin Proc Children's Hospital National Medical Center 35:171, 1979.

40. American Dietetic Association. The American Dietetic Association standards of professional practice for dietetics professionals. J Am Diet Assoc 98:83, 1998.

41. Eck LH, Slawson DL, Williams R, et al. A model for making outcomes research standard practice in clinical dietetics. J Am Diet Assoc 98:451, 1998.

42. Naglak M, Mitchell DC, Kris-Etherton P, et al. What to consider when conducting a cost-effectiveness analysis in a clinical setting. J Am Diet Assoc 98:1149, 1998.

43. Lucas B, Feucht S, eds. Cost Considerations: The Benefits of Nutrition Services for a Case Series of Children with Special Health Care Needs in Washington State. Olympia: Washington State Department of Health, 1998.

44. Gallagher-Allred C, Voss AC, Gussler JD. Nutrition Intervention and Patient Outcomes: A Self-study Manual. Columbis, Ohio: Ross Products Division, Abbott Laboratories, 1995.

45. Ireton-Jones CS, Gottschlich MM, Bell SJ. Practice-Oriented Nutrition Research—An Outcomes Measurement Approach. Gaithersburg, Md.: Aspen Publishers, 1998.

46. Fenton TR, Geggie JH, Warners JN, et al. Nutrition services in Canadian neonatal intensive care: the role of the dietitian. Canadian J Dietet Pract Res, in press, 2000.

47. Olsen IE, Richardson DK, Schmid C, et al. Variation in growth of premature infants among neonatal intensive care units (NICUs). Pediatr Res 47:422A, 2000.

48. Kuzma-O'Reilly BA. Effectiveness of nutrition support appraisal in the NICU. Pediatr Res 47:409A, 2000

Appendix B

Establishing and Developing the Position of Neonatal Nutritionist

Melody Thompson, MS, RD, LD

Creating the Position

Creating a neonatal nutritionist position involves research, justification, persuasion, and general hard work. In the era of shrinking health care resources, a great deal of effort may be required to convince hospital decision-makers to establish a new position. Someone (a dietitian, physician, or nurse) must spearhead the effort. Depending on the institution, the support of a neonatologist is anywhere from helpful to indispensable. With input from several individuals who have worked to create a neonatal registered dietitian (RD) position, the following step-by-step process was developed:[1]

- Recognize the need for nutrition services in the neonatal intensive care unit (NICU)
- Discuss the idea of an RD's involvement in the NICU with department directors (and other personnel) in the departments of nutrition services and neonatology to determine their attitudes
- Gather resources from:
  — Reviewing literature
  — Surveying other medical centers/pediatric facilities regarding RD services in the NICU
  — Reviewing patients' medical charts to determine levels of nutritional risk and potential outcome with RD involvement

- Develop proposal and job description for a neonatal RD. Include financial justification, such as revenue generation by charging for RD's services and/or savings from shorter patient stays, owing to improvement in nutrition status. A succinct, one-page justification may have an impact on decision-makers (see Figure B.1).
- Present proposal to directors of nutrition services, neonatology, and hospital administration. (Letters and verbal support from MDs, RDs, RNs, and other team members can be extremely helpful at this step)
- Conduct ongoing quality assurance studies to document that high-risk patients are not receiving adequate nutrition services
- Gain approval for the position
- Recruit and hire

Training Options

The Food and Nutrition Board of the National Academy of Sciences defines a neonatal nutritionist as a registered dietitian (licensed, where required) with either advanced pediatric training that includes clinical neonatal nutrition or clinical experience in the care of critically ill newborns.[2] Some neonatal RDs pursue formal education—from a one-week training program to a fellowship training lasting several months.[3] These formal programs are typically high-quality, standardized, and organized approaches to training. Formal education in neonatal nutrition is highly desirable and provides a good base for further development with work experience (see Figure B.2.).

Most currently practicing neonatal RDs have obtained at least part of their training by attending neonatal nutrition conferences.[4] These conferences are generally of high quality, with respected researchers and practitioners in the field as program participants. Local or on-the-job training is obtained by many neonatal nutritionists, presumably because of the convenience and low cost.[4] Although time away from work is minimized by local training, the quality of the training varies considerably with the time spent, resources available, and the knowledge and experience of the instructors. Due to the complexity of nutrition intervention needed by infants in NICUs, most neonatal RDs require a year or more of clinical experience before they can feel confident in their knowledge and experience base, regardless of the training option chosen.

Figure B.1. Cost-Effectiveness of the Neonatal Nutritionist

Rapidly advancing technology in the neonatal intensive care unit (NICU) has enabled smaller and smaller babies to survive the neonatal period.[1] These tiny babies pose complex nutrition issues for the medical team. The National Research Council recommends that dietitians be involved in the care of hospitalized neonates.[2] The council specifically recommends that the staff of level III NICUs include a registered dietitian with either advanced pediatric training that includes clinical neonatal nutrition or clinical experience in the nutrition care of critically ill newborn infants.

Studies have shown that recommendations and surveillance provided by neonatal dietitians resulted in improved weight gain,[3,4] improved energy intake,[3] faster initiation and progression of enteral feedings,[5] and decreased hospital stay[4,6] for high-risk infants. In the latter two studies, hospital stay was reduced by six days[4] and seven days,[6] respectively.

Using an estimated cost of $1,000 per day (for neonatal step-down care) and a decreased length of stay of (conservatively) three days for 300 infants in the NICU, the hospital could theoretically save close to $1 million by utilizing the intensive services of a neonatal nutritionist (i.e., $1,000 x 3 x 300 = $900,000).

References:

1. Phelps DL, et al. 28-day survival rates of 6676 neonates with birth weights of 1250 grams or less. Pediatrics 87:7, 1991.
2. Committee on Nutrition Status during Pregnancy and Lactation, Food and Nutrition Board. Nutrition services in perinatal care. 2d ed. Washington, D.C.: National Academy Press, 1992.
3. Price PT et al. Identifying priorities for a nutrition support team in a neonatal intensive care unit. ASPEN 14th Clinical Congress nutrition practice poster 81, Jan 28-31, 1990
4. LaBarre DJ et al. Effect of monitored feeding protocol on VVLBW infants. J Am Diet Assoc 87:A-58, 1987.
5. Valentine C, Schanler RJ. Neonatal nutritionist intervention improves nutritional support and promotes cost containment in the management of low birth weight infants. ASPEN 17th Clinical Congress nutrition practice poster 46, Feb 14-17, 1993.
6. Stave VS, et al. A comparison of growth rates of premature infants prior to and after close nutritional monitoring. Clin Proc Children's Hospital National Medical Center 35:171, 1979.

Figure B.2.   Neonatal Nutrition Training Programs

Neonatal nutrition training programs are available at two sites in the United States. Both programs are funded by federal grants from the Maternal and Child Health Bureau of Health and Human Services. Both offer:
• Neonatal nutrition fellowship programs
• One-week neonatal nutrition update practicums
• Annual neonatal nutrition conferences

More information about these programs is available from

Diane M. Anderson, PhD, RD, CSP, FADA
Associate Professor of Pediatrics
Neonatal Nutrition Training Program
Baylor College of Medicine/Section of Neonatology
1 Baylor Plaza
Houston, TX 77030

Karyl Rickard, PhD, RD, CSP, FADA
Professor of Nutrition and Dietetics
Neonatal Nutrition Training Program
J.W. Riley Hospital for Children
702 Barnhill Drive, Room 1010
Indianapolis, IN 46202

Establishing Role Priorities

Although a model job description is included in Appendix A, the neonatal RD's role actually may vary considerably from setting to setting. It is important to determine what the role expectations are in a particular institution. The neonatologists and clinical nutrition services manager may have specific role expectations in mind. Their attitudes and general philosophies should be identified and at least one or two areas in which the neonatal RD can have some immediate impact should be determined. Some negotiation on what should and should not be included in the neonatal RD's role may be necessary. Alternative personnel to perform tasks not appropriate for the neonatal RD may need to be specified. Job sharing between two experienced pediatric RDs may also be possible in an NICU.[5] The new neonatal RD may be expected to have a primary role in direct patient care and in education of health care professionals. It may be helpful to attend teaching rounds daily in the NICU to hear the terminology used, understand the physicians' priorities and perspectives, see the roles of other team members, get to know the patients' needs, and gradually begin to offer input on nutrition issues. If the NICU is large, the neonatal RD may not be able to see every patient every day. It is helpful to start out small and gradually increase patient load. This can be done by using inpatient screening criteria to prioritize care in the unit.[6-8] Weekly screening is usually recommended and may be completed by a dietetic technician, if available.[8,9] Infants who meet any of the criteria should receive a complete nutritional assessment and individualized care plan by a registered dietitian. No set of criteria will yield all of the at-risk infants. The goal is to have reasonable parameters that can be quickly assessed and that will reveal most of the patients who require nutritional intervention. The screening criteria shown in Table B.1, developed by the Ohio Neonatal Nutritionists, are meant to be used as a model subject to modification to suit the needs of the particular unit. Sample nutrition screening and assessment tools and policies are included in Chapter 7 (Figures 7.1, 7.2, and 7.3).

The following steps in establishing and developing the neonatal RD's role were devised with the input of several neonatal RDs who were the first to provide such services in their hospitals.[10]

- Meet with the chief of neonatology, NICU nurse manager, manager of neonatal nurse practitioners (NNPs), and clinical nurse specialists (CNSs) with the objectives of
    — Determining their expectations of the neonatal RD's role
    — Identifying their philosophies of patient nutrition management
    — Acquainting them with services that a neonatal RD can provide
- Meet other staff and team members who work in the NICU (e.g., clinical pharmacist, developmental therapist, lactation consultant)
- Observe the current system by engaging in these activities:
    — Review current nutrition policies, procedures, protocols
    — Read patient charts and bedside flow sheets
    — Attend medical rounds with the team
    — Collect data on growth and nutrient intake (including feeding methods and advancement) to identify where intervention is most needed
    — Evaluate the appropriateness of parenteral nutrition, formula, human milk, and supplement use
    — Evaluate the appropriateness of growth measurement techniques, tools, and growth charts
    — Review discharge and follow-up policies and procedures
- Verify your perceptions or interpretations with other team members
- Identify and prioritize nutrition issues that need to be addressed, updated, or changed
- Prioritize patient care levels (see Table B.1 for sample screening criteria); develop criteria specific to the needs of the patients and priorities of health care providers in the setting

- Draft and present proposals for changes in policies, procedures, protocols
  — Ask for the input of other team members to be incorporated into the second or final draft
  — Implement and monitor the impact of changes in policies, procedures, and protocols
- Educate MDs (neonatologists, fellows, residents, medical students), RNs (nurse manager, CNSs, NNPs, staff nurses), pharmacists, developmental therapists, lactation consultants, and other team members on neonatal nutrition issues
  — Present inservice programs, lectures, and formal and informal consultation
  — Provide booklets, pocket reference cards, and other educational materials.
- Develop research ideas and projects
- Exchange information with other neonatal nutritionists

This process may be facilitated by establishing specific goals. One new neonatal RD's goals included the following:[11]

Near-term goals: 1. Human milk fortifier will be ordered for all VLBW infants receiving human milk. 2. Preterm formula rather than standard formula will be ordered for all very low birth weight (VLBW) infants.

Intermediate goals: 1. RD will revise parenteral nutrition (PN) protocols with team input. 2. RD will start monthly nutrition rounds with MDs, NNPs, RNs, and RPh. 3. RD will develop referral criteria for RNs to use in seeking consultations in nutrition intervention.

Long-term goals: 1. RD will propose a study to monitor outcomes of infants followed by the RD versus those not followed by the RD. 2. RD will exchange information with public health nurses in follow-up of NICU graduates.

Another neonatal nutritionist updated PN policies and procedures during her first year in the neonatal RD role.[12] Her interventions included obtaining I.V. infusion pumps that accommodate infusion rates of < 1 ml/hour; formulating a laboratory monitoring protocol; changing from standard to pediatric amino acid product; increasing from two to six the options for standard house PN solutions; changing from a 10% to 20% I.V. fat emulsion; dosing pediatric parenteral vitamins according to patient weight; maximizing calcium and phosphorus content of solutions; and updating and including PN guidelines on the back of the PN order form.

Yet another neonatal RD developed a multidisciplinary neonatal nutrition task force.[13] The task force meets quarterly to review any proposed changes in neonatal nutrition protocols in their NICU. Task force members from each discipline are responsible for representing the viewpoint(s) of their discipline during discussion. These same members are also responsible for educating others in the nurs-

Table B.1. **Ohio Neonatal Nutritionists Screening Criteria for Identifying Neonatal Inpatients at Highest Nutritional Risk**

< 1 wk of age	(a) > 15% weight loss from birth weight
	(b) < 1 kg birth weight
1-2 wk of age	(a) < 60 kcal/kg
	(b) Any continued weight loss
> 2 wk of age	(a) < 2/3 expected caloric requirement, i.e.,
	< 60 kcal/kg (all I.V.)
	< 70 kcal/kg (I.V./enteral)
	< 80 kcal/kg (all enteral)
	(b) < 10 g/kg/d weight gain (< 38 wk GA)
	or < 1/2 expected g/d weight gain (> 38 wk GA)
	(c)* Prealbumin < 7.0 mg/dl, or albumin < 2.5 g/dl
	Direct bilirubin > 2.0 mg/dl
	Serum phosphorus < 4.0 mg/dl
	Alkaline phosphatase > 600 U/L
> 2 mo of age	Any of the above for > 2 wk of age plus
	(a) No source of dietary iron
	(b) Continued total parenteral nutrition

Any infant with newly diagnosed NEC, BPD, osteopenia, cardiac disorders, neurologic problems, G.I. surgical anomalies, or metabolic aberrations.

Any infant with birth weight of < 1.5 kg (and current weight of < 2 kg) on full feedings but not receiving fortified human milk or preterm formula

GA = gestational age; NEC = necrotizing enterocolitis; BPD = bronchopulmonary dysplasia

* Include as criteria only if screening can be done in some time-efficient manner for entire unit; use values only as guide—compare to institutional normal ranges.

ery and for promoting the benefits of proposed changes. One such change implemented by this task force was a switch to routine use of iron-fortified formulas (as opposed to low-iron formulas) for all formula-fed infants.

In summary, creating a neonatal nutritionist position involves a step-by-step process that leads from recognizing the need for nutrition services in the NICU to hiring a neonatal RD. Developing the newly created neonatal RD role is a similar process. Extensive clinical experience in neonatal nutrition is necessary to obtain competence, regardless of the neonatal RD's training. Developing specific, measurable goals may facilitate the process of establishing the role and measuring the neonatal RD's impact.

References

1. Personal communications from: M Girten, St. Christopher's Hospital for Children, Philadelphia, PA; RD Guthrie, Magee-Women's Hospital, Pittsburgh, PA; AA Sinden, University of Virginia Health Sciences Center, Charlottesville, VA; GB Smith, Arnold Palmer Hospital for Children and Women, Orlando, FL.

2. National Academy of Sciences Food and Nutrition Board. Nutrition Services in Perinatal Care. 2nd ed. Washington, D.C.: National Academy Press, 1992; 86.

3. Pittard WB, Anderson DA. Neonatal nutrition training. J Am Diet Assoc 83:471, 1983.

4. Ohio Neonatal Nutritionists. Nutrition services in neonatal intensive care: A national survey (conducted in April 1990).

5. Swiontek P, Chorba D. Job sharing a neonatal intensive care nutritionist position. J Am Diet Assoc 95:A-74, 1995.

6. Puangco MA, Schanler RJ. Nutritional risk screening in the neonatal intensive care unit (NICU). ASPEN 23rd Clinical Congress nutrition practice poster 26. Jan 31-Feb 3, 1999.

7. Smith S, Henry B, Sajous C. Development and efficacy of nutritional screening criteria for neonatal ICU patients. ASPEN 23rd Clinical Congress nutrition practice poster 28. Jan 31-Feb 3, 1999.

8. Zeringue DE, Valentine C. Screening indicators identify neonates at high nutritional risk. J Am Diet Assoc 95:A-32, 1995.

9. Wheeler RE, Rippetoe LR, Meyers BM. Dietetic technicians (DT) in the neonatal intensive care unit (NICU). J Am Diet Assoc 90:A-76, 1990.

10. Personal communications from: J Correll, Deaconess Medical Center, Spokane WA; D McNevich, Crozer-Chester Medical Center, Upland, PA; J Sentipal-Walerius, Magee-Women's Hospital, Pittsburgh, PA; P Sisk, Forsyth Memorial Hospital, Winston-Salem, NC; R Smith, Children's Hospital of Orange County, Orange, CA; C Valentine, Baylor College of Medicine—Texas Children's Hospital, Houston, TX; J Waldron, Ventura County Medical Center, Ventura, CA.

11. Personal communication from J Waldron, Ventura County Medical Center, Ventura, CA.

12. Personal communication from J Sentipal-Walerius, Magee Women's Hospital, Pittsburgh, PA.

13. Personal communication from L Rallison Vanatta, Phoenix Children's Hospital, Phoenix, AZ.

Appendix C

Atomic Weights/Valences
and Conversion Tables

Units of measure given for electrolyte and mineral intake recommendations often vary from product information given for formulas or compounds used to meet these recommendations. The conversion equations for milliequivalents (mEq), millimoles (mM), and milligrams (mg) and molecular weights are given below.

$$mEq = \frac{mg \times valence}{atomic\ or\ molecular\ weight}$$

$$mg = \frac{mEq \times atomic\ or\ molecular\ weight}{valence}$$

$$mM = atomic\ or\ molecular\ weight$$

$$mg = mM \times atomic\ or\ molecular\ weight$$

Element	Atomic weight	Valence
Sodium	23	1
Potassium	39	1
Chlorine	35	1*
Calcium	40	2
Phosphorus	31	3,5
Magnesium	24	2

* Chlorine may also have valences of 3, 5, and 7, but for prectical purposes, has a valence of 1 for most nutritional compunds

Conversion Table: Nutrient Content per Gram of Compound

Nutrient	Compound	mg*	mEq*	mMol*
calcium	calcium chloride (27.3% calcium by weight)	273	13.6	6.8
	calcium gluceptate (8.2% calcium by weight)	82	4.1	2.0
	calcium gluconate (9.3% calcium by weight)	93	4.7	2.3
chloride	calcium chloride (72.7% chloride by weight)	727	21	21
	potassium chloride (47.7% chloride by weight)	477	13.6	13.6
	sodium chloride (60.3% chloride by weight)	603	17.2	17.2
copper#	copper chloride (37.4% copper by weight)	374	—	—
	copper sulfate (25.5% copper by weight)	255	—	—
magnesium	magnesium sulfate (20.2% magnesium by weight)	202	16.8	8.4
potassium	potassium acetate (39.8% potassium by weight)	398	10.2	10.2
	potassium chloride (52.3% potassium by weight)	523	13.4	13.4
	dibasic potassium phosphate (44.9% potassium by weight)	449	11.5	11.5
	monobasic potassium phosphate (28.5% potassium by weight)	285	7.3	7.3
phosphorus	di-/monobasic potassium phosphate (17.2% phosphorus by wt)	172	—	5.5
	sodium phosphate (23.8% phosphorus by weight)	238	—	7.7
sodium	sodium acetate (17% sodium by weight)	168	7.3	7.3
	sodium bicarbonate (27.4% sodium by weight)	274	11.9	11.9
	sodium chloride (39.7% sodium by weight)	397	17.2	17.2
	sodium phosphate (31.2% sodium by weight)	312	13.5	13.5
zinc#	zinc chloride (47.8% zinc by weight)	478	—	—
	zinc gluconate (14.3% zinc by weight)	143	—	—
	zinc sulfate anhydrous (40.1% zinc by weight)	401	—	—
	zinc sulfate heptahydrate (23% zinc by weight)	225	—	—

* amount of nutrient in compound in milligrams (mg), milliequivalents (mEq), or millimoles (mM)

copper and zinc dosage range is in micrograms (mcg) per kg body weight if administered parenterally and < 10 mg/d enterally.

Conversion Table: Nutrient Content per 1 mL of Solution

Nutrient	Compound	mg*	mEq*	mMol*
calcium	calcium chloride 10% (1 gm/10 mL)	27.3	1.4	0.7
	calcium gluceptate 22% (1.1 gm/5 mL)	18	0.9	0.4
	calcium gluconate 10% (1 gm/10 mL)	9.3	0.5	0.2
chloride	calcium chloride 10% (1 gm/10 mL)	72.7	2.1	2.1
	potassium chloride (14.8%)	70	2.0	2.0
	sodium chloride (14.6%)	87.5	2.5	2.5
	sodium chloride (23.4%)	140	4.0	4.0
copper	copper chloride (1.07 mg copper chloride)	0.4	—	—
	copper sulfate (1.57 mg copper sulfate)	0.4	—	—
	copper sulfate (7.85 mg copper sulfate)	2.0	—	—
magnesium	magnesium sulfate heptahydrate 10%	9.6	0.8	0.4
	magnesium sulfate heptahydrate 12.5%	12	1.0	0.5
	magnesium sulfate heptahydrate 50%	48	4.0	2.0
phosphorus	potassium phosphate	93	—	3.0
	sodium phosphate	93	—	3.0
potassium	potassium acetate	39	1	1
	potassium chloride 7.4% (0.74 gm/10 mL)	39	1	1
	potassium chloride 14.8% (1.48 gm/10 mL)	78	2	2
	potassium phosphate	172	4.4	4.4
sodium	sodium acetate 8.2%	23	1	1
	sodium acetate 16.4%	46	2	2
	sodium bicarbonate 4.2%	11.5	0.5	0.5
	sodium bicarbonate 5%	13.8	0.6	0.6
	sodium bicarbonate 7.5%	20.7	0.9	0.9
	sodium bicarbonate 8.4%	23	1.0	1.0
	sodium acetate 32.8%	92	4	4
	sodium chloride 5.8%	23	1	1
	sodium chloride 14.6%	57.5	2.5	2.5
	sodium chloride 23.4%	92	4	4
zinc	zinc chloride (2.09 mg zinc chloride)	1	—	—
	zinc sulfate (4.39 mg heptahydrate or 2.46 mg anhydrous)	1	—	—
	zinc sulfate (21.95 mg zinc sulfate)	5	—	—

* amount of nutrient in compound or solution in milligrams (mg), milliequivalents (mEq),
   or millimoles (mM)

Appendix D

Growth Charts

Dancis Postnatal Growth Chart

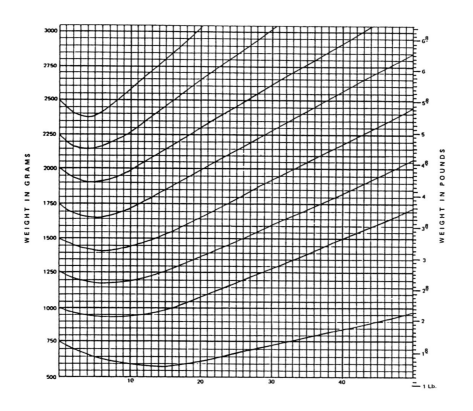

From Dancis J, O'Connell JR, Holt LE. A grid for recording the weight of premature infants. J Pediatr 33:570, 1948. Reprinted by permission of C.V. Mosby Co.

Hall/Shaffer Postnatal Growth Chart

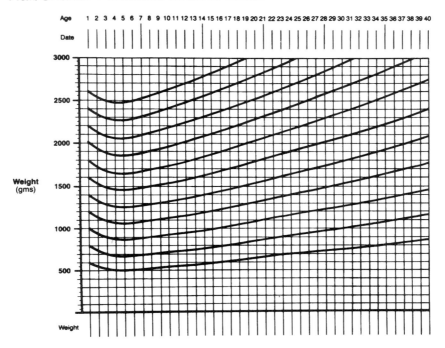

Reprinted with permission of Robert T. Hall, MD, and Stanley Shaffer, MD, © 1988.

Wright Postnatal Growth Grid

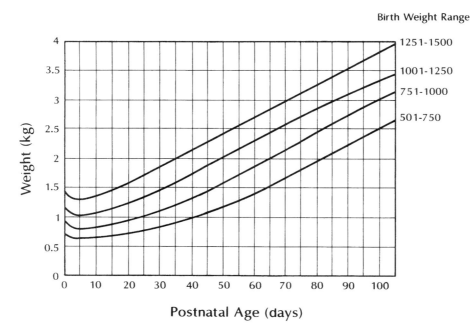

Adapted with permission from Wright K, Dawson JP, Fallis D, et al. New postnatal grids for very low birth weight infants. Pediatrics 91:922, 1993.

Shaffer/Wright Postnatal Growth Chart

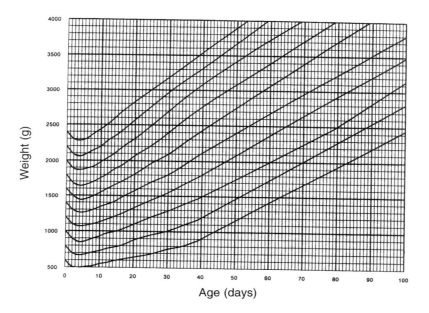

Combined data from Shaffer SG, et al., Pediatrics 79:702-5, 1987; and Wright K, et al., Pediatrics 91:922-6, 1993; calculated growth rate of 10 g/kg/d for infants > 1500 g birthweight but < 2500 g over 40 days of age.

Lair and Kennedy Neonatal Growth Charts

Reprinted with permission. Lair CS, Kennedy KA. Monitoring postnatal growth in the neonatal intensive care unit. Nutr Clin Pract 12:124, 1997.

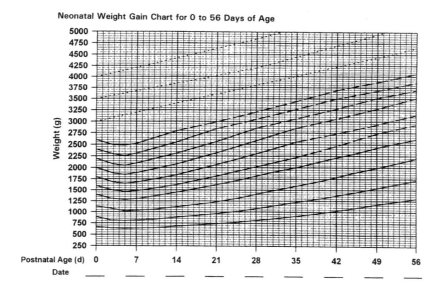

Neonatal Weight Gain Chart for 0 to 56 Days of Age

———— = Shaffer et al., Pediatrics 1987, and Wright et al., Peditrics 1993.
— — = Calculated for growth rate of 15 g/kg/d for infants < 2,500 g, 10 g/kg/d for infants 2,500-3,500 g, and 7 g/kg/d for infants > 3,500 g.
- - - - = Babson and Benda, J Pediatr 1976.

Lair and Kennedy Neonatal Growth Charts (continued)

Reprinted with permission. Lair CS, Kennedy KA. Monitoring postnatal growth in the neonatal intensive care unit. Nutr Clin Pract 12:124, 1997.

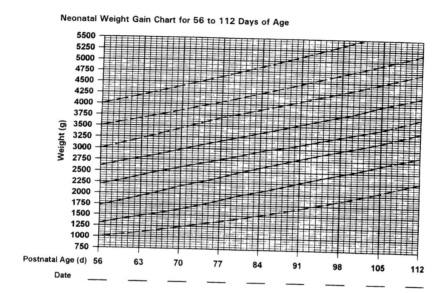

Neonatal Weight Gain Chart for 56 to 112 Days of Age

——— = Wright et al., Pediatrics 1993.
— — = Calculated for growth rate of 15 g/kg/d for infants < 2,500 g, 10 g/kg/d for infants 2,500-3,500 g, and 7 g/kg/d for infants > 3,500 g.

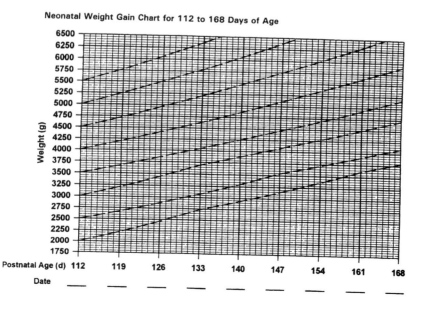

Neonatal Weight Gain Chart for 112 to 168 Days of Age

— — = Calculated for growth rate of 15 g/kg/d for infants < 2,500 g, 10 g/kg/d for infants 2,500-3,500 g, and 7 g/kg/d for infants > 3,500 g.

Lair and Kennedy Neonatal Growth Charts (continued)

Reprinted with permission. Lair CS, Kennedy KA. Monitoring postnatal growth in the neonatal intensive care unit. Nutr Clin Pract 12:124, 1997.

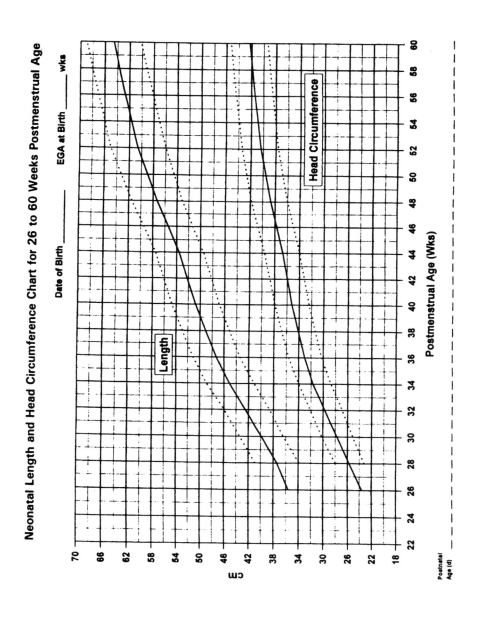

———— = 50th %ile Babson and Benda, J Pediatr 1976.
------- = 2SD Babson and Benda, J Pediatr 1976.

National Institute of Child Health and Human Development Neonatal Research Network Postnatal Growth Charts

Reprinted with permission. Ehrenkranz RA, Younes N, Lemons JA, et al. Longitundinal growth of hospitalized very low birth weight infants. Pediatr 104:280-289, 1999.

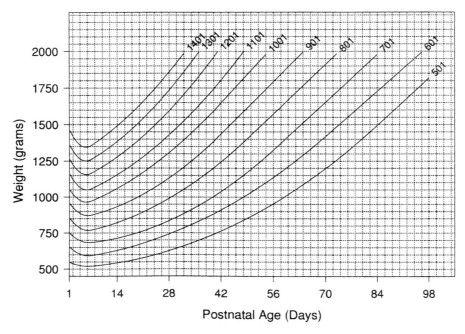

Average daily body weight versus postnatal age in days for infants stratified by 100-g birth weight intervals.

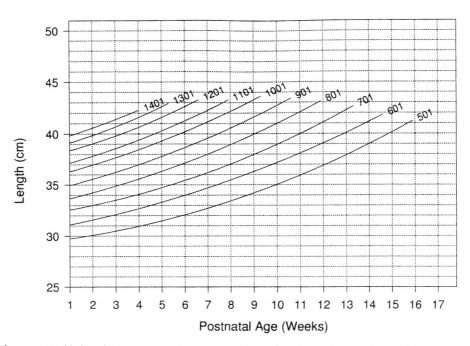

Average weekly length versus postnatal age in weeks for infants stratified by 100-g birth weight intervals.

National Institute of Child Health and Human Development Neonatal Research Network Postnatal Growth Charts (continued)

Reprinted with permission. Ehrenkranz RA, Younes N, Lemons JA, et al. Longitundinal growth of ospitalized very low birth weight infants. Pediatr 104:280-289, 1999.

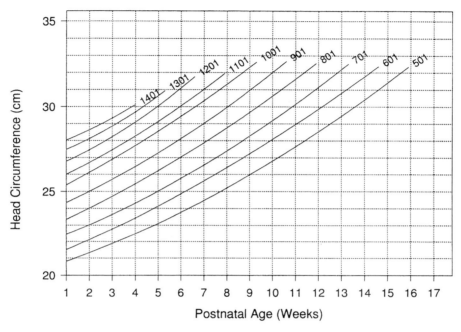

Average weekly head circumference versus postnatal age in weeks for infants stratified by 100-g birth weight intervals.

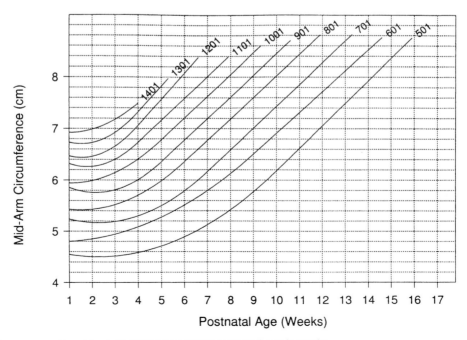

Average weekly midarm circumference versus postnatal age in weeks for infants stratified by 100-g birth weight intervals.

Lubchenco Intrauterine Growth Chart

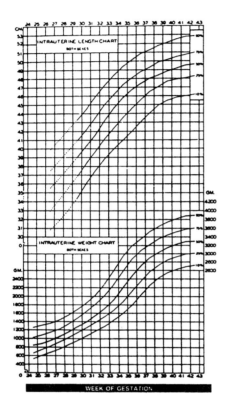
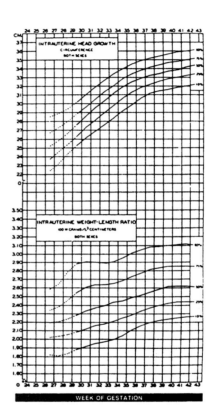

From Lubchenco LO, Hansman C, Boyd E. Intrauterine growth in length and head circumference as estimated from live births at gestational ages from 26 to 42 weeks. Pediatrics 37:403, 1966. ©American Academy of Pediatrics 1966.

Babson/Benda Intrauterine and Postnatal Growth Chart

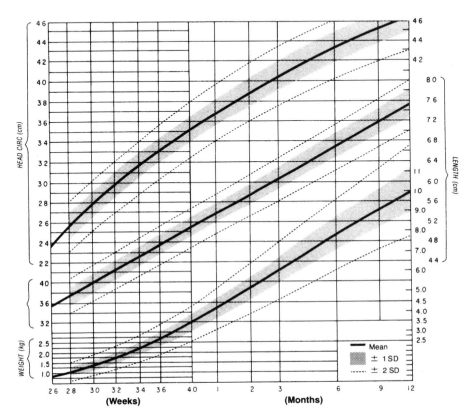

Babson SG, Benda GI. Growth graphs for the clinical assesment of infants of varying gestational age. J Pediatr 89:815, 1976. Reprinted with permission of C.V. Mosby Co. and Ross Laboratories.

Infant Health and Development Program Growth Percentiles: VLBW Premature Girls

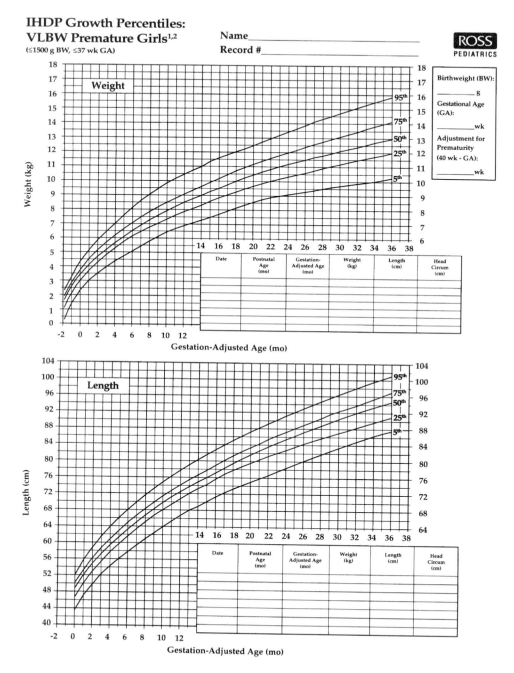

Used with permission of Ross Products Division, Abbott Laboratories, Inc., Columbus, OH 43216. From IHDP Growth Percentiles: VLBW Premature Girls, 1999 Ross Products Division, Abbott Laboratories, Inc.

Infant Health and Development Program Growth Percentiles: VLBW Premature Girls (continued)

IHDP Growth Percentiles: VLBW Premature Girls[1,2]

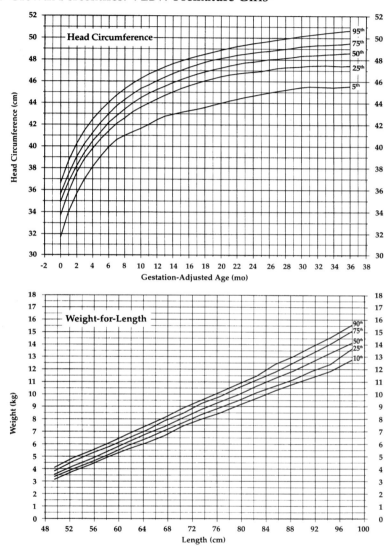

Infant Health and Development Program Growth Percentiles: VLBW Premature Boys

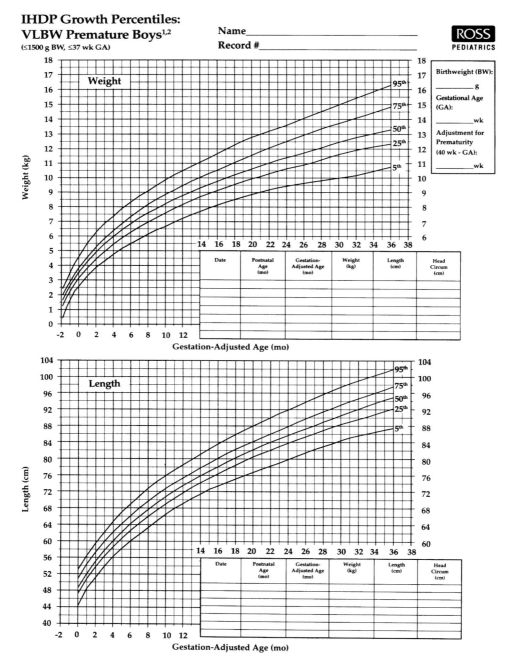

Used with permission of Ross Products Division, Abbott Laboratories, Inc., Columbus, OH 43216. From IHDP Growth Percentiles: VLBW Premature Boys, 1999 Ross Products Division, Abbott Laboratories, Inc.

Infant Health and Development Program Growth Percentiles: VLBW Premature Boys (continued)

IHDP Growth Percentiles: VLBW Premature Boys[1,2]

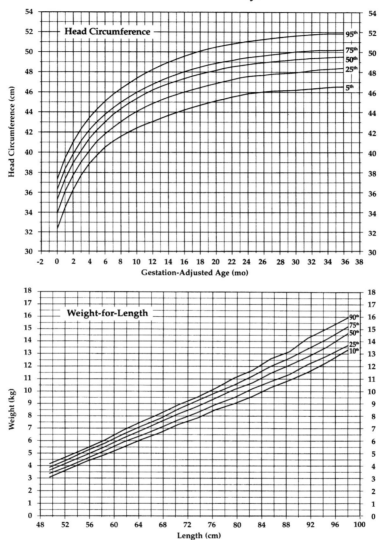

Infant Health and Development Program Growth Percentiles: LBW Premature Girls

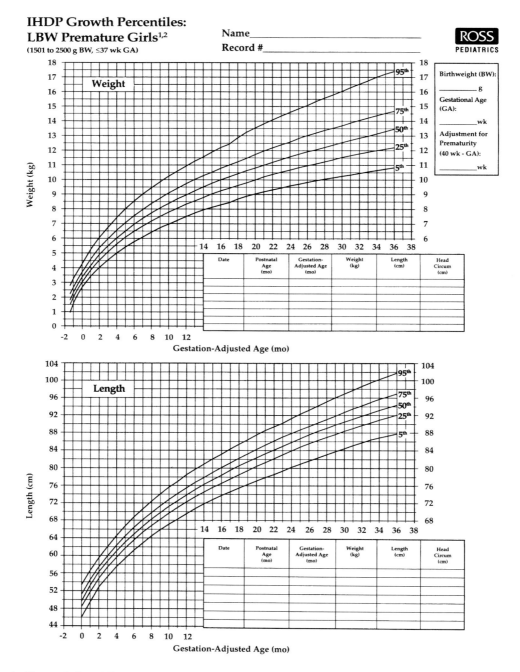

Used with permission of Ross Products Division, Abbott Laboratories, Inc., Columbus, OH 43216. From IHDP Growth Percentiles: LBW Premature Girls, 1999 Ross Products Division, Abbott Laboratories, Inc.

Infant Health and Development Program Growth Percentiles: LBW Premature Girls (continued)

IHDP Growth Percentiles: LBW Premature Girls[1,2]

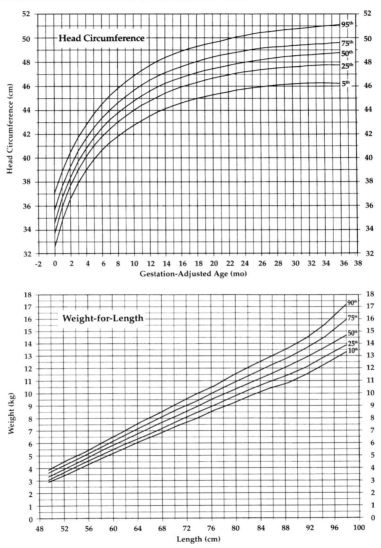

Infant Health and Development Program Growth Percentiles: LBW Premature Boys

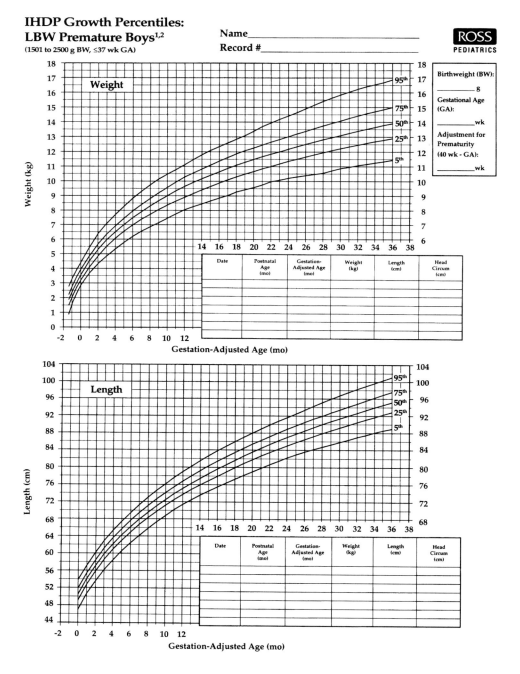

Used with permission of Ross Products Division, Abbott Laboratories, Inc., Columbus, OH 43216. From IHDP Growth Percentiles: LBW Premature Boys, 1999 Ross Products Division, Abbott Laboratories, Inc.

Infant Health and Development Program Growth Percentiles: LBW Premature Boys (continued)

IHDP Growth Percentiles: LBW Premature Boys[1,2]

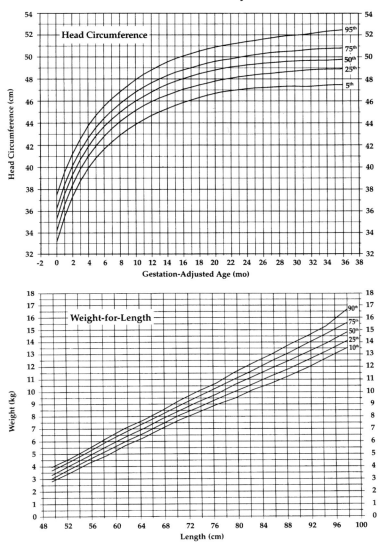

Appendix E
Drug/Nutrient Interactions

Gerri Keller, MEd, RD, LD

Drug	Use	Comments
Amphotericin[1,2]	Treatment of systemic fungal infections	Decreases renal blood flow and GFR. Injures tubular epithelium with resultant urinary loss of K, decreased reabsorption of Na, and renal tubular acidosis. Monitor BUN, creatinine, and electrolytes closely
Antibiotics[1,2]	Treatment of bacterial infection	May alter gut flora and subsequently ⇩ vitamin K synthesis. Nutrient effects vary with the antibiotic chosen
Chlorothiazide[1,2]	Diuretic Antihypertensive	Increases urinary loss of Na, K, Cl, Mg, P, Zn, riboflavin, and bicarbonate. May ⇧ serum glucose due to the inhibition of pancreatic insulin release. Renal excretion of Ca is ⇩; caution with Ca supplementation. Serum bilirubin may be ⇧ due to displacement from albumin. Minotir urine output, serum electrolytes, and serum glucose

Drug	Use	Comments
Cholestyramine[1]	Treatment of elevated serum cholesterol Bile acid binder	May ⇩ absorption of Ca, Fe, vitamins A, D, K, and B_{12}, folacin, MCT oil, and glucose. Iron stores may be ⇩ with chronic use. May ⇧ serum triglycerides, alkaline phosphatase, P, SGOT, and Cl. May ⇩ serum Ca, K, Na, B_{12}, and vitamins A, D, and K
Dexamethasone[1,2]	Anti-inflammatory	Increases urinary loss of K, Ca, Zn, vitamin C, and glucose. May cause hyperglycemia, hypokalemia, hypocalcemia, hypertension, and Na retention. Caution with K-depleting medications. Decreases absorption of Ca and P; may lead to osteoporosis. May inhibit growth. May lead to altered protein metabolism. May cause G.I. ulceration and/or hemorrhage
Digoxin[1,2]	Cardiotonic Antiarrhythmic	May cause feeding intolerance. Monitor serum electrolytes for imbalance especially if receiving diuretics and/or Amphotericin. Caution with Ca and vitamin D supplements, as hypercalcemia may potentiate drug effects and result in cardiac arrhythmias
Erythropoietin	Stimulates erythropoiesis	Protein intakes of 3.1 to 3.5 gm/kg/d may improve response as may increased intake of iron up to 6 mg/kg/d orally or 0.2-1.0 mg/kg/d parenterally, depending on estimated iron stores, iron losses, and estimated iron administered from blood transfusions.[6-8] Iron losses are approximately 0.34 mg/ml of blood loss (when hemoglobin concentration is 10 gm/dl). Packed red cells contain approximately 0.75 mg iron per ml[9]
Ferrous sulfate[1,2]	Iron supplement	In preterm infants, providing iron before adequate stores of vitamin E have been established may cause hemolysis. Vitamin C may ⇧ iron absorption. Monitor hemoglobin and reticulocytes. May cause nausea, black stools

Drug	Use	Comments
Fluoride[3]	Supplement	Do not add to infant formula, milk or milk products, or give with Ca supplements. Simultaneous ingestion may lead to formation of poorly absorbed Ca/fluoride compounds
Furosemide[1,2]	Diuretic	Increases urinary loss of Na, K, Cl, Mg, and Ca. Chronic therapy may cause renal calculi. Monitor urine output, serum electrolytes, and weight. May ⇧ serum glucose
Indomethacin[1,2,4]	Closure of ductus arteriosus	Monitor serum BUN, creatinine, and liver enzymes. May cause G.I. bleeding, which can lead to anemia. G.I. feedings may be withheld during treatment. Bolus doses of this drug are associated with necrotizing enterocolitis and G.I. perforation, possibly due to vasoconstriction of the splanchnic vascular bed and significantly reduced velocity of the superior mesenteric artery blood flow
Insulin[2]	To maintain euglycemia	May rapidly induce hypoglycemia in VLBW infants. Monitor serum glucose closely. Enhances synthesis of fat and cellular uptake of K. Inhibits lipolysis and conversion of protein to glucose
Phenobarbital[1,2]	Anticonvulsant	May ⇩ serum Ca, Mg, and vitamins B_6, B_{12}, C, and folacin. Vitamin B_6 supplements may ⇩ drug effects. May ⇧ turnover of vitamins D and K. May cause decreased bone density and osteomalacia
Phenytoin sodium[1,2]	Anticonvulsant	Ca supplements may ⇩ bioavailability of both drug and mineral; vitamin B_6 supplements may ⇩ effects of drug; folic acid supplements may alter drug response. Tube feedings ⇩ bioavailability of drug. May ⇧ turnover of vitamins D and K; may lead to rickets or osteomalacia. Hyperglycemia. May ⇧ serum alkaline phosphatase, GGT, and Cu. May ⇩ serum Ca, Mg, and vitamins B_6, B_{12}, D, and folacin. Bilirubin will displace drug from protein-binding sites, resulting in increased levels of free drug

Drug	Use	Comments
Potassium chloride[1,2]	K replacement	May cause malabsorption of Vitamin B_{12}. G.I. irritation is common, and symptoms may include diarrhea, vomiting, and bleeding. Use with caution in infants receiving potassium-sparing diuretics
Sodium bicarbonate[1-2]	Treatment of metabolic acidosis or bicarbonate deficiency	May cause hypocalcemia and hypernatremia. Concurrent intake with iron may ⇩ iron absorption; concurrent intake with K may ⇩ serum K
Spironolactone[1,2]	Diuretic	Increases urinary loss of Na, Cl, Mg, and Ca. Potassium-sparing effect. Monitor serum K closely, especially with supplementation
Theophylline[1,2]	Bronchodilator Reduces neonatal apnea	May cause G.I. irritation, feeding intolerance, and hyperglycemia. Avoid extremes of dietary protein and carbohydrate
Valproic acid[1,5]	Anticonvulsant	Decreases plasma Ca and P; may lead to bone changes. May ⇧ serum alkaline phosphatase, SGOT, SGPT, and bilirubin. May mimic carnitine deficiency
Vitamin supplements		Many multivitamin liquids and single vitamin or mineral solutions are hyperosmolar. Monitor tolerance closely. Symptoms such as diarrhea may occur

References

1. Adapted with permission of Ann Moore Allen. In: Allen AM, Powers DE. Food-medication interactions, 7th ed., Pottstown, Pa.: Food-Medication Interactions, 1991.
2. Adapted with permission of Thomas E. Young. In: Young TE, Mangum OB. Neofax: A manual of drugs used in neonatal care. 4th ed. Columbus, Ohio: Ross Laboratories, 1991.
3. Physicians' desk reference, 46th ed. Oradell, N.J.: Medical Economics Co., 1992.
4. Coombs RC, Morgan MEI, Durbin GM, Booth IW, McNeish AS. Gut blood flow velocities in the newborn: Effects of patent ductus arteriosus and parenteral indomethacin. Arch Dis Child 65:1067, 1990.
5. Cowlter DL. Carnitine, valporate, and toxicity. J Child Neurol 6:7-14, 1991.
6. Brown MS, Shapiro H. Effect of protein intake on erythropoiesis during erythropoietin treatment of anemia of prematurity. J Pediatr 128:512, 1996.
7. Carnielli VP, DaRiol R, Montini G. Iron supplementation enhances response to high doses of recombinant human erythropoietin in preterm infants. Arch Dis Child Fetal Neonatal Ed 79:F44, 1998.
8. American Academy of Pediatrics Committee on Nutrition. Pediatric nutrition handbook. 4th ed. Elk Grove Village, Il.: AAP, 1998; 62.
9. Meyer MP, Haworth C, Meyer JH, et al. A comparison of oral and intravenous iron supplementation in preterm infants receiving recombinant erythropoietin. J Pediatr 129:258-63, 1996.

Appendix F

Characteristics of Intravenous Fluids[1]

Pamela T. Price, PhD, RD, CNSD

| | | Cations | | Anions | | |
Type of Fluid	Na (mEq/L)	K (mEq/L)	Ca (mEq/L)	Cl (mEq/L)	HOC3* (mEq/L)	Osmolarity (mOsm/L)[†]
Dextrose in water solutions						
D_5W						252
$D_{10}W$						505
$D_{20}W$						1,010
$D_{50}W$						2,525
Dextrose in saline solutions						
D_5W & 0.2% NaCl	34			34		320
D_5W & 0.45 NaCl	77			77		406
D_5W & 0.9% NaCl	154			154		559
$D_{10}W$ & 0.9% NaCl	154			154		812
Saline solutions						
1/2 NS (0.45% NaCl)	77			77		154
NS (0.9% NaCl)	154			154		308
3% NaCl	513			513		1,026
Multiple electrolyte solutions						
Ringer's solution	147	4	5	155		309
Lactated Ringer's	130	4	3	109	28	273
D_5W in lactated Ringer's	130	4	3	109	28	524

* Or its equivalent in lactate acetate, or citrate
† Osmolarity of the blood is 285-295 mOsm/L

Discussion

Isotonic solutions are calculated on the basis of the molecular weight of the solute. The molecular weight of sodium chloride is 58. One mole (58 g) of NaCl in 1 L of water constitutes a 2-osmolar solution, because sodium chloride forms 2 ions and each ion contributes one osmolar unit. Fifty-eight milligrams of NaCl in 1 L of water is a 2-milliosmolar solution (2 mOsm/L). Body fluids are an approximately 300-milliosmolar solution (2 mOsm/L). Therefore, it would take 150 times the 58 mg of NaCl (300 divided by the 2 mOsm of NaCl) or 8,700 mg (150 x 58) NaCl/L to have a solution isotonic with body fluids. Therefore, 8,700 mg (150 x 58) NaCl/L would be isotonic with body fluids. Converting to grams, 8,700 mg/L = 8.7 g/L = 0.87 g/100 ml. For simplification, 0.9 g is generally used instead of 0.87. Thus, 0.9 g of NaCl/100 ml (0.9 g%) is normal, or isotonic, saline.[1]

The molecular weight of dextrose is 180. Since dextrose does not dissociate, 180 g of dextrose contributes one osmolar unit of solute. The amount of dextrose needed to form a solution that is isotonic with body fluid is the molecular weight of dextrose, 180, times the 300 mOsm in body fluids: 180 x 300 = 54,000 mg. Converting milligrams to grams, 54,000 mg/L = 54 g/L, or 5.4 g/100 ml. Thus, for purposes of simplification, a 5% solution of dextrose is isotonic.[1]

An easy way to *approximate* the osmolarity of an I.V. fluid is to consider that for each 1% dextrose there are 50 mOsm/L, for each 1% amino acids there are 100 mOsm/L, and for each 1% NaCl there are 340 mOsm/L. Therefore:

a) for $D_{10}W$ and 0.45% NaCl (1/2 NS) there would be

$D_{10}W$ = 10 x 50 =	500 mOsm / L
0.45% NaCL = 0.45 x 340 =	153 mOsm / L
Total	653 mOsm / L

b) for a PN solution with 12.5% dextrose and 17 g amino acids/L (or 1.7 g amino acids per 100 ml or 1.7% amino acids), there would be

$D_{12.5}W$ = 12.5 x 50 =	625 mOsm / L
1.7% AA = 1.7 x 100 =	170 mOsm / L
Total	795 mOsm / L

Electrolytes, vitamins, and minerals add 300-400 mOsm/L. Intravenous fat is isotonic at about 300 mOsm/L.[2]

References

1. Reed GM, Sheppard VF. Regulation of fluid and electrolyte balance: A programmed instruction in clinical physiology. 2d ed. Philadelphia: Saunders, 1977; 85-86.
2. Zeman FJ. Clinical nutrition and dietetics. 2nd ed. New York: MacMillan, 1991; 140.

Appendix G

Enteral Nutrient Needs:
Summary Table

Amy L. Sapsford, RD, CSP, LD

Table G.1 Enteral Nutrient Needs Preterm/Low-Birth-Weight Infants (per 100 kcal except as noted)

		Tsang, Lucas, Uauy, Zlotkin[1]	Tsang, Lucas, Uauy, Zlotkin[1]	AAP-CON[2]	CPS[3]	CPS[3]	ESPGAN-CON[4]
Reference Criteria:		<1,000 g	≥1,000 g	Stable, growing preterm infants	Stable, growing (stabilization to discharge)†	Postdischarge (1 yr following discharge)†	General guidelines for preterm infants
Water	ml	125-167	125-167	...	120-200/kg	120-160/kg	115-154
Energy	kcal	100	100	100	100	100	100
Protein	g	3.00-3.16	2.5-3.0	2.9-3.3	<1,000 g: 2.9-3.3; ≥1,000 g: 2.5-3.0	1.8	2.25-3.10
Carbohydrate	g						
Lactose	g	3.16-9.50	3.16-9.80	9-13	6.25-12.9	6.25-12.9	7-14
Oligomers	g	0-7.0	0-7.0	...	...	...	...
Fat	g	...	...	4.5-6.0	3.8-5.7	3.7-6.1	3.6-7.0
Linoleic	g	0.44-1.70	0.44-1.70	0.4+	0.44-0.56	0.44-0.56	0.5-1.4
Linolenic	g	0.11-0.44	0.11-0.44	...	0.11	0.11	>0.055
C18:2/C18:3		≥5	≥5	...	...	...	5-15
Vitamin A	IU	583-1,250	583-1,250	75-225	<1,000 g: 1,250; ≥1,000 g: 555-1,250	1,110	300-500‡
Lung Disease	IU			...	Cannot Recommend	Cannot Recommend	...
Vitamin D	IU	1,250-2,333; 125-333; Aim = 400 IU/d	1,250-2,333; 125-333; Aim = 400 IU/d	270	400/d; 800 IU/d in black or Asian descent or low plasma 25-OH vit D (10-20 ng/ml)	400/d	800-1,600/d
Vitamin E	IU	5-10	5-10	>1.1	0.4-0.8	0.4	0.6-10.0
Suppl to HM	IU	2.9	2.9	...	...	...	...
Vitamin K	µg	6.66-8.33	6.66-8.33	4	5.0-8.3	16.7	4-15
Ascorbate	mg	15-20	15-20	35	1,000 IM at birth	1,000 IM at birth	7-40
Thiamin	µg	150-200	150-200	>40	33.3-41.7	41.7	20-250
Riboflavin	µg	200-300	200-300	>60	300-383	417	60-600
Pyridoxine	µg	125-175	125-175	>35	15/g protein	15/g protein	35-250
Niacin	mg	3-4	3-4	>0.25	0.7	0.7	0.8-5.0
Pantothenate	mg	1.0-1.5	1.0-1.5	>0.3	0.7-1.1	0.7-1.1	>0.3
Biotin	µg	3-5	3-5	>1.5	1.3	1.3	>1.5
Folate	µg	21-42	21-42	33	50/d	25/d	>60

	Units	Tsang, Lucas Uauy, Zlotkin[1]	Tsang, Lucas Uauy, Zlotkin[1]	AAP-CON[2]	CPS[3]	CPS[3]	ESPGAN-CON[4]
Vitamin B_{12}	µg	0.25	0.25	>0.15	0.15/d	0.15/d	>0.15
Sodium	mg	38-58	38-58	48-67	48.0-76.7	38.3-57.5	23-53
Potassium	mg	65-100	65-100	66-98	81.4-114.0	81.4-114.0	90-152
Chloride	mg	59-89	59-89	…	74.0-118.3	59.2-88.8	57-89
Calcium	mg	100-192	100-192	175	133-200	252/d (breast-fed) 376/d (formula-fed)	70-140
Phosphorus	mg	50-117	50-117	91.5	64.6-98.0	105.4/d (breast-fed) 272.8/d (formula-fed)	50-87
Magnesium	mg	6.6-12.5	6.6-12.5	…	4-8	4-12	6-12
Iron	mg	1.67	1.67	1.7-2.5	<1,000 g: 2.5-3.3 ≥1,000 g: 1.7-2.5 Start 6-8 wks. after birth	<1,000 g: 2.5-3.3 ≥1,000 g: 1.7-2.5	1.5
Zinc	µg	833	833	>500	420-670	817	550-1,100
Copper	µg	100-125	100-125	90	60-100	60-100	90-120
Selenium	µg	1.08-2.50	1.08-2.50	…	2.6-4.0	2.6-4.0	…
Chromium	µg	0.083-0.420	0.083-0.420	…	0.042-0.083	0.042-0.083	…
Manganese	µg	6.3	6.3	>5	0.46-0.92	0.46-0.92	1.5-7.5
Molybdenum	µg	0.25	0.25	…	0.16-0.32	0.16-0.32	…
Iodine	µg	25-50	25-50	5	26.4-52.9	26.4-52.9	10-45
Taurine	mg	3.75-7.50	3.75-7.50	…	…	…	…
Carnitine	mg	~2.4	~2.4	…	…	…	>1.2
Inositol	mg	27.0-67.5	27.0-67.5	…	…	…	…
Choline	mg	12.0-23.4	12.0-23.4	…	…	…	…

References:

1. Tsang RC, Lucas A, Uauy R, Zlotkin S, eds. Concensus Recommendations. Nutritional Needs of the Preterm Infant: Scientific Basis and Practical Guidelines. Baltimore: Williams and Wilkins, 1993.
2. Committee on Nutrition, American Academy of Pediatrics (AAP-CON). Nutritional needs of preterm infants. In: Kleinman RE, ed. Pediatric Nutrition Handbook, 4th ed. Elk Grove Village, IL: AAP, 1998; p 56.
3. Nutrition Committee, Canadian Paediatric Society (CPS): Nutrient needs and feeding of premature infants. Can Med Assoc J 152(11): 1765, 1995
4. Committee on Nutrition of the Preterm Infant, European Society of Paediatric Gastroenterology and Nutrition (ESPGAN-CON). Nutrition and feeding of preterm infants. Acta Paediatr Scand 336 (suppl): 1, 1987.
† Data published per kg. Used 120 kcal/kg for conversion to 100 kcal.
‡ Supplement of 666-3300 IU/d to human milk may be required.

Table G.2 Enteral Nutrient Needs Infants 0-6 months (per day except as noted)

		Recommended Dietary Allowances (RDA)[1]	Dietary Reference Intakes (RDI)[2-5] Adequate Intake (AI)	Tolerable Upper Intake Level (UL)
Water	ml	1.5 ml/kcal	...[a]	...[a]
Energy	kcal	108 kcal/kg (± 20%)	...[a]	...[a]
Protein	g	13	...[a]	...[a]
Vitamin A	IU	1,250	...[a]	...[a]
Vitamin D	IU	300	200†	1,000
Vitamin E		4.5 IU	4 mg α Tocopherol	ND
Vitamin K	µg	5.0	...[a]	...[a]
Vitamin C	mg	30	40	ND
Thiamin	µg	300	200	ND
Riboflavin	µg	400	300	ND
Pyridoxine	µg	300	100	ND
Niacin	mg	5	2‡	ND
Pantothenate	mg	2[b]	1.7	ND
Biotin	µg	10[b]	5	ND
Choline	mg	...	125††	ND
Folate	µg	25	65‡‡	ND
Vitamin B$_{12}$	µg	0.3	0.4	ND
Sodium	mg	120[b]	...[a]	...[a]
Potassium	mg	500[b]	...[a]	...[a]
Chloride	mg	180[b]	...[a]	...[a]
Calcium	mg	400	210	ND
Phosphorus	mg	300	100	ND
Magnesium	mg	40	30	ND
Iron	mg	6	...[a]	...[a]
Zinc	µg	5,000	...[a]	...[a]
Copper	µg	400-600[b]	...[a]	...[a]
Selenium		10 µg	15 µg	45 mg
Chromium	µg	10-40[b]	...[a]	...[a]
Manganese	µg	300-600[b]	...[a]	...[a]
Molybdenum	µg	15-30[b]	...[a]	...[a]
Iodine	µg	40	...[a]	...[a]
Fluoride	mg	0.1-0.5[b]	0.01	0.7

Footnotes:

[a] RDI not yet issued

[b] Estimated safe and adequate intake; see reference for details

† In the absence of adequate exposure to sunlight.

‡ As preformed niacin, not niacin equivalents (NE).

‡‡ As dietary folate equivalent (DFE). 1 DFE = 1 µg food folate = 0.6 µg folic acid (from fortified food supplement) consumed with food = 0.5 µg synthetic (supplemental) folic acid taken on an empty stomach.

†† Although AIs have been set for choline, there are few data to assess whether a dietary supply of choline is needed at all stages of life cycle, and it may be that the choline requirement can be met by endogenous synthesis at some of these stages.

ND Not determinable due to lack of data of adverse effects in this age group and concerns with regard to lack of ability to handle excess amounts.

References:

1. National Research Council, Food and Nutrition Board. Recommended Dietary Allowances. 10th ed. Washington, D.C.: National Academy of Sciences, 1989.

2. Yates AA, Schlicker SA, Suitor CW. Dietary Reference Intakes: The new basis for recommendations for calcium and related nutrients, B vitamins and choline. JADA 98:699, 1998.

3. Institute of Medicine, Food and Nutrition Board. Dietary reference intakes for calcium, phosphorus, magnesium, vitamin D and fluoride. www.nap.edu

4. Institute of Medicine, Food and Nutrition Board. Dietary reference intakes for thiamin, riboflavin, niacin , vitamin B-6, folate, vitamin B12, pantothenic acid, biotin, and choline. www.nap.edu

5. Institute of Medicine, Food and Nutrition Board. Dietary reference intakes for Vitamin C, Vitamin E, selenium, and carotenoids. www.nap.edu

Appendix H

Potential Renal Solute Load and Osmolality

Amy L. Sapsford, RD, CSP, LD
and Sharon Groh-Wargo, MS, RD, LD

I. Potential Renal Solute Load

Potential renal solute load (PRSL) is expressed as mOsm/L or as mOsm/100 kcal. Upper limits of 277 mOsm/L and 30-35 mOsm/100 kcal have been proposed for infant formulas.[1-4] PRSL can be calculated using the following equation:

PRSL equation: PRSL (mOsm/L) =

$$\{\text{protein (g/L)} \div 0.175^{\#}\} + \{\text{Na (mEq/L)} + \text{K (mEq/L)} + \text{Cl (mEq/L)}\} + \{\text{P}_a{}^* \text{(mg/L)} \div 31\}$$

\# This factor assumes that all dietary N from protein is converted to urea. The protein part of the equation can also be calculated as mg N/L ÷ 28 mg N/mOsm.[1,3]

*P_a = Available phosphorus; assumed to be total phosphorus of human milk and milk-based formulas, and two-thirds of the phosphorus of soy-based formulas.[3]

Sample calculations of PRSL:

1. Mature, term human milk: composition per liter[5]

Energy (kcal)	699
Protein (g)	9.1
Sodium (mEq)	7.9
Potassium (mEq)	14.8
Chloride (mEq)	11.8
Phosphorus (mg)	147

$$\text{PRSL (mOsm/L)} = \{\text{protein (9.1 g/L)} \div 0.175\} + \{\text{Na (7.9 mEq/L)} + \text{K(14.8 mEq/L)} + \text{Cl (11.8 mEq/L)}\} + \{P_a(147 \text{ mg/L}) \div 31\}$$

$$\text{PRSL (mOsm/L)} = 52 + 34.5 + 4.74 = 91 \text{ mOsm/L}$$

$$\text{PRSL (mOsm/100 kcal)} = \frac{91 \text{ mOsm}}{699 \text{ kcal}} \cdot \frac{x}{100 \text{ kcal}} = 13 \text{ mOsm/100 kcal}$$

2. Formula for preterm infant Similac Special Care$_{24}$ (Ross): Composition per liter[5]

Energy (kcal)	806
Protein (g)	21.8
Sodium (mEq)	15.1
Potassium (mEq)	26.6
Chloride (mEq)	18.4
Phosphorus (mg)	806

$$\text{PRSL (mOsm/L)} = \{\text{protein (21.8g/L)} \div 0.175\} + \{\text{Na(15.1mEq/L)} + \text{K(26.6mEq/L)} + \text{Cl(18.4mEq/L)}\} + \{P_a(806 \text{mg/L}) \div 31\}$$

$$\text{PRSL (mOsm/L)} = 125 + 60 + 26 = 211 \text{ mOsm/L}$$

$$\text{PRSL (mOsm/100 kcal)} = \frac{211 \text{ mOsm}}{806 \text{ kcal}} \cdot \frac{x}{100 \text{ kcal}} = 26 \text{ mOsm/100kcal}$$

II. Estimated Actual Renal Solute Load and Urine Osmolality

An estimated urine osmolality can be calculated using the PRSL of the feeding (as shown), along with figures for estimated *actual* renal solute load and water available for urine (as follows):

Calculation of estimated actual renal solute load:

A. PRSL of Intake (mOsm/d) = {PRSL of formula (mOsm/L) x intake of formula (ml/d)} ÷ 1,000
B. Approximate renal solute load deposited into new tissue (mOsm/d)[1] = 0.9 mOsm/g weight gain x weight gain (g/d)
C. Estimated actual renal solute load (mOsm/d): A – B = C

Calculation of water available for urine (two methods):

Method 1: Full-term newborns and young infants
A. Intake of milk (ml/d)
B. Water content of milk (ml/d)*
C. Nonrenal water losses (stool + insensible plus water requirement for growth (normal environmental temperature) = 345 ml/d; nonrenal water losses (hot environmental temperature) = 620 ml/d
D. Water available for urine (ml/d): B – C = D

Method 2: Preterm infants
A. Intake of milk (ml/d)
B. Water content of milk (ml/d)*
C. Stool water losses = 10 ml/kg per day[2]
D. Insensible or evaporative water losses = 70 ml/kg per day[6]
E. Water for growth = 7% of (C + D)[1]
F. Water available for urine (ml/d): B – (C + D + E) = F

\# Water content of milk[1,5]
    Human milk = 950 g water/1,000 ml milk
    20 kcal/oz formula = 900-910 g water/1,000 ml formula
    24 kcal/oz formula = 870-890 g water/1,000 ml formula

Calculation of estimated urine osmolality:

Calculations for urine osmolality are based on volume of water available for urine (ml water/d), but values are expressed as mOsm/kg water, ignoring the slight error incurred in making the conversion.

A. Estimated urine osmolality (mOsm/kg water) =
$$\frac{\text{Estimated actual renal solute load (mOsm/d)}}{\text{Water available for urine (ml/d)}} \bullet 1000$$

B. Approximate possible urine osmolality, term: 700-900 mOsm/kg water[7,8]

Approximate possible urine osmolality, preterm: 200-600 mOsm/kg water[7,8]

(Note: Goal is to stay below or within these ranges)

Sample calculations of estimated actual renal solute load and urine osmolality:

1. Full-term breast-fed infant @ 1 mo of age
   - Weight: 4.0 kg
   - Average weight gain past 7 days: 30 g/d
   - Intake of human milk (estimated): 600 ml/d

Estimated actual renal solute load:

A. {91(mOsm/L) x 600 (ml/d) } ÷ 1000 = 54.6 mOsm/d
B. 0.9 mOsm/g weight gain x 30 g/d = 27 mOsm/d
C. 54.6 mOsm/d – 27 mOsm/d = 27.6 mOsm/d

Water available for urine:
A. 600 ml/d human milk
B. (600 ml/d x 950 g water/1,000 ml milk) ÷ 1,000 = 570 ml/d
C. 345 ml/d nonrenal water losses plus water for growth (normal environmental temperature)
D. 570 ml/d – 345 ml/d = 225 ml/d

Estimated urine osmolality:
A. $\dfrac{27.6 \text{ mOsm/d}}{225 \text{ ml/d}}$ • 1000 = 123 mOsm/kg water
B. This estimated urine osmolality is well below the approximate possible urine osmolality for term infants of 700-900 mOsm/kg water and, therefore, suggests no risk for dehydration.

2. Preterm formula-fed infant @ 1 mo of age
   - Weight: 1.2 kg
   - Average weight gain past 7 days: 20 g/d
   - Intake Similac Special Care$_{24}$ (Ross): 15 ml q 2° or 180 ml/d

Estimated actual renal solute load:
A. {211 (mOsm/L) x 180 (ml/d)} ÷ 1000 = 38 mOsm/d
B. 0.9 mOsm/g weight gain x 20 g/d = 18 mOsm/d
C. 38 mOsm/d – 18 mOsm/d = 20 mOsm/d

Water available for urine:
A. 180 ml/d Similac Special Care$_{24}$
B. (180 ml/d x 880 g water/1,000 ml formula) ÷ 1,000 = 158 ml/d
C. 10 ml/kg/d x 1.2 kg = 12 ml/d
D. 70 ml/kg/d x 1.2 kg = 84 ml/d
E. (12 + 84) x 7% = 6.7 ml/d
F. 158 – (12 + 84 + 6.7) = 55 ml/d

Estimated urine osmolality:

A. $\dfrac{20 \text{ mOsm/d}}{55 \text{ ml/d}} \bullet 1000 = 364 \text{ mOsm/kg water}$

B. This estimated urine osmolality is well within the approximate possible urine osmolality for preterm infants of 200-600 mOsm/kg water and, therefore, suggests no risk for dehydration.

III. Osmolality

The American Academy of Pediatrics recommends that formulas have concentrations of no greater than 450 mOsm/kg water.[9] Osmolality of medications and supplements commonly used in the intensive care nursery can alter the osmolality of infant feedings. The osmolality of mixtures of human milk, formulas, medication, and/or vitamin/mineral supplements can be estimated using the equation below along with the osmolality values for human milk and formulas listed in Appendix J and Appendix K, and the osmolality values for medications and supplements listed in Table H.1.

Equation for calculating final osmolality of a mixture of medications/supplements, and formula:[10]

$$O_M = \frac{O_D(V_D) + O_F(V_F)}{V_{D+F}}$$

Where

O_M is the osmolality of the mixture of medication/supplement and formula

O_D is the osmolality of the drug or medication/supplement

O_F is the osmolality of the formula

V_D is the volume of the medication/supplement in ml

V_F is the volume of the formula in ml

Sample calculation of final osmolality:

- Preterm infant 1.2 kg
- Similac Special Care$_{24}$ 15 ml q 2°
- Caffeine citrate solution 0.72 ml PO QD
- Vitamin ADC solution 0.5 ml PO QD

Table H.1. Osmolality of Selected Medications and Vitamin/Mineral Supplements[10]

Generic name	Brand name	Concentration	Manufacturer	mOsm/kg
Caffeine citrate solution	Generic	10mg/1ml	Armend/CHOP*	89
Calcium carbonate suspension[†]	Generic	500mg/5 ml Ca	Roxane	3140
Calcium glubionate syrup	Neo-Calglucon	1.8g/5 ml	Sandoz	2043
Cisapride suspension[†]	Propulsid	1 mg/1 ml	Janssen/CHOP*	4323
Dexamethasone solution[†]	Generic	1 mg/1 ml	Roxane	10,737
Ergocalciferol solution[†]	Calciferol	8000 U/1 ml	Schwarz Pharma	16,277
Ferrous sulfate drops[†]	Generic	25 mg/1 ml	Barre	4587
Furosemide solution[†]	Lasix	10 mg/1 ml	Hoechst	4037
Multivitamin solution[†]	Poly-vi-sol	NA	Mead-Johnson	11,173
Phenobarbital elixir[†]	Generic	4 mg/1 ml	Rugby	7417
Ranitidine syrup[†]	Zantac	15 mg/1 ml	G. Wellcome	2360
Theophylline solution	Generic	2 mg/1 ml	Roxane/CHOP*	28
Vitamins ADC solution[†]	Tri-vi-sol	NA	Mead-Johnson	7010
Vitamin E drops[†]	Aquasol E	50 mg/1 ml	Astra	4083

* Children's Hospital of Philadelphia (CHOP) formulation
† Measurements performed with medication/supplement diluted 10-fold

	Osmolality (mOsm/kg)	Volume of dose (ml)
Similac Special Care$_{24}$	280	15
Caffeine citrate solution	89	0.72
Tri-vi-sol	7,010	0.5

$$O_M = \frac{89\ (0.72) + 7010\ (0.5) + 280\ (15)}{0.72\ +\ 0.5\ +\ 15}$$

$$= \frac{64.1 + 3505 + 4200}{16.22}$$

$$= 479\ mOsm\ /\ kg$$

Comment: This final osmolality exceeds the recommended maximum of 450 mOsm/kg. Changing the Tri-vi-sol to BID results in a more physiological final osmolality.

References

1. Fomon SJ, Ziegler EE. Water and renal solute load. In: Fomon SJ, ed. Nutrition for normal infants. St Louis: Mosby, 1993.
2. Ziegler EE, Fomon SJ. Potential renal solute load of infant formulas. J Nutr 119:1785, 1989.
3. Fomon SJ, Ziegler EE. Renal solute load and *potential* renal solute load. J Pediatr 134:11, 1999.
4. LSRO Assessment of nutrient requirements for infant formulas. J Nutr 128:2059S, 1998.
5. Ross Pediatrics: Composition of feedings for infants and young children. Ross ready reference. (A7368), June 1999.
6. Fanaroff AA, Wald M, Gruber HS, et al. Insensible water loss in low birth weight infants. Pediatrics 50:236, 1972.
7. Hay WW. Nutritional needs of the extremely low-birth-weight infant. Semin Perinatol 15:482, 1991.
8. Bergmann KKE, Ziegler EE, Fomon SJ. Water and renal solute load. In: Fomon SF, ed. Infant nutrition. 2nd ed. Philadelphia: Saunders, 1974; 24.
9. American Academy of Pediatrics Committee on Nutrition. Commentary on breastfeeding and infant formula, including proposed standards for formulas. Pediatrics 57:278, 1976.
10. Jew RK, Owen D, Kaufman D, et al. Osmolality of commonly used medications and formulas in the neonatal intensive care unit. Nutr Clin Prac 12:158, 1997.

Appendix I

Preparing Formulas with Various Caloric Densities

Barbara Kuzma-O'Reilly, RD, LD, LPCC

The osmolality of a formula will increase by approximately the same percentage as the caloric increase. Attention should be paid to the increase in renal solute load and in osmolality when concentrating formulas beyond 24 kcal/oz. The caloric density of formulas prepared from powder may vary significantly due to different techniques used in measuring powder. For this reason, it is strongly recommended that liquid formula concentrates be used whenever possible to make formula of higher caloric density. Scoops provided in cans of infant formula powders and standard household measuring devices are recommended for preparing infant formulas.

Preparation of Fortified Human Milk Using Similac NeoSure or EnfaCare Powder

Desired concentration, kcal/oz	Powder (tsp.*)	Expressed human milk (oz)	Final volume (oz) (approximate)
24 (0.80 kcal/cc)	1/2	1.5	1.5
27 (0.90 kcal/cc)	1	1.5	2.0
30 (1.00 kcal/cc)	1 + 1/2	1.5	2.5

* Use level packed measuring teaspoon for EnfaCare and level unpacked measuring teaspoon for Similac NeoSure

Preparation of Selected* Infant Formulas Using Liquid Concentrate

Desired concentration, kcal/oz	Liquid concentrate (oz)	Water (oz)	Final volume (oz)
10 (0.34 kcal/cc)	13	39	52
15 (0.50 kcal/cc)	13	22	35
20 (0.67 kcal/cc)	13	13	26
24 (0.80 kcal/cc)	13	9	22
27 (0.90 kcal/cc)	13	6	19
30 (1.00 kcal/cc)	13	4	17

Concentrated liquid infant formula contains 40 kcal/oz (1.35 kcal/cc).
* Standard and soy formulas; Nutramigen and Lactofree

Small Volume Preparation of Selected* Infant Formulas Using Powder

Desired concentration, kcal/oz	Powder (scoops)	Water (oz) (approximate)	Final volume (oz)
10 (0.34 kcal/dd)	1	4.0	4.5
15 (0.50 kcal/cc)	2	5.5	6.0
20 (0.67 kcal/cc)	4	8.0	9.0
24 (0.80 kcal/cc)	3	4.5	5.5
27 (0.90 kcal/cc)	5	7.0	8.0
30 (1.00 kcal/cc)	6	7.5	9.0

Use *packed* scoop for Nutramigen, Pregestimil and Portagen
* Standard and soy formulas; Nutramigen, Pregestimil, Portagen, Similac PM 60/40, Lactofree, and Similac Lactose Free

Larger Volume Preparation of Selected* Infant Formulas Using 1 Cup Powder

Desired concentration, kcal/oz	Powder (cup[†])	Water (oz) (approximate)	Final volume (oz)
20 (0.67 kcal/cc)	1	29	32
24 (0.80 kcal/cc)	1	22	26
27 (0.90 kcal/cc)	1	20	24
30 (1.00 kcal/cc)	1	18	22

* See above
† One level measuring cup of powdered infant formula contains approximately 640 kcal. One cup of formula powder displaces approximately 3-4 oz. of water, so water volumes are approximate. Preparation of large volumes of formula should be done by adding water to the powder to equal desired final volume. Use packed household measures for Nutramigen and Portagen.
Adapted with permission from Cox JH, Nutrition manual for at-risk infants and children. Chicago: Precept Press, 1997.

Preparation of Neocate Small Volumes

Desired concentration, kcal/oz	Powder (scoops)	Water (oz) (approximate)	Final volume (oz)
10 (0.34 kcal/cc)	4	7.5	8
15 (0.50 kcal/cc)	3	3.5	4
20 (0.67 kcal/cc)	4	3.5	4
25 (0.84 kcal/cc)	5	3.0	4

Larger Volume Preparation of Neocate

Desired concentration, kcal/oz	Powder (g)	Water (oz) (approximate)	Final volume (oz)
20 (0.34 kcal/cc)	152	28.0	32
24 (0.50 kcal/cc)	183	27.5	32
27 (0.67 kcal/cc)	205	26.5	32
30 (1.00 kcal/cc)	228	26.0	32

Approximate Household Measures of Neocate Powder

1 cup = 115 g	1 scoop = 4.75 g
1/2 cup = 55 g	1 tbsp = 7 g
1/3 c. = 35 g	1 tsp = 2 g
1/4 c. = 30 g	1/2 tsp = 1 g

Preparation of Similac NeoSure to Varying Caloric Densities

Desired concentration, kcal/oz	Neosure Powder (scoops)	Water (oz) (approximate)	Final volume (oz)
10 (0.34 kcal/cc)	1	4.5	5.0
15 (0.50 kcal/cc)	2	6.0	6.5
20 (0.67 kcal/cc)	2	4.5	5.0
22 (0.73 kcal/cc)	2	4.0	4.5
24 (0.80 kcal/cc)	3	5.5	6.0
27 (0.90 kcal/cc)	3	4.5	5.5
30 (1.00 kcal/cc)	3	4.0	5.0

Large Volume Preparation of Similac NeoSure

Desired concentration, kcal/oz	NeoSure Powder (packed cups)	Water (oz) (approximate)	Final volume (oz)
20 (0.67 kcal/cc)	1	29	32.0
22 (0.73 kcal/cc)	1	26	29.0
24 (0.80 kcal/cc)	1	23	27.0
27 (0.90 kcal/cc)	1	20	24.0
30 (1.00 kcal/cc)	1	18	21.5

Preparation of EnfaCare to Varying Caloric Densities

Desired concentration, kcal/oz	EnfaCare powder (packed scoops)	Water (oz) (approximate)	Final volume (oz)
10 (0.34 kcal/cc)	1	4.5	5.0
15 (0.50 kcal/cc)	2	6.0	6.5
20 (0.67 kcal/cc)	3	6.5	7.0
22 (0.73 kcal/cc)	3	6.0	6.5
24 (0.80 kcal/cc)	3	5.5	6.0
27 (0.90 kcal/cc)	3	5.0	5.5
30 (1.00 kcal/cc)	3	4.5	5.0

Large Volume Preparation of EnfaCare Powder

Desired concentration, kcal/oz	EnfaCare powder (packed cups)	Water (oz) (approximate)	Final volume (oz)
20 (0.67 kcal/cc)	1 cup + 2 tbsp	29	32
22 (0.73 kcal/cc)	1 1/4 cups	29	32
24 (0.80 kcal/cc)	1 1/3 cups	29	32
27 (0.90 kcal/cc)	1 1/2 cups	28	32
30 (1.00 kcal/cc)	1 2/3 cups	28	32

Printed with permission of Mead Johnson Nutritionals, Evansville, Ind.

Simple Guidelines for Preparation of 24 kcal/oz Selected Infant Formulas:

Those with Liquid Concentrate = 40 kcal/oz and Powder = 44 kcal/scoop

Powder

Rule of thumb for concentrating formula to 24 kcal/oz is to identify a specific volume and then multiply that by **0.6** to get the number of scoops required. For example:

> Desired volume is 12 oz.
> 0.6 x 12 = 7 scoops of powder (rounded off)
> Start with 7 scoops and add water to the 12-ounce level to yield a final
> volume of 12 ounces

Amount of powder	Water	Final volume
3 scoops	fill to 5 oz. level after adding powder	5 oz.
12 scoops	fill to 20 oz. level after adding powder	20 oz.

Liquid Concentrate

Rule of thumb for concentrating formula to 24 kcal/oz is to identify a specific volume and then multiply that by 0.6 to get the number of oz. of liquid concentrate required. For example:

> Desired volume is 24 oz.
> 0.6 x 24 = 14 oz. of liquid concentrate (rounded off)
> Mix 14 oz. of liquid concentrate with 10 oz. of water to yield a final volume
> of 24 oz.

Amount of liquid concentrate	Water	Final volume
3 oz.	2 oz.	5 oz.
13 oz.	9 oz.	22 oz.

Reprinted with permission from the Pediatric Practice Group of the Oregon Dietetic Association, Guidelines for Selecting and Concentrating Infant Formula, 1997.

Dilution Equations for Concentrated and Powdered Formulas

From liquid concentrate

$$\frac{a \times b}{c} - a = y$$

Example: $\frac{13 \times 40}{24} - 13 = 9$

Where   a = amount of formula to be diluted (constant 13 oz.)
        b = caloric density of the formula (concentrate liquid is 40 kcal/oz)
        c = desired caloric density (24 kcal/oz)
        y = amount of added water needed (oz)

From powder

$$\frac{a}{b} - c = x$$

Example: $\frac{44}{24} - 0.2 = 1.6$

Where   a = calories per scoop (44 calories)
        b = desired concentration of formula (24 kcal/oz)
        c = water displacement per oz (constant 0.2/oz)
        x = amount of water to use per scoop (oz)

Reprinted with permission of Mead Johnson Nutritionals, Evansville, IN.

Scoop Information for Powdered Infant Formulas

Formula	Weight (g) (per scoop)	Calories (kcal) (per scoop)	Displacement volume (mL) (per scoop)
EnfaCare*	9.80	48.5	6.10
Enfamil with Iron*	8.50	44.0	6.10
Enfamil AR*	8.70	44.0	6.10
Isomil†	8.70	44.6	6.20
Neocate‡	4.75	20.0	3.75
Nutramigen*	9.08	44.0	6.30
Pregestimil*	8.80	44.0	6.10
Prosobee*	8.80	44.0	6.10
Similac NeoSure†	9.60	49.4	7.40
Similac with Iron†	8.50	44.4	6.20

* Mead Johnson Nutritionals, Evanston, Illinois
† Ross Products Division of Abbott Laboratories, Columbus, Ohio
‡ SHS (Scientific Hospital Supplies) Inc, Gaithersburg, Maryland

Appendix J

High-Calorie Formula Recipes and Nutrient Analyses

Barbara Kuzma-O'Reilly, RD, LD, LPCC

Nutrient analysis based on 100 ml		30 kcal/oz formulas			
		1	2	3	4
ENERGY	kcal	99	100	100	100
VOLUME	ml	100	100	100	100
PROTEIN	g	2.39	2.69	2.12	2.29
FAT	g	5.35	5.45	5.62	5.54
CARBOHYDRATE	g	10.6	10.5	10.6	10.5
Calcium	mg	148	164	141	124
Phosphorus	mg	75	92	78	65
Magnesium	mg	9.2	11.3	9.4	8.9
Iron	mg	1.01	1.80	1.41	0.67
Zinc	mg	1.14	1.43	1.17	0.98
Manganese	µg	8.7	11.6	9.4	7.8
Copper	µg	175	221	195	143
Iodine	µg	6	8	5	12
Sodium	mg	34	41	36	35
Potassium	mg	117	132	101	116
Chloride	mg	73	80	69	73
Vitamin A	IU	501	632	531	501
Vitamin D	IU	108	132	117	79
Vitamin E	IU	3.5	3.9	3.1	2.7
Vitamin K	µg	10.1	11.8	9.4	7.9
Thiamin (B-1)	µg	179	243	195	170
Riboflavin (B-2)	µg	401	517	484	299
Vitamin B-6	µg	161	217	195	135
Vitamin B-12	µg	0.41	0.52	0.43	0.35
Niacin	µg	3161	4329	3906	2560
Folic Acid	µg	26.6	34.4	28.9	23.8
Pantothenic acid	µg	1224	1658	1484	1049
Biotin	µg	21.9	30.8	28.9	17.1
Vitamin C	mg	23.9	32.2	28.9	20.5
Choline	mg	12.6	11.3	7.8	12.7
Inositol	mg	5.1	5.6	4.3	11.0
Linoleic Acid	mg	827	711	547	675
Carnitine	mg	3.9	5.9	4.6	4.0
Taurine	mg	6.6	6.9	5.2	6.6
Water	g	85	85	85	84
Osmolality	mOsm/kg	423	399	270	451
E:PUFA		1.7	3.1	2.5	2.9
RSL (term)	mOsm	16.1	18.1	14.6	15.7
PROTEIN % kcal	%	9.7	10.7	8.5	9.2
FAT % kcal	%	48.7	49.0	50.7	50.0
CARB % kcal	%	42.8	42.1	42.4	42.1

Nutrient analysis by NEONOVA Nutrition Optimizer Version 4.1. Ross Products Division, Abbott Laboratories, Columbus, Ohio. Fluid osmolality measured by St. Vincent Mercy Medical Center Pathology Department, Toledo, Ohio.

Nutrient analysis based on 100 ml		27 kcal/oz formulas		
		5	6	7
ENERGY	kcal	90	89	90
VOLUME	ml	100	100	100
PROTEIN	g	2.65	2.01	2.42
FAT	g	4.61	4.96	4.89
CARBOHYDRATE	g	9.9	9.4	9.5
Calcium	mg	142	114	178
Phosphorus	mg	72	59	90
Magnesium	mg	6.3	7.9	10.5
Iron	mg	1.61	0.46	0.48
Zinc	mg	1.31	0.85	1.32
Manganese	µg	6.0	6.7	10.6
Copper	µg	111	131	211
Iodine	µg	21	10	6
Sodium	mg	34	31	38
Potassium	mg	96	100	117
Chloride	mg	75	65	72
Vitamin A	IU	1039	453	588
Vitamin D	IU	222	72	126
Vitamin E	IU	5.4	2.3	3.6
Vitamin K	µg	7.5	6.7	10.7
Thiamin (B-1)	µg	181	145	222
Riboflavin (B-2)	µg	253	286	508
Vitamin B-6	µg	129	125	209
Vitamin B-12	µg	0.24	0.31	0.48
Niacin	µg	3374	2364	4174
Folic Acid	µg	30.3	21.2	32.0
Pantothenic acid	µg	1034	968	1592
Biotin	µg	4.1	16.2	30.3
Vitamin C	mg	17.4	19.0	30.9
Choline	mg	11.1	11.0	9.6
Inositol	mg	14.1	10.4	5.0
Linoleic Acid	mg	918	594	635
Carnitine	mg	0.6	3.3	5.3
Taurine	mg	0.7	5.8	6.1
Water	g	86	86	87
Osmolality	mOsm/kg	348	362	331
E:PUFA		5.3	2.4	2.8
RSL (term)	mOsm	16.7	13.8	16.4
PROTEIN % kcal	%	11.8	9.0	10.8
FAT % kcal	%	46.3	50.0	48.9
CARB % kcal	%	44.0	42.2	42.3

Nutrient analysis by NEONOVA Nutrition Optimizer Version 4.1. Ross Products, Division, Abbott Laboratories, Columbus, Ohio. Fluid osmolality measured by St. Vincent Mercy Medical Center Pathology Department, Toledo, Ohio.

Formula Recipes Provided by Members of the Ohio Neonatal Nutritionists

Formula 1   30 kcal/oz

Similac Concentrated Liquid 40 Cal Improved (Ross)	60 ml
Similac Natural Care (Ross)	120 ml

This recipe is designed to meet the nutrient needs of an infant who requires fluid restriction (100-130 ml/kg/day). Additional iron and vitamin D supplementation may be necessary with intakes < 350 ml/day. Fluid osmolality is 423 mOsm/kg, approaching the American Academy of Pediatrics (AAP) suggested maximum of 450 mOsm/kg

Formula 2   30 kcal/oz

Similac Special Care w/Iron 24 (Ross)	180 ml
Similac NeoSure Powder (Ross)	8 g

This recipe is designed to meet the nutrient needs of an infant who requires fluid restriction (100-130 ml/kg/day). Additional vitamin D supplementation may be required with intakes < 300 ml/day. Fluid osmolality is 399 mOsm/kg, approaching the AAP suggested maximum of 450 mOsm/kg

Formula 3   30 kcal/oz

Similac Special Care w/Iron 24 (Ross)	120 ml
Polycose Powder (Ross)	3 g
MCT Oil (Mead Johnson)	2 ml

This recipe may be used when fluid restriction is mild (150 ml/kg/day) and caloric needs are high. This formula should provide adequate vitamins for a growing premature or term infant at 150 ml/kg/day

Formula 4   30 kcal/oz

Human milk	60 ml
Similac Natural Care (Ross)	60 ml
Similac NeoSure Powder (Ross)	7 g

This recipe is designed to increase the caloric density of human milk for infants who require a fluid restriction (100-130 ml/kg/day). Additional iron and vitamin D supplementation may be necessary with intakes < 350 ml/day. Fluid osmolality is 451 mOsm/kg, which is at the AAP suggested maximum of 450 mOsm/kg

Formula 5	27 kcal/oz
Enfamil Premature Formula w/Iron 24 (Mead Johnson)	200 ml
Similac NeoSure Powder (Ross)	4 g

This recipe is designed to increase a base formula to 27 cal/oz for use with infants who require fluid restriction (130-150 mil/kg/day). Additional vitamin and mineral supplementation is not needed with intakes > 300 ml/day

Formula 6	27 kcal/oz
Human milk	60 ml
Similac Natural Care (Ross)	60 ml
Similac NeoSure Powder (Ross)	4 g

This recipe is designed to increase the caloric density of human milk to 27 cal/oz for use with infants who require fluid restriction (130-150 ml/kg/day). Additional supplementation of iron, vitamin D, and zinc may be necessary for intakes < 350 ml/day

Formula 7	27 kcal/oz
Similac Natural Care (Ross)	240 ml
Similac NeoSure Powder (Ross)	5 g

This recipe is designed for infants who require fluid restriction (130-150 ml/kg/day). Additional iron is necessary at all intake volumes, and vitamin D supplementation may be necessary with intakes < 350 ml/day

Appendix K

Composition of Human Milk and Selected Enteral Products

Amy L. Sapsford, RD, CSP, LD

Human Milk and Human Milk Fortifiers	Calories	Carbohydrate		Protein		Fat		Na	K	Ca	P	Mg	Fe	Osmolality	Indications
	kcal/dl	Source	g/dl	Source	g/dl	Source	g/dl	mEq/dl		mg/dl			U/fl	mOsm/kg H2O	
Human Milk (Mature)†	68	Lactose	7.2	human milk (whey predominant)	1.05	human milk	3.9	.78	1.34	28	14	3.5	.03/ na	290	Ideal for growing infant; preterm, LBW infant may need fortifier
Human Milk (Preterm)†	67	Lactose	6.6	human milk (whey predominant)	1.4	human milk	3.9	1.09	1.46	25	13	3.1	0.12/ na	290	Ideal for initial feedings; preterm, LBW infant may need fortifier
Enfamil Human Milk Fortifier 4 packets (w/o HM) (Mead Johnson) Powder	14	corn syrup solids and lactose	2.7	whey protein concentrate, sodium caseinate (60:40)	0.7	-	< 0.1	0.3	0.4	90	45	1	0	~varies	4 packets powder supplement to be added to 100 ml mother's milk beginning at 2-4 weeks of age in rapidly growing premature infants
Similac Human Milk Fortifier 4 packets (w/o HM) (Ross) Powder	14	corn syrup solids	1.8	whey protein concentrate, nonfat dry milk (60:40)	1.0	MCT oil	0.4	0.6	1.6	117	67	7.0	.035	varies	4 packets powder supplement to be added to 100 ml mother's milk as a nutritional supplement for low birth weight infants
Similac Natural Care Human Milk Fortifier (Ross) Ready to Feed	81	lactose and glucose polymers	8.5	nonfat milk and whey (60:40)	2.2	MCT, soy, and coconut oils	4.4	1.52	2.69	169	85	9.7	0.3/ na	280	For mixing with human milk or for feeding alternately with human milk to LBW infants
Human Milk (Preterm) mixed 1:1 with Similac Natural Care (Ross)	74	human milk, lactose and glucose polymers	7.6	human milk, nonfat milk and whey	1.8	human milk, MCT, soy, and coconut oils	4.2	1.3	2.07	98	49	6.6	0.21/ na	285	For preterm, LBW infant on human milk with increased needs for protein, vitamins, minerals and calories
Human Milk (Preterm) mixed with 4 packets Enfamil Human Milk Fortifier (Mead Johnson)	80	human milk lactose, corn syrup solids and lactose	9.3	human milk, whey protein concentrate, sodium caseinate	2.1	human milk	3.5	1.5	1.72	115	60	4.3	0.09	410 - 440	For preterm, LBW infant on human milk with increased needs for protein, vitamins, minerals and calories
Human Milk (Preterm) mixed with 4 packets Similac Human Milk Fortifier (Ross)	80	human milk lactose, corn syrup solids	8.2	human milk, whey protein concentrate, non fat dry milk	2.4	human milk, MCT oil	4.1	1.7	3.0	138	78	9.8	0.46	374-384	For balanced fortification of pretem, low birth weight infants receiving human milk

Infant Formulas for Preterm Infants in the Hospital	Calories	Carbohydrate		Protein		Fat		Na	K	Ca	P	Mg	Fe	Osmolality	Indications
	kcal/dl	g/dl	Source	g/dl	Source	g/dl	Source	mEq/dl		mg/dl			U/fl	mOsm/kg H₂0	
Enfamil Premature 20 (Mead Johnson) Ready to Feed	68	7.5	corn syrup solids, lactose	2.0	whey protein concentrate and nonfat milk (60:40)	3.5	MCT, soy and coconut oils	1.17	1.79	112	56	4.6	0.17/ 1.2	260	For rapidly growing LBW infants
Similac Special Care 20 (Ross) Ready to Feed	68	7.17	lactose and glucose polymers	1.83	nonfat milk and whey (60:40)	3.67	MCT, soy and coconut oils	1.26	2.23	122	68	8.1	0.25/ 1.2	235	For rapidly growing LBW infants
Enfamil Premature 24 (Mead Johnson) Ready to Feed	81	9.0	corn syrup solids, lactose	2.4	whey protein concentrate and nonfat milk (60:40)	4.1	MCT, soy and coconut oils	1.39	2.1	134	67	5.5	0.2/ 1.5	310	For rapidly growing LBW infants
Similac Special Care 24 (Ross) Ready to Feed	81	8.61	lactose and glucose polymers	2.2	nonfat milk and whey (60:40)	4.41	MCT, soy and coconut oils	1.52	2.69	146	81	10	0.3/ 1.5	280	For rapidly growing LBW infants

Enriched Preterm Discharge Formulas	Calories	Carbohydrate		Protein		Fat		Na	K	Ca	P	Mg	Fe	Osmolality	Indications
	kcal/dl	gm/dl	Source	gm/dl	Source	gm/dl	Source	mEq/dl		mg/dl			U/fl	mOsm/kg H₂0	
Similac NeoSure (Ross) Ready to Feed for Hospital Use; Powder	74	7.6	lactose and glucose polymers	1.9	whey protein concentrate and nonfat milk (50:50)	1.9	Soy, coconut, and MCT oils (25%) (Ready to Feed) Soy, Safflower, Coconut and MCT Oils (25%) (Powder)	1.04	2.7	77.7	45.9	6.7	na/ 1.3	290	Nutritionally complete infant formula designed to meet the special nutritional needs of premature infants after discharge from the hospital and throughout the first year of life. Mix 1 scoop powder to 2 oz water = 22 kcal/oz
EnfaCare (Mead Johnson) Ready to Feed for Hospital Use; Powder	74	8.2	Liquid: maltodextrin and lactose Powder: Corn syrup solids and lactose	1.9	whey protein concentrate and nonfat milk (60:40)	3.8	High oleic sunflower oil, soy oil, MCT oil and coconut oil	1.1	2.2	93	51	5.4	Na/ 1.3	Liquid: 230 Powder: 260	Enriched formula for conditions such as prematurity. Mix 1 scoop powder to 2 oz water = 22 kcal/oz

Cow Milk-based Infant Formula	Calories	Carbohydrate		Protein		Fat		Na	K	Ca	P	Mg	Fe	Osmolality	Indications
	kcal/dl	g/dl	Source	Source	g/dl	Source	g/dl	mEq/dl		mg/dl			µ/l	mOsm/kg H₂O	
Enfamil 20 (Mead Johnson) Ready To Feed, Concentrated Liquid, Powder	68	7.0	lactose	reduced minerals whey and nonfat milk (60:40)	1.52	palm olein, soy, coconut and high oleic sunflower oils	3.8	0.8	1.87	51.9	37.9	5.3	0.34/1.28	300	For feeding full-term infants or as a supplement to breast-feeding
Similac 20 (Ross) Ready To Feed, Concentrated Liquid, Powder	68	7.2	lactose	nonfat milk (70:30)	1.45	High oleic safflower oil, coconut oil, soy oil	3.65	0.8	1.81	49	38	4.1	0.15/1.2	300	For feeding full-term infants or as a supplement to breast-feeding; nucleotides have been added
Generic Store Brand Formerly SMA (Wyeth Nutritionals)	68	7.2	lactose	nonfat milk and whey protein concentrate (60:40)	1.5	Oleo, coconut, high oleic safflower and soy oils	3.6	0.65	1.43	42	28	4.5	na/1.2	300	For feeding full-term infants or as a supplement to breast-feeding
Enfamil Lactofree (Mead Johnson) Concentrated Liquid, Powder	68	7.0	corn syrup solids	milk protein isolate (18:82)	1.49	Palm olein, soy, coconut and high oleic sunflower oils	3.7	0.87	1.9	55	37	5.4	na/1.2	200	An alternative lactose-free formula containing casein predominant milk protein.
Similac PM 60/40 (Ross) Powder	68	6.9	lactose	whey and caseinate (60:40)	1.58	Soy and coconut oils* *plus corn oil in powder	3.76	0.7	1.48	38	19	4.1	0.15/na	280	For feeding infants who require lower mineral levels; 2:1 calcium:phosphorus ratio
Similac Lactose Free (Ross) Concentrated Liquid, Powder	68	7.23	corn syrup solids and sucrose	milk protein isolate	1.45	Soy and coconut oils	3.65	0.9	1.85	56.8	37.8	4.1	na/1.2	230	A complete infant feeding that is an alternative to standard milk-based and soy-based formulas when lactose is a concern and a milk-based formula is preferred
Carnation Good Start (Nestle) Powder	68	7.4	lactose, maltodextrin	whey hydrolysate	1.6	Palm olein, soy, coconut, and high oleic safflower oils	3.4	.7	1.67	43	24	4.46	na/1	265	For feeding full term infants or as a supplement to breast-feeding

Soy Infant Formulas	Calories	Carbohydrate		Protein		Fat		Na	K	Ca	P	Mg	Fe	Osmolality	Indications
	kcal/dl	Source	g/dl	Source	g/dl	Source	g/dl	mEq/dl			mg/dl		↓/↑	mOsm/kg H₂O	
Carnation Alsoy (Nestle) Powder	68	corn maltodextrin, sucrose	7.5	soy protein isolate, L-methionine	1.9	Palm olein, soy, coconut and high oleic safflower oil	3.4	1	2.2	71.4	41.5	7.5	1.2	296	For potential sensitivity to cow's milk protein, when lactose should be avoided, or for vegetarian families
Isomil (Ross) Ready to Feed, Concentrated Liquid, Powder	68	corn syrup and sucrose	6.96	soy protein isolate, L-methionine	1.66	High oleic safflower oil, coconut oil, soy oil	3.7	1.3	1.87	71	51	5.1	na/ 1.2	240	For potential sensitivity to cow's milk protein, when lactose should be avoided, or for vegetarian families Contains two carbohydrate sources using two absorptive pathways to enhance absorption
Isomil DF (Ross) Ready to Feed	68	corn syrup and sucrose	6.83	soy protein isolate, L-methionine	1.66	High oleic safflower oil, coconut oil, soy oil	3.69	1.3	1.87	71	5.1	51	na/ 1.2	240	Formulated as a short-term feeding for the dietary management of diarrhea in infants and toddlers, contains soy fiber, 0.12% or 6 g/L
Prosobee (Mead Johnson) Ready to Feed, Concentrated Liquid, Powder	68	corn syrup solids	6.8	soy protein isolate, L-methionine	2.0	Palm olein, soy, coconut, and high oleic sunflower oils	3.6	1.04	2.1	64	7.4	50	na/ 1.28	200	For potential sensitivity to cow's milk protein, when sucrose and lactose should be avoided, or for vegetarian families
Generic Store Brand Formerly Nursoy (Wyeth Nutritionals) Ready to Feed, Concentrated Liquid, Powder	68	sucrose (liquid) sucrose and corn syrup solids (powder)	6.9	soy protein isolate, L-methionine	1.8	Oleo, coconut, high oleic safflower, and soy oils	3.6	0.87	1.79	60	6.7	42	na/ 1.2	296	For potential sensitivity to cow's milk protein, when lactose should be avoided, or for vegetarian families

Elemental and Semi-Elemental Formulas for Infants and Children over 1 year	Calories	Carbohydrate		Protein		Fat		Na	K	Ca	P	Mg	Fe	Osmolality	Indications
	kcal/dl	g/dl	Source	g/dl	Source	g/dl	Source	mEq/dl		mg/dl			U/l	mOsm/kg H₂0	
Alimentum (Ross) Ready to Feed	68	6.89	sucrose and modified tapioca starch	1.86	Casein hydrolysate, L-cystine, L-tyrosine, L-tryptophan	3.75	MCT, safflower and soy oils 50% MCT oil	1.3	2.05	71	51	5.1	na/ 1.2	370	For sensitivity to cow milk protein or other intact proteins, pancreatic insufficiency, severe malabsorption disorder, short gut, gastrointestinal immaturity, cystic fibrosis, cholestasis, etc.
Nutramigen (Mead Johnson) Ready to Feed, Concentrated Liquid, Powder	68	7.4	corn syrup solids, modified cornstarch	1.89	Casein hydrolysate, L-cystine, L-tyrosine, L-tryptophan	3.4	Palm olein, soy, coconut and high oleic sunflower oils 0% MCT oil	1.39	1.89	64	43	7.4	na/ 1.22	320	For sensitivity to cow milk and other proteins, colic and diarrhea, due to milk protein allergy, lactose and sucrose intolerance, 11/94 new fat blend
Pregestimil (Mead Johnson) Ready to Feed for Hospital Use Powder	68	6.9	corn syrup solids, modified cornstarch and dextrose	1.9	Casein hydrolysate, L-cystine, L-tyrosine, L-tryptophan	3.8	MCT, corn, high-oleic sunflower and soy oils 55% MCT oil	1.17	1.89	64	43	7.4	na/ 1.28	320	For sensitivity to cow milk protein or other intact proteins, pancreatic insufficiency, severe malabsorption disorder, gastrointestinal immaturity, cystic fibrosis, cholestasis, etc.
Neocate (SHS) Powder	68	7.09	Corn syrup solids	2.23	L-amino acids	2.74	Hybrid safflower oil, coconut and soy oils 5% MCT oil	1	2.7	75	56	7.5	Na/ 1.2	342	Powder formula for infants with protein allergy. Prepare 1 scoop to 1 oz water. To prepare 32 oz, mix 1 1/3 unpacked level cup with 28 oz water.
Neocate One + (SHS) Ready to Feed, Powder	100	14.6	Corn syrup solids, sucrose	2.5	L-amino acids	3.5	Coconut oil, canola oil, hybrid safflower oil 35%MCToil	.87	2.4	62	62	9	0.77	610 powder 835 liquid	Unflavored powder and flavored liquid in brick packs; for children over 1 year of age with food protein intolerance
Nutren Junior (Nestle) Ready to Feed	100	12.7	maltodextrin, sucrose	3.0	isolated casein and whey proteins	4.2	soybean oil, 25% MCT oil, canola oil	2	3.4	100	80	20	1.4	350	Complete liquid nutrition supplement formulated to meet needs of children 1 – 10 yrs able to tolerate intact protein
Peptamen Jr. (Nestle) Ready to Feed	100	13.8	Maltodextrin, corn starch	3.0	Hydrolyzed whey protein	3.85	Coconut oil, sunflower oil 60% MCT oil	2	3.8	100	80	20	1.4	365	Vanilla flavored liquid formula for children with protein intolerance
Vivonex Pediatric (Novartis) Powder	80	13.0	Maltodextrin, modified starch	2.4	L-amino acids	2.4	MCT, soybean oil 68% MCT oil	1.7	3.1	97	80	20	1.0	360	Powder elemental formula for children over 1 year of age; for G.I. disorders such as short gut or intractable diarrhea.
EleCare (Ross) Powder	100	10.7	corn syrup solids	3.0	Free amino acids	4.76	high oleic safflower oil, MCT oil, Soy Oil	1.97	3.85	108	81	8.4	na/ 1.8	596 364 for 20 cal/oz.	Powder formula to meet nutrition needs of children 1 year of age and older who need an amino acid-based medical food or who cannot tolerate intact protein

Formulas for special needs	Calories	Carbohydrate		Protein		Fat		Na	K	Ca	P	Mg	Fe	Osmolality	Indications
	kcal/dl	Source	g/dl	Source	g/dl	Source	g/dl	mEq/dl		mg/dl			↓/fl	mOsm/kg H₂O	
Portagen (Mead Johnson) Powder	68	corn syrup solids, sucrose	7.8	sodium caseinate	2.4	MCT, corn oil	3.3	1.61	2.2	64	48	13.6	na/ 1.28	230	When long-chain triglycerides are poorly digested, absorbed, utilized; lactose intolerance. 85% of calories from fat derived from MCT
RCF (1:1 dilution with water without added carbohydrate) (Ross) Concentrated Liquid	41	type and amount selected to meet needs	0	soy protein isolate, L-methionine	2.0	soy and coconut oils	3.6	1.3	1.87	70	50	5.0	.15/ na	74* *varies	Carbohydrate free concentrated liquid; carbohydrate (CHO) and water must be added before feeding. 52 g CHO + 12 fl oz water + 13 fl oz Concentrate = 20 kcal/fl oz.
Mono- and Disaccharide-Free Diet Powder (Product 3232A) (Mead Johnson) Powder	43 without added CHO	type and amount selected to meet needs	0* *2.31 gm starch	casein hydrolysate	1.9	MCT, corn oils	2.85	1.26	1.9	63	42	7.4	na/ 1.27	250* *varies	Mono- and disaccharide-free diet powder, contains 37% modified tapioca starch; carbohydrate (CHO) must be added before feeding 59 g CHO + 81 g powder + water to = 1 qt = 20 kcal/fl oz
Enfamil AR (Added Rice) (Mead Johnson) Ready to Feed	68	lactose, rice starch, maltodextrin	7.5	nonfat milk 20:80	1.7	palm olein, soy, coconut, and high oleic sunflower	3.5	1.2	2.1	53	36	5.4	1.2	230	Viscosity increases to levels similar to formula with added rice cereal when in acid environment; Specifically contraindicated in preterm infants due to reports of bezoar formation
ProViMin (Ross) Powder	68	must be added	7.0	casein, L-amino acids	2.2	must be added	3.6	1.6	2.5	77	58	12	1.3	200	To prepare 1 L of formula, add 30 gm ProViMin, 69 g CHO, and 35 g fat. Add water to make 1 L

Formula for older infants/children	Calories kcal/dl	Carbohydrate G/dl	Carbohydrate Source	Protein g/dl	Protein Source	Fat g/dl	Fat Source	Na mEq/dl	K mEq/dl	Ca mg/dl	P mg/dl	Mg mg/dl	Fe U/fl	Osmolality mOsm/kg H₂O	Indications
Carnation Follow-Up Formula (Nestle) Powder	68	8.8	corn syrup and lactose	1.8	Cow milk casein predominant	2.8	palm olein, soy, coconut, and high oleic safflower oils	1.13	2.3	90	60	5.6	na/ 1.3	326	For babies on solid foods 6 months to 1 year of age
PediaSure (Ross) Ready to Feed	100	11	corn syrup solids and sucrose	3.0	Low lactose whey protein and sodium caseinate	5.0	high oleic safflower and soy oils, and 20% medium chain triglycerides	1.65	3.35	97	80	20	na/ 1.4	310	Vanilla, strawberry, chocolate or banana flavored; nutritionally complete, balanced, isotonic formula designed for tube or oral feeding of children 1 to 10 years of age; available in 8 oz cans
PediaSure With Fiber (Ross) Ready to Feed	100	11	corn syrup solids and sucrose	3.0	Low lactose whey protein and sodium caseinate	5.0	high oleic safflower and soy oils, and 20% medium chain triglycerides	1.65	3.35	97	80	20	na/ 1.4	310	Contains soy fiber that provides 0.5 g/dl total dietary fiber; vanilla flavored, nutritionally complete, balanced, isotonic formula designed for tube or oral feeding of children 1 to 10 years of age; available in 8 oz cans
Kindercal (Mead Johnson) Ready to Feed	100	13.5	maltodextrin and sugar	3.4	Calcium caseinate, sodium caseinate	4.4	canola oil, 20% medium chain triglycerides, corn oil, and high oleic sunflower oil	1.6	3.36	85	85	21	na/ 1.06	isotonic	Contains soy fiber that provides 0.63 g/dl dietary fiber, isotonic formulation with 20% MCT oil. 100% of NAS-NRC in <950 ml for 1 - 10 year old children, available in 8 oz cans
Carnation Instant Breakfast mixed with 2% milk (Nestle) Powder	93	14.4	Maltodextrin, sugar, lactose	4.4	Nonfat dry milk, cow milk	1.8	Butterfat	3.9	6.3	185	111	37	na/ 3.3	661-747	Milk based oral supplement not for tube feeding; for infants >12 months
Cow milk and Goat milk															
Whole Milk	63	4.85	lactose	3.39	Cow milk casein predominant	3.44	Butterfat	2.2	4.0	123	96	13.4	0.05	285	For feeding infants >12 months old
2% Milk	52	4.95	lactose	3.43	Cow milk casein predominant	1.98	Butterfat	2.2	4.0	126	98	14.4	0.05	na	Acceptable for feeding children >2 years old
Skim Milk	36	4.95	lactose	3.52	Cow milk casein predominant	0.19	Butterfat	2.3	4.38	127	104	11.3	0.04	na	Not recommended for infants or young children
Goat's Milk	71	4.6	lactose	3.7	Goat's milk	4.3	Butterfat	2.2	5.4	138	114	-	0.05	na	Multivitamin with iron and folic acid supplementation may be indicated

Modular Supplements Protein	Calories	Calcium	Phos	Protein		Indications
	Kcal	mg	mg	Source	g	
Casec Powder (Mead Johnson)	3.7/g 17/Tbsp.	66 mg/Tbsp	38 mg/Tbsp	Soluble calcium caseinate from skim milk	8.8 g/10 g powder 1 Tbsp. = 4.7 g = 17 kcal	Provides extra protein for children and adults unable to meet protein needs in a normal diet; powder mixes easily with formula, food or beverages.
ProMod Powder (Ross)	4.2/g 28/scoop (6.6 g) 1 Tbsp. = 4 g = 16.8 kcal	44 mg/scoop	33 mg/scoop	whey protein concentrate	5 g/6.6 g powder (1 scoop)	Provides extra protein for children and adults unable to meet protein needs in a normal diet; powder mixes easily with formula, food or beverages.

Modular Supplements Carbohydrate	Calories	Carbohydrate		Indications
	kcal	Source	g	
Karo Syrup (Many brands available)	3.9 kcal/ml 1 Tbsp. = 15 ml = 20 g = 58 kcal	polysaccharides, glucose, maltose, fructose	1 g/ml	Hyperosmolar, may cause diarrhea, sweet taste, contains sodium approximately 1 mEq/Tbsp light syrup and 1.7 mEq/Tbsp dark syrup
Moducal Powder (Mead Johnson)	30/Tbsp. 1 Tbsp = 8 g	glucose polymers	95/100 g powder	For additional calories solely from carbohydrate, minimal sweetness, low in electrolytes; best form for home use as liquid must be refrigerated and discarded 24 hours after opening
Polycose Liquid (Ross)	2/ml 60/1 fl oz	glucose polymers	50 g/100 ml	For additional calories solely from carbohydrate, minimal sweetness, low in electrolytes; unused portion of 4 fl oz bottle must be refrigerated and discarded after 24 hours
Polycose Powder (Ross)	3.8/g 8/tsp = 2 g 23/Tbsp = 6 g	glucose polymers	94 g/100 g powder	For additional calories solely from carbohydrate, minimal sweetness, low in electrolytes; best form for home use as liquid must be refrigerated and discarded 24 hours after opening

Modular Supplements Fat	Calories	Fat		Indications
	kcal	Source	g	
Corn Oil or Safflower Oil (Many brands available)	9/g, 8.3/ml	corn or safflower oil	1 Tbsp. = 15 ml = 14 g	Readily available source of long chain fats for patients who require additional calories, source of essential fatty acids and fat soluble vitamins
Microlipid (Mead Johnson)	4.5/ml	safflower oil	0.5 g/ml	Emulsified fat source providing essential fatty acids and fat-soluble vitamins; stays in solution without separating
MCT Oil (Mead Johnson)	8.3/g, 7.6/ml	fractionated coconut oil	1 Tbsp. = 15 ml = 14 g	Increases calories in foods for patients who cannot easily digest long chain fats, provides no essential fatty acids, packaged in 1 quart bottle

Oral Electrolyte Solutions	Calories	Carbohydrate		Na	K	Cl	Osmolality	Indications
	kcal/dl	g/dl	Source		mEq/dl		mOsm/kg H20	
Pedialyte (Ross)	10	2.5	Dextrose, citrate	4.5	2.0	3.5	250	To replenish fluids and electrolytes lost in diarrhea and vomiting
Rehydralyte (Ross)	10	2.5	dextrose, citrate	7.5	2.0	6.5	305	To replace water and electrolytes lost during moderate to severe diarrhea
Infalyte (Mead Johnson)	12.6	3.24	rice syrup solids, citrate	5.0	2.5	4.5	200	To replenish fluids and electrolytes lost in diarrhea and vomiting
EqualYTE (Ross)	10	3.0	dextrose, fructooligo-saccharides	7.8	2.5	6.1	290	Enteral rehydration solution; Sodium equal to half-normal saline

†Ross Products Division: Neonova Nutrition Optimizer, Version 4.5, 1999. Compiled from "Composition of Mature Preterm Human Milk Based on Values Obtained in the Literature", Ross Medical Department.

Manufacturers

Mead Johnson Nutritionals, U.S.
2400 West Lloyd Expressway
Evansville, IN 47721-0001
812-429-5000
812-429-6199
www.meadjohnson.com

Nestle Clinical Nutrition
Three Parkway North
Suite 500
PO Box 760
Deerfield, IL 60015-0760
1-800-422-2752
1-800-633-2330 ext. 4887
(no website)

Novartis Nutrition Corporation
PO Box 370
Minneapolis, MN 55440-0370
1-800-999-9978
Pharmaceuticals: 1-800-526-0175
www.novartis.com

Ross Product Division, Abbott Laboratories
625 Cleveland Avenue
Columbus, OH 43215
614-227-3333
1-800-515-7677
www.welcomeaddition.com

SHS North America
PO Box 117
Gaithersburg, MD 20884-0117
1-800-NEOCATE
www.shsna.com

Wyeth Nutritionals, Inc.
PO Box 7447
Philadelphia, PA 19101-7447
1-800-272-5095
www.parentschoiceformula.com
www.babymil.com

Appendix L

Selected Vitamin and Mineral Supplements

Amy L. Sapsford, RD, CSP, LD

Product (Manufacturer)	Amount	Vitamin A (IU)	Vitamin D (IU)	Vitamin E (IU)	Vitamin K (mg)	Vitamin C (mg)	Thiamin (mg)	Riboflavin (mg)	Niacin (mg)	Vitamin B6 (mg)	Vitamin B12 (mcg)	Iron (mg)	Fluoride (mg)
ADC DROPS													
Tri-Vi-Sol* (Mead Johnson)	1.0 ml	1,500	400			35							
Vi-Daylin ADC Drops* (Ross)	1.0 ml	1,500	400			35							
ADC WITH FLUORIDE DROPS													
Tri-Vi-Flor 0.25 mg Drops† (Mead Johnson)	1.0 ml	1,500	400			35							0.25
Tri-Vi-Flor 0.5 mg Drops† (Mead Johnson)	1.0 ml	1,500	400			35							0.5
Vi-Daylin/F ADC Drops† (Ross)	1.0 ml	1,500	400			35							0.25
ADC WITH IRON DROPS													
Tri-Vi-Sol with Iron Drops* (Mead Johnson)	1.0 ml	1,500	400			35						10	
Vi-Daylin ADC with Iron Drops* (Ross)	1.0 ml	1,500	400			35						10	
ADC WITH FLUORIDE AND IRON DROPS													
Tri-Vi-Flor 0.25 mg with Iron Drops† (Mead Johnson)	1.0 ml	1,500	400			35						10	0.25
Tri-Vi-Flor 0.5 mg with Iron Drops† (Mead Johnson)	1.0 ml	1,500	400			35						10	0.5
Vi-Daylin/F ADC Drops with Iron† (Ross)	1.0 ml	1,500	400			35						10	0.25
MULTIVITAMIN DROPS													
Poly-Vi-Sol Drops* (Mead Johnson)	1.0 ml	1,500	400	5		35	0.5	0.6	8	0.4	2		
Vi-Daylin Drops* (Ross)	1.0 ml	1,500	400	5		35	0.5	0.6	8	0.4	1.5		
MULTIVITAMIN WITH FLUORIDE DROPS													
Poly-Vi-Flor 0.25 mg Drops† (Mead Johnson)	1.0 ml	1,500	400	5		35	0.5	0.6	8	0.4	2		0.25
Poly-Vi-Flor 0.5 mg Drops† (Mead Johnson)	1.0 ml	1,500	400	5		35	0.5	0.6	8	0.4	2		0.5
Vi-Daylin/F Drops† (Ross)	1.0 ml	1,500	400	5		35	0.5	0.6	8	0.4	2		0.25
MULTIVITAMIN WITH IRON DROPS													
Poly-Vi-Sol With Iron Drops* (Mead Johnson)	1.0 ml	1,500	400	5		35	0.5	0.6	8	0.4	2	10	
Vi-Daylin with Iron Drops* (Ross)	1.0 ml	1,500	400	5		35	0.5	0.6	8	0.4	2	10	
MULTIVITAMIN WITH FLUORIDE AND IRON DROPS													
Poly-Vi-Flor 0.25 mg with Iron Drops† (Mead Johnson)	1.0 ml	1,500	400	5		35	0.5	0.6	8	0.4	2	10	0.25
Poly-Vi-Flor 0.5 mg with Iron Drops† (Mead Johnson)	1.0 ml	1,500	400	5		35	0.5	0.6	8	0.4	2	10	0.5
Vi-Daylin/F with Iron Drops† (Ross)	1.0 ml	1,500	400	5		35	0.5	0.6	8	0.4	2	10	0.25
FAT SOLUBLE MULTIVITAMIN													
ADEKs Pediatric Drops* (ScandiPharm)	1 ml	1,500	400	40	0.1	45	0.5	0.6	6	0.6	4	0	0

** Also contains 15 mcg biotin, 3 mg pantothenic acid, 5 mg zinc and 1 mg beta carotene

Product (Manufacturer)	Amount	Vitamin D IU	Vitamin E IU	Vitamin C mg	Iron mg	Fluoride mg	Calcium mg	Phosphorus mg	Sodium mEq	Potassium mEq	Chloride mEq	Bicarbonate mEq
SINGLE NUTRIENT SUPPLEMENTS												
Drisdol Drops† (Sanofi Winthrop) Ergocalciferol (D₂)	1.0 ml	8000										
	1 drop	200										
Aquasol E Drops* (Astra)	1.0 ml		50									
Ce-Vi-Sol* (Mead Johnson)	0.6 ml			35								
Fer-in Sol Drops* (Mead Johnson)	0.6 ml				15							
Fer In Sol Syrup* (Mead Johnson)	5.0 ml				18							
Pediaflor Drops†(Ross)	1.0 ml					0.5						
Luride Drops† (Colgate)	1 drop					0.125						
Neocalglucon* (Novartis) Calcium glubionate 6.5%	5 ml						115					
DiCalD Tablets*(Abbott)	1 tab	133					117	90				
Sodium Chloride† (Injection)	1 ml								2.5		2.5	
Potassium Chloride† (Injection)	1 ml									2	2	
BiCitra† (Baker Norton)	1 ml								1			1
Polycitra† (Baker Norton)	1 ml								1	1		2

* Over the counter
† Prescription required
Reference: Nutritional Products. In: Kastrup, EK, ed. Facts and Comparisons. St. Louis: Wolters Kluwer Co. 1999; p. 1 – 233 and selected product information.

Manufacturers

Abbott Hospital Products
Abbott Laboratories
1 Abbott Park Road
Abbott Park, IL 60064-3500
1-800-633-9110
www.abbott.com

Astra Pharmaceutical Products, Inc.
50 Otis
Wesyborough, MA 01581
508-366-1100
www.astra.com

Baker Norton/IVAX
4400 Biscayne Blvd.
Miami, FL 33137
1-800-347-4774
www.ivax.com

Colgate Oral Pharmaceuticals
1 Colgate Way
Canton, MA 02021
781-821-2880
www.colgate.com

Mead Johnson Nutritionals, U.S.
2400 West Lloyd Expressway
Evansville, IN 47721-0001
814-429-5000
812-429-6199
www.meadjohnson.com

Novartis Pharmaceutical Division
59 T. 10
East Hanover, NJ 07936
1-800-526-0175
www.pharma.us.novartis.com

Ross Products Division, Abbott Laboratories
625 Cleveland Avenue
Columbus, OH 43215
614-227-3333
1-800-515-7677
www.welcomeaddition.com

Sanofi Winthrop Pharmaceuticals
90 Park Avenue
New York, NY 10016
212-551-4000
1-800-446-6267
www.sanofi-synthelabo.fr

ScandiPharm
22 Inverness Parkway
Birmingham, AL 35242
1-800-950-8085
www.scandipharm.com

Appendix M
Breast-Feeding Resources

Joy G. Kubit, BSN, RN, IBCLC

Pump rental companies

Medela, Inc.
P.O. Box 660
4610 Prime Parkway
McHenry, IL 60050
(800) 435-8316
FAX: (800) 995-7867
www.Medela.com

Hollister, Inc. (Ameda-Egnell)
2000 Hollister Drive
Libertyville, IL 60048-3781
(800) 323-4060
(847) 680-1017
www.Hollister.com

Written information

Gotsch G. Breastfeeding your premature baby. Schaumburg, IL: LaLeche League International, 1999.

Harrison H. The premature baby book. New York: St. Martin's Press, 1983.

O'Leary M. You can breastfeed your preterm infant. Health Sciences Center for Educational Resources, SB-56, University of Washington, Seattle, WA 98195 (video and pamphlets), 1989, (206) 545-1186.

Ludington-Hoe. Kangaroo care: The best you can do to help your preterm infant. New York: Battan, 1993.

Danner S, Cerutti E. Pamphlets (1990):
     Nursing your premature baby
     Nursing your baby with Down syndrome
     Nursing your baby with a cleft palate or cleft lip
     Nursing your neurologically impaired baby.

     Available from   Childbirth Graphics
                             P.O. Box 21207
                             Waco, TX 76702-1207
                             (800) 299-3366 ext 287

LaLeche Pamphlets:
     Nursing my baby with a cleft of the soft palate (1996)
     Breastfeeding a baby with Down syndrome (1997)
     Tips for breastfeeding twins (1998)
     Breastfeeding the baby with reflux (1999)

     Available from   LaLeche League International
                             1400 N Meacham Road
                             Schaumburg, IL 60173-4826
                             (847) 519-7730
                             www.LaLecheLeague.org

Twins

Gromada K. Mothering multiples: Breastfeeding and caring for twins. Franklin Park, IL: LaLeche League International, 1999.

Noble E. Having twins. New York: Houghton-Mifflin, 1991.

Locating a lactation consultant

International Lactation Consultant Association
4101 Lake Boone Trail
Suite 201
Raleigh, NC 27607

LaLeche League International
P.O. Box 4079
Schaumburg, IL 60168-4079
(847) 519-7730

Relaxation tapes

Medela, Inc.
Box 600
McHenry, IL 60050
(800) 435-8316

Nursing supplementers

Medela SNS
Box 660
McHenry, IL 60050
(800) 435-8316

Lact-Aid International Inc.
Box 1066
Athens, TN 37371
(423) 744-9090
www.lact-aid.com

Parent support organizations

LaLeche League International
P.O. Box 4079
Schaumburg, IL 60168-4079
(847) 519-7730

Parents for Prematures
Box 3046
Kirkland, WA 98083-3046
(206) 283-7466

Additional resources

Hand Expressing and Cup Feeding (Video; 30 min)
Nursing Mothers' Association of Australia
Suzanne Pratt NMAA
45 Garrison Drive
Glen Waverly 3150
Australia

Human Milk Banking Association of North America, Inc.
    For publications and association business:
    Mothers' Milk Bank, Denver,
    Denver, CO (303) 869-1888

    For questions about donating or receiving banked milk:
    Triangle Mothers' Milk Bank
    Raleigh, NC (919) 250-8599

National Commission on Donor Milk Banking
8 Jan Sebastian Way #11
Sandwich, MA 02563
Lois D. W. Arnold, MPH, IBCLC, President
(508) 833-2272
(508) 833-9933
milkbank@capecod.net

Appendix N

Tube Feeding: Nutrition Assessment of the Discharged Infant

Amy L. Sapsford, RD, CSP, LD

Questions to ask for nutrition assessment	Recommended intervention if infant is not meeting growth expectations	Recommended intervention if infant is exceeding growth expectations (catch-up growth excluded)
What formula is infant receiving?	Consider composition of macronutrients and micronutrients and determine whether it is appropriate. Recommend change in formula as appropriate.	Consider composition of macronutrients and micronutrients and determine whether it is appropriate. Recommend change in formula as appropriate.
What caloric density is the formula?	If infant is able to tolerate, increase the caloric density of the formula by concentrating the formula. Gradual progression of caloric density to 30 calories per ounce with resulting increased osmolility should be well tolerated in most infants. If increased potentil renal solute load is contraindicated, modular carbohydrate and fat supplements can be used. If the tube diameter is small, the extent or method of increasing caloric density *may* need to be limited. To avoid clogging the tube, powdered formulas *may* need to be mixed with a blender or whisk.	If infant has been on increased caloric density formula, begin gradual wean. If infant is already on 20 cal/oz formula, consider decreasing caloric density, keeping in mind how dilution affects other nutrients. Evaluate readiness to wean volume, frequency, or rate. Evaluate readiness to progress to oral feedings. Supplement protein, minerals, electrolytes, and vitamins if needed to maintain adequate intake at lower energy intakes.
What volume is the infant receiving?	If infant has no contraindications, increase the volume of feedings offered. Contraindications for increasing volume include medical need for a fluid restriction, limited gastric capacity, severe reflux, or sensitivity to volume increases as in G.I. problems that may result in dumping syndrome.	If total volume infant is receiving exceeds fluid needs, consider decreasing. For a continuous feeding, this can be accomplished by decreasing the rate or by giving a "window" of time off the pump. For bolus feeds, recommend discontinuing a night feeding in attempt to normalize schedule. If volume is inadequate to meet fluid needs, explore other sources of oral calories or caloric density of formula being given.
Are the tube feedings being administered by continuous pump?	If infant has been given a "window" of time-off feedings to allow freedom from the pump, consider establishing 24-hr feedings again until growth needs are met. Also consider increasing volume and caloric density to provide nutrition needed. Examine other factors, including those that may cause increased energy expenditure that could contribute to poor growth.	If infant can tolerate attempts at oral feedings, give a 1-hr. "window" during which time the infant may nipple the volume that would have been received in that hour. Increase number of "windows" to expose infant to more practice at nippling. Since nippling requires energy expenditure, this may help an infant gaining weight too rapidly. An infant who cannot tolerate oral feedings but requires continuous infusion can be progressed to an extended "window" of 4-6 hr off the pump if fluid needs are met and those calories are no longer required.

Questions to ask for nutrition assessment	Recommended intervention if infant is not meeting growth expectations	Recommended intervention if infant is exceeding growth expectations (catch-up growth excluded)
Are the tube feedings being given by intermittent boluses?	If infant has progressed to an every-4-hr feeding schedule, consider increasing the frequency of feeding to try to get in 1-2 extra feedings per day. Also consider continuing bolus feedings during the day and placing infant on a continuous pump at night. This method allows for infant to receive additional volume at night given over 8-10 hr while not disturbing sleep pattern.	If infant is being fed through the night, begin to normalize schedule by eliminating night feedings. If infant already has been weaned off of night feedings, begin eliminating bolus feedings during the day. Make "mealtimes" normal by feeding bottles or solid foods if developmentally appropriate.
Is infant on oral feedings during the day and continuous pump feedings at night?	Attempt to maximize the feedings at night to improve overall intake.	Begin to normalize schedule. If oral feedings are accepted, consider setting pump to turn off 4 hr prior to when infant will take first bottle or breakfast. This period of "fasting" will allow infant to feel hungry on awakening.
Is the infant able to take anything by mouth?	Encourage oral feedings, keeping in mind that the infant will likely burn more calories when oral feedings begin. Alter volume and caloric density as needed to support growth as the infant learns to nipple-feed. If infant is not able to feed orally, consider other issues to provide additional nutrition.	Encourage oral feedings, keeping in mind that the infant will likely burn more calories when oral feedings begin. Alter volume and caloric density as needed to minimize excessive growth as the infant learns to nipple-feed. If infant is not able to feed orally, consider other issues to limit excessive nutrition.
Is the infant getting the nutrition it needs from an infant formula?	As infant progesses beyond a weight-age or adjusted age of 1 yr, changing to a prepared pediatric tube feeding formula may be indicated and accepted. Careful analysis of infant's or child's nutrition needs should meet the child's needs within the family's financial contraints.	As infant progresses beyond an adjusted age of 1 yr, changing to a prepared pediatric tube-feeding formula may be indicated and accepted. Dilution by addition of water may provide nutrition to achieve lower calorie goals, but may result in need to add vitamin/mineral supplements. Careful analysis of infant's or child's nutrition needs should be evaluated and formula choice individualized to meet the child's needs within the family's financial constraints.
How long has infant required nasogastric tube feedings and what is the probability of progressing to oral feedings?	If infant is on nasogastric tube feedings with limited ability to feed orally, consider evaluation for gastrostomy tube placement for long-term use. This should be a team decision, with parents an integral part of decision-making process. Parents should be given complete information to assist them in making a well-informed decision.	If infant is on nasogastric tube feedings with limited ability to feed orally, consider evaluation for gastrostomy tube placement for long-term use. This should be a team decision, with parents an integral part of decision-making process. Parents should be given complete information to assist them in making a well-informed decision.

Appendix O

Oral Feeding:
Outpatient Nutrition
Assessment
of the Infant
with Special Needs

Amy L. Sapsford, RD, CSP, LD

Questions to ask for nutrition assessment	Recommended intervention if infant is not meeting growth expectations	Recommended intervention if infant is exceeding growth expectations (catch-up growth excluded)
Is infant nursing?	Consider potential problems that could affect weight gain in nursing infant (see Chapter 17). If necessary, use supplements with increased caloric density formula offered by bottle or supplemental lactation device.	Continue nursing and examine intake for other sources of calories. Review infant's hunger and satiety cues with parents.
How often is infant bottle-feeding?	Increase number of feeds given per day, such as an every-3-hr feeding schedule. Encourage parent to hold infant during feedings.	Decrease number of feeds given per day. Progress to every-4-hr feeding schedule. Encourage parent to hold infant during feedings. Review hunger and satiety cues with parents.
Is infant taking bottle-feedings around the clock?	Introduce nighttime feeds to increase frequency of feedings. Remind parent to avoid use of bottle in bed to decrease risk of dental caries.	Attempt to wean nighttime feeds and establish daytime schedule.
How much is infant taking in each bottle?	Increase volume and instruct parent to gradually increase weekly.	Maintain volume of feedings offered if volume is not excessive. If infant is clearly being offered excessive volume, recommend reducing amount given.
What is the caloric density of the formula?	Increase the caloric density of the formula by concentrating. Modular supplements can be used but require additional purchase and mixing, and they alter nutrient balance.	If infant has been on increased caloric density formula, begin gradual wean back to 20 cal/oz formula.
What type of nipple is the infant using?	If infant is medically compromised, changing to another nipple may be beneficial. Evaluation by therapist is indicated if feeding is a problem.	Continue with nipple infant prefers to use.
Is infant taking other liquids of low nutrient value such as juice or water?	Discontinue use of these supplements and reassure parent there is "water" in the formula. Continue full-strength juice if used to treat constipation.	Continue use of dilute juice or water if age appropriate. Older infant may be able to take juice or water from a cup.

Questions to ask for nutrition assessment	Recommended intervention if infant is not meeting growth expectations	Recommended intervention if infant is exceeding growth expectations (catch-up growth excluded)
If infant is taking solid foods, what types are being offered?	Once infant has demonstrated tolerance of single-ingredient foods, offer "high-calorie" commercial baby foods such as deserts and dinners. Suggest parent read labels of baby food jars. Home-prepared baby foods may contain more calories and less water than commercial baby foods. Supplement foods with glucose polymers or sugar, margarine or desired oil, infant formula powder, additional meats or other creative supplements, if indicated.	Continue use of single-ingredient foods while maintaining variety. Avoid offering the baby foods such as deserts and dinners that are supplemented with sugar and starch. Avoid adding extra calories in home-prepared baby foods.
How are solid foods being given?	Recommend use of spoon for feding solids. Do not encourage solids in bottle or feeder. If infant is not accepting spoon, reassure parent that majority of infant's nutrition is from formula. If regular spoon is not accepted, try a plastic-coated spoon or a soft plastic spoon. Evaluation by a therapist is recommended if infant has aversion to solid foods.	Make sure infant is taking foods by spoon and not by a bottle or a feeder. Use of these devices can contribute to overfeeding. Remind parent that taking solids by spoon is a developmental milestone. Infant does not need to take large volumes by bottle for "success" at taking solids.
What other factors are affecting infant's nutrition needs?	Explore other reasons why infant may not be gaining weight, such as respiratory problems; acute illnesses, including diarrhea, otitis media, or colds, which may affect appetite and intake; medications; clinical condition; and activity. Refer to physician for follow-up of medical concerns.	Explore other reasons why infant may be gaining too quickly. If neurological status is affected, infant may have limited movement abilities. Fluid status should be evaluated to ensure infant is not retaining fluid. In other instances, accelerated growth may be desired to achieve some catching up.
When should I reassess the infant?	Infant should have a weight check in about 1-2 wk. This could be accomplished by pediatrician who is following closely. Registered dietitian should reassess in 1 mo to monitor growth and intake and make additional recommendations or referrals. These infants require regular "fine-tuning." If possible, follow-up phone contacts with parent are helpful, especially if there are transportation limitations.	Infant should have a weight check in about 2 wk. This could be accomplished by pediatrician who is following closely. Registered dietitian should assess in 1 mo to monitor growth and intake and make additional recommendations or referrals. If possible, follow-up phone contacts with parent are helpful, especially if there are transportation limitations.

Appendix P

Recommended Library

Barbara Kuzma-O'Reilly RD, LD, LPCC

American Academy of Pediatrics Committee on Nutrition. Kleinman RE, ed. Pediatric Nutrition Handbook. 4th ed. Elk Grove Village, IL: AAP, 1998.

American Dietetic Association. Pediatric Nutrition Dietetic Practice Group, eds. Pediatric Manual of Clinical Dietetics. Chicago: ADA, 1997.

American Society of Parenteral and Enteral Nutrition. Clinical Guidelines Handbook: Abridged Version of Guidelines for the Use of Parenteral and Enteral Nutrition in Adult and Pediatric Patients. Silver Springs, MD: ASPEN, 1994.

Atkinson SA, Lemons JA, eds. Human Milk for Very-Low-Birth-Weight Infants. In: Report of the 108th Ross Conference on Pediatric Research. Columbus, OH: Ross Products Division, Abbott Laboratories, 1999.

Baker RD, Baker S, Davis A. Pediatric Parenteral Nutrition. New York: Chapman & Hall, 1997.

Baker S, Baker RD, Davis A. Pediatric Enteral Nutrition. New York: Chapman & Hall, 1994.

Blackburn ST, Lopez DL. Maternal, Fetal and Neonatal Physiology: A Clinical Perspective. Philadelphia: Saunders, 1992.

Briggs GG, Freeman RK, Yaffe SL, eds. Drugs in Pregnancy and Lactation. 4th ed. Baltimore: Williams and Wilkins, 1994.

Carlson S. Neonatal Nutrition Handbook. Iowa City: University of Iowa Hospitals Dietary Department, 1994.

Cowett RM, ed. Nutrition and Metabolism of the Micropremie. Clinics in Perinatology, Philadelphia: Saunders, March, 2000.

Cox JH, ed. Nutrition Manual for At-Risk Infants and Toddlers. Chicago: Precept Press, 1997.

Fanaroff AA, Martin RJ. Neonatal-Perinatal Medicine: Disease of the Fetus and Infant. 6th ed. St. Louis: Mosby, 1997.

Feldhausen J, Thomson C, Duncan B, Taren D. Pediatric Nutrition Handbook. New York: Chapman & Hall, 1996.

Fomon SJ. Nutrition of Normal Infants. St. Louis: Mosby, 1993.

Gaull GE, ed. Pediatric Nutrition. Pediatric Clinics of North America, Philadelphia: Saunders, August 1995.

Groh-Wargo S, Thompson M, Cox JH, eds. Nutritional Care for High-Risk Newborns. 3d ed. Chicago: Precept Press, 2000.

Hay WW, Lucas A, eds. Posthospital Nutrition in the Preterm Infant. In: Report of the 106th Ross Conference on Pediatric Research. Columbus, OH: Ross Products Division, Abbott Laboratories, 1996.

Hay WW. Neonatal Nutrition and Metabolism. St. Louis: Mosby Year Book, 1990.

Helms KK. Pediatric Nutrition Self Study Course. Gaithersburg: Aspen, 1994.

Helms KK. Self Study Guide for High Risk Newborns. Lake Dallas, TX: Helm Seminar Publishing, 1996.

Huggins KH. The Nursing Mother's Companion. 4th ed. Boston: Harvard Common Press, 1999.

Jensen RG, ed. Handbook of Milk Composition. San Diego: Academic Press, 1995.

Klaus MH, Fanaroff AA. Care of the High Risk Neonate. 4th ed. Philadelphia: Saunders, 1993.

Lawrence RA, Lawrence RM. Breastfeeding: A Guide for the Medical Profession, 5th ed. St. Louis: Mosby, 1999.

Lebenthal E, ed. Pediatric Gastroenterology. Pediatric Clinics of North America. Philadelphia: Saunders, Feb, April 1996.

Manual of Clinical Dietetics. Chicago: American Dietetic Association, 1996.

Meier PP. Professional Guide to Breastfeeding Premature Infants. Columbus, Ohio: Ross Products Division, Abbott Laboratories, 1997, (60003).

Meites S, ed. Pediatric Clinical Chemistry. Washington D.C.: American Association for Clinical Chemistry, 1989.

Morris SE, Klein MD. Pre-Feeding Skills. Tuscon: Therapy Skill Builders, 1987.

National Academy of Science Institute of Medicine, Food and Nutrition Board Committee on Nutritional Status During Pregnancy and Lactation. Nutrition services in perinatal care. Washington D.C.: National Academy Press, 1992.

Neu J, ed. Neonatal Gastroenterology. Clinics in Perinatology, Philadelphia: Saunders, June 1996.

Pereira GR, Georgieff MK, eds. Neonatal/Perinatal Nutrition. Clinics in perinatology, Philadelphia: Saunders, March 1995.

Polin RA, Fox WW, eds. Fetal and Neonatal Physiology. 2d ed. Philadelphia: Saunders, 1998.

Queen PM, Helm KK, Lang CE, eds. Pediatric Nutrition Handbook. 2nd ed. Rockville MD: Aspen, 1999.

Riordan J, Auerbach KG, eds. Breastfeeding and Human Lactation, 2nd ed. Boston: Jones and Bartlett Publishers, 1999.

Satter E. Child of mine: Feeding with Love and Good Sense. Palo Alto, Calif.: Bull Publishing, 1992.

Silverman A, Roy CC. Pediatric Clinical Gastroenterology. 4th ed. St. Louis: Mosby, 1995.

Stoll BJ, Kliegman RM, eds. Necrotizing Enterocolitis. Clinics in perinatology, Philadelphia: Saunders, June 1994.

Suskind RM, Lewinter-Suskind L, eds. Textbook of Pediatric Nutrition, 2nd ed. New York: Raven Press, 1993.

Taketomo CK, Hodding JH, Kraus D, eds. Pediatric Dosage Handbook. 6th ed. Hudson, Ohio: Lexi-Comp Inc., 1999.

Trahms CM, Pipes PP. Nutrition in Infancy and Childhood. 6th ed. St. Louis: WCB/McGaw Hill, 1997.

Tsang RC, Lucas A, Uauy R, Zlotkin S, eds. Nutritional Needs of the Preterm Infant: A Scientific and Practical Guide. Baltimore: Williams and Wilkins, 1992.

Tsang RC, Zlotkin SH, Nichols BL, Hansen JW, eds. Nutrition During Infancy: Principles and Practice, 2d ed. Cincinnati, Ohio: Digital Educational Publishing, 1997.

Walker WA, Watkins JB, eds. Nutrition in Pediatrics: Basic Science and Clinical Applications. London: BC Decker, 1997.

Walker WA, Durie PR, Hamilton JR, Walker-Smith JA, Watkins, JB, eds. Pediatric Gastrointestinal Disease: Pathophysiology, Diagnosis, Management, 2d ed. St. Louis: Mosby, 1996.

Wooldridge NH, Spinozzi N, eds. Quality Assurance Criteria for Pediatric Nutrition Conditions: A Model. Chicago: American Dietetic Association, 1990.

Ziegler EE, Lucas A, Moro GE, eds. Nutrition of the Very Low Birthweight Infant. Nestle Nutrition Workshop Series, Paediatric Programme, Vol 43. Hagerstown, MD: Lippincott Williams and Wilkins, 2000.

INDEX